FRANK

RUTLEDGE

Diseases of the Liver and Biliary System

Diseases of the Liver and Biliary System

SHEILA SHERLOCK

DBE MD(Edin.) MD(Lisbon)(Hon) DSc(Hon) FRCP FRCPE
FRCCP(Hon) FRCPI(Hon) FACP(Hon)

Professor of Medicine
Royal Free Hospital School of Medicine
University of London

SIXTH EDITION

Blackwell Scientific Publications

OXFORD LONDON EDINBURGH
BOSTON MELBOURNE

© 1963, 1968, 1975, 1981 by
Blackwell Scientific Publications
Editorial offices:
Osney Mead, Oxford OX2 0EL
8 John Street, London WC1N 2ES
9 Forrest Road, Edinburgh EH1 2QH
52 Beacon Street, Boston,
  Massachusetts 02108, USA
214 Berkeley Street, Carlton
  Victoria 3053, Australia

First published 1955
Reprinted 1956
Second edition 1958
Reprinted 1959, 1961
Third edition 1963
Reprinted 1965, 1966
Fourth edition 1968
Reprinted 1969, 1971
Fifth edition 1975
Sixth edition 1981

Printed and bound in
Great Britain by
Butler & Tanner Ltd
Frome and London

DISTRIBUTORS
USA
  Blackwell Mosby Book Distributors
  11830 Westline Industrial Drive
  St Louis, Missouri 63141

Canada
  Blackwell Mosby Book Distributors
  120 Melford Drive
  Scarborough, Ontario M1B 2X4

Australia
  Blackwell Scientific Book
    Distributors
  214 Berkeley Street, Carlton
  Victoria 3053

German third edition 1965
Greek fourth edition 1972
Japanese fourth edition 1973
  (fifth edition in preparation)
Spanish fifth edition 1976
Portuguese third edition 1978
Italian fifth edition in preparation

British Library
Cataloguing in Publication Data

Sherlock, Sheila
    Diseases of the Liver and Biliary System.—6ed.
    1. Biliary tract—Diseases
    I. Title
    616.3′6   RC849   80–42405
  ISBN 0–632–00766–4

Contents

6. Investigation of the Biliary Tract

7. Hepato-cellular Failure

8. Hepatic Encephalopathy

9. Acute (Fulminant) Hepatic Failure

10. Ascites

11. The Portal Venous System and Portal Hypertension

12. The Hepatic Artery and Hepatic Veins: the Liver in Circulatory Failure

13. Jaundice

Contents

14. Cholestasis

15. Virus Hepatitis

16. Chronic Hepatitis

17. Drugs and the Liver

18. Hepatic Cirrhosis

19. Alcohol and the Liver

20. Iron Overload States

21. Wilson's Disease

22. Nutritional and Metabolic Liver Diseases

23. The Liver in Infancy and Childhood

24. The Liver in Pregnancy

25. Cysts and Congenital Biliary Abnormalities

26. The Liver in Systemic Disease; Hepatic Trauma

27. The Liver in Infections

28. Hepatic Tumours

29. Gall-stones and Inflammatory Gall Bladder Diseases

30. Benign Stricture of the Bile Ducts

31. Disease of the Ampulla of Vater and Pancreas

32. Tumours of the Gall Bladder and Bile Ducts

33. Hepatic Transplantation

Preface

This is more than a new sixth edition, for a gap of six years has meant that the book has had to be re-written. Exciting and fundamental advances come under three headings—new techniques of investigation, fresh concepts and new treatments.

The new techniques include hepato-biliary scanning, advances in percutaneous and endoscopic cholangiography; these have warranted new chapters. Advances in virology, particularly viral markers, have meant complete re-writing of the section on virus hepatitis.

Fresh concepts of cholestasis, primary biliary cirrhosis and sclerosing cholangitis have outdated our older views of these disorders. Chronic hepatitis has been re-classified to make it more understandable.

New treatments are following apace as there have been advances in immunosuppression, immunostimulation, anti-viral prophylaxis and chemotherapy. The management of our patients during this coming decade will outmode many of the treatments of the 1970s. New antibiotics for the immunosuppressed cirrhotic and praziquantel for the treatment of schistosomiasis are but two examples of these changes.

These advances have necessitated drastic pruning of outmoded views and ruthless elimination of old references to make way for new material. There are 151 new figures and 1080 new references. Further figures will be found in *A Colour Atlas of Liver Disease* (1979) published by Wolfe Medical Publications Ltd., in which John A. Summerfield is my co-author.

I owe much to my colleagues. Professor P. J. Scheuer has kept me up to date with histopathology, and Dr Robert Dick, likewise with radiology.

Nowadays a clinician is only as good as these essential services, and in this respect we are particularly blessed at the Royal Free Hospital, London.

I would also like to express my indebtedness for help to Dr Leslie Berger, Professor Barbara Billing, Dr Roger Chapman, Dr James Dooley, Dr Owen Epstein, Professor H. M. Gilles, Dr Jenny Heathcote, Professor Neil McIntyre, Dr Marsha Morgan, Dr Gray Smith-Laing, Dr John Summerfield, Dr Anthony Tavill and Dr Howard Thomas.

Mrs Maggie Pettifer has been an excellent editor, and has double-checked everything. Miss Aileen Duggan has made light of the secretarial burden. Miss P. Fear, chief librarian at the Royal Free Hospital, has given meticulous advice on the references. Additional artistic work is that of our medical artist, Miss Janice Cox.

The production of this largely re-written edition with its new format owes much to the co-operation of Mr Peter Saugman and Mr Jony Russell of Blackwell Scientific Publications.

My daughters, Amanda and Auriole, have continued to give me the solid support which was essential if this edition was to be completed. They have now outgrown the days when they chased proofs along windy beaches, for they are now committed to their own academic endeavours. After thirty years of marriage, my husband, Dr D. Geraint James, remains the perfect consort for an academic wife.

Sheila Sherlock

London
January 1981

xiii

Preface to the First Edition

My aim in writing this book has been to present a comprehensive and up-to-date account of diseases of the liver and biliary system, which I hope will be of value to physicians, surgeons and pathologists and also a reference book for the clinical student. The modern literature has been reviewed with special reference to articles of general interest. Many older more specialized classical contributions have therefore inevitably been excluded.

Disorders of the liver and biliary system may be classified under the traditional concept of individual diseases. Alternatively, as I have endeavoured in this book, they may be described by the functional and morphological changes which they produce. In the clinical management of a patient with liver disease, it is important to assess the degree of disturbance of four functional and morphological components of the liver—hepatic cells, vascular system (portal vein, hepatic artery and hepatic veins), bile ducts and reticulo-endothelial system. The typical reaction pattern is thus sought and recognized before attempting to diagnose the causative insult. Clinical and laboratory methods of assessing each of these components are therefore considered early in the book. Descriptions of individual diseases follow as illustrative examples. It will be seen that the features of hepato-cellular failure and portal hypertension are described in general terms as a foundation for subsequent discussion of virus hepatitis, nutrition liver disease and the cirrhoses. Similarly blood diseases and infections of the liver are included with the reticulo-endothelial system, and disorders of the biliary tract follow descriptions of acute and chronic bile duct obstruction.

I would like to acknowledge my indebtedness to my teachers, the late Professor J. Henry Dible, the late Professor Sir James Learmonth and Professor Sir John McMichael, who stimulated my interest in hepatic disease, and to my colleagues at the Postgraduate Medical School and elsewhere who have generously invited me to see patients under their care. I am grateful to Dr A. G. Bearn for criticizing part of the typescript and to Dr A. Paton for his criticisms and careful proof reading.

Miss D. F. Atkins gave much assistance with proof reading and with the bibliography. Mr Per Saugman and Mrs J. M. Green of Blackwell Scientific Publications have co-operated enthusiastically in the production of this book.

The photomicrographs were taken by Mr E. V. Willmott, FRPS, and Mr C. A. P. Graham from sections prepared by Mr J. G. Griffin and the histology staff of the Postgraduate Medical School. Clinical photographs are the work of Mr C. R. Brecknell and his assistants. The black and white drawings were made by Mrs H. M. G. Wilson and Mr D. Simmonds. I am indebted to them all for their patience and skill.

The text includes part of unpublished material included in a thesis submitted in 1944 to the University of Edinburgh for the degree of M.D., and part of an essay awarded the Buckston-Browne prize of the Harveian Society of London in 1953. Colleagues have allowed me to include published work of which they are jointly responsible. Dr Patricia P. Franklyn and Dr R. E. Steiner have kindly loaned me radiographs. Many authors have given me permission to reproduce illustrations and detailed acknowledgments are given in the text. I wish also to thank the editors of the following journals for permission to include illustrations: *American Journal of Medicine, Archives of Pathology, British Heart Journal, Circulation, Clinical Science, Edinburgh Medical Journal, Journal of Clinical Investigation, Journal of Laboratory and Clinical Investigation, Journal of Pathology and Bacteriology, Lancet, Postgraduate Medical Journal, Proceedings of the Staff Meetings of the Mayo Clinic, Quarterly Journal of Medicine, Thorax* and also the following publishers: Butterworth's Medical Publications, J. & A. Churchill Ltd, The Josiah Macy Junior Foundation and G. D. Searle & Co.

Finally I must thank my husband, Dr D. Geraint James, who, at considerable personal inconvenience, encouraged me to undertake the writing of this book and also criticized and rewrote most of it. He will not allow me to dedicate it to him.

Chapter 1
Anatomy of the Liver and
Biliary Tract

The liver, the largest organ in the body, weighs 1200–1500 g and comprises one-fiftieth of the total adult body weight. It is relatively larger in infancy, comprising one-eighteenth of the birth weight. This is mainly due to a large left lobe.

Sheltered by the ribs in the right upper quadrant, it is shaped like a pyramid whose apex reaches the xiphisternum (figs. 1, 2, 3). The upper border lies approximately at the level of the nipples. There are two anatomical lobes, the right being about six times the size of the left. Lesser segments of the right lobe are the *quadrate lobe*, on its inferior surface, and the *caudate lobe* on the posterior surface. The right and left lobes are separated anteriorly by a fold of peritoneum called the falciform ligament, inferiorly by the fissure for the ligamentum teres, and posteriorly by the fissure for the ligamentum venosum.

The liver has a double blood supply. The *portal vein* brings venous blood from the intestines and spleen and the *hepatic artery*, coming from the coeliac axis, supplies the liver with arterial blood. These vessels enter the liver through a fissure, the *porta hepatis*, which lies far back on the inferior surface of the right lobe. Inside the porta, the portal vein and hepatic artery divide into branches to the right and left lobes, and the right and left hepatic bile ducts join to form the common hepatic duct. The *hepatic nerve plexus* contains fibres from both sympathetic ganglia T7 to T10 which synapse in the coeliac plexus, the right and left vagi and the right phrenic nerve. It accompanies the hepatic artery and bile ducts into their finest ramifications, even to the portal tracts and hepatic parenchyma.

The *ligamentum venosum*, a slender remnant of the ductus venosus of the foetus, arises from the left branch of the portal vein and fuses with the inferior vena cava at the entrance of the left hepatic vein. The *ligamentum teres*, a remnant of the umbilical vein of the foetus, runs in the free edge of the falciform ligament from the umbilicus to the inferior border of the liver and joins the left branch of the portal vein. Small veins accompanying it connect the portal vein with veins around the umbilicus. These become prominent when the portal venous system is obstructed inside the liver.

The venous drainage from the liver is into the *right* and *left hepatic veins* which emerge from the back of the liver and at once enter the inferior vena cava very near its point of entry in the right auricle.

Lymphatic vessels terminate in small groups of glands around the porta hepatis. Efferent vessels drain into glands around the coeliac axis. Some superficial hepatic lymphatics pass through the diaphragm in the falciform ligament and finally reach the mediastinal glands. Another group accompanies the inferior vena cava into the thorax and ends in a few small glands around the intrathoracic portion of the inferior vena cava.

The *inferior vena cava* makes a deep groove to

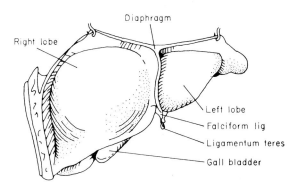

Fig. 1. Anterior view of the liver.

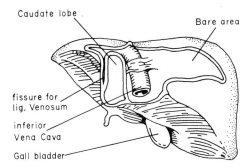

Caudate lobe

Bare area

fissure for
lig. Venosum

inferior
Vena Cava

Gall bladder

Fig. 2. Posterior view of the liver.

the right of the caudate lobe about an inch from the mid-line.

The *gall bladder* lies in a fossa extending from the inferior border of the liver to the right end of the porta hepatis.

The liver is completely covered with peritoneum except in three places. It comes into direct contact with the diaphragm through the bare area which lies to the right of the fossa for the inferior vena cava. The other areas without peritoneal covering are the fossae for the inferior vena cava and gall bladder.

The liver is kept in position by peritoneal ligaments and by the intra-abdominal pressure transmitted by the tone of the muscles of the abdominal wall.

Segmental anatomy [11] (fig. 4)

One lobar fissure is in line with the fissure of the inferior vena cava above and the fossa of the gall bladder below. This fissure takes an oblique course from left to right to the porta hepatis and divides

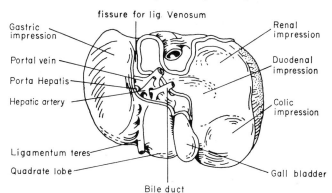

fissure for lig. Venosum

Gastric
impression

Portal vein

Porta Hepatis

Hepatic artery

Renal
impression

Duodenal
impression

Colic
impression

Ligamentum teres

Quadrate lobe

Gall bladder

Bile duct

Fig. 3. Inferior view of the liver.

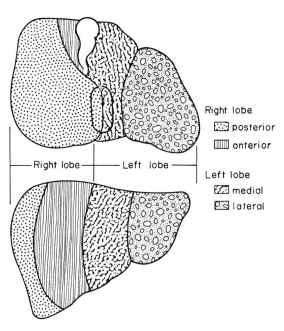

Right lobe
[··] posterior
[ⅢⅢ] anterior

Left lobe
[▨] medial
[▨] lateral

Right lobe — Left lobe

Fig. 4. The segments of the human liver (Healey 1970).

the liver into two anatomical left and right lobes. The left segmental fissure divides the two left lobes into medial and lateral segments. The right segmental fissure divides the right lobe into an anterior and a posterior segment. Knowledge of this anatomy is particularly valuable in planning hepatic surgery.

Anatomy of the biliary tract (fig. 5)

The *right and left hepatic ducts* emerge from the right and left lobes of the liver and unite in the porta hepatis to form the *common hepatic duct*. This is soon joined by the *cystic duct* from the gall bladder to form the common bile duct.

The *common bile duct* runs between the layers of the lesser omentum, lying anterior to the portal vein and to the right of the hepatic artery. Passing behind the first part of the duodenum in a groove on the back of the head of the pancreas, it enters the third part of the duodenum. The duct runs obliquely through the posteromedial duodenal wall about its middle, usually joining the main pancreatic duct to form the *ampulla of Vater* (1720). The ampulla makes the mucous membrane bulge inwards to form an eminence, the *duodenal papilla*. In about 30% of subjects the bile and pancreatic ducts open separately into the duodenum. The common bile duct, measured at operation, is about 0.5–1.5 cm diameter.

The duodenal portion of the common bile duct

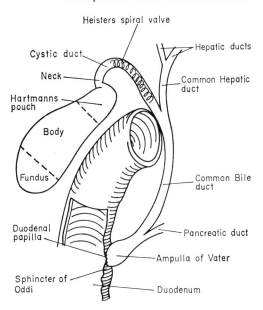

Fig. 5. Gall bladder and biliary tract.

Labels on figure:
Heisters spiral valve
Cystic duct
Hepatic ducts
Neck
Common Hepatic duct
Hartmanns pouch
Body
Common Bile duct
Fundus
Duodenal papilla
Pancreatic duct
Ampulla of Vater
Sphincter of Oddi
Duodenum

is surrounded by a thickening of both longitudinal and circular muscle fibres derived from the intestine. This is called the *sphincter of Oddi* (1887).

The *gall bladder* is a pear-shaped bag 9 cm long with a capacity of about 50 ml. Any decrease in concentrating power is accompanied by a lowering of the powers of expansion. The fundus is the broad end and is directed forward: this is the part palpated when the abdomen is examined. The body extends into a narrow neck which continues into the cystic duct. The *valves of Heister* are spiral folds of mucous membrane in the wall of the cystic duct and neck of the gall bladder. *Hartmann's pouch* is a sacculation at the neck of the gall bladder; this is a common site for a gall-stone to lodge.

The wall consists of a musculo-elastic network without definite layers, the muscle being particularly well developed in the neck and fundus. The mucous membrane is in delicate closely woven folds; instead of glands there are deep indentations of mucosa, the *crypts of Luschka*, which penetrate into the muscular layer. There is no sub-mucosa or muscularis mucosae.

The *Rokitansky–Aschoff sinuses* are branching evaginations from the lumen into the mucosa and muscularis of the gall bladder. They play an important part in acute cholecystitis and gangrene of the gall bladder wall.

The gall bladder receives blood from the *cystic artery*. This branch of the hepatic artery is large, tortuous and variable in its anatomical relationships. The bile ducts also have a variable arterial supply [15]. Smaller blood vessels enter from the liver through the gall bladder fossa. The venous drainage is into the *cystic vein* and thence into the portal venous system.

There are many *lymphatic vessels* in the submucous and subperitoneal layers. These drain through the cystic gland at the neck of the gall bladder to glands along the common bile duct, where they anastomose with lymphatics from the head of the pancreas.

Nerve supply. The gall bladder and bile ducts are liberally supplied with nerves, from both the parasympathetic and the sympathetic system.

Functional divisions of the liver

The functional division into right and left lobes with respect to biliary drainage and vascular supply differs from the anatomically accepted right and left lobes. The line of functional division lies to the right of the attachment of the falciform ligament and follows an irregular line from the inferior vena cava obliquely across the upper surface of the liver to the tip of the gall bladder. The functional right and left lobes are supplied by the right and left hepatic ducts and portal venous branches and drained by corresponding hepatic veins.

Development of the liver and bile ducts

The liver begins as a hollow endodermal bud from the foregut (duodenum). The bud separates into two parts. The hepatic section forms the hepatic duct and its branches and the main mass of liver cells. It is met by ingrowing capillary plexuses from the vitelline veins which will form the sinusoids. The biliary part forms the gall bladder and extrahepatic bile ducts.

ANATOMICAL ABNORMALITIES OF THE LIVER

Accessory lobes [5]. The liver of the pig, dog and camel is divided into distinct and separate lobes by strands of connective tissue. Occasionally the human liver may show this reversion and up to sixteen lobes have been reported. This abnormality is rare and without clinical significance. The lobes are small and usually on the under surface of the liver so that they are not detected but noted incidentally at scanning, operation or necropsy.

Rarely they are intrathoracic. An accessory lobe may have its own mesentery containing hepatic artery, portal vein, bile duct and hepatic vein [18]. This may twist and demand surgical intervention.

Riedel's lobe [21] is fairly common and is a downward tongue-like projection of the right lobe of the liver. It is a simple anatomical variation; it is not a true accessory lobe. The condition is more frequent in women. It is detected as a mobile tumour on the right side of the abdomen, which descends with the diaphragm and on respiration. It may come down as low as the right iliac region. It is easily mistaken for other tumours in this area, especially a visceroptotic right kidney. It does not cause symptoms and treatment is not required. Scanning may be used to identify Riedel's lobe and other anatomical abnormalities.

Cough furrows on the liver are parallel grooves on the convexity of the right lobe. They are one to six in number and run anteroposteriorly, being deeper posteriorly. They are said to be associated with a chronic cough.

Atrophy of the left lobe [1, 4]. Severe atrophy confined to the functional left lobe of the liver is not uncommon at post mortem. The lobe is decreased in size, with wrinkling and thickening of the capsule, fibrosis and prominent biliary and vascular markings. Histologically, the portal areas seem crowded together.

The usual cause is interference with the left branch of the portal vein. At the time of birth the left lobe loses its blood and oxygen supply when

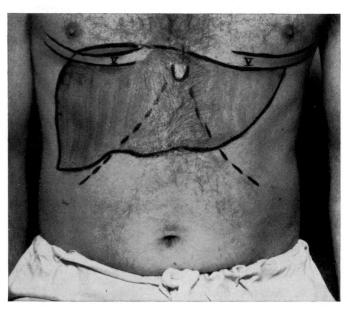

Fig. 6. Surface marking of the liver. The 5th ribs are outlined.

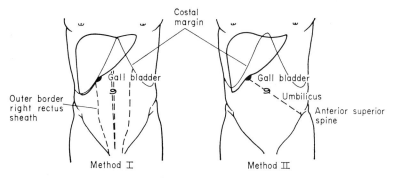

Surface markings of the Gall Bladder

Fig. 7. Surface markings of the gall bladder.
Method I: the gall bladder is found where the outer border of the right rectus abdominis muscle intersects the 9th costal cartilage.

Method II: a line drawn from the left anterior superior iliac spine through the umbilicus intersects the costal margin at the site of the gall bladder.

the ductus venosus is obliterated; degenerative changes follow. This atrophy may persist into adult life. Later, compression of the left hepatic duct or the left branch of the portal vein or the left branch of the hepatic artery, for instance by malignant disease, can result in atrophy of the left lobe.

Anatomical abnormalities of gall bladder and biliary tract (see Chapter 25).

Surface marking (figs. 6, 7)

Liver. The upper border of the right lobe is on a level with the 5th rib at a point 2 cm medial to the right mid-clavicular line (1 cm below the right nipple). The upper border of the left lobe corresponds to the upper border of the 6th rib at a point in the left mid-clavicular line (2 cm below the left nipple). Here only the diaphragm separates the liver from the apex of the heart.

The lower border passes obliquely upwards from the 9th right to the 8th left costal cartilage. In the right nipple line it lies between a point just under to 2 cm below the costal margin. It crosses the mid-line about mid-way between the base of the xiphoid and the umbilicus and the left lobe extends only 5 cm to the left of the sternum.

Gall bladder. The fundus lies at the outer border of the right rectus abdominis muscle at its junction with the right costal margin (9th costal cartilage) (fig. 7). In an obese subject it may be difficult to identify the outer border of the rectus sheath and the gall bladder may then be located by the Grey–Turner method. A line is drawn from the left anterior superior iliac spine through the umbilicus; its intersection with the right costal margin indicates the position of the gall bladder.

METHODS OF EXAMINATION

Liver. The lower edge should be determined by palpation just lateral to the right rectus muscle. This avoids mistaking the upper intersection of the rectus sheath for the liver edge.

The liver edge moves 1–3 cm downwards with deep inspiration. It is usually palpable in normal subjects inspiring deeply. The edge may be tender, regular or irregular, firm or soft, thickened or sharp. The lower edge may be displaced downwards by a low diaphragm, for instance in emphysema. Movements may be particularly great in athletes or singers. Some patients with practice become very efficient at 'pushing down' the liver. The normal spleen can become palpable in a similar fashion. Common causes of a liver palpable below the umbilicus are malignant deposits, or polycystic Hodgkin's disease, amyloidosis, congestive cardiac failure, and gross fatty change. Rapid change in liver size may occur when congestive cardiac failure is corrected, cholestatic jaundice relieved, severe diabetes controlled, or when fat is dispersed. The surface can be palpated in the epigastrium and any irregularity or tenderness noted.

Pulsation of the liver, usually associated with tricuspid valvular incompetence, is felt by manual palpation with one hand over the right lower ribs posteriorly and the other anteriorly on the abdominal wall.

The upper edge is determined by fairly heavy percussion passing downwards from the nipple-line. The lower edge is recognized by very light percussion passing upwards from the umbilicus towards the costal margin. Percussion is a valuable method of determining liver size and is the only clinical method of determining a small liver.

The anterior, hepatic, linear projection is obtained by measuring the vertical distance between uppermost and lowermost points of hepatic dullness by percussion in the right mid-clavicular lines. This is usually 12–15 cm. Results agree with hepatic size obtained by scanning.

Friction may be palpable and audible, usually due to recent biopsy, tumour or perihepatitis [6]. The venous hum of portal hypertension is audible between the umbilicus and the xiphisternum. An arterial murmur over the liver may indicate a primary liver cancer or acute alcoholic hepatitis.

The gall bladder is palpable only when it is distended. It is felt as a pear-shaped cystic mass usually about 3 inches long. In a thin person, the swelling can sometimes be seen through the anterior abdominal wall. It moves downwards on inspiration and is mobile laterally but not downwards. The swelling is dull to percussion and directly impinges on the parietal peritoneum, so that the colon is rarely in front of it. Gall bladder dullness is continuous with that of the liver.

Abdominal tenderness should be noted. Inflammation of the gall bladder causes a positive *Murphy's sign*. This is the inability to take a deep breath when the examining fingers are hooked up below the liver edge. The inflamed gall bladder is then driven against the fingers and the pain causes the patient to catch his breath.

The enlarged gall bladder must be distinguished from a *visceroptotic right kidney*. This, however, is more mobile, can be displaced towards the pelvis and has the resonant colon anteriorly. A *regenerative* or *malignant nodule* feels much firmer.

Radiology. A plain film of the abdomen, including the diaphragms, may be used to assess liver size and in particular to decide whether a palpable liver is due to actual enlargement or to downward displacement. On moderate inspiration the normal level of the diaphragm, on the right side, is opposite the 11th rib posteriorly and the 6th rib anteriorly.

HEPATIC MORPHOLOGY [14]

Kiernan (1833) [12] introduced the concept of hepatic lobules as the basic architecture. He described circumscribed pyramidal lobules consisting of a central tributary of the hepatic vein and at the periphery a portal tract containing bile duct,

portal vein radicle and hepatic artery branch. Columns of liver cells and blood-containing sinusoids extended between these two systems.

Stereoscopic reconstructions [3] and scanning electron microscopy [9] have shown the human liver as columns of liver cells radiating from a central vein, and interlaced in orderly fashion by sinusoids (fig. 8).

The liver tissue is pervaded by two systems of tunnels, the portal tracts and the hepatic central canals which dovetail in such a way that they never touch each other; the terminal tunnels of the two systems are separated by about 0.5 mm (fig. 9). As far as possible the two systems of tunnels run in planes perpendicular to each other. The sinusoids are irregularly disposed, normally in a direction perpendicular to the lines connecting the central veins. The terminal branches of the portal vein discharge their blood into the sinusoids and the direction of flow is determined by the higher pressure in the portal vein than in the central vein.

The *central hepatic canals* contain radicles of the hepatic vein and their adventitia. They are surrounded by a limiting plate of liver cells.

The *portal triads* (syn. portal tracts, Glisson's capsule) contain the portal vein radicle, the hepatic arteriole and bile duct with a few round cells and a little connective tissue (fig. 10). They are surrounded by a limiting plate of liver cells.

The liver has to be divided functionally. Traditionally the unit is based on a central hepatic vein and its surrounding liver cells. However, Rappaport [19] envisages a series of functional acini, each centred on the portal triad with its terminal branch of portal vein, hepatic artery and bile duct (fig. 11). These interdigitate, mainly perpendicularly with terminal hepatic veins of adjacent acini. The circulatory peripheries of acini (adjacent to terminal hepatic veins) suffer most from injury whether viral, toxic or anoxic. Bridging necrosis is located in this area. The regions closer to the axis formed by afferent vessels and bile ducts survive longer and may later form the core from which regeneration will proceed. The contribution of each acinar zone to liver cell regeneration depends on the acinar location of damage [16, 20].

Cells in zone 1 may participate, particularly in oxidative phosphorylation, while those in zone 3 may be particularly important in glycolysis.

The liver cells (*hepatocytes*) comprise about 60%

Fig. 8 (*facing*) Synopsis of the structure of the normal human liver.

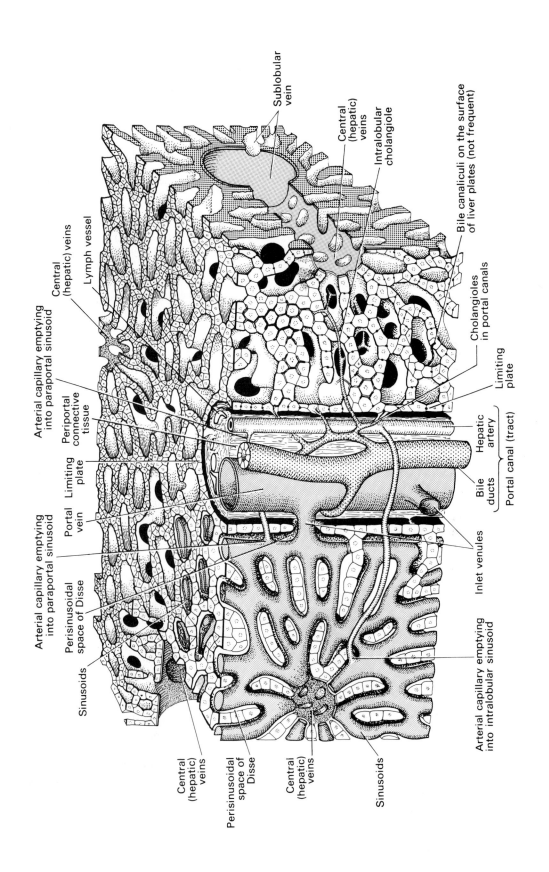

Sublobular vein

Central (hepatic) veins

Intralobular cholangiole

Bile canaliculi on the surface of liver plates (not frequent)

Cholangioles in portal canals

Limiting plate

Hepatic artery

Bile ducts

Portal canal (tract)

Inlet venules

Arterial capillary emptying into intralobular sinusoid

Sinusoids

Central (hepatic) veins

Perisinusoidal space of Disse

Central (hepatic) veins

Sinusoids

Perisinusoidal space of Disse

Portal vein

Limiting plate

Periportal connective tissue

Lymph vessel

Central (hepatic) veins

Arterial capillary emptying into paraportal sinusoid

Arterial capillary emptying into paraportal sinusoid

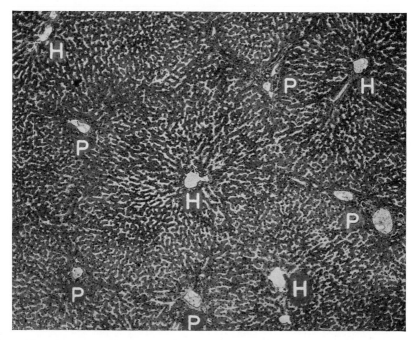

Fig. 9. Normal hepatic histology. H=terminal
hepatic vein; P=portal tract. Stained H & E, ×60.

of the liver. They are polygonal and approximately
$30\,\mu$m in diameter. The nucleus is single or, less
often, multiple and divides by mitosis. The life span
of liver cells is about 150 days in experimental
animals. The hepatocyte has three surfaces: one
facing the sinusoid and space of Disse, the second
facing the canaliculus and the third facing neighbouring hepatocytes. There is no basement
membrane.

The walls of the sinusoids consist of endothelial
and phagocytic cells of the reticulo-endothelial
system. The flat cell components are known as
Kupffer cells. These cells play an important part
in the production of immune bodies, in phagocy-
tosis and in blood formation. Kupffer cells may
come from the bone-marrow [13].

There are approximately 202×10^3 cells in each
milligramme of normal human liver of which

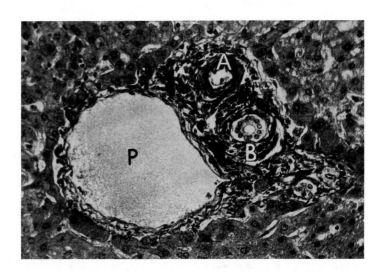

Fig. 10. Normal portal tract.
B=bile duct; P=portal
vein; A=hepatic artery.
Stained elastic tissue, ×220.

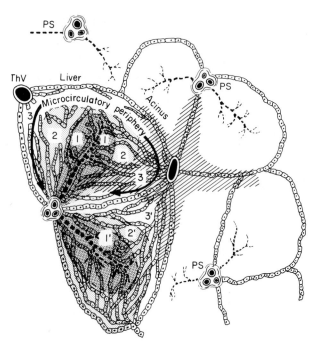

Fig. 11. Blood supply of the simple liver acinus, zonal arrangements of cells and the microcirculatory periphery. The acinus occupies adjacent sectors of neighbouring hexagonal fields. Zones 1, 2 and 3 respectively represent areas supplied with blood of first, second and third quality with regard to oxygen and nutrient contents. These zones centre about the terminal afferent vascular branches, bile ductules, lymph vessels and nerves (PS) and extend into the triangular portal field from which these branches crop out. Zone 3 is the microcirculatory periphery of the acinus since its cells are as remote from their own afferent vessels as from those of adjacent acini. The *perivenular* area is formed by the most peripheral portions of zone 3 of several adjacent acini. In injury progressing along this zone, the damaged area assumes the shape of a seastar (heavy. cross-hatching around a ThV in the centre). 1, 2, 3 = microcirculatory zones; 1′, 2′, 3′ = zones of neighbouring acinus; - - - - afferent vessels of acini outlining the hexagons (Rappaport 1976).

171×10^3 are parenchymatous and 31×10^3 littoral (sinusoidal including Kupffer cells) [8].

The *space of Disse* is a tissue space between hepatocytes and sinusoidal lining cells. It contains tissue fluid which flows outwards into lymphatics in the portal triads. The *hepatic lymphatics* are found in the periportal connective tissue and are lined throughout by endothelium. Tissue fluid seeps through the endothelium into the lymph vessels.

The branch of the hepatic arteriole forms a plexus around the bile ducts and supplies the structures in the portal tracts. It empties into the sinusoidal network at different levels. There are no direct hepatic–arteriolar–portal–venous anastomoses.

The excretory system of the liver begins with the *bile canaliculi* (figs. 186, 188). These have no walls but are simply grooves on the contact surfaces of liver cells. Their surfaces are covered by microvilli.

The plasma membrane is reinforced by microfilaments forming a supportive cytoskeleton (fig. 186). The canalicular surface is separated from the rest of the intercellular surface by junctional complexes including tight junctions, gap junctions and desmosomes. The intra-lobular canalicular networks drain into thin-walled terminal bile ducts or cholangioles (*canals of Hering; ductules*), and these terminate in larger (*inter-lobular*) bile ducts in the portal canals [10].

ELECTRON MICROSCOPY AND HEPATO-CELLULAR FUNCTION
(figs. 12, 13, 14) [22]

The liver cell margin is straight except for a few anchoring pegs (desmosomes). From it, equally sized and spaced microvilli project into the lumen of the bile canaliculi. Along the sinusoidal border,

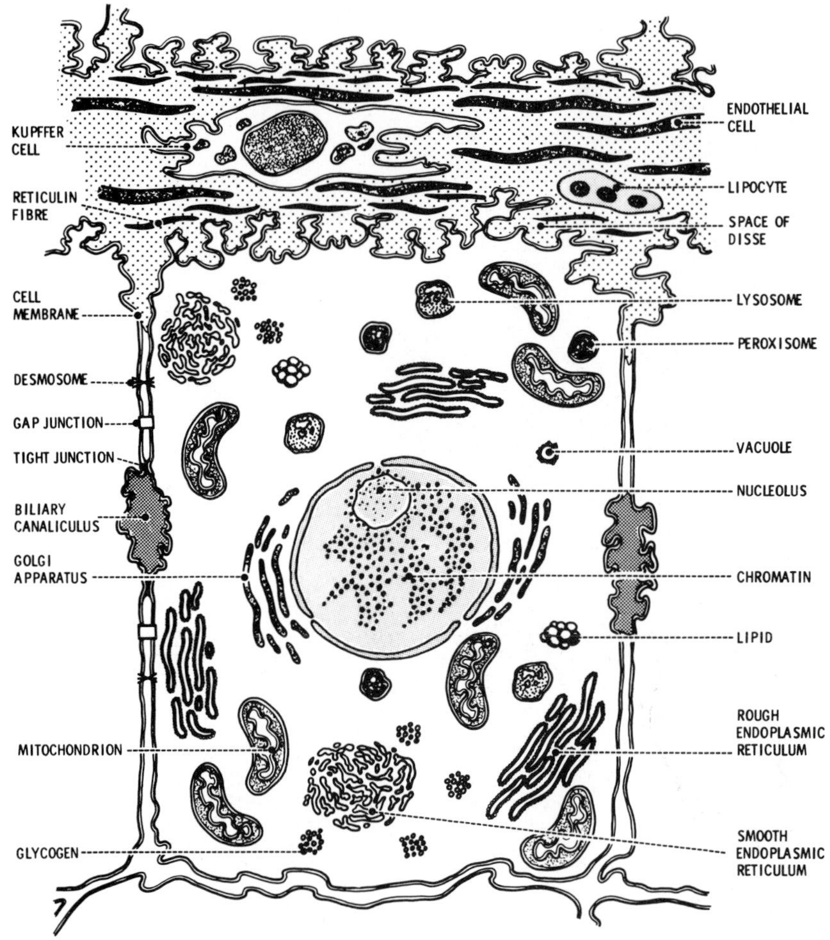
KUPFFER CELL
RETICULIN FIBRE
CELL MEMBRANE
DESMOSOME
GAP JUNCTION
TIGHT JUNCTION
BILIARY CANALICULUS
GOLGI APPARATUS
MITOCHONDRION
GLYCOGEN
ENDOTHELIAL CELL
LIPOCYTE
SPACE OF DISSE
LYSOSOME
PEROXISOME
VACUOLE
NUCLEOLUS
CHROMATIN
LIPID
ROUGH ENDOPLASMIC RETICULUM
SMOOTH ENDOPLASMIC RETICULUM

Fig. 12. The organelles of the liver cell.

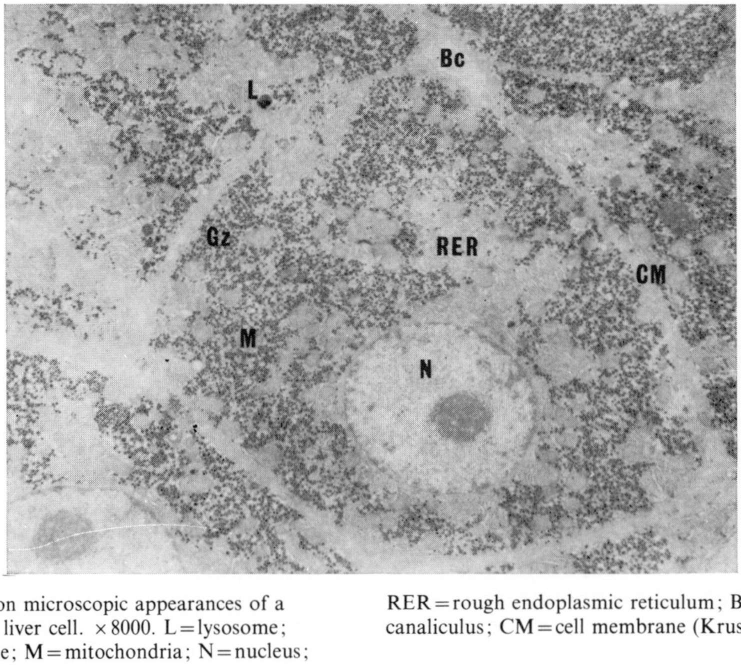
Bc
L
Gz
RER
CM
M
N

Fig. 13. Electron microscopic appearances of a normal human liver cell. ×8000. L=lysosome; Gz=Golgi zone; M=mitochondria; N=nucleus; RER=rough endoplasmic reticulum; Bc=bile canaliculus; CM=cell membrane (Krustev 1967).

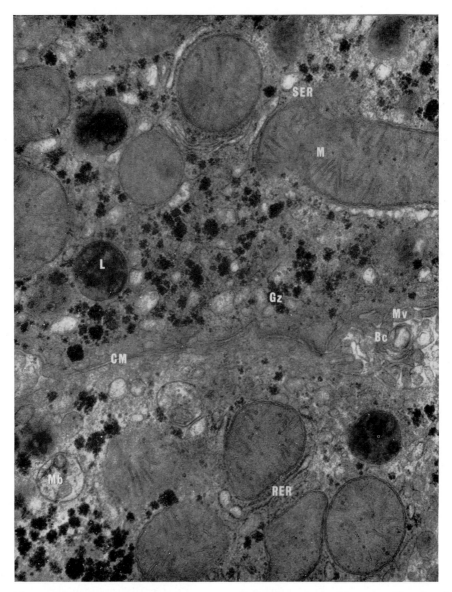

Fig. 14. Electron microscopic appearances of a normal human liver cell: the zone around the bile canaliculus. × 102 000. M = mitochondria; L = lysosome; Mb = microbody; Bc = bile canaliculus; CM = cell membrane; Mv = microvillus; Gz = Golgi zone; SER = smooth endoplasmic reticulum; RER = rough endoplasmic reticulum (Krustev 1967).

irregularly sized and spaced microvilli project into the perisinusoidal tissue space. This microvillous structure indicates active secretion or absorption, mainly of fluid.

The *nucleus* contains deoxyribonucleoprotein. Human liver after puberty also contains tetraploid nuclei and, at about age 20, in addition, octoploid nuclei are found. Increased polyploidy has been regarded as precancerous. In the chromatin net-work one or more nucleoli are embedded. The nucleus has a double contour with pores allowing interchange with the surrounding hyaloplasm.

The *mitochondria* also have a double membrane, the inner being invaginated to form grooves or cristae. An enormous number of energy-providing processes take place within them, particularly those involving oxidative phosphorylation. They contain many enzymes, particularly those of the citric acid cycle and those involved in β oxidation of fatty acids. They can transform energy so released into ADP. Haem synthesis occurs here.

The *rough endoplasmic reticulum (RER)* is seen as lamellar profiles lined by ribosomes. These are responsible for basophilia under light microscopy. They synthesize specific proteins, particularly albumin, those used in blood coagulation and enzymes. They may adopt a helix arrangement, as polysomes, for co-ordination of this function. Glucose-6-phosphatase is synthesized. Triglycerides are synthesized from free fatty acids and complexed with protein to be secreted by exocytosis as lipoprotein. The RER may participate in glycogenesis [2].

The *smooth endoplasmic reticulum (SER)* forms tubules and vesicles. It contains the microsomes. It is the site of bilirubin conjugation and the detoxification of many drugs and other foreign compounds. Steroids are synthesized. These include cholesterol and the primary bile acids which are conjugated with the amino acids glycine and taurine. The SER is increased by enzyme inducers such as phenobarbital.

Peroxisomes are distributed near the SER and glycogen granules. Their function is unknown.

The *lysosomes* are pericanalicular dense bodies adjacent to the bile canaliculi. They contain many hydrolytic enzymes which, if released, could destroy the cell. They are probably intracellular scavengers which destroy organelles with shortened life spans. They are the site of deposition of ferritin, lipofuscin, bile pigment and copper. Pinocytic vacuoles may be observed in them. Some pericanalicular dense bodies are termed *microbodies*.

The *Golgi apparatus* consists of a system of particles and vesicles again lying near the canaliculus. It may be regarded as a 'packaging' site for excretion into the bile. This entire group of lysosomes, microbodies and Golgi apparatus is a means of sequestering any material which was ingested and has to be excreted, secreted or stored for metabolic processes in the hyaloplasm. The Golgi apparatus, lysosomes and canaliculi are concerned in cholestasis (Chapter 14).

The intervening *hyaloplasm* contains granules of glycogen, lipid and fine fibrils.

Microtubules and microfilaments (fig. 186) provide a supporting cytoskeleton [7]. They may control cell movement and shape and may be concerned with movement of secretory granules.

The *sinusoidal wall* consists of three types of cells: endothelial cells, Kupffer cells and fat-stor-

ing cells or lipocytes. The Kupffer cells and endothelial cells are littoral cells in contact with the lumen of the sinusoids. The lipocytes lie in the space of Disse between the hepatocytes and the littoral cells [23].

The *Kupffer cells* are elongated structures having an irregular outline, crenated nucleus, few mitochondria and varying numbers of lysosomes. They contain phagocytosed material.

Lipocytes (Ito cells) located in the perisinusoidal space probably represent undifferentiated mesenchymal cells or resting fibroblasts [17].

Pit cells are found in the sinusoidal wall. They contain granules and may have an endocrine function [24].

The *bile ductules* have a basement membrane with surrounding collagen fibres. The lumen is indented by microvilli.

REFERENCES

1. BENZ E.J., BAGGENSTOSS A.H. & WOLLAEGER E.E. (1952) Atrophy of the left lobe of the liver. *Arch. Path.* **53,** 315.
2. BERNAERT D., WANSON J.C., DROCHMANS P. *et al* (1977) Effect of insulin on ultrastructure and glycogenesis in primary cultures of adult rat hepatocytes. *J. cell Biol.* **74,** 878.
3. ELIAS H. (1952) Morphology of the liver. *Trans. 11th Conf. on Liver Injury,* p. 111. New York, Josiah Macy Jr Foundation.
4. EMERY J.L. (1952) Degenerative changes in the left lobe of the liver in the newborn. *Arch. Dis. Childh.* **27,** 558.
5. FRASER C.G. (1952) Accessory lobes of the liver. *Ann. Surg.* **135,** 127.
6. FRED H.L. & BROWN G.R. (1962) The hepatic friction rub. *New Engl. J. Med.* **266,** 554.
7. FRENCH S.W. & DAVIES P.L. (1975) Ultrastructural localisation of actin-like filaments in rat hepatocytes. *Gastroenterology* **68,** 765.
8. GATES G.A., HENLEY K.S., POLLARD H.M. *et al* (1961) The cell population of human liver. *J. Lab. clin. Med.* **57,** 182.
9. GRISHAM J.W., NOPANITAY W. & COMAGNO J. (1976) Scanning electron microscopy of the liver: a review of methods and results. In *Progress in Liver Disease,* ed. H. Popper & F. Schaffner, vol. 5. Grune and Stratton, New York.
10. HANZON V. (1952) Liver cell secretion under normal and pathologic conditions studied by fluorescence microscopy on living rats. *Acta physiol. Scand.* **28,** suppl. 101.
11. HEALEY J.E. Jr (1970) Vascular anatomy of the liver. *Ann. NY Acad. Sci.* **170,** 8.
12. KIERNAN F. (1833) The anatomy and physiology of the liver. *Philos. Trans. London* **123,** 711.
13. Leading article (1980) Bone-marrow origin of Kupffer cells. *Lancet* i, 130.

14. MacSween R.N.M. & Scothorne R.J. (1979) Developmental anatomy and normal structure. In *Pathology of the Liver*, eds. R.N.M. MacSween, P.P. Anthony & P.J. Scheuer. Churchill Livingstone, Edinburgh.

15. Northover J.M.A. & Terblanche J. (1979) A new look at the arterial supply of the bile duct in man and its surgical implications. *Br. J. Surg.* **66**, 379.

16. Nostrant T.J., Miller D.L., Appleman H.D. *et al* (1978) Acinar distribution of liver cell regeneration after selective zonal injury in the rat. *Gastroenterology* **75**, 181.

17. Popper H. & Udenfriend S. (1970) Hepatic fibrosis. *Am. J. Med.* **49**, 707.

18. Pujari B.D. & Deodhare S.G. (1976) Symptomatic accessory lobe of liver with a review of the literature. *Postgrad. med. J.* **52**, 234.

19. Rappaport A.M. (1963) Acinar units and the pathophysiology of the liver. In *The Liver. Morphology, Biochemistry, Physiology*, vol. 1, p. 265, ed. C. Rouiller. Academic Press, New York.

20. Rappaport A.M. (1976) The microcirculatory acinar concept of normal and pathological hepatic structure. *Beitr. Path. Bd.* **157**, 215.

21. Reitemeier R.J., Butt H.R. & Baggenstoss A.H. (1958) Riedel's lobe of the liver. *Gastroenterology* **34**, 1090.

22. Rouiller C. & Jézéquel A-M. (1963) Electron microscopy of the liver. In *The Liver*, vol. I, p. 195, ed. C. Rouiller. Academic Press, New York.

23. Wisse E. (1972) An ultrastructural characterisation of the endothelial cell in the rat liver sinusoid under normal and various experimental conditions as a contribution to the distinction between endothelial and Kupffer cells. *J. ultrastr. Res.* **38**, 528.

24. Wisse E., Van't Noordende J.M., V.D. Meulen J. *et al* (1976) The pit cell: description of a new type of cell occurring in the rat liver sinusoids and peripheral blood. *Cell Tiss. Res.* **173**, 423.

Chapter 2
Biochemical Assessment
of Liver Function

SELECTION OF BIOCHEMICAL TESTS

Biochemical methods in the patient with liver disease are needed for accurate diagnosis, to estimate the severity, to assess prognosis and to evaluate therapy (table 1).

The multiple functions of the liver (fig. 15) are only exceeded by the number of biochemical methods designed to test them. There is no 'magic' test and a large number of methods are unnecessary. The more investigations are multiplied, the greater chance there is of biochemical deficiency being demonstrated. This type of 'shotgun' investigation adds to the confusion. A few simple tests of established value should be used.

Tests most useful in the *diagnosis of jaundice* (Chapter 13) are the serum alkaline phosphatase

level, electrophoresis of the serum proteins and serum transaminase values. Daily inspection of the stools is useful. An isolated rise in serum unconjugated bilirubin suggests Gilbert's syndrome or haemolysis.

Assessment of the *severity of liver cell damage* is done by serial serum total bilirubin, albumin, transaminase and prothrombin after vitamin K estimations.

The diagnosis of *minimal hepato-cellular damage*, due to well-compensated cirrhosis or alcoholic liver damage, may be attempted by noting minimally elevated serum bilirubin and serum transaminase values. Similar changes will be seen in conditions such as fever or circulatory failure. Serum γ-glutamyl transpeptidase (γ-GT) is useful for diagnosing minimal alcoholic liver damage.

Hepatic infiltrations such as primary or secon-

Table 1. Essential serum methods in hepatobiliary disease.

Test	Normal range	International/l	Value
Bilirubin			
total	0.3–1.0 mg/dl	5–17 mmol	Diagnosis jaundice. Assess severity
conjugated	< 0.3 mg/dl	< 5 mmol	Gilbert's disease, haemolysis
Alkaline phosphatase	3–13 KA/dl, 1.5–4 Bodansky/dl	21–100	Diagnosis jaundice, hepatic infiltrations
Aspartate transaminase (AST SGOT)		5–15	Early diagnosis, hepato-cellular disease, follow progress
Alanine transaminase (ALT SGPT)		5–30	ALT relatively lower than AST in alcoholism
Gamma glutamyl transpeptidase		7–30 10–48	Diagnosis alcohol abuse, marker biliary phosphatase
Albumin	3.5–5.0 g/dl	35–50 g	Assess severity
γ-globulin	0.5–1.5 g/dl	5–15 g	Diagnosis chronic hepatitis and cirrhosis—follow course
Prothrombin time (PTT)	10–14 sec		After vitamin K Assess severity

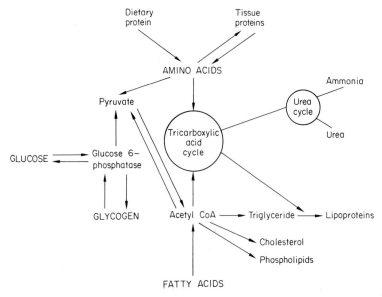

Fig. 15. The important metabolic pathways of protein, carbohydrate and fat in the liver.

dary cancer, amyloid disease or the reticuloses are suggested by an elevated serum alkaline phosphatase value without jaundice.

Immunological tests are of particular value, especially the smooth muscle antibody for the diagnosis of chronic active hepatitis (page 282) and the mitochondrial antibody for primary biliary cirrhosis (page 230). Specific serum markers for virus hepatitis are now available (Chapter 15).

These immunological and virological tests, together with the wider use of needle liver biopsy and better imaging using scanning, ultrasound, arteriography and percutaneous and endoscopic cholangiography, have made diagnosis much more precise. The diagnostic role of the standard liver function tests has therefore been reduced. They remain useful for initial screening for hepatobiliary disease, for detecting severity and for following progress [1, 2].

REFERENCES

1. GOLDBERG D.M. & ELLIS G. (1978) Mathematical and computer assisted procedures in the diagnosis of liver and biliary tract disorders. *Adv. clin. Chem.* **20,** 50.
2. STERN R.B., KNILL-JONES R.P. & WILLIAMS R. (1975) Use of computer programme for diagnosing jaundice in district hospitals and specialised liver units. *Br. med. J.* ii, 659.

BILE PIGMENTS

BILIRUBIN

Bilirubin metabolism is described in detail in Chapter 13.

Serum bilirubin estimations are based on the van den Bergh reaction whereby a direct reaction at 15 minutes gives an estimate of the conjugated bilirubin present. The total bilirubin is determined in the presence of an accelerator such as caffein–benzoate or methanol [6]. An approximate value for the unconjugated (indirect) bilirubin is obtained by subtracting the value for conjugated from that for the total bilirubin.

Inspection of *faeces* is an important investigation in jaundice. Clay-coloured stools indicate biliary obstruction or, rarely, very severe bilirubin glucuronyl-transferase deficiency. Quantitative determinations of faecal urobilinogen are rarely performed nowadays.

Bilirubin cannot be detected in the *urine* of normal subjects or patients with unconjugated hyperbilirubinaemia. In cholestatic patients a small fraction of the conjugated bilirubin in plasma is dialysable and therefore filtered by the glomerulus, some is re-absorbed by the tubules and the remainder gives the dark colour to the urine.

Tablets and dipsticks impregnated with diazo agents are commercially available, easy to use and give satisfactory results for the detection of con-jugated *bilirubin* in urine.

Uses. In acute virus hepatitis bilirubin appears in the urine before urobilinogen or before jaundice. In an undiagnosed febrile illness, bilirubinuria favours the diagnosis of hepatitis. Bilirubinuria is an early sign that an agent is having a hepato-toxic effect.

URÓBILIN(OGEN)

Urobilinogen can be detected in freshly voided urine using dipsticks or Ehrlich's aldehyde agent.

Uses. An increase of urobilinogen in the urine is found when hepato-cellular function is in-adequate to re-excrete all bilirubin absorbed from the intestines. It is therefore a sensitive index of *hepato-cellular dysfunction*, often when other tests are normal. It is a good indication of alcoholic liver damage, well-compensated cirrhosis or malignant disease of the liver. It is also raised with the mild liver dysfunction of pyrexia and circula-tory failure, and haemolytic disease.

In *virus hepatitis* the early appearance of urobilinogen in the urine represents liver cell dysfunction. At the height of the jaundice, in most instances, the liver excretes little if any bili-rubin, and urobilinogen disappears from the urine. Convalescence is heralded by its reappearance, and complete recovery by its final disappearance.

In *cholestatic jaundice* urobilinogen disappears from the urine. Its absence strongly suggests com-plete biliary obstruction due to malignant disease. Partial obstruction due to gall-stones or biliary stricture is usually associated with intermittent increases in urobilinogen in the urine.

Bromsulphalein

The dye bromsulphalein (BSP) is rapidly removed by the liver and excreted in the bile, 67–100% being recovered at two hours after injection. Extra-hepatic removal is probably greatest in the pre-sence of jaundice and at high plasma BSP levels [5]. The BSP is tightly bound to plasma albumin [2].

The standard BSP test consists of slow in-travenous injection of 5 mg/kg of the dye followed by a sampling from the opposite arm at 30 or 45 minutes. The normal is 0–10% retention at 30 minutes and 0–3% at 45 minutes. BSP removal de-creases with age [8]. Obese subjects may show in-creased retention. The test is used to assess liver dysfunction in the absence of jaundice. However,

in view of the cost, the occasional side-effects (which may be fatal [1]), and the inconvenience it is rarely performed nowadays.

In patients who are suspected of Dubin–John-son hyperbilirubinaemia a blood sample is taken not only at 45 minutes after injection but also at two hours. A higher level at two hours than at 45 minutes is diagnostic and reflects release of con-jugated BSP back into the blood stream after a normal initial uptake [7].

Indocyanine green

This dye is removed from the circulation specific-ally by the liver. It is not conjugated and there is no extra-hepatic removal or entero-hepatic circu-lation [4]. It is safer, more expensive and more spe-cific than BSP. It is not routinely used to test liver function but may be valuable for liver blood flow studies [3].

REFERENCES

1. ASTIN T.W. (1965) Systemic reaction to brom-sulphthalein. *Br. med. J.* ii, 408.
2. BAKER K.J. & BRADLEY S.E. (1966) Binding of sul-fobromophalein (BSP) sodium by plasma albu-min. Its role in hepatic BSP extraction. *J. clin. In-vest.* **45**, 281.
3. CAESAR J., SHALDON S., CHIANDUSSI L. *et al* (1961) The use of indocyanine green in the measurement of hepatic blood flow and as a test of hepatic func-tion. *Clin. Sci.* **21**, 43
4. CHERRICK G.R., STEIN S.W., LEEVY C.M. *et al* (1960) Indocyanine green: observations on its physical properties, plasma decay, and hepatic extraction. *J. clin. Invest.* **39**, 592.
5. GIGES B. (1951) Prolonged retention of bromsulfa-lein in patients with regurgitation jaundice. *J. lab. clin. Med.* **38**, 210.
6. MALLOY H.T. & EVELYN K.A. (1937) The determi-nation of bilirubin with the photoelectric colori-meter. *J. biol. Chem.* **119**, 481.
7. MANDEMA E., DE FRAITURE W.H., NIEWIG H.O. *et al* (1960) Familial chronic idiopathic jaundice (Dubin–Sprinz disease) with a note on bromsul-phalein metabolism in this disease. *Am. J. Med.* **28**, 42.
8. THOMPSON E.N. & WILLIAMS R. (1965) Effect of age on liver function with particular reference to bromsulphalein excretion. *Gut* **6**, 266.

LIPID AND LIPOPROTEIN METABOLISM [1, 2, 3]

Several types of lipid are carried in plasma in rela-tively large amounts—cholesterol and cholesterol esters, phospholipids and triglycerides.

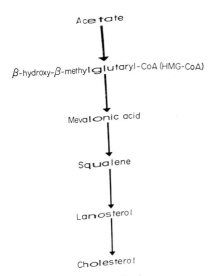

Acetate

↓

β-hydroxy-β-methyl glutaryl-CoA (HMG-CoA)

↓

Mevalonic acid

↓

Squalene

↓

Lanosterol

↓

Cholesterol

Fig. 16. Cholesterol biosynthesis.

Cholesterol is found in almost all cell membranes and is a precursor of bile acids and steroid hormones. It is synthesized in the liver, small intestine and in other tissues. Synthesis takes place mainly from acetate in the microsomal fraction and in cell sap (fig. 16). Hepatic synthesis is inhibited by cholesterol feeding and by fasting, and synthesis is increased by a biliary fistula or bile duct ligation and also by an intestinal lymph fistula. The rate limiting step is the conversion of HMG–CoA to mevalonate; the mechanism controlling this process is uncertain. Cholesterol in membranes and in bile is present almost exclusively as free sterol. In plasma and in certain tissues such as the liver, adrenal and skin, cholesterol esters (cholesterol esterified with long-chain fatty acids) are also found. Cholesterol esters are more nonpolar than free cholesterol and therefore even less soluble in water. Esterification is carried out in plasma by the enzyme lecithin cholesterol acyl transferase (LCAT) which is synthesized in the liver.

Phospholipids are a heterogeneous group of compounds. They contain one or more phosphoric acid groups and another polar group. This may be a heterogeneous base such as choline or ethanolamine. In addition there are one or more long-chain fatty acid residues. The phospholipids are much more complex in terms of chemical reactivity than cholesterol and cholesterol esters. They are important constituents of cell membranes and take part in a large number of chemical reactions. The most abundant phospholipid in plasma and most cellular membranes is phosphatidyl choline or lecithin.

Triglycerides are simpler compounds than the phospholipids. They have a backbone of glycerol, the hydroxy groups of which have been esterified with fatty acids. Naturally-occurring triglycerides contain a variety of fatty acids; they act as a store of energy and also as a method of transport of energy from the gut and liver to peripheral tissues.

Lipoproteins. Cholesterol, phospholipids and triglycerides are insoluble in water and would not exist in plasma in free solution. Two major groups of lipoproteins are involved in lipid transport. One migrates in an electrical field with α_1 globulins (HDL) and the other with β globulins (LDL). A third fraction, very low density lipoprotein (VLDL), is also recognized. The fourth type of lipoprotein is the chylomicron which is a large triglyceride-rich particle originating from the gut and appearing in plasma after the ingestion of a fatty meal. The chemical and physical differences between the various lipoproteins are due partly to their differing lipid composition and partly to variations in their protein content.

A number of different protein sub-units are present in plasma lipoproteins; in their delipidated form they are called apoproteins. Apoprotein APO-A1 activates plasma LCAT; apoprotein APO-C1 activates lipoprotein lipase.

Changes in liver disease (fig. 17)

The increase in total serum cholesterol level in cholestasis is not due simply to the retention of cholesterol normally excreted in the bile. The mechanism is uncertain but it might be related to regurgitation into plasma of biliary phospholipid [1]. Whereas slight increases to 1.5–2 times normal are sometimes seen in acute cholestasis, very high values are found in chronic conditions, especially postoperative stricture and primary biliary cirrhosis. Values of over five times the upper limit of normal are associated with skin xanthomas. Malnutrition lowers the serum cholesterol so that values may be normal in carcinomatous biliary obstruction. Increased values are seen during recovery from virus hepatitis, in fatty liver and in some patients with gall-stones.

In cirrhosis total serum cholesterol values are usually normal. Low results indicate malnutrition or decompensation.

In hepato-cellular disease and in obstructive jaundice the plasma triglycerides tend to be in-

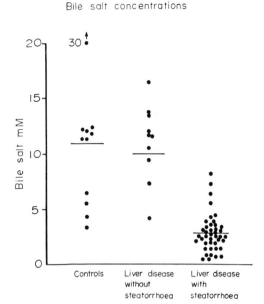

Fig. 20. Patients with chronic, non-alcoholic liver disease and steatorrhoea show a reduced bile salt concentration in their aspirated intestinal contents compared with control subjects and patients with chronic liver disease without steatorrhoea (Badley *et al* 1970).

and monoglyceride or fatty acid, so allowing cholesterol to be absorbed.

Bile salts help to emulsify dietary fat and probably also play a part in the mucosal phase of absorption. Diminished secretion leads to steatorrhoea (fig. 20). They assist pancreatic lipolysis. They release gastro-intestinal hormones.

Disordered intra-hepatic metabolism of bile salts may be important in the pathogenesis of cholestasis (page 211). They may have a role in the causation of the pruritus of cholestasis, although this is controversial.

They may be responsible for target cells in the peripheral blood of jaundiced patients (page 36) and for the secretion of conjugated bilirubin in urine.

When deconjugated or dehydroxylated by intestinal bacteria, bile acids are ineffective in absorption. This may partly explain the malabsorption complicating diseases with stasis and bacterial overgrowth in the small intestine.

Removal of the terminal ileum interrupts the entero-hepatic circulation and allows large amounts of primary bile acids to reach the colon and be dehydroxylated by bacteria, so reducing the body's bile salt pool. The altered bile salts in the colon excite a profound electrolyte and water loss with diarrhoea [6].

Lithocholic acid is mostly excreted in the faeces and only slightly absorbed. It is cirrhogenic to experimental animals and can be used to produce experimental gall-stones. Taurolithocholic acid can also cause intra-hepatic cholestasis perhaps by interfering with the bile salt-independent fraction of bile flow.

Serum bile acids

Total serum bile acid concentrations may be assayed by an enzymatic method using hydroxy-steroid dehydrogenase. Gas–liquid chromatography allows individual bile acids to be distinguished [12]. Enzymatic fluorometry is a simple modification of this technique [8]. Radio-immunoassay adds to the sensitivity, and assays for conjugates of cholic, chenodeoxycholic and deoxycholic acids have been described [11, 13, 14].

The concentration of total serum bile acids indicates the fraction re-absorbed from the intestine that escaped extraction on its first passage through the liver. Increases in both hepato-cellular and cholestatic jaundice limit their diagnostic effectiveness. Serum bile acids have, however, been recommended for detecting minimal liver cell damage, for instance in viral hepatitis or drug toxicity, and for following the response to treatment in chronic active hepatitis [9]. Normal serum bile acids are found in Gilbert's syndrome [7]. Diagnostic kits for serum bile acids are now available. It seems unlikely, however, that this estimation will replace simpler and less costly biochemical tests of liver function.

A refinement is the estimation of serum bile acids two hours after a meal (post-prandial bile acids) and this is a most sensitive test of hepato-cellular function [2, 7].

Estimations of individual bile acids show that in cholestasis the ratio of serum trihydroxy to dehydroxy acid increases [10]. Patients with hepato-cellular failure usually have a low ratio, the main bile acid being chenodeoxycholic acid.

The serum cholic:chenodeoxycholic acid ratio can discriminate between normal subjects, patients with extra-hepatic cholestasis and cirrhosis [11]. It is unlikely to be widely applied because of the complexity of the analytical techniques.

An intravenous isotopic *bile acid tolerance test* has been used [16]. Abnormalities reflect poor

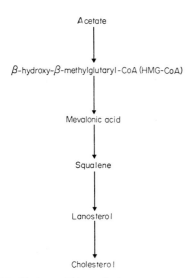

Fig. 16. Cholesterol biosynthesis.

Cholesterol is found in almost all cell membranes and is a precursor of bile acids and steroid hormones. It is synthesized in the liver, small intestine and in other tissues. Synthesis takes place mainly from acetate in the microsomal fraction and in cell sap (fig. 16). Hepatic synthesis is inhibited by cholesterol feeding and by fasting, and synthesis is increased by a biliary fistula or bile duct ligation and also by an intestinal lymph fistula. The rate limiting step is the conversion of HMG–CoA to mevalonate; the mechanism controlling this process is uncertain. Cholesterol in membranes and in bile is present almost exclusively as free sterol. In plasma and in certain tissues such as the liver, adrenal and skin, cholesterol esters (cholesterol esterified with long-chain fatty acids) are also found. Cholesterol esters are more non-polar than free cholesterol and therefore even less soluble in water. Esterification is carried out in plasma by the enzyme lecithin cholesterol acyl transferase (LCAT) which is synthesized in the liver.

Phospholipids are a heterogeneous group of compounds. They contain one or more phosphoric acid groups and another polar group. This may be a heterogeneous base such as choline or ethanolamine. In addition there are one or more long-chain fatty acid residues. The phospholipids are much more complex in terms of chemical reactivity than cholesterol and cholesterol esters. They are important constituents of cell membranes and take part in a large number of chemical reactions. The most abundant phospholipid in plasma and

most cellular membranes is phosphatidyl choline or lecithin.

Triglycerides are simpler compounds than the phospholipids. They have a backbone of glycerol, the hydroxy groups of which have been esterified with fatty acids. Naturally-occurring triglycerides contain a variety of fatty acids; they act as a store of energy and also as a method of transport of energy from the gut and liver to peripheral tissues.

Lipoproteins. Cholesterol, phospholipids and triglycerides are insoluble in water and would not exist in plasma in free solution. Two major groups of lipoproteins are involved in lipid transport. One migrates in an electrical field with α_1 globulins (HDL) and the other with β globulins (LDL). A third fraction, very low density lipoprotein (VLDL), is also recognized. The fourth type of lipoprotein is the chylomicron which is a large triglyceride-rich particle originating from the gut and appearing in plasma after the ingestion of a fatty meal. The chemical and physical differences between the various lipoproteins are due partly to their differing lipid composition and partly to variations in their protein content.

A number of different protein sub-units are present in plasma lipoproteins; in their delipidated form they are called apoproteins. Apoprotein APO-A1 activates plasma LCAT; apoprotein APO-C1 activates lipoprotein lipase.

Changes in liver disease (fig. 17)

The increase in total serum cholesterol level in cholestasis is not due simply to the retention of cholesterol normally excreted in the bile. The mechanism is uncertain but it might be related to regurgitation into plasma of biliary phospholipid [1]. Whereas slight increases to 1.5–2 times normal are sometimes seen in acute cholestasis, very high values are found in chronic conditions, especially post-operative stricture and primary biliary cirrhosis. Values of over five times the upper limit of normal are associated with skin xanthomas. Malnutrition lowers the serum cholesterol so that values may be normal in carcinomatous biliary obstruction. Increased values are seen during recovery from virus hepatitis, in fatty liver and in some patients with gall-stones.

In cirrhosis total serum cholesterol values are usually normal. Low results indicate malnutrition or decompensation.

In hepato-cellular disease and in obstructive jaundice the plasma triglycerides tend to be in-

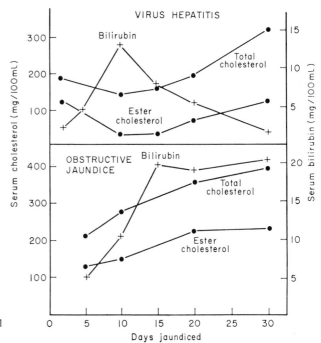

Fig. 17. Serum ester and total cholesterol levels in virus hepatitis and cholestasis.

creased, the excess being found in the low density lipoprotein (LDL) fraction. In both conditions the percentage of cholesterol esters is decreased due to LCAT deficiency related to impaired formation and, in obstructive jaundice, due to a marked increase in free cholesterol. Lipoprotein electrophoresis shows absence of pre-β and a wide, deeply staining β band.

In *cholestasis* an abnormal lipoprotein, lipoprotein X, very rich in free cholesterol and lecithin, is found which appears on electron microscopy as bilamellar discs (Chapter 14).

LCAT deficiency is a marked feature, perhaps due to decreased synthesis. This would result in a rise in free cholesterol with a reduction in the esters.

The haematological changes of cholestasis can be related to abnormalities in cholesterol and lipoprotein.

Serum cholesterol esters, lipoproteins, and LCAT are not estimated routinely.

REFERENCES

1. McIntyre N., Harry D.S. & Pearson A.J.G. (1975) The hypercholesterolaemia of obstructive jaundice. *Gut* **16**, 379.
2. McIntyre N. (1978) Plasma lipids and lipoproteins in liver disease. *Gut* **19**, 526.
3. Sabesin S.M., Ragland J.B. & Freeman M.R. (1979) Lipoprotein disturbances in liver disease. In *Progress in Liver Disease*, vol. VI, eds H. Popper & F. Schaffner, p. 243. Grune and Stratton, New York.

BILE ACIDS [5]

Bile acids are synthesized only in the liver, 0.3–0.7 g being produced and lost in the faeces daily (Chapter 29).

The primary bile acids, cholic acid and chenodeoxycholic acid, are formed in the liver from cholesterol (fig. 18). Synthesis may be controlled by the amount of bile acid returning to the liver in the entero-hepatic circulation [4]. When the primary bile salts come into contact with bacteria in the colon, or elsewhere in the intestine if there is bacterial overgrowth, 7α dehydration takes place with production of the secondary bile acids, deoxycholic and lithocholic acids. Very little lithocholic acid is formed. In human bile the amount of the trihydroxy acid (cholic acid) roughly equals the sum of the two dihydroxy acids (chenodeoxycholic and deoxycholic).

The bile acids are conjugated in the liver, through a peptide bond, with the amino acids glycine or taurine forming the bile salts. Glycine con-

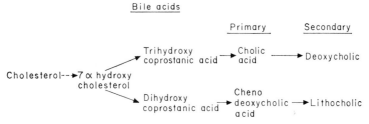

Fig. 18. Production of primary and secondary bile acids.

jugates predominate. Bacteria are also capable of hydrolysing the bile salts to bile acid and glycine or taurine.

Bile salts are excreted into the biliary canaliculus against an enormous concentration gradient between liver and bile. The process depends on a carrier-mediated, active transport system. At that point the bile salts enter into micellar association with cholesterol and phospholipids (fig. 395). In the upper small intestine the bile salt micelles are too large and too polar to be absorbed. They are intimately concerned with the digestion and absorption of lipids. It is not until the terminal ileum and proximal colon that absorption takes place by a special transport process found only in the ileum. The absorbed bile salts enter the portal venous blood and reach the liver where they are taken up

with great avidity by the hepatocytes. Synthesis is under negative feedback control. In the liver cell, they are reconjugated and re-excreted into the bile. Lithocholic acid is not re-excreted. This *enterohepatic circulation* of bile salts takes place two to five times daily (fig. 19).

Changes in disease

Bile salts increase the biliary excretion of water, lecithin, cholesterol and conjugated bilirubin (fig. 189).

Altered biliary excretion with defective biliary micelle formation is important in the pathogenesis of gall-stones (fig. 395) and in the steatorrhoea of cholestasis [1].

They form a micellar solution with cholesterol

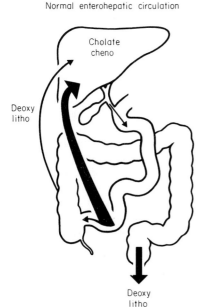

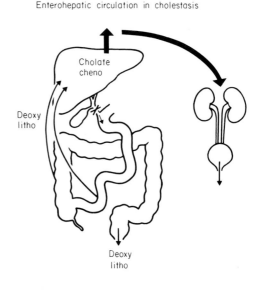

Fig. 19. The entero-hepatic circulation of bile acids in normal subjects and in cholestasis.

Bile salt concentrations

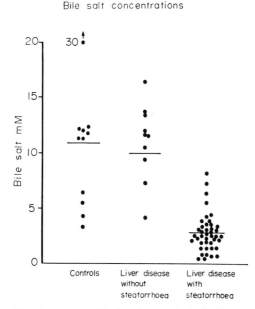

Fig. 20. Patients with chronic, non-alcoholic liver disease and steatorrhoea show a reduced bile salt concentration in their aspirated intestinal contents compared with control subjects and patients with chronic liver disease without steatorrhoea (Badley *et al* 1970).

and monoglyceride or fatty acid, so allowing cholesterol to be absorbed.

Bile salts help to emulsify dietary fat and probably also play a part in the mucosal phase of absorption. Diminished secretion leads to steatorrhoea (fig. 20). They assist pancreatic lipolysis. They release gastro-intestinal hormones.

Disordered intra-hepatic metabolism of bile salts may be important in the pathogenesis of cholestasis (page 211). They may have a role in the causation of the pruritus of cholestasis, although this is controversial.

They may be responsible for target cells in the peripheral blood of jaundiced patients (page 36) and for the secretion of conjugated bilirubin in urine.

When deconjugated or dehydroxylated by intestinal bacteria, bile acids are ineffective in absorption. This may partly explain the malabsorption complicating diseases with stasis and bacterial overgrowth in the small intestine.

Removal of the terminal ileum interrupts the entero-hepatic circulation and allows large amounts of primary bile acids to reach the colon and be dehydroxylated by bacteria, so reducing the body's bile salt pool. The altered bile salts in the colon excite a profound electrolyte and water loss with diarrhoea [6].

Lithocholic acid is mostly excreted in the faeces and only slightly absorbed. It is cirrhogenic to experimental animals and can be used to produce experimental gall-stones. Taurolithocholic acid can also cause intra-hepatic cholestasis perhaps by interfering with the bile salt-independent fraction of bile flow.

Serum bile acids

Total serum bile acid concentrations may be assayed by an enzymatic method using hydroxysteroid dehydrogenase. Gas–liquid chromatography allows individual bile acids to be distinguished [12]. Enzymatic fluorometry is a simple modification of this technique [8]. Radioimmunoassay adds to the sensitivity, and assays for conjugates of cholic, chenodeoxycholic and deoxycholic acids have been described [11, 13, 14].

The concentration of total serum bile acids indicates the fraction re-absorbed from the intestine that escaped extraction on its first passage through the liver. Increases in both hepato-cellular and cholestatic jaundice limit their diagnostic effectiveness. Serum bile acids have, however, been recommended for detecting minimal liver cell damage, for instance in viral hepatitis or drug toxicity, and for following the response to treatment in chronic active hepatitis [9]. Normal serum bile acids are found in Gilbert's syndrome [7]. Diagnostic kits for serum bile acids are now available. It seems unlikely, however, that this estimation will replace simpler and less costly biochemical tests of liver function.

A refinement is the estimation of serum bile acids two hours after a meal (post-prandial bile acids) and this is a most sensitive test of hepatocellular function [2, 7].

Estimations of individual bile acids show that in cholestasis the ratio of serum trihydroxy to dehydroxy acid increases [10]. Patients with hepato-cellular failure usually have a low ratio, the main bile acid being chenodeoxycholic acid.

The serum cholic:chenodeoxycholic acid ratio can discriminate between normal subjects, patients with extra-hepatic cholestasis and cirrhosis [11]. It is unlikely to be widely applied because of the complexity of the analytical techniques.

An intravenous isotopic *bile acid tolerance test* has been used [16]. Abnormalities reflect poor hepato-cellular function and portal–systemic shunting. There is much overlap between hepato-cellular and cholestatic jaundice and the test is not a practical proposition.

The *radio-active glycocholate breath test* for the diagnosis of small bowel bacterial overgrowth is a research tool.

In cholestasis bile acids are excreted in the *urine* by active transport and passive diffusion [3]. The pattern is similar to that in the serum, but sulphate esters account for a larger proportion of the total bile acids [15].

REFERENCES

1. BADLEY B.W.D., MURPHY G.M., BOUCHIER I.A.D. *et al* (1970) Diminished micellar phase lipid in patients with chronic nonalcoholic liver disease and steatorrhea. *Gastroenterology* **58**, 781.
2. BARNES S., GALLO G.A., TRASH D.B. *et al* (1975) Diagnostic value of serum bile acid estimations in liver disease. *J. clin. Path.* **28**, 506.
3. BARNES S., GOLLAN J.L. & BILLING B.H. (1977) The role of tubular reabsorption in the renal excretion of bile acids. *Biochem J.* **164**, 65.
4. GRUNDY S.M., HOFMANN A.F., DAVIGNON J. *et al* (1966) Human cholesterol synthesis is regulated by bile acids. *J. clin. Invest.* **45**, 1018.
5. HAZLEWOOD G.A.D. (1978) *The Biological Importance of Bile Salts.* North Holland, Amsterdam.
6. HOFMANN A.F. (1967) The syndrome of ileal disease and the broken enterohepatic circulation: cholerheic enteropathy. *Gastroenterology* **52**, 752.
7. JAVITT N.B. (1977) Diagnostic value of serum bile acids. *Clin. Gastroenterol.* **6**, 219.
8. KOBAYISHI K., ALLEN R.M., BLOOMER J.R. *et al* (1979) Enzymatic fluorometry for estimating serum total bile acid concentration. *J. Am. med. Assoc.* **241**, 2043.
9. KORMAN M.G., HOFMANN A.F. & SUMMERSKILL W.H.J. (1974) Assessment of activity in chronic active liver disease: serum bile acids compared with conventional tests and histology. *New Engl. J. Med.* **290**, 1399.
10. OSBORN E.C., WOOTTON I.D.P., DA SILVA L.C. *et al* (1959) Serum-bile-acid levels in liver disease. *Lancet* ii, 1049.
11. PENNINGTON C.R., BAQIR Y.A., ROSS P.E. *et al* (1979) Measurement of serum primary bile acid ratio by gas liquid chromatography and radioimmunoassay. *J. clin. Path.* **32**, 565.
12. ROSS P.E., PENNINGTON C.R. & BOUCHIER I.A.D. (1977) Gas liquid chromatographic assay of serum bile acids. *Analytic Biochem.* **80**, 458.
13. SCHALM S.W., BERGE-HENEGOUWEN G.P. VAN, HOFMANN A.F. *et al* (1977) Radioimmunoassay of bile acids: development, validation and preliminary application of an assay for conjugates of chenodeoxycholic acid. *Gastroenterology* **73**, 285.
14. SIMMONDS W.J., KORMAN M.G., GO V.L.W. *et al* (1973) Radioimmunoassay of conjugated cholyl bile acids in serum. *Gastroenterology* **65**, 705.
15. SUMMERFIELD J.A., CULLEN J., BARNES S. *et al* (1977) Evidence for renal control of urinary excretion of bile acid and bile acid sulphates in the cholestatic syndrome. *Clin. Sci. molec. Med.* **5**, 51.
16. THJODLEIFSSON B., BARNES S., CHITRANUKROH A. *et al* (1977) Assessment of the plasma disappearance of cholyl-1-^{14}C-glycine as a test of hepatocellular disease. *Gut* **18**, 697.

AMINO ACID AND PROTEIN METABOLISM

Amino acids derived from the diet and from tissue breakdown arrive at the liver for metabolism. Some are transaminated or deaminated to keto-acids which are metabolized by many pathways including the tricarboxylic acid cycle (Krebs–citric acid cycle). Others are metabolized to ammonia and urea (Krebs–Henseleit urea cycle). The maximal rate of urea synthesis in chronic liver disease is markedly reduced [9]. However, experimentally, at least 85% of liver must be removed before this mechanism fails significantly and before blood and urinary amino acid levels increase [5]. A low blood urea concentration is a rare accompaniment of fulminant liver failure. A rise in blood ammonia level also represents a failure of the Krebs–Henseleit cycle and this increase has been related to hepatic encephalopathy.

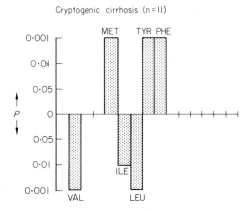

Fig. 21. The plasma amino acid pattern in cryptogenic cirrhosis (mean of 11 patients). The aromatic amino acids are increased while the branched chain ones are decreased. Blocks represent increases or decreases in amino acid values. MET= methionine, TYR=tyrosine, PHE=phenyl alanine, VAL=valine, ILE=isoleucine, LEU=leucine (Morgan *et al* 1980).

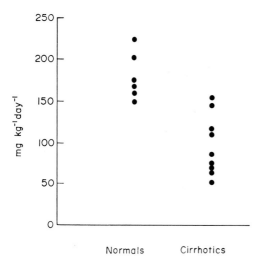

Fig. 22. The absolute synthesis of serum albumin (^{14}C carbonate method) in cirrhosis is reduced (Tavill *et al* 1971).

The aromatic amino acids tyrosine, phenylalanine and tryptophan are increased in all forms of hepato-cellular disease, perhaps due to failure of hepatic deamination. The branched chain amino acids, valine, leucine and isoleucine, are decreased perhaps due to increased catabolism in skeletal muscle (fig. 21) [6].

In fulminant hepatitis there is marked generalized amino-aciduria involving particularly cystine and tyrosine and this carries a bad prognosis.

The hepatectomized animal cannot synthesize albumin [10]. The human liver synthesizes albumin

[8, 11], fibrinogen, prothrombin, haptoglobin, glycoprotein, transferrin and ceruloplasmin. The immunoglobulins are synthesized by immunocytes. These observations support the clinical findings that liver disease is associated with failure to maintain serum albumin values whereas immunoglobulins tend to be increased. Albumin production is enhanced by more intense activity of each liver cell rather than a rise in the number of cells. The liver also catabolizes albumin.

Normals make about 10 g albumin daily; hypoalbuminaemic patients with cirrhosis can synthesize only about 4 g daily [12] (fig. 22). About 2 g fibrinogen and 1 g transferrin are also produced.

The normal half-life of serum albumin is 20–26 days. In cirrhosis it is increased and albumin turnover is correspondingly decreased, reflecting impaired synthesis [13]. A rise or fall in plasma protein concentration may reflect changes not only in hepatic production but also in plasma volume. Total exchangeable albumin pool is not depleted in cirrhosis. When ascites is present, however, the extravascular albumin pool is expanded at the expense of the intravascular one [13] (fig. 23).

Corticosteroids increase the rate of synthesis of albumin. Protein loss into the gut is not increased in cirrhosis.

CLINICAL SIGNIFICANCE

Changes are slow and do not immediately reflect acute liver damage. Even complete cessation of albumin production results in only 25% decrease

Fig. 23. The turnover of plasma albumin in a 70 kg adult seen in the context of the daily protein economy of the gastro-intestinal tract and overall nitrogen balance. The total exchangeable albumin pool of about 300 g is distributed between the intravascular and extravascular compartments in a ratio of approximately 2:3. In this simplified schema the balance sheet is expressed in terms of g of protein ($=6.25\times$g of N). Losses do not include relatively minor routes, e.g. 2 g per day from the skin (Tavill 1972).

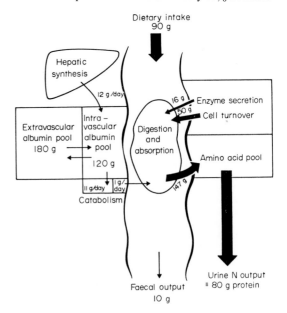

in serum levels after eight days. Thus patients with severe virus hepatitis may have normal serum albumin values. Similarly, serum protein levels are usually normal in early biliary obstruction when the liver cells are relatively unaffected, but with continuing cholestasis, serum albumin falls. Malnutrition and fever will also tend to lower the serum albumin. Serum levels of clotting proteins, such as prothrombin, with a short half-life, are rapidly reduced following acute liver damage (fig. 96).

The characteristic change in chronic liver disease is a fall in serum albumin and a rise in globulin levels. Albumin and globulin reflect different functions; the albumin–globulin ratio is therefore meaningless.

'Normal' values depend on the analytical methods used. Auto-analytical procedures tend to give low serum albumin values.

In severe, prolonged, virus hepatitis and in cirrhosis, serum albumin levels bear a close relation to the clinical state and are helpful prognostically and in following treatment. Serum values may be normal in well-compensated cirrhosis and are of little value diagnostically.

Hyperglobulinaemia is a feature of acute and chronic hepato-cellular disease. It reflects a reticulo-endothelial reaction to antigens, largely of gut origin (fig. 312). Extremely high values characterize chronic active hepatitis, levels falling only in the later stages or with corticosteroid treatment.

Electrophoretic pattern of the serum proteins

Paper electrophoresis gives the proportions of the various serum proteins (fig. 24).

In cirrhosis albumin is reduced and in acute hepatitis these changes are much less conspicuous.

The α_1-globulins contain glycoproteins and tend to be low in hepato-cellular disease, falling in parallel with the serum albumin. An increase accompanies acute febrile illnesses and malignant disease. An absent α_1-globulin may indicate α_1 anti-trypsin deficiency.

The α_2- and β-globulins contain lipoproteins (page 17). In cholestasis the increase in α_2- and β-globulin components (fig. 24) correlates with the height of serum lipids. This pattern may be useful in distinguishing biliary from non-biliary cirrhosis. High lipoprotein components strongly support a biliary aetiology.

Haptoglobins are reduced in chronic hepato-cellular disease [7] and raised in cholestasis. Ceruloplasmin is increased in alcoholic cirrhosis and chronic active hepatitis. Transferrin is reduced in alcoholic cirrhosis [7].

The γ-globulins rise in hepatic cirrhosis due to increased production [3]. The increased numbers of plasma cells in marrow, and even in the liver itself, may be the source. The γ-globulin peak in hepato-cellular disease shows a wide base (*polyclonal gammopathy*). *Monoclonal gammopathy* is rare [14] and may be age rather than chronic liver

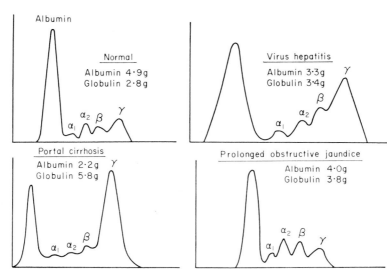

Fig. 24. Electrophoretic pattern of the serum proteins. Note the raised γ- and, to a lesser extent, β- and α_2-globulins in virus hepatitis. In cirrhosis the albumin is depressed and there is an increase in the globulin fraction. In cholestasis the α_2- and β-globulins are raised.

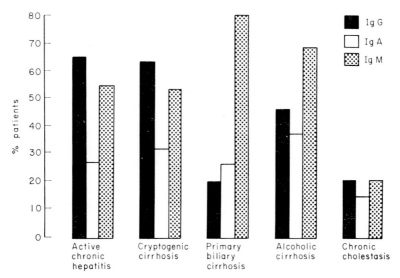

Fig. 25. Incidence of raised serum immunoglobulin levels in liver disease. In active chronic hepatitis the pattern of elevated IgG, IgA and IgM is very similar to that seen in cryptogenic cirrhosis. In primary biliary cirrhosis IgM increase is the commonest abnormality although about one-quarter of patients also show increases in IgG and IgA. In cirrhosis of the alcoholic, IgM elevation is the commonest abnormality but IgA and IgG can also be increased. In chronic cholestasis (obstructive jaundice) a percentage of serum immunoglobulins in one or other component. The test cannot be used diagnostically (Feizi 1968).

disease-related [1]. The dip between β- and γ-globulins tends to be bridged.

Immunoglobulins (fig. 25). IgG is markedly increased in chronic active hepatitis and cryptogenic cirrhosis. There is a slow and sustained increase in viral hepatitis and it is also increased in cirrhosis of the alcoholic [4].

IgM is markedly increased in primary biliary cirrhosis (fig. 25) and to a lesser extent in viral hepatitis and cirrhosis, whether chronic active or cryptogenic.

IgA is markedly increased in cirrhosis of the alcoholic but also in primary biliary and cryptogenic cirrhosis.

In chronic active hepatitis and cryptogenic cirrhosis the pattern is surprisingly similar, with increases in IgG, IgM and to a lesser extent IgA [4].

About 10% of patients with chronic cholestasis due to large bile duct obstruction show increases in all three main immunoglobulins.

Patterns are not diagnostic of any one disease but only give suggestive evidence.

REFERENCES

1. ELLMAN L.L., PACHAS W.N., PINALS R.S. *et al* (1969) M-components in patients with chronic liver disease. *Gastroenterology* **57**, 138.

2. FEIZI T. (1968) Serum immunoglobulins in liver disease. *Gut* **9**, 193.

3. HAVENS W.P. Jr, DICKENSHEETS J., BIERLY J.N. *et al* (1954) The half-life of I^{131} labeled normal human gamma globulin in patients with hepatic cirrhosis. *J. Immmunol.* **73**, 256.

4. LEE F.I. (1965) Immunoglobulins in viral hepatitis and active alcoholic liver-disease. *Lancet* ii, 1043.

5. MANN F.C. (1927) The effects of complete and of partial removal of the liver. *Medicine* **6**, 419.

6. MORGAN M.Y., MILSOM J.P. & SHERLOCK S. (1981) Plasma amino acid patterns in liver disease. *Gut.* In press.

7. MURRAY-LYON I., CLARKE H.G.M., MCPHERSON K. *et al* (1972) Quantitative immunoelectrophoresis of serum proteins in cryptogenic cirrhosis, alcoholic cirrhosis and active chronic hepatitis. *Clin. chim. Acta* **39**, 215.

8. ROTHSCHILD M.A., ORATZ M. & SCHREIBER S.S. (1972) Albumin synthesis. *N. Engl. J. Med.* **286**, 748.

9. RUDMAN D., DIFULCO T.J., GALAMBOS J.T. *et al* (1973) Maximal rates of excretion and synthesis of urea in normal and cirrhotic subjects. *J. clin. Invest.* **52**, 2241.

10. TARVER H. & REINHARDT W.O. (1947) Methionine labelled with radioactive sulfur as an indicator of protein formation in the hepatectomized dog. *J. biol. Chem.* **167**, 395.

11. TAVILL A.S. (1972) The synthesis and degradation of liver-produced proteins. *Gut* **13**, 225.

12. TAVILL A.S., CRAIGIE A. & ROSENOER V.M. (1968) The measurement of the synthetic rate of albumin in man. *Clin. Sci.* **34**, 1.

13. WILKINSON P. & MENDENHALL C.L. (1963) Serum albumin turnover in normal subjects and patients with cirrhosis measured by ^{131}I-labelled human albumin. *Clin Sci.* **25**, 28.
14. ZAWADZKI Z.A. & EDWARDS G.A. (1970) Dysimmunoglobulinemia associated with hepato-biliary disorders. *Am. J. Med.* **48**, 196.

SERUM ENZYME TESTS

These tests will usually diagnose the type of liver injury, whether hepato-cellular or cholestatic, but cannot be expected to diagnose one form of hepatitis from another or to determine whether cholestasis is intra- or extra-hepatic. Only a few tests are necessary and the combination of a serum aspartate transaminase (SGOT) and alkaline phosphatase (with occasionally serum alanine transaminase, SGPT) will usually detect a patient with liver disease.

The phosphatases

SERUM ALKALINE PHOSPHATASE [5, 8]

Alkaline phosphatase is a phosphomonoesterase. The level rises in cholestasis and to a lesser extent when the liver cells are damaged. The increased serum alkaline phosphatase is of hepatic origin and the alkaline phosphatase of bile is derived from the liver. Experimentally, bile duct ligation results in a seven-fold increase in hepatic alkaline phosphatase and a two-and-a-half-fold increase in serum concentration [5]. Both rises are prevented by inhibitors of protein synthesis, suggesting that the increase in hepatic alkaline phosphatase is due to *de novo* hepatic protein synthesis and that it is hepatic enzyme which appears in the serum [5]. The enzyme is tightly bound to lipid membranes, particularly those in the canalicular area. Any disorder interfering with bile flow, whether intra- or extra-hepatic, increases synthesis. Bile acids may be the stimulus for the increase [3]. It is uncertain how the enzyme reaches the serum. It is solubilized before doing so, presumably by the detergent action of retained bile acids on lipid membranes. Alkaline phosphatase has a serum half-life of seven days. It therefore tends to remain elevated after the serum bilirubin has returned to normal. It is probably destroyed in the liver.

Serum hepatic alkaline phosphatase may be distinguished from bony phosphatase by fractionation into iso-enzymes on polyacrylamide gel or cellulose acetate, but this is not a routine method [7, 9].

Clinical significance

In cholestatic jaundice levels are usually four times the upper limit of normal whereas in hepato-cellular jaundice they are less than this; anomalies occur. Low values are unusual in obstructive jaundice. Incomplete cholestasis, due to such causes as biliary stricture or primary biliary cirrhosis, is associated with a particularly high phosphatase level, out of proportion to the serum bilirubin. Serum alkaline phosphatase is a more sensitive index of cholestasis.

Raised levels are sometimes observed with primary or secondary tumours, even without jaundice or involvement of bone. Increased values are also found with other space-occupying hepatic lesions such as amyloid, abscess, leukaemia or granulomas. These increases are presumably due to obstruction of many small bile channels in many parts of the liver.

Serum phosphatase determinations do not reflect liver cell damage. In active cirrhosis without jaundice, especially in children, phosphatase values may be raised sometimes to very high levels; they may be normal in well-compensated cirrhosis. Increased values are found in bone disease. Increases are also seen in growing children, and values about one-and-a-half times normal are found after the fifth decade of life. Non-specific mild elevations are seen in a variety of conditions, including Hodgkin's disease and heart failure.

SERUM 5-NUCLEOTIDASE

The enzyme is an alkaline phosphomonoesterase which specifically hydrolyses nucleotide attached to the 5 position of the pentose.

Values are normal in bone disease and raised in hepato-biliary conditions, especially cholestatic jaundice. Its main value is in deciding whether a raised serum alkaline phosphatase level is due to bone or hepato-biliary disease.

SERUM GAMMAGLUTAMYL TRANSPEPTIDASE (γ-GT)

This enzyme is found in many tissues. Three isoenzymes are found in normal serum and five in the cholestatic [10]. Serum values are increased in both cholestasis and hepato-cellular disease [11]. It parallels serum alkaline phosphatase in cholestasis and may be used to confirm that a raised serum phosphatase is of hepato-biliary origin. Levels are increased with hepatic metastases but not consistently and this estimation cannot be used for pre-operative detection.

Serum levels are raised in patients with alcohol abuse and these are useful for screening [6]. Increases may be due to microsomal enzyme induction by alcohol.

Values may remain raised for many months after hepatitis and particularly after mononucleosis [4].

The transaminases

Glutamic oxaloacetic transaminase (GOT) (aspartate transaminase) is a mitochondrial enzyme present in large quantities in heart, liver, skeletal muscle and kidney, and the serum level of the enzyme increases whenever these tissues are acutely destroyed, presumably due to release from damaged cells. Very high values are found with hepato-cellular necrosis or myocardial infarction.

Glutamic pyruvic transaminase (GPT) (alanine transaminase) is a cytosol enzyme also present in liver and although the absolute amount is less than GOT a greater proportion is present there compared with heart and skeletal muscles. A serum increase is therefore more specific for liver damage than SGOT.

In practice, differentiation of myocardial infarction from acute hepatitis is not a clinical problem and it is sufficient to measure only the SGOT. The GPT is less stable in stored serum.

USE OF TRANSAMINASE DETERMINATIONS

These are useful in the early diagnosis of virus hepatitis, particularly in epidemics and in detecting the non-icteric case. Measurements must be made early for normal values may be reached within a week of the onset. The patient may develop fatal acute hepatic necrosis in spite of falling transaminase values. Serial estimations are essential. Very high values in viral hepatitis and mononucleosis do not correlate with the degree of liver damage. Very high levels may be seen in the early stages of acute choledocholithiasis.

Routine auto-analyser screening may show unexpectedly raised transaminase levels. These are often due to alcohol abuse or heart failure. Transaminase determinations are helpful in screening for liver injury due to drugs.

Results vary in cirrhosis, being particularly high in chronic active hepatitis. The value falls with corticosteroid treatment. Very high levels are unusual in alcoholic liver disease. Moderate increases, usually about five times the upper limit of normal, are noted in cholestasis and primary or secondary hepatic tumours. A high ratio of SGOT to SGPT (greater than two) may be useful in diagnosing alcoholic hepatitis and cirrhosis [2].

Other serum enzymes

None of these have gained acceptance for routine use.

Lactic dehydrogenase (LDH) is a relatively insensitive index of hepato-cellular injury, but marked increases are found in patients with neoplasms, especially with hepatic involvement.

Isocitric dehydrogenase (ICD). Raised values are found with hepato-cellular damage and normal ones with myocardial infarction and in the myopathies. The estimation is believed to be more specific for hepatic disease than SGOT [1].

Choline esterase is a non-specific esterase synthesized by the liver. Decreases in hepato-cellular disease, especially cirrhosis, reflect diminished synthesis and also poor nutrition. In malnutrition, the serum level parallels that in the liver. Decreases may be useful in detecting hepatotoxicity due to chemicals.

REFERENCES

1. BELL J.L., SHALDON S. & BARON D.N. (1962) Serum isocitrate dehydrogenase in liver disease and some other conditions. *Clin. Sci.* **23**, 57.
2. COHEN J.A. & KAPLAN M.M. (1975) The SGOT/ SGPT ratio in liver disease. *Gastroenterology* **69**, 813.
3. HATOFF D.E. & HARDISON W.G.M. (1979) Induced synthesis of alkaline phosphatase by bile acids in rat liver cell culture. *Gastroenterology* **77**, 1062.
4. HORWITZ C.A., BURKE M.D., HENLE W.W. *et al* (1977) Late persistence of serum γ-glutamyl transpeptidase activity after mononucleosis. *Gastroenterology* **72**, 1322.
5. KAPLAN M.M. (1972) Alkaline phosphatase. *Gastroenterology* **62**, 452.
6. ROSALKI S.B. (1975) Gamma-glutamyl transpeptidase. *Adv. clin. Chem.* **17**, 53.
7. SIMON F.R. & SUTHERLAND E. (1977) Hepatic alkaline phosphatase isoenzymes: isolation, characterisation and differentiation alteration. *Enzyme* **22**, 80.

8. WARNES T.W. (1972) Alkaline phosphatase. *Gut* **13**, 926.
9. WARNES T.W., HINE P. & KAY G. (1976) Poly-acrylamide gel disc electrophoresis of alkaline phosphatase isoenzymes in bone and liver disease. *J. clin. Path.* **29**, 782.
10. WENHAM P.R., PRICE C.P. & SAMMONS H.G. (1979) Serum γ-glutamyl transferase isoenzymes in extra-hepatic biliary obstruction. *J. clin. Path.* **32**, 902.
11. WHITFIELD J.B., POUNDER R.E., NEALE G. *et al* (1972) Serum γ-glutamyl transpeptidase activity in liver disease. *Gut* **13**, 702.

CARBOHYDRATE METABOLISM

The liver occupies a key position in carbohydrate metabolism [1, 7] (fig. 15).

In fulminant acute hepatic necrosis the blood glucose level may be low (page 111). This is rare in chronic liver disease. The oral and intravenous glucose tolerance tests may, however, show impairment and there is relative insulin resistance (Chapter 22).

Galactose tolerance is also impaired in hepato-cellular disease and oral and intravenous tests have been devised. Results are independent of insulin secretion. Galactose removal by the liver has been used to measure hepatic blood flow.

REFERENCES

1. SAMOLS E. & HOLDSWORTH D. (1968) Disturbance in carbohydrate metabolism in liver disease. In *Carbohydrate metabolism*, vol. 2, p. 289, eds F. Dickens, P.J. Randle & W.J. Whelan. Academic Press, New York.
2. SHERLOCK S. (1970) Carbohydrate changes in liver disease. *Am. J. clin. Nutr.* **23**, 462.

Chapter 3
Needle Biopsy of the Liver

Needle biopsy was first employed by Paul Ehrlich in 1883 to study the glycogen content of the diabetic liver [3]. The method did not achieve early popularity because of the undoubted risks involved. The elaboration of the technique, the clearer definition of indications and contraindications and the introduction of safer needles have resulted in needle biopsy being accepted in most large hospitals. This does not imply that it is always without risk. Needle biopsy should always be regarded as potentially fatal. Five hundred may be performed without incident only for the 501st to be complicated by massive intraperitoneal haemorrhage demanding immediate treatment.

Selection and preparation of the patient [29]

The biopsy should be performed in hospital, preferably in the morning when after-care is easy. Out-patient biopsies can be done in good-risk patients if they can be observed for three hours and are staying near the hospital where medical support is available [20]. If the intercostal route is used, the patient must be co-operative and able to control his respiration, otherwise the liver capsule may tear.

Care should be taken if there is spontaneous bruising or bleeding, especially if the patient is jaundiced. Prothrombin time should always be done. If the patient is jaundiced, vitamin K (10 mg i.m.) should be administered for two days. If prothrombin time is more than three seconds increased over control the biopsy should not be performed. The platelet count should exceed 80 000, although the dangers of thrombocytopenia have been over-emphasized [13]. If a biopsy is urgently indicated it may be performed under cover of fresh-frozen plasma, prothrombin-complex concentrates and platelet infusions [15]. Patients with haemophilia frequently suffer from hepatitis; biopsy is possible under cover of factor VIII concentrates [10, 21].

The patient's blood group should be known and facilities for blood transfusion must always be available.

A mild sedative such as 0.2 g sodium amytal is given 30 minutes before puncture.

Biopsy should not be done with tense ascites as a specimen will not be obtained.

If the liver is small it may not be penetrated by the needle and distortion may result in puncture of the gall bladder or large blood vessels in the hilum. A plain X-ray of the abdomen and scanning may be necessary to assess liver size and the height of the diaphragm.

Hydatid cyst is an absolute contraindication, for puncture may result in fatal anaphylaxis or peritoneal dissemination. Suspected haemangioma, right empyema or subphrenic abscess are also contraindications. Biopsy may be done in the presence of deep cholestatic jaundice (see table 2); it should not be performed with deep hepato-cellular jaundice.

Position and local anaesthesia

The patient lies supine with the right side as near the edge of the bed as possible. A firm pillow may be placed under the left side so that the body is slightly tilted to the right. The right arm is placed behind the head and the patient looks to the left. The skin is anaesthetized. A long (8 cm) fine-bore needle is used to infiltrate the pleura and is then passed through the diaphragm to anaesthetize the peritoneum and the capsule of the liver. At least 5 ml of local anaesthetic is needed.

Site of puncture

The intercostal technique provides the whole transverse depth of the right lobe for puncture; intra-abdominal viscera are avoided. It does involve puncture of the pleural cavity. The site chosen is the 8th, 9th or 10th intercostal space in the mid axillary line. The place is that of maximum dullness to percussion.

The subcostal method is confined to livers enlarged below the right costal margin. A specific lesion may be aimed at. Otherwise the site chosen is below and to the right of the xiphoid process in the mid-clavicular line, the needle being directed to the right and cephalad. Scanning or even ultra-sonic scanning may be used to select the site for puncture.

The transjugular (transvenous) approach uses a needle inserted through a catheter placed in the hepatic vein from the jugular vein. This is then introduced into the liver tissue by transfixing the hepatic venous wall [8]. The method is used in those in whom a coagulation defect would preclude trans-hepatic liver biopsy. The technique is not easy and specimens tend to be small and fragmented. This type of liver biopsy is really necessary in those with poor clotting. If required, such biopsies can usually be done intercostally after infusion of the requisite clotting factors.

Technique of puncture

The biopsy may be obtained either by aspiration such as in the Menghini [17] technique or by predominantly a puncture procedure such as in the Vim–Silverman (Trucut) method. The method should be undertaken only by the well-trained. The novice should practise on the cadaver before attempting it on the patient. The aspiration of blood from the liver should not occasion alarm.

Menghini 'one second' needle biopsy [17] (figs. 26, 27). The 1.4mm diameter needle is used routinely. A short needle is available for paediatric use. The tip of the needle is oblique and slightly convex towards the outside. This results in an excellent cut of the biopsy specimen without any need to rotate the needle. The needle is also fitted within its shaft with a blunt nail, 3 cm long and 0.2 mm diameter smaller than the internal diameter of the cannula. The diameter of the flattened head of the nail is larger than that of the cannula and also than that of the internal diameter of the insertion of the aspirating syringe. This prevents the nail from falling into the cannula and also from being aspirated into the syringe. This internal block prevents the biopsy from being fragmented or distorted by violent aspiration into the syringe.

Three ml of sterile solution are drawn into the syringe which is inserted through the anaesthetized track down to but not through the intercostal space. Two ml of solution are injected to clear the needle of any skin fragments. Aspiration is now commenced and maintained. This is the slow part of the procedure. With the patient holding his breath in expiration, the needle is rapidly introduced perpendicular to the skin into the liver substance and extracted. This is the quick part of the procedure. The tip of the needle is now placed under saline in a flat-bottomed glass receptacle. It may be necessary to gently inject a little of the remaining saline from the syringe to free the biopsy.

This method has the advantage that the needle is only briefly in the liver, only slightly more than the 'one second' claimed by the originator [16]; this increases safety. The method is also extremely easy to perform. Discomfort to the patient is less than that with other techniques. The instrument is simple and inexpensive. The main disadvantage is that in fibrotic livers the failure rate is high and the specimens obtained may be small. Menghini has now performed his method on more than 2000 occasions without fatality.

Vim–Silverman method. The instrument (fig. 28) consists of a short trocar and cannula. The trocar is removed and the biopsy is punched out by the introduction of a longer cannula split longitudinally, both halves of which tend to spring apart. The short cannula is then advanced until the tips of both are level. The apparatus is rotated to break off the end of the biopsy and withdrawn. Suction is not necessary. This method has a high success rate in the presence of cirrhosis. The sample is large but may be distorted.

After-care

After biopsy a small dose of an analgesic such as pethidine (Demarol) may be necessary. A further sedative such as soluble barbitone may be given

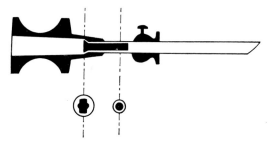

Fig. 26. Longitudinal section of the Menghini liver biopsy needle. Note the nail in the shaft of the needle (Menghini 1958).

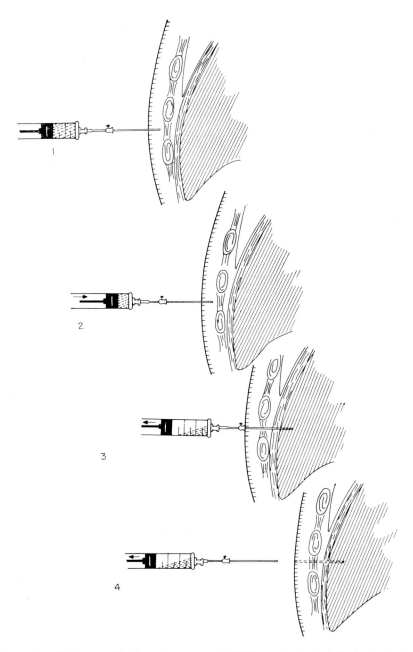

Fig. 27. Stages of needle biopsy of the liver using the Menghini technique (Menghini 1958).
1   The biopsy needle with attached syringe is pushed into the subcutaneous tissue.
2   1 ml of saline is injected to expel any tissue fragments from the needle.

3   While aspiration is maintained and the patient holds his breath in expiration, the needle is quickly inserted through the intercostal space and into the liver.
4   Aspiration being maintained, the needle is quickly withdrawn.

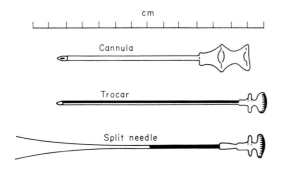

Fig. 28. Vim–Silverman liver biopsy needle.

in the evening. The pulse rate is charted hourly for the first 24 hours and the physician should be called if a rise is observed. Routine visits should be paid four and eight hours after biopsy. A very careful watch must be kept on the patient. Rest in bed is essential for 24 hours.

During the puncture the patient may complain of a drawing feeling across the epigastrium. Afterwards, some patients have a slight ache in the right side for about 24 hours and some complain of pain referred from the diaphragm to the right shoulder.

Difficulties

Failures arise in patients with cirrhosis, especially with ascites, for the tough liver is difficult to pierce and a few liver cells may be extracted, leaving the fibrous framework behind. Another source of difficulty may be pulmonary emphysema; the liver is then pushed downwards by the low diaphragm so that the trocar passes above it.

Failure is often due to the needle not being sharp enough to penetrate the capsule. Also, the trocar may be withdrawn before the instrument has pierced the capsule. Disposable needles are an advantage for they are sharp.

The percentage of successes increases with diameter of the needle used but so does the complication rate and one must be weighed against the other. The 1 mm Menghini needle, for instance, which is extremely safe, often fails to procure adequate hepatic tissue for diagnosis. The Vim–Silverman needle causes more haemorrhages.

A 0.7 simple 22-gauge needle has been used to obtain tissue for electron microscopy and cytology [14]. Tissue diagnosis is usually impossible. The method may be useful for the diagnosis of cancer.

The question of a second puncture on the same occasion, if the first fails, is a difficult one. Provided the patient is not jaundiced, the operator is experienced, and the Menghini technique is being used, this is justifiable.

Liver biopsy in paediatrics

The Menghini technique may be employed. In infants a local anaesthetic, with 15–60 mg pentobarbital 30 minutes before the biopsy, is adequate. The child is restrained by adhesive strapping across the upper thighs and chest and the subcostal approach used [6]. If the liver is small then the intercostal route is employed, the assistant compressing the chest at the end of expiration to arrest respiration [5].

In older children general anaesthesia is generally preferred, depending on the co-operation of the child. If splenic venography is necessary, the two procedures can be performed under the same anaesthetic.

Risks and complications

In a review of 20 016 needle biopsies the mortality was stated to be 0.17% [31, 32]. Deaths from haemorrhage were usually in those with a hopeless prognosis. Fatalities are even less if only the Menghini method is used. In one combined European series of 23 382 biopsies the mortality was only 0.017% [30] and in another of 79 381 only 0.015% [11].

Pleurisy and perihepatitis

A friction rub caused by fibrinous perihepatitis or pleurisy may be heard on the next day. It is of little consequence and pain subsides with analgesics. Chest X-ray may show a small pneumothorax.

Haemorrhage

Bleeding from the puncture wound usually consists of a thin trickle lasting 10–60 seconds and the

total blood loss is only 5–10 ml. Serious haemorrhage is usually intraperitoneal but may be
intrathoracic from an intercostal artery. The
bleeding results from perforation of distended
portal or hepatic veins or aberrant arteries. In
some cases a tear of the liver follows deep breathing during the intercostal procedure. Severe hae-
mothorax usually responds to blood transfusion
and chest aspiration. Haemorrhage is extremely
rare in the non-jaundiced. It is most common in
severe hepato-cellular disease and where this is
suspected biopsy should be avoided. Patients with
cholestatic jaundice, after vitamin K therapy,
tolerate liver biopsy well [18].

Intra-hepatic haematomas

These can often be detected if post-biopsy hepatic
scans or angiography are performed [24]. They are
usually asymptomatic but can cause fever, rises in
serum transaminases, a fall in haematocrit and,
if large, right upper quadrant tenderness and
an enlarging liver. Surgical drainage is rarely
necessary.

Intra-hepatic arteriovenous fistula

This may follow needle biopsy or percutaneous
cholangiography [19]. This is rarely large enough
to be clinically significant and may close spontaneously.

Biliary complications

Using the intercostal approach, the gall bladder
should be avoided, but if it is punctured the resultant *biliary peritonitis* may require surgical
drainage.

A large bile duct may be punctured in patients
with extra-hepatic cholestasis. This has led to liver
biopsy being contraindicated in such patients. It
is, however, a very small risk and the puncture usually seals itself off (table 2). Needle biopsy is being

performed less often in such cases now that dilated
intra-hepatic ducts may be identified by ultrasound or percutaneous or endoscopic cholangiography.

Haemobilia is marked within three days of
biopsy by gastro-intestinal haemorrhage, biliary
colic and bilirubinuria. The diagnosis is confirmed
by gastro-duodenoscopy and selective hepatic
arteriography [9].

Transient septicaemia can complicate biopsy
particularly in those with cholangitis. The organisms are usually Gram-negative. Occasionally a
septicaemic shock may develop [12].

Menghini needle fracture

The distal fragment lodges in the liver substance
particularly when the patient breathes suddenly
with a needle *in situ* [22]. Before use the biopsy
needle should be carefully scrutinized for defects.

Puncture of other viscera

This is very rare. The colon or the kidney may be
biopsied, but this is not usually dangerous. Pancreatic puncture can be serious.

Reliability of needle biopsies as representative

It is surprising that such a small biopsy should so
often be representative of changes in the whole
liver [1]. The lesions of cholestasis, steatosis, virus
hepatitis and the reticuloses are fortunately diffuse. This is also true of most cirrhoses, although
in macronodular cirrhosis it is possible to aspirate
a large nodule and find normal architecture [26].
There is sampling variability in the diagnosis of
cirrhosis in the presence of acute hepatitis or
chronic active hepatitis. The focal granulomatous
diseases such as sarcoidosis, tumours, deposits and
abscesses may be missed, but infrequently if serial
sections are cut.

Misdiagnosis is often due to smallness of

Table 2. Needle liver biopsy in surgical cholestasis
(Morris *et al* 1975). Royal Free Hospital, London.

Serum bilirubin (mg/100 ml)	No. patients	Complications		
		cholangitis	pleural effusion	pain
> 10	18	1	0	1
< 10	39	1	1	0

sample, especially failure to obtain portal zones, the focal nature of the disease process and particularly inexperience of the interpreter.

Fibrous tissue is increased under the capsule in operative biopsies and this may give a false impression of the liver as a whole. Operative biopsies may also show artefactual changes such as patchy loss of glycogen, haemorrhages and polymorph infiltration, all due to the effects of trauma and the anaesthetic.

A combination of peritoneoscopy with needle liver biopsy enables the surface of the liver to be visualized and the biopsy taken directly from any focal abnormality. More than one biopsy may be taken. In experienced hands peritoneoscopy adds little to the time taken or to the discomfort involved. With less practised operators, however, the increase in extent of the procedure and the time taken does not compensate for the information obtained.

Naked eye appearances

A satisfactory biopsy is 1–4 cm long and weighs 10–50 mg.

The cirrhotic liver tends to crumble into fragments of irregular contour. The fatty liver has a pale greasy look and floats in the formol–saline fixative. The liver containing malignant deposits is dull white in colour. The liver from a patient with Dubin–Johnson hyperbilirubinaemia is diffusely chocolate-coloured (fig. 182).

In cholestatic jaundice, the greenish central areas contrast with the less green periphery. The vascular centres of lobules in hepatic congestion may be obvious.

Fixation and preparation of specimen [26]

After the biopsy the specimen is gently expelled on to filter paper and placed as quickly as possible into fixative, usually 10% formol–saline. If methods other than routine light microscopy are to be used the specimen may need special handling or fixation and such methods must be planned beforehand. They include electron microscopy, chemical analysis and preparation of frozen sections.

Normal histological techniques are applied. The processes of fixation, dehydration and clearing can be much shorter than for large tissue blocks. Routine stains should include haematoxylin and eosin, a stain for iron and a good connective tissue stain

or stains. A variety of histochemical methods can be applied to paraffin sections, including methods for copper, glycogen and hepatitis B surface antigen. Frozen sections are occasionally used for rapid diagnosis and histochemical enzyme methods and increasingly for immunofluorescent studies. Electron microscopy is valuable in storage diseases, and chemical analysis in these as well as in Wilson's disease (copper) and haemochromatosis (iron). Micro-enzyme analysis includes the measurement of glucuronyl transferase activity in patients with suspected Gilbert's disease.

Serial sections are important for the diagnosis of lesions such as granulomas which may be scattered through the liver.

Cytological preparations are made by smearing the aspirated tissue core on a slide. These are useful in the diagnosis of cancer.

Normal histological appearances

The portal zones bear a regular relation to the central areas. This may be difficult to establish in small biopsies especially if no portal zones have been obtained, but this orientation is an essential first step. Each portal zone consists of one or two bile ductules, a branch of the hepatic artery and of the portal vein, a few mononuclears and an occasional fibroblast. The liver cell plates are one cell thick and contain abundant glycogen. Mitoses are not seen in the liver cells which are usually mononucleate and of regular size. The sinusoids are lined by Kupffer cells and can be seen converging upon the central vein.

Isolated sinusoidal dilatation prompts a search for a tumour or a disease associated with granulomas [2].

Indications [26, 28] (table 3)

Jaundice. This is a major indication when the diagnosis is difficult but the method carries extra risk in this group.

The cirrhoses (Chapter 18) and chronic hepatitis [25] (Chapter 16).

Alcoholic liver injury. Diagnosis of type and extent of involvement may be possible only after needle biopsy.

Congenital hepatic fibrosis (Chapter 25).

Hepatic tumours (Chapter 28).

Reticulo-endothelial diseases (Chapter 4).

Miliary granulomas of the liver (Chapter 26).

Table 3. Indications for needle liver biopsy.

Acute and chronic jaundice
Acute hepatitis and its sequelae
Cirrhosis and portal hypertension
Drug-related liver disease
Liver disease in the alcoholic
Unexplained hepatomegaly or abnormalities of liver
  function
Storage diseases
Infective and other systemic diseases
Screening of relatives of patients with familial
  diseases

Infections. These include tuberculosis, brucelo-
sis, syphilis, histoplasmosis, coccidioidomycosis,
pyogenic infection, leptospirosis icterohaemor-
rhagica and amoebiasis. When indicated, the
appropriate stains for the causative organism
should be applied and a portion of the biopsy
cultured.

Storage diseases. These include amyloidosis
and glycogen disease (Chapter 22).

Assessment of therapy, for instance, corticosteroids, venesection in haemochromatosis.

Other indications include obscure hepatomegaly
or splenomegaly, abnormal biochemical tests of
liver function of uncertain cause and in the eluci-
dation of chronic sequelae of viral hepatitis.

Needle liver biopsy in clinical research

Histochemical techniques have been widely
applied. Bile canaliculi may be beautifully shown
by staining for adenosine triphosphatase (ATPase),
and staining for glucose-6-phosphatase may be
used. Conjugated and unconjugated bilirubin may
be shown by a modified diazo technique [23]. Electron microscopy may be combined with histochemistry. ATPase is localized to the microvilli of
the canaliculi and 5-nucleotidase to the microvilli
of the sinusoidal border. Acid phosphatase is
found in Kupffer cells, degenerating foci and
regenerating nodules; alkaline phosphatase
defines cholangioles.

The distribution of hepatitis viral antigens may
be shown by appropriate staining and immunofluorescent methods.

Quantitative analysis of liver biopsy specimens
is made inaccurate by sampling difficulties and by
failure to find a suitable standard of reference. In
the liver with normal structure, results are reasonably reliable. For instance, the glycogen content
of the diabetic liver has been shown to be normal

[4]. The lipid composition can be estimated [7].
Difficulties arise particularly in biopsies from cirrhotic livers where the proportion of fibrous tissue
is uncertain. Chemical analysis for DNA, which
is confined to the nucleus, probably represents the
best reference base although this may be valueless
where the proportion of cells of different types is
variable. Alternatively the substance being investigated may be referred to dry weight or to total
nitrogen content of the biopsy.

Many quantitative studies of hepatic enzymes
have been made. The enzymes of mitochondrial,
lysosomal, membrane-bound and cytoplasmic
fractions of the biopsy can be estimated [27].

REFERENCES

1. ABDI W., MILLAN J.C. & MEZEY E. (1979) Sampling
   variability on percutaneous liver biopsy. *Arch.
   intern. Med.* **139,** 680.
2. BRUGUERA M., ARANGUIBEL F., ROS E. *et al*
   (1978) Incidence and clinical significance of sinusoidal dilatation in liver biopsies. *Gastroenterology*
   75, 474.
3. FRERICHS F.T. VON (1884) *Über den Diabetes.*
   Hirschwald, Berlin.
4. HILDES J.A., SHERLOCK S. & WALSHE V. (1949)
   Liver and muscle glycogen in normal subjects in
   diabetes mellitus and in acute hepatitis. *Clin. Sci.*
   7, 287.
5. HONG R. & SCHUBERT W.K. (1960) Menghini
   needle biopsy of the liver. *Am. J. Dis. Child.* **100,**
   42.
6. KAYE R., KOOP C.E., WAGNER B.M. *et al* (1959)
   Needle biopsy of the liver. An aid in the differential
   diagnosis of prolonged jaundice in infancy. *Am. J.
   Dis. Child.* **98,** 699.
7. LAURELL S. & LUNDQUIST A. (1971) Lipid composition of human liver biopsy specimens. *Acta med.
   Scand.* **189,** 65.
8. LEBREC D., DEGOTT C., RUEFF B. *et al* (1978)
   Transvenous (transjugular) liver biopsy. An experience based on 100 biopsies. *Am. J. dig. Dis.* **23,**
   302.
9. LEE S.P., TASMAN-JONES C. & WATTIE W.J. (1977)
   Traumatic hemophilia: a complication of percutaneous liver biopsy. *Gastroenterology* **72,** 941.
10. LESESNE H.R., MORGAN J.E., BLATT P.M. *et al*
    (1977) Liver biopsy in hemophilia. A. *Ann. intern.
    Med.* **86,** 703.
11. LINDNER H. (1967) Grenzen und Gefahren der per-
    kutanen Leberbiopsie mit der Menghini-Nadel:
    Erfahrungen bei 80,000 Leberbiopsien. *Dtsch.
    Med. Wschr.* **92,** 1751.
12. LOIUDICE J., BUHAC I. & BALINT J. (1977) Septi-
    cemia as a complication of percutaneous liver
    biopsy. *Gastroenterology* **72,** 949.
13. LOSOWSKY M.S. & WALKER B.E. (1968) Liver
    biopsy and splenoportography in patients with
    thrombocytopenia. *Gastroenterology* **54,** 241.

14. LUNDQUIST A. (1970) Liver biopsy with a needle of 0.7 mm outer diameter. Safety and quantitative yield. *Acta med. Scand.* **188,** 471.

15. MANNUCCI P.M., FRANCHI F. & DIOGUARDI N. (1976) Correction of abnormal coagulation in chronic liver disease by combined use of fresh-frozen plasma and prothrombin complex concentrates. *Lancet* ii, 542.

16. MENGHINI G. (1958) One-second needle biopsy of the liver. *Gastroenterology* **35,** 190.

17. MENGHINI G. (1970) One-second biopsy of the liver—problems of its clinical application. *New Engl. J. Med.* **283,** 582.

18. MORRIS J.S., GALLO G.A., SCHEUER P.J. *et al* (1975) Percutaneous liver biopsy in patients with bile duct obstruction. *Gastroenterology* **68,** 750.

19. OKUDA K., MUSHA H., NAKAJIMA Y. *et al* (1978) Frequency of intrahepatic arteriovenous fistula as a sequela to percutaneous needle puncture of the liver. *Gastroenterology* **74,** 1204.

20. PERRAULT J., McGILL D.B., OTT B.J. *et al* (1978) Liver biopsy: complications in 1000 patients and outpatients. *Gastroenterology* **74,** 103.

21. PRESTON F.E. (1978) Percutaneous liver biopsy and chronic liver disease in haemophiliacs. *Lancet* ii, 592.

22. PUROW E., GROSBERG S.J. & WAPNICK S. (1977) Menghini needle fracture after attempted liver biopsy. *Gastroenterology* **73,** 1404.

23. RAIA S. (1970) Histochemical separation of conjugated and unconjugated bilirubin and its assessment by thin layer chromatography. *J. Histochem. Cytochem.* **18,** 153.

24. RAINES D.R., VANHEERTUM R.L. & JOHNSON L.F. (1974) Intrahepatic hematoma: a complication of percutaneous liver biopsy. *Gastroenterology* **67,** 284.

25. SCHEUER P.J. (1979) Chronic hepatitis. In *Pathology of the Liver*, eds R.N.M. MACSWEEN, P.P. ANTHONY & P.J. SCHEUER, p. 248. Churchill Livingstone, Edinburgh.

26. SCHEUER P.J. (1980) *Liver Biopsy Interpretation*, 3rd edn. Baillière Tindall, London.

27. SEYMOUR C.A. & PETERS T.J. (1977) Enzyme activities in human liver biopsies: assay methods and activities of some lysosomal and membrane-bound enzymes in control tissue and serum. *Clin. Sci. mol. Biol.* **52,** 229.

28. SHERLOCK S. (1945) Aspiration liver biopsy, technique and diagnostic application. *Lancet* ii, 397.

29. SHERLOCK S. (1962) Needle biopsy of the liver: a review. *J. clin. Path.* **15,** 291.

30. THALER H. (1964) Über vorteil und Risiko der leberbiopsie methode nach Menghini. *Wien. Klin. Wchschr.* **29,** 533.

31. ZAMCHECK N. & SIDMAN R.L. (1953) Needle biopsy of the liver: I. Its use in clinical and investigative medicine. *New Engl. J. Med.* **249,** 1020.

32. ZAMCHECK N. & KLAUSENSTOCK O. (1953) Liver biopsy: IIII. The risk of needle biopsy. *New Engl. J. Med.* **249,** 1062.

Chapter 4
The Haematology of Liver Disease

GENERAL FEATURES

Hepato-cellular failure, portal hypertension and jaundice may affect the blood picture. Chronic liver disease is usually accompanied by 'hypersplenism'. Diminished erythrocyte survival is frequent. In addition both parenchymal hepatic disease and cholestatic jaundice may be associated with blood coagulation defects. Dietary deficiencies, alcoholism and difficulties in hepatic synthesis of proteins used in blood formation or coagulation add to the complexity of the problem.

BLOOD VOLUME

Plasma volume is frequently increased in patients with cirrhosis, especially with ascites [8] and also with longstanding obstructive jaundice or with hepatitis. This hypervolaemia may partially, and sometimes totally, account for a low peripheral haemoglobin or erythrocyte level. Total circulating haemoglobin is reduced in only about half the patients.

Erythrocyte changes

The red cells are usually *hypochromic*. This is often due to gastro-intestinal bleeding. In portal hypertension anaemia follows gastro-oesophageal bleeding and is enhanced by thrombocytopenia and disturbed blood coagulation. In cholestasis or cirrhosis of the alcoholic, haemorrhage may be from a duodenal ulcer. Epistaxis, bruising and bleeding gums add to the anaemia.

The erythrocytes are usually *normocytic*. This is a combination of the microcytosis of chronic blood loss and the macrocytosis inherent in patients with liver disease. *Spherocytes* represent increased splenic sequestration. The ratio of red cell membrane cholesterol to phospholipids (CP ratio) is changed and this results in various morphological abnormalities including thin macrocytes, target cells and spur cells [6, 7].

Thin macrocytes are frequent and associated with a macronormoblastic marrow. These resolve when liver function improves.

Target cells are also thin macrocytes. They are found in both hepato-cellular and cholestatic jaundice. They are flat, macrocytic and have an increased surface area and increased resistance to osmotic lysis. They are particularly prominent in cholestasis where a rise in bile acids may contribute by inhibiting lecithin cholesterol acyl transferase (LCAT) activity [5]. The membrane LCAT activity is decreased.

Spur cells are cells with unusual thorny projections. They are also termed '*burr*' cells or *acanthocytes*. They are associated with far advanced liver disease usually in alcoholics. Severe anaemia and haemolysis is also found [4, 9, 10]. Their appearance is a bad prognostic sign. The membrane CP ratio is markedly increased due to increased membrane cholesterol; total phospholipid remains normal. They have a shortened survival. Their rigid membranes make them particularly susceptible to being filtered in the spleen.

Alcoholics show genuine *thick macrocytes* probably related to the toxic effect of alcohol on the bone marrow. Folic acid and B_{12} deficiency may contribute.

Erythrocytosis may complicate primary liver cancer (Chapter 28).

Bone marrow of chronic hepato-cellular failure is hyperplastic and macronormoblastic. In spite of this, erythrocyte volume is depressed and the marrow therefore does not seem able to compensate completely for the anaemia (relative marrow failure).

Folate and B_{12} metabolism

The liver stores folate and converts it to its active storage form, tetrahydrofolate [3]. Folate deficiency may accompany chronic liver disease usually in the alcoholic. This is largely due to dietary deficiency [18]. Serum folate levels are low. Folate therapy is useful. The liver also stores vitamin B_{12}. Hepatic levels are reduced in liver disease. When hepatocytes become necrotic the vitamin is released into the blood and high serum B_{12} levels are recorded. This is shown in hepatitis, active cirrhosis and with primary liver cancer. Values in cholestatic jaundice are normal.

The blood levels of vitamin B_{12} and folate correlate with the hepatic content. Megaloblastic anaemia is rare with chronic liver disease and vitamin B_{12} therapy is rarely needed.

Erythrocyte survival and haemolytic anaemia

Increased red cell destruction is almost constant in hepato-cellular failure and jaundice of all types [20]. This is reflected in erythrocyte polychromasia and reticulocytosis.

The mechanism is extremely complex. In cirrhosis it is in part related to splenomegaly and to reticulo-endothelial hyperplasia generally. In many instances, however, the spleen is not the site of erythrocyte destruction. Splenectomy or corticosteroid therapy have little effect [20].

Haemolysis may be acute in patients with alcoholic hepatitis who also have hypercholesterolaemia (*Zieve's syndrome*) [25] and with spur cell anaemia.

Very rarely an auto-immune haemolytic anaemia with a positive Coombs' test is seen in chronic active hepatitis and primary biliary cirrhosis.

Aplastic anaemia is a rare complication of acute virus hepatitis [15].

Changes in the leucocytes and platelets

Leucopenia and thrombocytopenia are commonly found in patients with cirrhosis, usually with a mild anaemia ('*hypersplenism*').

The leucopenia is of the order of 1500–3000 cells per mm³, the depression mainly affecting polymorphs. Occasionally it may be more severe. The thrombocytopenia is rarely severe, the platelet count being between 60 000 and 120 000 per mm³. Occasionally there may be purpura even when the platelet count is only slightly lowered. The thrombocytopenia in congestive splenomegaly is largely due to a greatly increased splenic platelet pool [1]. Increased destruction of platelets is minimal. Platelet half-life is normal.

These changes are also found in other diseases with splenomegaly. Similar haematological changes occur with thrombosis of the portal vein.

Abnormal platelet aggregation due to intravascular coagulopathy may be important in severe liver failure [24].

Alcohol impairs platelet function.

Splenectomy is often recommended for the hypersplenism of cirrhosis. This may be followed by a rise in leucocytes and platelets; the response of the red cells is disappointing. The mortality of splenectomy in patients with liver disease is high. Splenectomy in patients with portal hypertension is liable to be followed by splenic and portal vein thrombosis which preclude later operations on the portal vein. Unless the patient is actually *suffering* from the leucopenia or from the thrombocytopenia the spleen should not be removed; mere demonstration of a low platelet or white cell count is not sufficient. The circulating platelets and leucocytes, although in short supply, are, in contrast to those of leukaemia, functioning well.

The haematological changes are not affected by portal–systemic shunts if the spleen is left *in situ*.

Other important changes include the leucocytosis of cholangitis, fulminant hepatitis, alcoholic hepatitis, hepatic abscess and malignant disease. Atypical lymphocytes are found in the peripheral blood in virus infections such as infectious mononucleosis and virus hepatitis.

Lupus erythematosus cells are found in chronic active hepatitis.

Patients with very high serum globulin values show plasmacytosis of the bone marrow.

THE LIVER AND BLOOD COAGULATION

Disturbed blood coagulation in patients with hepato-biliary disease is particularly complex. The liver manufactures most of the clotting factors. Failure of bile salt secretion into the intestine results in inadequate vitamin K absorption. The liver also clears activated clotting factors from the blood. Disseminated intravascular coagulation can follow acute hepato-cellular necrosis (fig. 29). Finally these coagulation difficulties often occur in combination with thrombocytopenia and an elevated portal venous pressure which predispose to gastro-intestinal bleeding.

The liver synthesizes fibrinogen and the vitamin K-dependent factors II, VII, IX and X, also labile factor V, contact factors XI and XII, and fibrin stabilizing factor XIII. Factor VIII is an immunoglobulin produced generally in the reticulo-endothelial system (including the liver) and levels are normal in cholestasis and hepato-cellular disease. The half-life of all these clotting proteins

Chapter 4

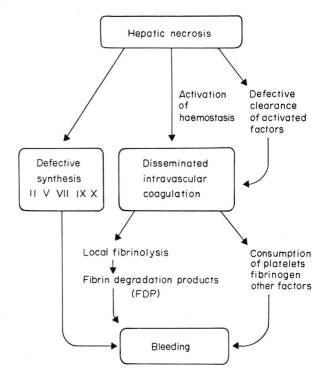

Fig. 29. Bleeding in hepato-cellular failure. Hepatic necrosis leads to defective synthesis of clotting factors II, V, VII, IX and X. Disseminated intravascular coagulation can follow activation of haemostasis by cell necrosis and defective clearance of activated factors by the necrotic liver. Platelets, fibrinogen and other factors are consumed and local fibrinolysis leads to fibrin degradation products (FDP). Bleeding is the end result.

is very short and hence reductions can follow very rapidly on acute hepato-cellular necrosis (fig. 29).

Vitamin K is fat-soluble and its absorption from the gut is facilitated by bile salts. It is essential for the production of factors II, VII, IX and X. Basic precursor proteins are first formed and vitamin K is essential for the second step, allowing the production of a unique amino acid, gammacarboxy glutamic acid, which confers coagulating activity on the precursor proteins [23]. In vitamin K deficiency the protein precursors known as PIVKA (proteins induced by vitamin K absence) accumulate and can be measured [23].

In hepato-cellular disease the factors most likely to be affected are VII, followed by II and X. IX is the last to be reduced. Synthesis of factors V and fibrinogen may be decreased but are less easily depressed than the others.

In addition the liver clears active clotting factors from the circulation and this includes thromboplastin. In hepato-cellular disease failure of this process adds to the bleeding.

Finally the liver cell is concerned with fibrinolysis (fig. 30). Plasminogen is probably synthesized by the liver cells and plasmin activator cleared by the liver. Antiplasmin is made by the liver. Primary fibrinolysis may develop in

patients with cirrhosis although it is difficult to distinguish from secondary fibrinolysis due to disseminated intravascular coagulation. Patients with primary liver cancer can synthesize an abnormal fibrinogen resembling that found in the foetus [11]. Dysfibrinogenaemia is also found in severe liver disease and may be a bad prognostic sign [14]. An abnormal fibrinolytic mechanism is also seen with cholestasis [17].

In patients with acute hepatic necrosis disseminated intravascular coagulation can be seen [21]. This is due to the cell necrosis activating haemostasis at the same time as defective clearance of activated factors. This coagulopathy is marked by depression of plasma fibrinogen, reduced survival

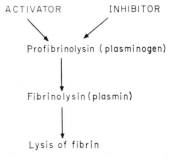

Fig. 30. Fibrinolytic enzyme system.

of circulating fibrinogen [21], reduced clotting factors and low platelets. Intravascular microthrombi form and circulating fibrinogen degradation products (FDP) can be shown. Activation of the fibrinolysis system is marked by low plasminogen activator and plasminogen levels (prolonged euglobulin lysis time). Such changes have been demonstrated in patients with fulminant hepatitis and drug-related acute hepatic necrosis [21]. However, in most instances the defect is a mild one, platelets are usually above 100000, FDP only moderately increased and fibrinogen only slightly reduced [16]. Moreover, examination of liver biopsy material shows only slight deposition of fibrin and this is related much more to areas of necrosis than to intravascular deposition. The severity of the bleeding seems unrelated to the degree of coagulopathy.

In chronic, stable alcoholic liver disease, fibrinogen turnover is not increased and mild consumptive coagulopathy is unlikely [2].

TESTS OF COAGULATION

The prothrombin time (PT) before and after 10 mg vitamin K intramuscularly is the most satisfactory test for a coagulation defect in patients with hepato-biliary disease. It is also a most sensitive indication of hepato-cellular necrosis and/or prognosis. The partial thromboplastin time (PTT) is sometimes performed and is slightly more sensitive than the PT. The thrombotest is less costly and is sensitive to the anticoagulant effect of PIVKA.

Estimation of individual clotting factors is rarely necessary although a fall of factor VII, which has the shortest half-life (about six hours), holds a particularly bad prognosis in fulminant hepatic failure [13].

Fibrinolysis and disseminated intravascular coagulation are diagnosed by marked prolongation of the PT, fibrinogen levels below 1.0 g per litre, FDPs greater than 100 g per litre and thrombocytopenia less than 100×10^9 per litre.

Spontaneous bleeding, bruising and purpura, together with a history of bleeding after minimal trauma, are more important indications of a bleeding tendency in patients with liver disease than are laboratory tests.

Management of coagulation defect

Vitamin K_1 should be given to all patients with a prolonged one-stage prothrombin time. The usual course is 10 mg vitamin K_1 by intramuscular injection for three days. This is effective in about three hours and will correct hypoprothrombinaemia related to bile salt deficiency. Defects predominantly due to hepato-cellular disease will not be restored by the vitamin K_1 treatment. Nevertheless even in patients with predominantly hepato-cellular jaundice there may be a component of bile salt secretory failure and the prothrombin time often improves by a few seconds [22]. A prolongation of the one-stage prothrombin time of more than three seconds or a thrombotest of less than 40% after intramuscular vitamin K_1 contraindicates such procedures as liver biopsy, splenic venography, percutaneous cholangiography or laparotomy. If such procedures are essential, the clotting defect may be corrected by fresh-frozen plasma or prothrombin-complex concentrate which correct the defect for a few hours [12, 19].

In general, apart from vitamin K_1 therapy, it is not necessary to restore blood coagulation to normal in patients with liver disease unless there is active bleeding. Stored blood transfusion will supply prothrombin, VII, VIII and X. Fresh blood also supplies factor V and platelets. Fresh-frozen plasma is a good source of clotting factors, especially V. It has a disadvantage in that the volume infused is large and fluid overload may develop. Prothrombin-complex concentrate is made up in a much smaller volume and supplies factors II, IX and X and variable quantities of VII. It has a disadvantage of transmission of viral hepatitis (B and non-A, non-B). Platelet infusions are of temporary benefit.

Patients with bleeding oesophageal varices may require enormous quantities of blood transfusion even up to 40 units during one hospital admission. This raises the possibility of citrate intoxication. This would be expected to be more common in those with hepatic disease for the liver metabolizes citrate. Very high concentrations of serum citrate have been observed during multiple transfusions in liver disease and these may depress the ionized calcium. Calcium supplements should be given. In general, however, this is a small risk provided blood is not infused at a rate greater than 1 unit per five minutes.

Disseminated intravascular coagulation is treated by control of trigger factors such as infection, shock and dehydration. Fresh blood is most useful but, if unavailable, fresh-frozen plasma and packed red blood cells may be used. DIC is never severe enough to merit heparin therapy.

Platelet-rich plasma concentrates are used if thrombocytopenia is a problem and may be given to cover a procedure such as liver biopsy in a severely thrombocytopenic patient.

REFERENCES

1. ASTER R.H. (1966) Pooling of platelets in the spleen: role of platelets in the pathogenesis of 'hypersplenic' thrombocytopenia. *J. clin. Invest.* **45**, 645.
2. CANOSO R.T., HUTTON R.A. & DEYKIN D. (1979) The hemostatic defect of chronic liver disease: kinetic studies using ^{75}Se-selenomethionine. *Gastroenterology* **76**, 540.
3. CHANARIN I., HUTCHINSON M., McLEAN A. *et al* (1966) Hepatic folate in man. *Br. med. J.* i, 396.
4. COOPER R.A. (1969) Anemia with spur cells: a red cell defect acquired in serum and modified in the circulation. *J. clin. Invest.* **48**, 1820.
5. COOPER R.A., ARNER E.C., WILEY J.S. *et al* (1975) Modification of red cell membrane structure by cholesterol-rich lipid dispersions; a model for the primary spur cell defect. *J. clin. Invest.* **55**, 115.
6. COOPER R.A., DILOY-PURAY M., LANDO P. *et al* (1972) An analysis of lipoproteins, bile acids, and red cell membranes associated with target cells and spur cells in patients with liver disease. *J. clin. Invest.* **51**, 3182.
7. COOPER R.A. & JANDL J.H. (1968) Bile salts and cholesterol in the pathogenesis of target cells in obstructive jaundice. *J. clin. Invest.* **47**, 809.
8. EISENBERG S. (1956) Blood volume in patients with Laennec's cirrhosis of the liver as determined by radioactive chromium-tagged red cells. *Am. J. Med.* **20**, 189.
9. GISSELBRECHT C., METREAU J-M., DHUMEAUX D. *et al* (1977) L'acanthocytose au cours des cirrhoses. *Gastroenterol. clin. Biol.* **1**, 621.
10. GRAHN E.P., DIETZ A.A., STEFANI S.S. *et al* (1968) Burr cells, hemolytic anemia and cirrhosis. *Am. J. Med.* **45**, 78.
11. GRALNICK H.R., GIVELBER H. & ABRAMS E. (1978) Dysfibrinogenemia associated with hepatoma: increased carbohydrate content of the fibrinogen molecule. *New Engl. J. Med.* **299**, 221.
12. GREEN G., DYMOCK I.W., POLLER L. *et al* (1975) The use of factor VII-rich prothrombin complex concentrate in liver disease. *Lancet* i, 1311.
13. GREEN G., POLLER L., THOMSON J.M. *et al* (1976) Factor VII as a marker of hepato-cellular synthetic function in liver disease. *J. clin. Path.* **29**, 971.
14. GREEN G., THOMSON J.M., DYMOCK I.W. *et al* (1976) Abnormal fibrin polymerisation in liver disease. *Br. J. Haematol.* **34**, 427.
15. HAGLAR L., PASTORE R.A., BERGIN J.J. *et al* (1975) Aplastic anemia following viral hepatitis. *Medicine (Baltimore)* **54**, 139.
16. HILLENBRAND P., PARBHOO S.P., JEDRYCHOWSKI A. *et al* (1974) Significance of intravascular coagulation and fibrinolysis in acute hepatic failure. *Gut* **15**, 83.
17. JEDRYCHOWSKI A., HILLENBRAND P., AJDUKIE-WICZ A.B. *et al* (1973) Fibrinolysis in cholestatic jaundice. *Br. med. J.* i, 640.
18. KLIPSTEIN F.A. & LINDENBAUM J. (1965) Folate deficiency in chronic liver disease. *Blood* **25**, 443.
19. MANNUCCI P.M., FRANCHI F. & DIOGUARDI N. (1976) Correction of abnormal coagulation in chronic liver disease by combined use of fast frozen plasma and prothrombin complex concentrates. *Lancet* ii, 542.
20. PITCHER C.S. & WILLIAMS R. (1963) Reduced red cell survival in jaundice and its relation to abnormal glutathione metabolism. *Clin. Sci.* **24**, 239.
21. RAKE M.O., FLUTE P.T., PANNELL G. *et al* (1970) Intravascular coagulation in acute hepatic necrosis. *Lancet* i, 533.
22. SHERLOCK S. & ALPERT L. (1965) Bleeding in surgery in relation to liver disease. *Proc. R. Soc. Med.* **58**, 257.
23. STENFLO J. (1974) Vitamin K and the biosynthesis of prothrombin. IV. *J. biol. Chem.* **249**, 5527.
24. THOMAS D.P., REAM V.J. & STUART R.K. (1967) Platelet aggregation in patients with Laennec's cirrhosis of the liver. *New Engl. J. Med.* **276**, 1344.
25. ZIEVE L. (1966) Hemolytic anemia in liver disease. *Medicine (Baltimore)* **45**, 497.

HAEMOLYTIC JAUNDICE

Haemoglobin is released in excessive amounts, increasing from the normal of 6.25 g to as much as 45 g daily [2]. Consequently there is an increase in the serum bilirubin, 85% of which is unconjugated. The rise in conjugated bilirubin is probably due to retention.

Even if bile pigment production reaches its maximum of 1500 mg daily (six times normal) serum bilirubin rises only to about 2–3 mg/100 ml. This is because of the great capacity of the liver to handle pigment. If patients with haemolytic jaundice show serum bilirubin values greater than 4–5 mg/100 ml there is probably the additional factor of hepato-cellular dysfunction. Anaemia itself will, of course, depress liver function.

Unconjugated bilirubin is not water-soluble and does not pass into the urine. A little bilirubin may be detected in the urine by sensitive tests if the conjugated level in the blood rises to values which are unusually high for haemolysis.

Bile pigment excretion is greatly increased and large quantities of stercobilinogen are found in the stools. Each milligramme of stercobilinogen corresponds to the breakdown of 24 mg haemoglobin. This estimate can only be approximate, for a significant proportion of the faecal haem pigment is derived from sources other than haemoglobin of mature erythrocytes.

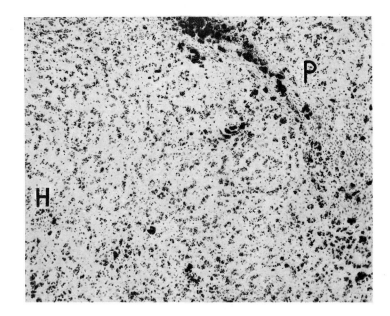

Fig. 31. Haemolytic jaundice. The hepatic architecture is normal. Increased amounts of iron are seen in the liver cells, Kupffer cells and especially the large macrophages of the portal tracts (P). H = hepatic vein. Stained ferro-cyanide, × 90.

PATHOLOGICAL CHANGES

The breakdown of haemoglobin yields iron. If it exceeds regeneration, iron will be deposited. *Tissue siderosis* is a feature of most types of haemolytic anaemia.

The *liver* is normal sized and is reddish-brown due to increased amounts of iron. Histology shows iron in Kupffer cells, large macrophages of the portal tracts, and to a lesser extent in hepatic parenchyma (fig. 31). In the severely anaemic, there is centrizonal sinusoidal distension with fatty change. Focal areas of liver cell necrosis are attributed to vascular obstruction of sinusoids by impacted cells undergoing lysis or to the direct effect of haemolysis on the liver cells. The Kupffer cells are generally swollen and hyperplastic; foci of erythropoiesis are uncommon. The *gall bladder* and *bile passages* contain dark viscid bile. Calcium bilirubinate pigment calculi are found in half to two-thirds of patients. Secondary cholecystitis may be followed by crops of multiple, faceted, mixed gall-stones.

The *spleen* is enlarged, fleshy and packed with erythrocytes. The *red bone marrow* is hyperplastic.

CLINICAL FEATURES

The picture varies with the cause, but certain symptoms and signs are common to all forms of haemolysis.

Anaemia depends on the rate of destruction compared with regeneration of red blood cells. It varies but increases rapidly with crises where the patient becomes ill with aching pains in the abdomen and limbs, fever, headache and sometimes even a fall in blood pressure and collapse.

Jaundice is usually mild and lemon yellow. The patients never acquire the greenish colour of prolonged cholestasis. It increases rapidly with haemolytic crises or if there is a coincidental difficulty in biliary excretion such as virus hepatitis or choledocholithiasis.

Pigment *gall-stones* may be associated with the features of chronic cholecystitis. Stones in the common bile duct may cause obstructive jaundice, and the co-existence of two types of jaundice provides a confusing clinical picture. Gall-stones in children always suggest a haemolytic aetiology.

Splenomegaly is present in the chronic forms.

Ulcers or pigmentation from healed ulcers, usually over the internal or external malleoli, occur in some types.

HAEMATOLOGICAL CHANGES

Anaemia is variable and the peripheral blood shows active regeneration [3]. Reticulocytes are increased to 20% or more of the total red cell count. Leucocytes are usually increased.

The sternal marrow is hyperplastic and the proportion of erythroid to leucopoietic cells rises.

The survival of labelled erythrocytes is reduced and increased uptake can be shown in the spleen.

FAECES AND URINE

The faeces are dark and stercobilinogen is increased. Urobilinogen is increased in the urine. Both of these quantitative tests may be unreliable.

Bilirubin is detected in the urine only rarely, when jaundice is deep. When blood destruction is rapid, free haemoglobin may be found in the urine and microscopy reveals pigmented casts.

SERUM BIOCHEMISTRY

Serum unconjugated bilirubin levels are raised but conjugated bilirubin is only slightly increased.

The serum alkaline phosphatase, albumin and globulin concentrations are normal. Serum haptoglobins are diminished. The serum cholesterol level is low.

If haemolysis is particularly acute methaemalbumin can be detected in the serum [3]. Serum ferritin is increased. Free haemoglobin may be detected.

DIFFERENTIAL DIAGNOSIS

The diagnosis of haemolytic from other forms of jaundice is usually easy. The absence of pain and pruritus and the dark colour of the stools are points of difference from cholestatic jaundice. The absence of other stigmata of hepato-cellular disease, the normal serum alkaline phosphatase and proteins distinguish it from virus hepatitis and cirrhosis.

Distinction from the congenital unconjugated hyperbilirubinaemias may be difficult particularly as many patients with Gilbert's disease show a decreased erythrocyte survival but not sufficient to account for the depth of jaundice reached.

THE LIVER IN HAEMOLYTIC ANAEMIAS

HEREDITARY SPHEROCYTOSIS

Jaundice is rarely noticed before school age or adolescence. Deep jaundice may, however, develop in the neonatal period and be associated with incipient kernicterus. All grades of severity occur but deep jaundice is rare; the mean serum bilirubin level is 2.0 mg (range 0.6–5.7 mg/100 ml). The spleen is enlarged. Symptoms of gall-stones occur in about half the patients.

Hereditary elliptocytosis is usually a harmless trait, the haemolysis being compensated. It may occasionally develop into active decompensated haemolytic anaemia.

VARIOUS ENZYME DEFECTS

Many of the hereditary non-spherocytic anaemias are now known to be due to various defects in the metabolism of the red cells. They include deficiency of pyruvate kinase or triosephosphate isomerase or deficiency in the pentose phosphate pathway such as glucose-6-phosphate-dehydrogenase. These conditions may be of particular importance in the aetiology of neonatal jaundice.

Viral hepatitis can precipitate destruction of glucose-6-phosphate-dehydrogenase deficient cells and so cause acute haemolytic anaemia [5].

SICKLE-CELL DISEASE

The abnormal haemoglobin crystallizes in the erythrocytes when the oxygen tension is reduced. There are crises of blood destruction with acute attacks of pain. Leg ulcers are frequent. The upper jaw is protuberant and hypertrophied. The fingers are clubbed. Bone deformities seen radiologically include rarefaction and narrowing of the cortex of the long bones and a 'hair-on-end' appearance in the skull.

Hepatic histology [12]

Active and healed areas of necrosis may have followed anoxia due to vascular obstruction by impacted sickle cells or by Kupffer cells swollen with phagocytosed erythrocytes following intrahepatic sickling. The widened sinusoids show a foam-like fibrin reticulum within their lumen. This intra-sinusoidal fibrin may later result in fibrous deposition in the space of Disse and narrowed sinusoids. Bile plugs are prominent. Fatty change is related to anaemia and haemosiderosis to multiple transfusions. There is an association with cirrhosis of macronodular type.

The excessive bilirubin load induces bilirubin conjugating enzymes [8].

Electron microscopy. The changes resemble those seen in hypoxia [11]. The nutrition of the hepatocyte is interfered with by sinusoidal aggregates of sickled erythrocytes, fibrin and platelets with increased collagen and occasional basement membranes in the space of Disse.

Clinical features [7]

During a crisis the liver is enlarged and tender. The serum bilirubin rises higher than that usually seen in haemolytic jaundice. In some patients both serum conjugated and unconjugated bilirubin transaminases and alkaline phosphatase levels are increased and the faeces are pale [6, 11]. Sickle-cell disease seems to be one cause of intra-hepatic cholestasis. In some patients the crises may be precipitated by salmonella infections or by folic acid deficiency [9].

Serum bilirubin levels rise to extremely high values. This is due to intra-hepatic sickling [1] and is not serious. Concomitant viral hepatitis or obstructed bile ducts lead to exceptionally high serum bilirubin values. Similar very high levels are seen when viral hepatitis complicates glucose 6PD deficiency [5].

Gall-stones

The reported incidence of gall-stones in sickle-cell disease ranges from 6.5% to 37% [4]. About 55% are radio-opaque. The stones are usually in the gall bladder and duct calculi are rare [10]. The distinction between abdominal pain and jaundice due to choledocholithiasis from haemolytic crisis may be very difficult.

THALASSAEMIA

This condition is due to persistence of foetal haemoglobin into adult life. Crises of blood destruction and fever and the reactionary changes in bone are similar to those seen in sickle-cell disease. The liver shows siderosis and sometimes fibrosis. The haemosiderosis may progress to an actual haemochromatosis and indicate treatment by continuous desferrioxamine therapy (see Chapter 20). The stainable iron in the liver cells may be greater in those who have lost the spleen as a storage organ for iron. Episodes of intra-hepatic cholestasis of uncertain nature can also develop. Gall-stones may be a complication.

PAROXYSMAL NOCTURNAL HAEMOGLOBINURIA

This rare disease is due to an unknown defect in the red cells, which are sensitive to lysis when the pH of the blood becomes more acid during sleep.

During an acute episode the patients show a dusky reddish type of jaundice and the liver enlarges. Liver histology shows some centrizonal hepatic necrosis and moderate siderosis.

ACQUIRED HAEMOLYTIC ANAEMIA

The haemolysis is due to extra-corpuscular causes. Spherocytosis is slight and osmotic fragility only mildly impaired.

The patient is moderately jaundiced. The increased pigment is unconjugated, but in severe cases conjugated bilirubin increases and appears in the urine. This may be related to bilirubin overload in the presence of liver damage. Blood transfusion accentuates the jaundice for transfused cells survive poorly.

The haemolysis may be *idiopathic*. The increased haemolysis is then due to auto-immunization. Coombs' test is positive.

The *acquired* type may complicate other diseases, especially those involving the reticuloendothelial system. These include Hodgkin's disease, the leukaemias, reticulo-sarcoma, carcinomatosis and uraemia. The anaemia of hepatocellular jaundice is also partially haemolytic. Coombs' test is usually negative.

Auto-immune haemolytic anaemia is a rare complication of chronic active hepatitis and primary biliary cirrhosis.

HAEMOLYTIC DISEASE OF THE NEWBORN (Chapter 23)

INCOMPATIBLE BLOOD TRANSFUSION

Chills, fever and backache are followed by jaundice. Urobilinogen is present in the urine. Liver function tests give normal results. In severe cases free haemoglobin is detected in blood and urine. Diagnostic difficulties arise when a patient suffering from a disease that may be complicated by hepato-cellular failure or biliary obstruction becomes jaundiced after a blood transfusion.

REFERENCES

1. BUCHANAN G.R. & GLADER B.E. (1977) Benign course of extreme hyperbilirubinemia in sickle cell anemia: analysis of six cases. *J. Pediat.* **91**, 21.
2. CROSBY W.H. & AKEROYD J.H. (1952) The limit of hemoglobin synthesis in hereditary hemolytic anemia. *Am. J. Med.* **13**, 273.

3. DACIE J.V. (1960–67) *The Haemolytic Anaemias—Congenital and Acquired*, 2nd edn, vols I–IV. J. & A. Churchill, London.
4. FLYE M.W. & SILVER D. (1972) Biliary tract disorders and sickle cell disease. *Surgery* **72**, 361.
5. KATTAMIS C.A. & TJORTJATOU F. (1970) The hemolytic process of viral hepatitis in children with normal or deficient glucose-6-phosphate dehydrogenase activity. *J. Pediat.* **77**, 422.
6. KLION F.M., WEINER M.J. & SCHAFFNER F. (1964) Cholestasis in sickle cell anemia. *Am. J. Med.* **37**, 829.
7. KONOTEY-AHULU F.I.D. (1969) The liver in sickle-cell disease—clinical aspects. *Ghana med. J.* **8**, 104.
8. MADDREY W.C., CUKIER J.O., MAGLALANG A.C. *et al* (1978) Hepatic bilirubin UDP-glucuronyltransferase in patients with sickle cell anemia. *Gastroenterology* **74**, 193.
9. ONUAGULUCHI G. & AKANDE E.O. (1966) Severe crises with jaundice in young non-pregnant adults with sickle-cell haemoglobin-C disease. *Lancet* i, 737.
10. PERRINE R.P. (1973) Cholelithiasis in sickle cell anemia in a Caucasian population. *Am. J. Med.* **54**, 327.
11. ROSENBLATE H.J., EISENSTEIN R. & HOLMES A.W. (1970) The liver in sickle cell anemia. A clinical-pathologic study. *Arch. Path.* **90**, 235.
12. SONG Y.S. (1957) Hepatic lesions in sickle cell anemia. *Am. J. Path.* **33**, 331.

THE LIVER AND DISEASES OF THE RETICULO-ENDOTHELIAL SYSTEM

The reticulo-endothelial system produces reticulin fibres and forms an endothelial lining for blood spaces. The components in the liver are the primitive reticulum cells in the portal tracts and sinusoidal walls which differentiate into:

1. The stellate cells of Kupffer, which line the sinusoidal wall and are phagocytic. They are flat cells with large pale nuclei and abundant cytoplasm, sometimes extending into a star shape. Similar rounded macrophages are found in the portal spaces. Some differentiate into reticulin fibres which extend along the sinusoids and around the liver cords, giving them support. Under the electron microscope they show tube-like processes and have peroxidase activity.

2. Free, rounded stem cells in the sinusoidal wall and portal tracts. These are potential precursors of the red and white blood series. Under the electron microscope these show pinocytic vesicles.

3. The lymphoid tissue of the liver which is located in the portal tracts.

4. Lipocytes (Ito cells) are fat-storing cells in the sinusoids.

The cells of this system are sources of serum immunoglobulins.

The reticulo-endothelial system in the liver is involved in five groups of diseases: the primary reticuloses, diseases where there is excessive demand for new blood, reticulo-endothelial storage diseases, chronic hepatitis and infectious diseases which excite a reticulo-endothelial reaction.

PRIMARY RETICULOSES

Leukaemia

Myelogenous

The enlarged liver is smooth and firm, and the cut section shows small, pale nodules.

Microscopically (figs. 32, 33) both tracts and sinusoids are infiltrated with immature and mature cells of the myeloid series. The immature cells lie outside the sinusoidal wall, suggesting that they have been manufactured in the liver, i.e. the liver is actively haemopoietic rather than infiltrated.

The portal tracts are enlarged, with myelocytes and polymorphs, both neutrophil and eosinophil; round cells are also conspicuous. The liver cell cords are compressed by the leukaemic deposits.

Lymphocytic

Macroscopically, the liver is moderately enlarged, with pale areas on section.

Microscopically (fig. 34) the leukaemic infiltration involves only the portal tracts, the normal sites of lymphoid tissue in the liver. They are enlarged and contain both mature and immature cells of the lymphatic series. The sinusoids are not affected. The liver cells are normal.

Hairy cell leukaemia

This may present with splenomegaly and pancytopenia. Liver biopsy shows leukaemic cells infiltrating the portal cells and sinusoids. Angiomatous lesions, usually periportal, consist of blood spaces lined by hairy cells.

LONG-TERM SURVIVORS

Intensive cytotoxic therapy and marrow transplantation allow long-term survival particularly in

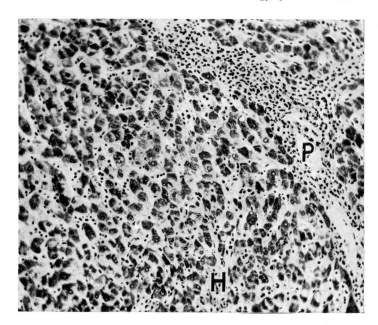

Fig. 32. Myelogenous leukaemia. Essential hepatic architecture is normal, but the sinusoids and a portal tract (P) contain increased numbers of cells of the myeloid series. Stained Best's carmine, × 70.

children with acute leukaemia. Such patients show marked portal zone fibrosis and portal hypertension [7].

BONE MARROW TRANSPLANTS

Recipients may develop graft-versus-host reactions which include chronic active hepatitis and bile duct lesions [3, 17]. Opportunist organisms may cause hepatitis.

Hodgkin's disease

Hepatic involvement occurs in about 70% of patients [11]. Typical Hodgkin's tissue is seen spreading out from the portal tracts, with lymphocytes, large pale epithelioid cells, eosinophils, plasma cells (fig. 35) and giant cells of the Dorothy Reed type. Later, fibroblasts are found in a supporting connective tissue reticulum. Occasionally only focal accumulations of Kupffer cells are seen and these may be difficult to differentiate from that of other reticuloses. More usually the picture is pleomorphic. Amyloidosis may be a complication.

Many reticuloses related to Hodgkin's disease affect the liver. In histiocytic medullary reticulosis, for instance, large numbers of reticulum cells fill the sinusoids and portal tracts. Occasionally the deposits may be single and large. Paraproteinaemia may be a complication.

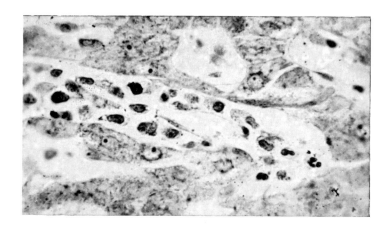

Fig. 33. Myelogenous leukaemia. Lining the sinusoid wall, but outside the endothelial lining, can be seen various cells of the myeloid and lymphocytic series. Stained Leishman, × 350.

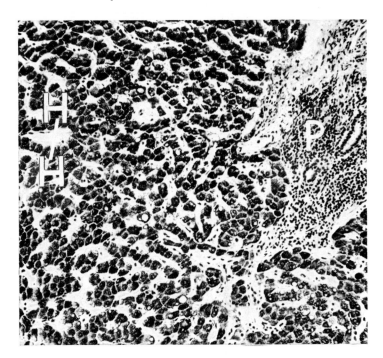

Fig. 34. Lymphocytic leukaemia. Essential hepatic architecture is normal, but a portal tract contains many cells of the lymphocyte series. The sinusoids are not affected. Stained Best's carmine, × 70.

Clinical features

Pyrexia, often of intermittent Pel–Ebstein type, is usual with abdominal Hodgkin's disease.

Jaundice [11] is usually mild and haemolytic. It is exacerbated by bilirubin overload following blood transfusion. Deep jaundice is most frequently related to intra-hepatic deposits and is terminal. Involvement of the main hepatic bile duct is rare [11]. Jaundice combined with exudative ascites is seen in about 15%.

Occasionally a most obscure intra-hepatic, usually cholestatic, jaundice may be seen [11]. It is unrelated to deposits in liver or bile ducts. Hepatic histology shows only canalicular stasis [10]. It is unrelated to drug therapy and is usually unaffected by treatment, although a trial of corticosteroids is worthwhile.

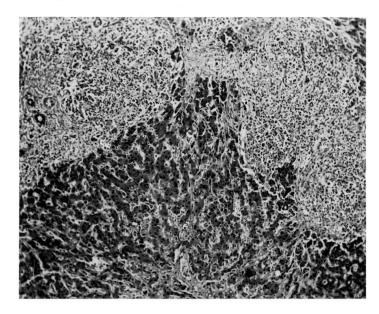

Fig. 35. Hodgkin's disease. The portal zones are infiltrated by Hodgkin's tissue. Stained H & E, × 70.

Diagnosis of hepatic involvement

The 'staging' of patients suffering from Hodgkin's disease has achieved great importance. Detection of hepatic involvement immediately places the patient in an advanced category. Fever, jaundice and splenomegaly increase the likelihood of liver involvement. Increases in serum-5-nucleotidase and transaminase values are suggestive although often non-specific [1].

Hepatic scintiscanning may be helpful [12]. Focal filling defects are always associated with Hodgkin's involvement although this is an infrequent finding. It is unusual for a needle biopsy of the liver to reveal Hodgkin's tissue if the scan is normal.

Needle biopsy cannot be regarded as excluding hepatic involvement if normal or non-specific reticulo-endothelial changes are seen. Laparotomy adds to the chance of a positive liver biopsy [1]. Peritoneoscopy or laparotomy with multiple needle biopsies double the yield over single, blind, needle ones [1].

Presentation as jaundice may provide great diagnostic difficulties. Hodgkin's disease should always be considered in patients with jaundice, fever and weight loss [18]. Liver biopsy may be helpful but can give normal appearances.

Lymphosarcoma

Nodules of lymphosarcomatous tissue may be found in the liver, especially in the portal tracts. Macroscopically they resemble metastatic carcinoma. The liver may also be involved in giant follicular lymphoma.

Multiple myeloma

The liver may be involved in plasma cell myeloma, the portal tracts and sinusoids being filled with plasma cells. Associated amyloidosis may involve the hepatic arterioles.

Angio-immunoblastic lymphadenopathy

This resembles Hodgkin's disease. The liver shows a pleomorphic portal zone infiltrate (lymphocytes, plasma cells and blast cells) without histiocytes or Dorothy Reed cells [8].

Myeloid metaplasia

The primitive reticulum cells of hepatic sinusoids and portal tracts possess the potential capacity to mature into adult erythrocytes, leucocytes or platelets. If the stimulus to blood regeneration is sufficiently strong, this function can be resumed. This is rare in the adult although myeloid metaplasia in the liver of the anaemic infant is not unusual. In the adult, it occurs with bone marrow replacement or irritation, and especially in association with secondary carcinoma of bone, myelofibrosis, myelosclerosis, multiple myeloma, and the marble bone disease of Albers-Schoenberg. It complicates all conditions associated with a leucoerythroblastic anaemia.

The condition is well exemplified by myelofibrosis and myelosclerosis, where the liver is enlarged, with a smooth firm edge. The spleen is enormous, and its removal results in even greater enlargement of the liver.

Microscopic features

The conspicuous abnormality is a great increase in the cellular content, both in the portal tracts and in the distended sinusoids (fig. 36). The cells are of all types and varying maturity. Myeloblasts and myelocytes are prominent. There are many reticulum cells and these may be converted into giant cells. The haemopoietic tissue may form discrete foci in the sinusoids.

Systemic mastocytosis

This can present with hepato-splenomegaly [5]. Liver biopsy, stained with haematoxylin and eosin, shows periportal, polygonal cells with eosinophil granules. On staining with Giemsa and toluidine blue, the typical metachromatic cytoplasmic granules may be identified.

PORTAL HYPERTENSION IN THE
RETICULOSES AND MYELOPROLIFERATIVE
SYNDROME

The myeloproliferative syndrome includes chronic myeloid leukaemia, polycythaemia rubra vera, myelosclerosis and haemorrhagic thrombocythaemia. Patients with these conditions or with Hodgkin's disease may suffer gastro-intestinal haemorrhage. In some this is due to peptic ulceration or gastro-intestinal erosions. In others it is secondary to hepatic, portal or splenic vein thrombosis related to the increased clotting tendency. Occasionally the portal hypertension is presinusoidal and seems to be secondary to infiltrative

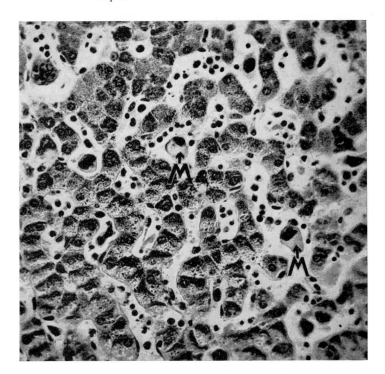

Fig. 36. Myeloid metaplasia secondary to bone marrow fibrosis. Giant cells resembling megakaryocytes (M), late erythroblasts, normoblasts and polymorphs are seen in the hepatic sinusoids. Stained Best's carmine, × 300.

lesions in the portal tracts and sinusoids (fig. 141). In systemic mastocytosis new fibre formation in the sinusoids may contribute [5]. Increased portal blood flow through the enlarged spleen may play a part. Portal fibrosis can be related to cytotoxic therapy.

LIPOID STORAGE DISEASES

The lipoidoses are disorders in which abnormal amounts of lipids are stored in the cells of the reti-culo-endothelial system. They may be classified according to the lipid stored (table 4).

PRIMARY AND SECONDARY XANTHOMATOSIS

Cholesterol is stored mainly in the skin, tendon sheaths, bone and blood vessels. The liver is rarely involved but there may be isolated nests of choles-terol-containing foamy histiocytes in the liver. Investigation of the liver is of little diagnostic value.

Table 4. The lipoid storage diseases.

Disease	Storage material	Liver involvement in lipoid storage
I Xanthomatosis	Cholesterol	
Primary essential		
Hyper-cholesterolaemic		Rare
Normo-cholesterolaemic		Rare
(Hand–Schuller–Christian)		
Secondary		
Essential hyperlipaemia		Rare
Diabetes mellitus		Rare
Obstructive jaundice		Rare
II Gaucher's disease	Cerebroside	Constant
III Niemann–Pick disease	Sphingomyelin (phospholipid)	Constant

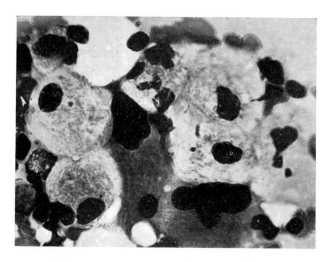

Fig. 37. Gaucher's disease. Smears of sternal marrow show large pale Gaucher cells with fibrillary cytoplasm and eccentric hyperchromatic nuclei. Stained Leishman, × 600.

CHOLESTERYL ESTER STORAGE DISEASE [2]

This rare, recessive, relatively benign disease is associated with symptomless hepato-splenomegaly. The liver is orange in colour and hepatocytes contain excess cholesteryl ester and neutral fat. A septate fibrosis is also present. The defect is in lysosomal acid lipase.

GAUCHER'S DISEASE

This rare, familial disease affects mainly Ashkenazi Jews [9]. A glucocerebroside, comprising sphingosine, fatty acid and glucose, is stored in cells of the reticulo-endothelial system. This accumulates due to a deficiency of the lysosomal enzyme, β-glucocerebrosidase in liver and spleen [14].

The characteristic Gaucher cell is approximately 70–80 μm in diameter, oval or polygonal in shape and with pale cytoplasm. It contains two or more peripherally placed hyperchromatic nuclei between which fibrils pass parallel to each other (fig. 37). It is quite different from the foamy cell of xanthomatosis or Niemann–Pick's disease.

Electron microscopy. The accumulated lysosomal β-glucocerebroside formed from degraded cell membranes actually precipitates within the lysosomes and forms long (200–400 Å), rod-like tubules. These are then seen by light microscopy. A somewhat similar cell is seen in chronic myeloid leukaemia and in multiple myeloma [15] due to increased turnover of β-glucocerebroside.

CHRONIC ADULT FORM

This is the common type. It commences insidiously, usually before the age of 30 years. It is very chronic and may be recognized in quite old people. It is inherited as an autosomal recessive.

The mode of presentation is variable, with unexplained hepato-splenomegaly (especially in children), spontaneous bone fractures, or bone pain with fever. Alternatively there may be a bleeding diathesis, with non-specific anaemia.

The clinical features include pigmentation which may be generalized or a patchy, brownish tan. The lower legs may have a symmetrical pigmentation, leaden grey in colour and containing melanin. The eyes show yellow pingueculae (fig. 38).

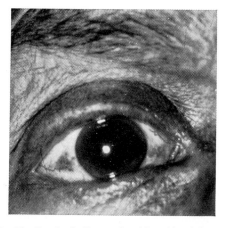

Fig. 38. Gaucher's disease. On either side of the pupil are wedge-shaped pingueculae consisting of yellow thickenings, fatty in appearance.

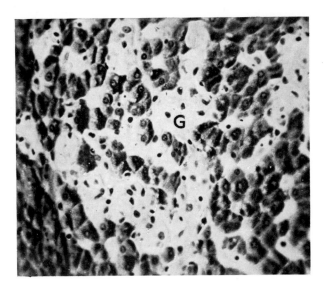

Fig. 39. Gaucher's disease. Liver sections show areas between the liver cell cords filled with large pale cells (G) with small dark nuclei. Stained Best's carmine, × 250.

The spleen is enormous and the liver is moderately enlarged, smooth and firm. Superficial lymph glands are not usually involved.

Portal hypertension is rare and of similar aetiology to that seen in other reticuloses It may be associated with ascites.

Bone X-rays. The long bones, especially the lower ends of the femora, are expanded, so that the waist normally seen above the condyles disappears. The appearance has been likened to that of an Erlenmeyer flask or hock bottle.

Sternal marrow shows the diagnostic Gaucher cells (fig. 37).

Aspiration liver biopsy should be performed if sternal puncture has yielded negative results. The liver is diffusely involved (fig. 39).

Peripheral blood changes. With diffuse bone-marrow involvement, a leucoerythroblastic picture may be seen. Alternatively leucopenia and thrombocytopenia with prolonged bleeding time may be associated with only a moderate hypochromic microcytic anaemia [16].

Leucocytes and fibroblasts in culture show reduced β-glucocerebrosidase activity.

Blood biochemical changes. The serum cholesterol level is normal. A persistently elevated serum acid phosphatase level not inhibited by L-tartrate may suggest Gaucher's disease. Serum angiotensin-converting enzyme is markedly increased.

Treatment

There is no specific therapy. Splenectomy is indicated for the very large spleen causing abdominal discomfort, and occasionally for thrombocytopenia or an acquired haemolytic anaemia. Replacement therapy, using the deficient enzyme encapsulated in liposomes, has been attempted [4].

Radiotherapy may be useful for severe bone pain.

Acute infantile Gaucher's disease

This acute form of the disease presents within the first six months of life and is usually fatal before two years. The child appears normal at birth. There is cerebral involvement, progressive cachexia and mental deterioration. The liver and spleen are enlarged and superficial lymph glands may also be palpable.

Autopsy shows Gaucher cells throughout the reticulo-endothelial system. They are, however, not found in the brain, where the pathological change is a degeneration of the cerebral cortex.

NIEMANN–PICK DISEASE

This rare, familial disease of unknown aetiology mainly affects the Jewish race. The deficiency is in the enzyme sphingo-myelinase, derived from cell membranes, in the lysosomes of the reticulo-endothelial system. The liver and spleen are predominantly involved.

The characteristic cell is pale, ovoid or round, 20–40 μm in diameter. In the unfixed state it is loaded with granules; when fixed in fat solvents the granules are dissolved, giving a vacuolated and foamy appearance. There are usually only one or two nuclei. Electron microscopy shows lysosomes containing the abnormal lipid.

Niemann–Pick disease occurs in infants, who die before the age of two years. The condition starts in the first three months, with anorexia, weight loss and retardation of growth. The liver and spleen enlarge, the skin becomes waxy and acquires a yellowish-brown coloration on exposed parts. The superficial lymph glands are enlarged. The patient is blind and deaf. In the terminal stages there is fever.

The fundus oculi may show a cherry-red spot at the macula.

The peripheral blood shows a microcytic anaemia and in the later stages the foamy Niemann–Pick cell may be found.

The disease may present as neonatal jaundice which remits. Inactive cirrhosis develops slowly. Progressive neurological deterioraion appears in late childhood [19].

Diagnosis is made by marrow puncture, which reveals characteristic Niemann–Pick cells.

SEA-BLUE HISTIOCYTE SYNDROME

This rare condition is characterized by histiocytes staining a sea-blue colour with Wright or Giemsa stain in bone marrow and in reticulo-endothelial cells of the liver. The cells contain deposits of phosphosphingolipid and glucosphingolipid. Clinically the liver and spleen are enlarged. The prognosis is usually good although thrombocytopenia and hepatic cirrhosis have been reported. It probably represents adult Niemann–Pick disease [13] which rarely involves the liver [6].

REFERENCES

1. BAGLEYK C.M. Jr, ROTH J.A., THOMAS L.B. *et al* (1972) Liver biopsy in Hodgkin's disease. Clinicopathologic correlations in 127 patients. *Ann. intern. Med.* **76,** 219.
2. BEAUDET A.L., FERRY G.D., NICHOLS B.L. Jr *et al* (1977) Cholesterol storage disease: clinical, biochemical and pathological studies. *J. Pediat.* **90,** 910.
3. BERK P.D., POPPER H., GERHARD R.F. *et al* (1979) Veno-occlusive disease of the liver after allogenic bone marrow transplantation. *Ann. intern. Med.* **90,** 158.
4. BRADY R.O., PENTCHEV P.G., GAL A.E. *et al* (1974) Replacement therapy for inherited enzyme deficiency: use of purified glucocerebrosidase in Gaucher's disease. *New Engl. J. Med.* **291,** 989.
5. CAPRON J-P., LEBREC C., DEGOTT C. *et al* (1978) Portal hypertension in systemic mastocytosis. *Gastroenterology* **74,** 595.
6. CHAN W.C., LAI K.S. & TODD D. (1977) Adult Niemann–Pick disease—a case report. *J. Path.* **121,** 177.
7. CRYER P.E. & KISSANE J.M. (1979) Pulmonary and hepatic disease after chemotherapy and bone marrow transplantation for acute leukaemia. *Am. J. Med.* **66,** 484.
8. FRIZZERA G., MORAN E.M. & RAPPAPORT H. (1975) Angio-immunoblastic lymphadenopathy: diagnosis and clinical course. *Am. J. Med.* **59,** 803.
9. GAUCHER E. (1882) De l'epithélioma primitif de la rate. Thèse de Paris.
10. JUNIPER K. (1963) Prolonged severe obstructive jaundice in Hodgkin's disease. *Gastroenterology* **44,** 199.
11. LEVITAN R., DIAMOND H.D. & CRAVER L.F. (1961) Jaundice in Hodgkin's disease. *Am. J. Med.* **30,** 99.
12. LIPTON M.J., NENARDO G.L., SILVERMAN S. *et al* (1972) Evaluation of the liver and spleen in Hodgkin's disease. 1. The value of hepatic scintigraphy. *Am. J. Med.* **52,** 356.
13. LONG R.G., LAKE B.D., PETTIT J.E. *et al* (1977) Adult Niemann–Pick disease: its relationship to the syndrome of the sea-blue histiocyte. *Am. J. Med.* **62,** 627.
14. PETERS S.P., LEE R.E. & GLEW R.H. (1977) Gaucher's disease, a review. *Medicine (Baltimore)* **56,** 425.
15. SCULLIN D.C. Jr, SHELBURNE J.D. & COHEN H.J. (1979) Pseudo-Gaucher cells in multiple myeloma. *Am. J. Med.* **67,** 347.
16. SHERLOCK S.P.V. & LEARMONTH J.R. (1942) Aneurysm of the splenic artery; with an account of an example complicating Gaucher's disease. *Br. J. Surg.* **30,** 151.
17. SHULMAN, H.M., SULLIVAN, K.M., WEIDEN, P.L. *et al* (1980) Chronic graft-versus-host syndrome in man. A long-term clinico pathologic study of 20 Seattle patients. *Am. J. Med.* **69,** 204.
18. TREWBY P.N., PORTMANN B., BRINKLEY D.M. *et al* (1979) Liver disease as presenting manifestation of Hodgkin's disease. *Q. J. Med.* **48,** 137.
19. WENGER, D.A., BARTH, G. & GITHENS, J.H. (1977) Nine cases of sphiogomyelin lipidosis, a new variant in Spanish-American children. Juvenile variant of Niemann–Pick disease with foamy and sea-blue histiocytes. *Am. J. Dis. Child.* **131,** 955.

Chapter 5
Imaging by Radio-isotopes, Ultrasound or Computerized Axial Tomography (CT)

RADIO-ISOTOPE SCANNING

An isotopically-labelled compound is injected and taken up by the liver. In some, such as [198]Au or [99m]technetium, the reticulo-endothelial system is the organelle concerned (see figs. 40, 41 in colour section). In others, such as [131]I Rose Bengal, the isotope is taken up by the liver cells and hence excreted in the bile.

[99m]Technetium is a gamma-emitting isotope which, when injected, is taken up by the reticulo-endothelial cells in the liver. It has a short half-life and gives a clear scan. The method is non-invasive. The use of a gamma camera lessens the time taken (fig. 42).

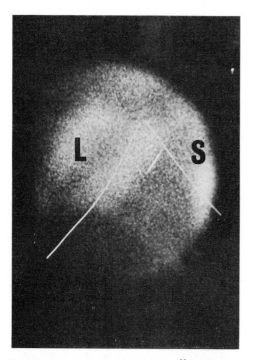

Fig. 42. Gamma camera scan using [99m]technetium in a patient with cirrhosis. Note patchy uptake in liver (L) and massive uptake of isotope in a large spleen (S).

The normal liver presents a fairly even distribution of activity (fig. 40) and the scintiscan gives a good index of liver size and shape unless there are infiltrative lesions invading the border of the liver. Liver mass may be estimated from the anterior or right lateral scan. Lesions which do not take up the isotope appear as filling defects (fig. 44). Primary or secondary tumours, cysts or abscesses may be localized by this means and the method can also be used to demonstrate deformities of the liver. Extrinsic lesions may also be suggested, for instance, a subphrenic abscess. The possibility of revealing a local lesion depends on its size and situation, for instance, those placed anteriorly are more easily shown than posterior ones. Lateral scanning helps in localization. The method is valuable in the diagnosis of space-occupying lesions larger than 2 cm but false-positive scans are a real problem.

Cirrhosis, or any generalized hepato-cellular disorder such as virus hepatitis or alcoholic hepatitis, is suggested by a generalized decrease in uptake, an irregular pattern and by uptake of technetium by the spleen and bone-marrow (figs. 41, 42). This picture may be useful diagnostically when a bleeding tendency contraindicates biopsy in a patient with hepato-cellular disease. Widespread metastases may produce a somewhat similar pattern to cirrhosis but without splenic uptake. Scanning may also be useful before liver biopsy to select the most suitable site for puncture.

In the presence of severe hepato-cellular disease, for instance acute viral or alcoholic hepatitis or advanced cirrhosis, the isotope is hardly taken up by the liver as the blood shunts past the reticulo-endothelial cells (fig. 43). In these circumstances space-occupying lesions cannot be identified.

[67]Gallium citrate accumulates in tissues that are actively synthesizing protein [22]. Lesions such as cysts or haemangiomas show as 'cold areas' with both technetium and gallium. A primary liver cancer or a liver abscess, which is synthesizing protein, is cold with technetium but takes up gallium

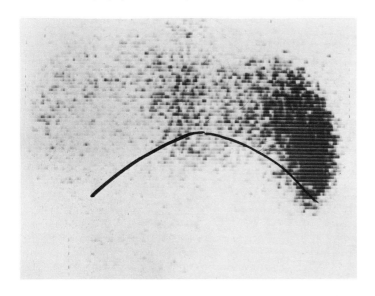

Fig. 43. In severe alcoholic hepatitis uptake of [99m]technetium by the liver may be negligible. Only splenic uptake is seen.

(fig. 45). [67]Gallium citrate is an awkward isotope to use for it has to be specially obtained and has a relatively short half-life.

Obstruction to the hepatic veins may be shown by preferential uptake by the caudate lobe (fig. 164). Obstruction to the bile ducts at the hilum of the liver is shown by filling defects resembling a hand (fig. 46).

Intra-hepatic haemangiomas or other vascular lesions may be detected by [113]indium which is bound by serum transferrin.

Serial scans may be useful in following the course of a lesion, for instance an amoebic abscess under treatment.

Observer error in the interpretation of radio-isotope scanning can be high and the scan should be used to create an index of suspicion rather than being regarded as diagnostic.

Biliary scanning

Compounds taken up by the liver cells and excreted in the bile can be labelled with an isotope [35]. These include [131]I Rose Bengal and the newer

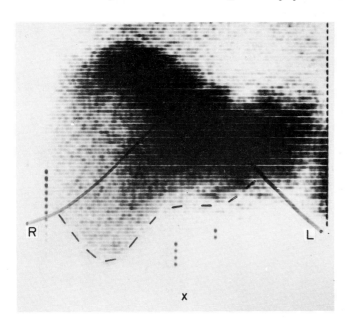

Fig. 44. Gamma camera scan using [99m]technetium in a patient with primary liver cancer shows a large filling defect in the right lobe of the liver (James *et al* 1974).

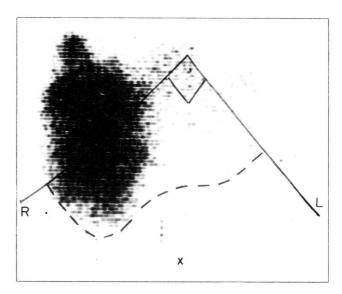

Fig. 45. Gallium citrate is taken up by the mass confirming that it is a malignant tumour (James *et al* 1974).

radiopharmaceuticals, [99m]Te pyridoxylidene glutamate, PG, and the imino-diacetic acid derivative, HIDA. Many others are being devised and evaluated [29].

HIDA is labelled with [99m]technetium and is rapidly extracted from the blood and excreted through the hepatocyte, giving early and high concentration in bile (fig. 47). HIDA is superior to [131]I Rose Bengal as a biliary scanner. Use of HIDA is applicable to all forms of jaundice provided that the total serum bilirubin level is less than 5 mg/dl [15]. It can be used to show that the cystic duct is patent, and is of particular value when acute cholecystitis is suspected. A non-visualized gall bladder within two hours of HIDA, with good visualization of the common bile duct,

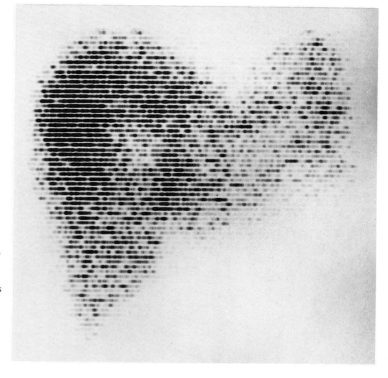

Fig. 46. Hepatic scan using [99m]technetium in a patient with carcinoma at the bifurcation of the hepatic ducts. This shows a filling defect at the hilum and into the right lobe with patchy uptake of the isotope into the left lobe: no secondaries were present on the left at autopsy. The hilar defect was due to dilated intra-hepatic bile ducts as the primary tumour was very small.

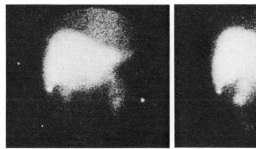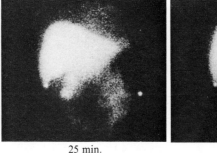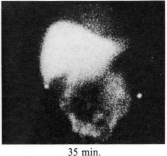

| 5 min. | 25 min. | 35 min. |

Fig. 47. ^{99m}Te-HIDA Gamma camera scan. Serial scans show the uptake of HIDA by the liver (5 min.) and into the common bile duct (25 min.) and finally into the duodenum (35 min.). This patient had acute cholecystitis. The gall bladder did not fill.

is diagnostic [10]. It is superior to ultrasonography and oral cholecystography in the circumstances [10]. Acute hepatitis must be excluded by estimating serum transaminase levels. HIDA can be used to detect post-operative and traumatic bile leaks and to verify the patency of biliary–enteric shunts whether made surgically or by prosthesis.

^{131}I Rose Bengal, or preferably HIDA, may be used in the differential diagnosis of neonatal hepatitis and biliary atresia. The excretion of the isotope into the duodenum is followed by sequential imaging using a gamma camera. Failure of excretion over several days implies atresia. The technique may be used to diagnose choledochal cysts [24].

ULTRASOUND [11, 30, 33]

This is a painless and harmless procedure particularly applicable to the liver. It is relatively inexpensive, costing 20 times less than the CT scan.

The principle is the reflexion of a fine beam of high frequency sound when it impinges on junctions of substances of different densities and elasticity. The echoes which then penetrate into the body are reflected back at different interfaces within the body. These are collected and recorded as electrical charges. They are dependent upon their electrical magnitude and are converted to shades of grey. The image is relayed to a TV monitor for display. Ultrasound enables the consistency of lesions, whether cystic or solid, to be evaluated. However, it does demand very special expertise in the interpretation and it is easy to read too much into the appearances. Failures occur when the diaphragm is high, the ribs low or with excessive upper abdominal gas in the bowel.

The normal ultrasound picture shows the liver as a large transonic area. The portal vein, inferior vena cava and aorta are shown (fig. 48). The normal biliary system is not seen.

Ultrasonography is an essential investigation in the patient with cholestatic jaundice (fig. 49) [31, 32]. The presence of dilated intra-hepatic bile ducts categorizes the cholestasis as due to large bile duct obstruction and is an important guide to further management. The bile ducts are seen as two fluid-filled structures in a para-sagittal plane. The dilated common duct assumes a humped or comma shape as it passes dorsally through the head of the pancreas [20]. The technique is 94% accurate if the serum bilirubin level exceeds 10 mg/dl [19]. False-negatives are seen if the cholestasis is of short duration and the ducts are less dilated. The whole common bile duct cannot be seen because of overlying gas.

The gall bladder is an ideal organ for sonographic analysis. It is useful where oral cholecystography has failed or is prohibited because of jaundice [23]. It may also be valuable in the pregnant woman [3]. The procedure is completed in one hour and may be more cost-effective than oral cholecystography [37]. Dilatation of the gall bladder may be shown [12]. Thickening of the gall bladder wall suggests cholecystitis [14]. Gallstones, 3 mm in size and upwards, may be seen as shadowing opacities which move. Specificity is high (97%) and sensitivity moderate (88%) [25] (fig. 50). Ultrasound has been recommended as a primary screening procedure in patients with acute, right upper quadrant pain [7]. Viscous bile or sludge may be observed with biliary obstruction or prolonged fasting.

The portal vein lies at the junction of the superior mesenteric and splenic veins, anterior to

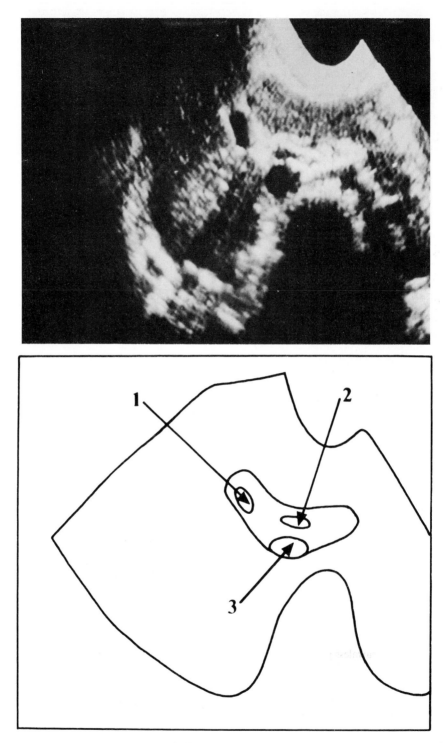

Fig. 48. Normal ultrasound appearances. The liver is shown as a large trans-sonic area. The portal vein (1), inferior vena cava (2) and aorta (3) are shown. The normal biliary system is not seen.

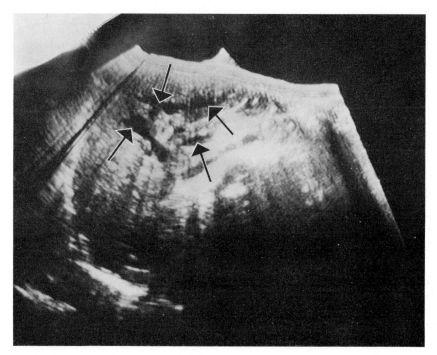

Fig. 49. Ultrasound shows dilated intra-hepatic bile ducts in a patient with carcinoma of the head of the pancreas.

the vena cava and slightly to the left of it (fig. 110). An obstructed portal vein may be visualized or, alternatively, dilatation may be noted. Ultrasound is a useful first investigation in a patient with bleeding oesophageal varices to determine whether or not the portal vein is patent [34]. Patency of a portal–systemic shunt can be confirmed by ultrasound.

In heart failure, a dilated hepatic vein and inferior vena cava can be observed (fig. 51). The hepatic artery is not well seen unless there is aneurysm formation.

Space-occupying lesions of about 2 cm in diameter, and even down to 1 cm under ideal circumstances, can be visualized. Metastases appear as dense, lucent or bull's eye deposits irrespective of site of primary or cell type [26]. Histological confirmation is still required. Primary liver cancer (fig. 52), hepatic cysts (fig. 53) or abscesses may be identified. Tumours of the gall bladder [8] or pancreas can also be seen. Ultrasonography may be useful in placing needles for liver biopsy or introducing instruments used to drain the biliary system or abscesses.

Ultrasonography also demonstrates ascites (fig.

51), although this is more conveniently done by less sophisticated methods.

False-negative and positive results are frequent in hepato-cellular disease, especially with macronodular cirrhosis [9, 13]. In the paediatric age group ultrasound has the advantage that ionizing radiation is not given. Congenital biliary anomalies such as Caroli's disease or choledochal cyst may be demonstrated.

COMPUTERIZED AXIAL TOMOGRAPHY (CT SCAN)
[1, 18, 21, 36]

This technique involves computerized tomographic reconstructions of multiple, intersecting gamma camera images and depicts the scan at three determined depths. The liver is envisaged as a series of sequential, contiguous, cross-sectional images, each representing a slice of tissue of a specified thickness (fig. 54). Typically, ten to twelve images are needed to examine the entire liver. A three-dimensional picture of a lesion is

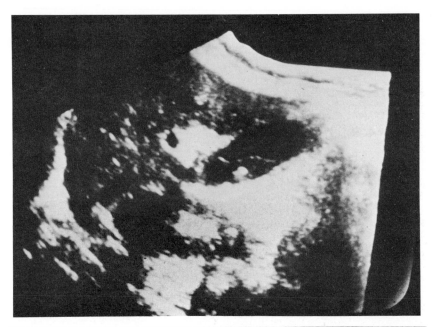

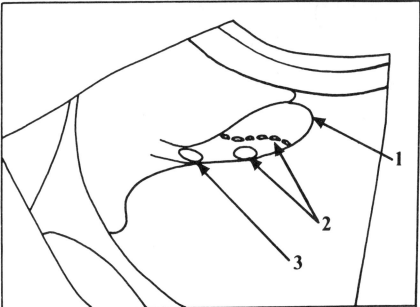

Fig. 50. Ultrasound in acute cholecystitis. A
distended gall bladder (1) contains stones (2). A
stone is impacted in the cystic duct (3).

built up and can be related to other structures such
as dilated ducts, veins in the porta hepatis or
lesions in adjacent organs. Fourteen 'cuts' give a
surface radiation of 3 rads.

The CT scan demonstrates detailed anatomy
across the whole abdomen at the level of the slice

(fig. 54). The identification of anatomical structures
may be facilitated by giving oral contrast material
to define the stomach and duodenum (gastrografin), or intravenous contrast to show blood
vessels, kidneys or bile ducts. As with ultrasound,
normal sized bile ducts are not shown. The CT

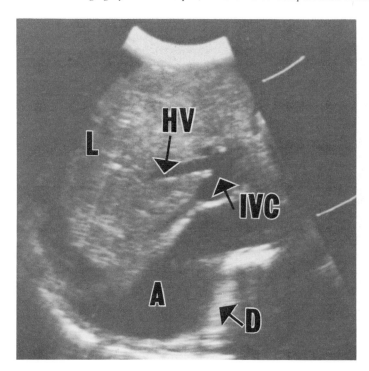

Fig. 51. Ultrasonography in congestive cardiac failure shows liver (L) with dilated hepatic vein (HV) and inferior vena cava (IVC). Ascites (A) and the diaphragm (D) are also shown.

scan has an advantage over ultrasound in the obese and where bowel gas is excessive.

The shape of the liver and any nodules on the surface may be noted. Liver volume can be calculated by obtaining the area of each of ten cross-sectional images. This represents the area of a slice of tissue of a specific thickness. Multiplying the area by the slice thickness gives slice volume, and finally a sum of the values of the slices gives liver volume [17]. Mass is obtained by multiplying liver volume by liver density.

CT scanning is valuable in defining the nature and extent of lesions that arise outside the liver and involve it extrinsically. Invasion of stomach, anterior abdominal wall and lung bases can be shown. The method is useful in surgical planning and in determining operability; similarly radiotherapy can be planned. CT scanning is particularly valuable in showing retro-peritoneal lesions such as those in the pancreas or in para-aortic lymph nodes (fig. 55).

In cholestatic jaundice, CT scanning will show dilated bile ducts where these exist. It distinguishes obstructive from non-obstructive jaundice with an accuracy rate of 90% [21]. Additionally, any pancreatic lesion causing biliary obstruction will be identified. It is more likely than ultrasound to give

the cause of cholestasis [16], but as a screening procedure in jaundiced patients it has no advantages over ultrasound, which is less costly.

CT scanning is of limited use in gall bladder disease as it will not consistently demonstrate gallstones and it is limited in its ability to visualize the thickness of the gall bladder wall.

It is a valuable method of detecting and differentiating circumscribed lesions, which it does with 87% success [21]. Metastases and primary liver cancer are less dense than normal tissue and cysts and abscesses are even less dense still (fig. 56). There is a 10% false-positive and negative rate [27]. Haemangiomas become denser after contrast infusion. CT scanning is useful for guided needle aspiration biopsy to obtain material for cytology. CT scanning is the most effective method of demonstrating space-occupying lesions [28] and only cost precludes its widespread use.

CT scanning is not well suited to the diagnosis of chronic liver disease [2]. Radionuclide scanning remains the preferred initial screening procedure in these circumstances [4].

The fatty liver shows a lower radiological density than normal (fig. 57). Mono-energetic CT can be used to assess liver fat content in alcoholic subjects. Results agree with chemical and hepatic

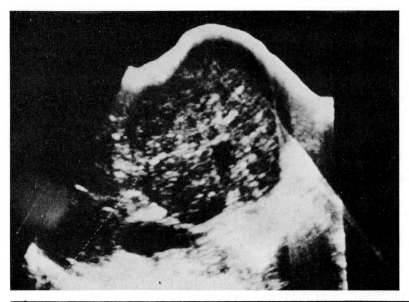

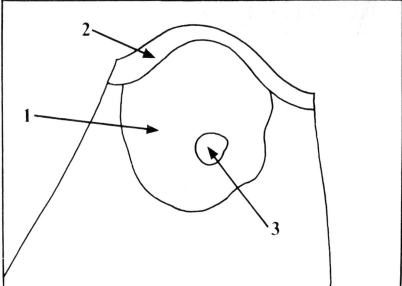

Fig. 52. Ultrasonography shows a large, round primary liver cancer (1) pushing out the anterior abdominal wall (2). A central necrotic cavity is seen (3).

histological assessment of liver fat [5]. The method may be useful in diagnosing fatty liver when liver biopsy is contraindicated.

In haemochromatosis, the radiological density is greater than normal. Dual-energetic CT may be used to estimate hepatic iron concentration in overload states [6]. Results correlate well with liver iron measured biochemically in liver biopsy specimens (fig. 58).

CONCLUSIONS

Choice of a technique for hepato-biliary imaging depends on many factors. Such considerations include the availability of the appropriate apparatus, the interpreter and the problem which has to be solved (table 5).

In general, radionuclide (isotope) scanning is the preferred screening technique because of the

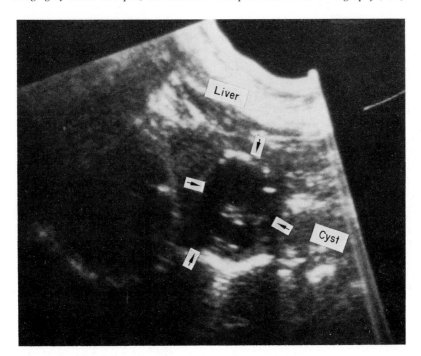

Fig. 53. Ultrasound shows multiple cysts in the liver.

high sensitivity and ease of performance. It is of particular value in screening for space-occupying lesions and for hepato-cellular disease. Weaknesses are the high false-positive or equivocal rate. Ultrasound is used to confirm and characterize equivocal isotope scan appearance.

CT scanning is often a tertiary procedure to confirm isotope or ultrasound appearances and to show fatty liver, peri-hepatic abscess, porta hepatis masses and to define tumour extent. The main disadvantages are the cost and the small ionizing radiation involved. In more affluent centres it often becomes the primary procedure.

For the diagnosis of jaundice, ultrasound is the preferred screening investigation. If necessary this may be followed by CT scanning to help in the

Table 5. Imaging in hepato-biliary disease.

	Radio-isotope	Ultrasound	CT
Cost of unit (approximate)	£60 000 ($138 000)	£35 000 ($80 500)	£300 000 ($690 000)
Operator skill	Minimal	Great	Minimal
Time (min.)	10–20	30	30–60
Morphological detail	Good	Good	Excellent
Interpretation	Easy	Many artefacts	Easy
Screening			
hepato-cellular disease	Good	Poor	Poor
tumours	Good	Good	Very good
dilated bile ducts	No	Very good	Very good
gall bladder disease	No	Very good	Poor
localization and disease spread	No	Good	Excellent
infiltrations (fat, iron)	No	No	Excellent

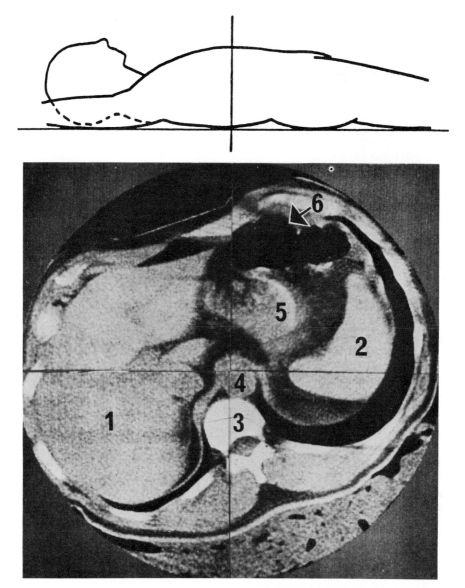

Fig. 54. Computerized tomography (CT) shows the liver (1) and spleen (2), vertebral body (3), aorta (4), pancreas (5) and stomach (6). The line drawing shows the level at which this CT scan was taken.

Fig. 55. CT scan shows enlarged para-aortic lymph nodes in abdominal Hodgkin's disease.
(1) Para-aortic glands, (2) vertebra, (3) liver, (4) kidney, (5) gastrografin in small intestine.

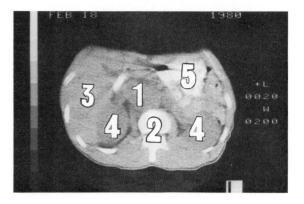

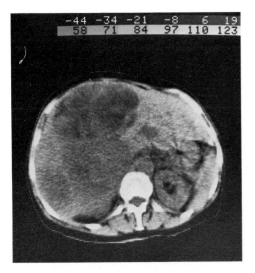

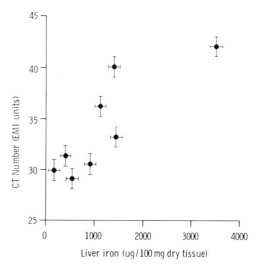

Fig. 56. CT scan in primary liver cancer shows multiple filling defects in the liver: the lesion is less dense than normal parenchyma.

Fig. 58. In primary haemochromatosis, values for liver iron estimated by CT correlate with liver iron determined biochemically on liver biopsy tissue (Chapman *et al* 1980).

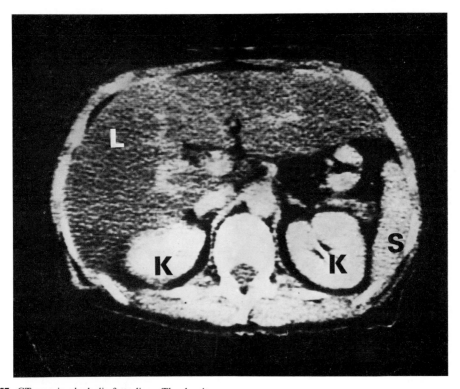

Fig. 57. CT scan in alcoholic fatty liver. The density of the enlarged liver (L) is lower than that of the kidney (K) or spleen (S) (Bydder *et al* 1980).

diagnosis of the cause of cholestasis and to show spread of disease.

For the diagnosis of gall-stones, oral cholecystography is the primary method of choice but in certain circumstances may be replaced by ultrasonography, particularly if jaundice is present or acute cholecystitis suspected. CT scanning is of little value in gall bladder disease.

HIDA scans provide a non-invasive method of determining bile duct patency in the presence of deep jaundice and for the diagnosis of acute cholecystitis.

REFERENCES

1. ABRAMS H.L. & MCNEIL B.J. (1978) Medical implications of computed tomography ('CAT scanning'). N. Engl. J. Med. 298, 255, 310.
2. ALFIDI R.J., HAAGA J.R., HAVRILLA T.R. et al (1976) Computed tomography of the liver. Am. J. Roentgenol. 127, 69.
3. BARTRUM R.J. Jr, CROW H.C. & FOOTE S.R. (1977) Ultrasonic and radiographic cholecystography. N. Engl. J. Med. 296, 538.
4. BIELLO D.R., LEVITT R.G., SIEGEL B.A. et al (1978) Computed tomography and radionuclide imaging of the liver: comparative evaluation. Radiology 127, 159.
5. BYDDER G., KREEL L., CHAPMAN R.W.G. et al (1980) Accuracy of computed tomography in diagnosis of fatty liver. Br. med. J. 281, 1042.
6. CHAPMAN R.W.G., WILLIAMS G., BYDDER G. et al (1980) Computed tomography for determining liver iron content in primary haemochromatosis. Br. med. J. i, 440.
7. CINTORA I., BEN-ORA A., MACNEIL R. et al (1979) Cholecystosonography for the decision to operate when acute cholecystitis is suspected. Am. J. Surg. 138, 818.
8. CRADE M., TAYLOR J.W., ROSENFIELD A.T. et al (1979) The varied ultrasonic character of gall-bladder tumour. JAMA 241, 2195.
9. DEWBURY K.C. & CLARK B. (1979) The accuracy of ultrasound in the detection of cirrhosis of the liver. Br. J. Radiol. 52, 945.
10. DOWN R.H.L., ARNOLD J., GOLDIN A. et al (1979) Comparison of accuracy of ^{99m}Tc-pyridoxylidene glutamate scanning with oral cholecystography and ultrasonography in diagnosis of acute cholecystitis. Lancet ii, 1094.
11. FERRUCCI J.I. Jr. (1979) Body ultrasonography. N. Engl. J. Med. 300, 590.
12. GONZALEZ A.C. & JOHNSON J.A. III (1978) Ultrasonic examination of the gall bladder: a review. Clin. Radiol. 29, 171.
13. GOSINK B.B., LEMON S.K., SCHEIBLE W. et al (1979) Accuracy of ultrasonography in diagnosis of hepatocellular disease. Am. J. Roentgenol. 133, 19.
14. HANDLER S.J. (1979) Ultrasound of gallbladder wall thickening and its relation to cholecystitis. Am. J. Roentgenol. 132, 581.
15. HARVEY E., LOBERG M., RYAN J. et al (1979) Hepatic clearance mechanisms of Tc-99m-HIDA and its effect on quantitation of hepatobiliary function: concise communication. J. nucl. med. Soc. 20, 310.
16. HAVRILLA T.R., HAAGA J.R., ALFID R.J. et al (1977) Computed tomography and obstructive biliary disease. Am. J. Roentgenol. 128, 765.
17. HEYMSFIELD S.B., FULENWIDER T., NORDLINGER B. et al (1979) Accurate measurement of liver, kidney and spleen volume and mass by computerised axial tomography. Ann. intern. Med. 90, 185.
18. KOROBKIN M. & GOLDBERG H.I. (1979) Computed tomography of the hepatobiliary system. Annu. Rev. Med. 30, 181.
19. LAPIS J.L., ORLANDO R.C., MITTELSTAEDT C.A. et al (1978) Ultrasonography in the diagnosis of obstructive jaundice. Ann. intern. Med. 89, 61.
20. LEE T.G., HENDERSON S.C. & EHRLICH R. (1977) Ultrasound diagnosis of common bile duct dilatation. Radiology 124, 793.
21. LEVITT R.G., SAGEL S.S., STANLEY R.J. et al (1977) Accuracy of computed tomography of the liver and kidney tract. Radiology 124, 123.
22. LOMAS F., DIBOS P.E. & WAGNER H.N. Jr (1972) Increased specificity of liver scanning with the use of ^{67}gallium citrate. N. Engl. J. Med. 286, 1323.
23. McCLUSKEY P.L., PRINZ R.A., GUICHO R. et al (1979) Use of ultrasound to demonstrate gallstones in symptomatic patients with normal oral cholecystograms. Am. J. Surg. 138, 655.
24. OSHIUMI Y., NAKAYAMA C., MORITA K. et al (1977) Serial scintigraphy of choledochal cysts using ^{131}I-rose-bengal and ^{131}I-bromsulphalein. Am. J. Roentgenol. 128, 769.
25. PRIAN G.W., NORTON L.W., EULE J. Jr et al (1977) Clinical indications and accuracy of gray scale ultrasonography in the patient with suspected biliary tract disease. Am. J. Surg. 134, 705.
26. SCHEIBLE W., GOSINK B.B. & LEOPOLD G.R. (1977) Gray scale echographic patterns of hepatic metastatic disease. Am. J. Roentgenol. 129, 983.
27. SCHERER U., ROTHE R., EISENBURG J. et al (1978) Diagnostic accuracy of CT in circumscript liver disease. Am. J. Roentgenol. 130, 711.
28. SNOW J.H. Jr, GOLDSTEIN H.M. & WALLACE S. (1979) Comparison of scintigraphy, sonography and computed tomography in the evaluation of hepatic neoplasms. Am. J. Roentgenol. 132, 915.
29. SPENNEY J.G., TOBIN M.M., MIHAS A.A. et al (1979) Utilisation of a radioiodinated bile salt for kinetic studies and hepatic scintigraphy. Gastroenterology 76, 272.
30. TAYLOR K.J.W. (ed.) (1979) Diagnostic Ultrasound in Gastrointestinal Disease (Clinics in Diagnostic Ultrasound I). Churchill Livingstone, Edinburgh.
31. TAYLOR K.J.W. & ROSENFIELD A.T. (1977) Grey-scale ultrasonography in the differential diagnosis of jaundice. Arch. Surg. 112, 820.
32. VALLON A.G., LEES W.R. & COTTON P.B. (1979) Grey-scale ultrasonography in cholestatic jaundice. Gut 20, 51.

33. VICARY F.R. (1977) Ultrasound and gastroenterology. *Gut* **18**, 386.
34. WEBB L.J., BERGER L.A. & SHERLOCK S. (1977) Grey-scale ultrasonography of portal vein. *Lancet* ii, 675.
35. WILLIAMS J.A.R., BAKER R.J., WALSH J.F. *et al* (1977) The role of biliary scanning in the investigation of the surgically jaundiced patient. *Surg. Gynecol. Obstet.* **144**, 525.
36. WITTENBERG J. & FERRUCCI J.T. Jr (1978) Computed body tomography. *Gastroenterology* **74**, 287.
37. WOLSON A.H. & GOLDBERG B.B. (1978) Gray-scale ultrasonic cholecystography: a primary screening procedure. *JAMA* **240**, 2073.

Chapter 6
Investigation of the Biliary Tract

Bile secretion

The liver secretes approximately 600 dl bile per day. There is a diurnal variation, more being excreted in the day than at night. Bile is secreted at a pressure of 15–25 cm H_2O and ceases when the pressure in the common bile duct rises to 35 cm H_2O. The sphincter of Oddi offers a resistance to bile flow of 10–25 cm H_2O. Protein is present in small amounts and there are variable amounts of mucin. The reaction of bile is neutral or slightly alkaline.

The cholesterol, phospholipid, bile salts and probably bilirubin form soluble macromolecular complexes or micelles. These allow the non-polar, insoluble cholesterol to be carried in solution (Chapter 29). Bile is usually sterile but occasionally *E. coli*, staphylococci or enterococci may be isolated.

The mechanisms and control of biliary secretion are discussed in Chapter 29. Secretion is largely by a bile salt-dependent mechanism and ductular flow is controlled by secretin. The place of nervous and vascular reflexes is unknown.

The entero-hepatic circulation of bile salts is discussed in Chapters 2 and 29.

FUNCTIONS OF BILE

Bile salts form micelles, solubilize triglyceride fat and assist in its absorption, together with calcium, cholesterol and fat-soluble vitamins, from the intestine.

Bile is the main route for excretion of bilirubin and cholesterol. The products of steroid hormones, particularly sex, thyroid and adrenal, are also excreted in bile.

Bile is the main route of excretion of some drugs and poisons such as the salts of heavy metals, atropine, strychnine and salicylates. This may be related to molecular size (fig. 279). Larger molecules, after being made soluble by such processes as conjugation, are excreted into the bile. Smaller molecules are excreted in the urine.

Bile salts absorbed from the intestine stimulate the liver to make more bile. Bile salts activate intestinal and pancreatic lipolytic and proteolytic enzymes.

Gall bladder function [8]

Hepatic bile is stored in the gall bladder where its volume is reduced by the absorption of an essentially isotonic NaCl, HCO_3 solution. The concentration of bile salts, bilirubin and cholesterol, for which the gall bladder wall is essentially impermeable, may increase 10-fold or more. This reduction is achieved by active transport of NaCl and HCO_3 along with a nearly isotonic amount of water from bile into the blood. The gall bladder mucosa is a typical leaky epithelium with high passive permeability to ions and water. The active ion transport by the gall bladder is related to an electrically neutral, coupled, NaCl influx process at the luminal membrane which ensures a one to one absorption of Na^+ and Cl^- and is partly responsible for the absent or low transepithelial potential difference.

The gall bladder is appreciably permeable to lipid-soluble molecules and this may lead to gradual but significant alteration of bile composition, by absorption of biliary lipids and of unconjugated bilirubin which have been formed by bacterial enzymatic breakdown of conjugated bilirubin [32]. Even some of the bile acids, particularly those conjugated with glycine or those which have undergone bacterial deconjugation, may be absorbed. This accelerated absorption of bile salts might promote gall-stone formation [23] (Chapter 29).

Because of micelle formation, the bile salts do not exert their expected osmotic activity. The concentrated bile therefore remains iso-osmotic with serum despite the fact that it has nearly twice the number of ionic particles per litre.

Motor functions of the biliary tract

The sphincter of Oddi [20] has a definite muscular layer which can act independently of the rest of the duodenal musculature. It is normally contracted and can withstand a pressure of 15–25 cm

H_2O in the common bile duct. Bile, produced by the liver, is therefore diverted into the cystic duct for storage in the gall bladder. When the gall bladder is full and if there is no specific stimulus for its evacuation, the sphincter relaxes and bile trickles into the duodenum.

Manometric studies at the time of endoscopic cholangiography show that the peak Oddi sphincter pressure is approximately 100 mmHg above the duodenal pressure. A high pressure zone with sphincter characteristics exists at the level of the choledocho-duodenal and pancreatico-duodenal junction, independent of duodenal dynamics. This sphincter creates a gradient between the bile or pancreatic ducts and the duodenum, and probably prevents reflux of duodenal content into these ducts [7]. Delivery of bile to the duodenum is wave-like and is predominantly controlled by the sphincter of Oddi [2]. The sphincter is responsive to enteric hormones [14]. Cholecystokinin and glucagon suppress sphincter of Oddi motor activity whereas pentagastrin increases it. Secretin causes a mixed response of excitation followed by inhibition. These phasic sphincter of Oddi contractions may have an important role in regulating biliary and pancreatic duct emptying.

Cholecystokinin (CCK), a peptide hormone, is released from the upper intestinal wall into the blood stream, in response to partly digested protein and fatty acids in the duodenum. This results in emptying of the gall bladder within one to two minutes and complete emptying within 15 minutes. The sphincter of Oddi is relaxed.

Gall bladder motility may be studied by timed aspiration of bile from the duodenum, but this lacks precision. Cine radiography of the biliary tract has been used to show peristalsis of the common bile duct. Gall bladder emptying can also be studied by cholescintography using $^{99m}Tc/HIDA$ [29].

Gall bladder stimulants include pituitrin. Atropine is a relaxant. The sphincter of Oddi is contracted by morphia, secretin and analgesics generally. Increased tone is little affected by the usual antispasmodics such as atropine. Amyl nitrite may relax the sphincter. Of the analgesics, pentazocine (Fortral) causes least rise in biliary pressure.

Duodenal intubation and drainage

These procedures are now rarely performed to assess biliary function although they continue to be used in pancreatic function tests.

Cholesterol crystals, calcium bilirubinate granules and microspheroliths are found in abnormal amounts in patients with gall bladder disease but also with other hepato-biliary and pancreatic abnormalities.

An increased bacterial flora may be found in patients with cholangitis and this may even produce a 'blind loop' syndrome [27].

The ^{14}C-glycocholic acid 'breath test' may also be used to detect colonization in the upper gastrointestinal tract in patients with cholangitis [18].

RADIOLOGY [4]

The shape and position of the gall bladder depend on the individual's somatotype; it may be found as high as the eleventh rib or below the iliac crest. It usually lies parallel to the spine, at the eleventh and twelfth ribs, and its body is cut by the shadow of the oblique lower margin of the liver. In one-quarter of normal subjects, part may overlap the shadow of the second and third lumbar vertebrae. The gall bladder always lies above the transverse colon and the fundus is usually in apposition to the duodenal cap. It overlies and is well anterior to the right renal shadow. Similarly, the more medially placed common bile duct overlies the pelvis of the kidney, but is anterior to it.

The common bile duct measured by intravenous cholangiography is usually less than 8 mm. Values greater than 15 mm are pathological; between 8 and 15 mm no conclusions can be drawn. The observed value is 3 mm larger by ERCP than by intravenous cholangiography [3].

PLAIN FILM OF THE ABDOMEN

This may reveal gall-stones, a calcified gall bladder wall or rarely the outline of a distended gall bladder. A soft tissue shadow may be seen in patients with carcinoma of the gall bladder.

With obstruction to the cystic duct, calcium carbonate may be excreted with the bile (milk of calcium bile or 'limey bile'). The wall of the gall bladder may also calcify (porcelain gall bladder).

Gas in the biliary tree (fig. 59) may be due to a spontaneous or post-operative biliary fistula. Gas may regurgitate through an incompetent sphincter of Oddi with cholecystitis, stricture or gall-stones or after sphincterotomy. Gas-gangrene infection is a very rare cause (emphysematous cholecystitis) [16].

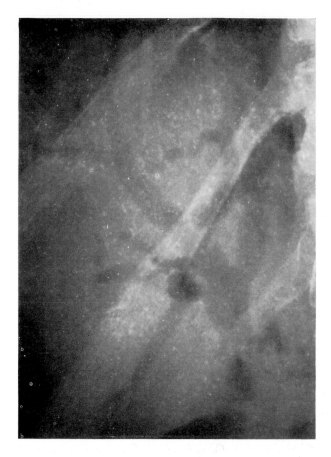

Fig. 59. Choledochojejunostomy.
Plain X-ray of the abdomen shows
gas outlining the biliary tract.

CHOLECYSTOGRAPHY AND CHOLANGIOGRAPHY

All the contrast materials are iodine-containing, conjugated and detoxicated by the liver, and excreted in the bile. With renal disease hepato-biliary excretion increases. Conversely, with hepato-cellular disease, renal excretion predominates and a pyelogram results. In such patients high blood levels of contrast are reached. Hypotension, shock and renal failure and coronary thrombosis may be precipitated [1].

ORAL CHOLECYSTOGRAPHY AND CHOLANGIOGRAPHY

This is the simplest and least expensive method of demonstrating the biliary tract. It should always precede intravenous techniques if the gall bladder is present. After a light evening meal, 14 hours before the examination, six tablets (3 g) of Ipodace (solu-biloptin) are taken. Next morning, three hours before the study, a further dose of 3 g solu-biloptin are taken. The gall bladder and common bile duct will be shown in 85% of patients. Films must be taken in both erect and prone positions. The erect position is particularly useful in demonstrating translucent stones which appear to float on the surface of the contrast (fig. 397).

Formerly a fatty meal was given to induce gall bladder contraction and increase opacification of cystic and common bile ducts. This has now been replaced by intravenous cholecystokinin octapeptide. An abnormal, positive test is shown by incomplete emptying or spasm of the gall bladder, the significance of which is uncertain. The patient's symptoms may be induced.

Normal visualization, without stones, gives a 95% probability that the gall bladder is normal.

Continued administration of solu-biloptin over four days has been used to show duct stones [26].

Minor reactions include nausea, vomiting and diarrhoea and a skin rash. Serious reactions such as anaphylactoid shock or renal failure are rare.

The contrast material has a uricosuric effect. Bilirubin is retained because the contrast material competes for hepatic excretion.

Cholecystography should not be undertaken if the serum conjugated bilirubin level is above 2 mg/ 100 ml. The radio-opaque dye will not be sufficiently concentrated to give satisfactory definition. Failure to fill within 14 hours may be due to defective gastro-intestinal absorption due to vomiting, diarrhoea or local disease. The gall bladder may have been previously removed, be diseased, or be intra-hepatic. The cystic duct may be obstructed. Hepato-cellular function may be so poor that insufficient dye is excreted into the ducts.

In the absence of jaundice or hepato-cellular failure, lack of visualization implies gall bladder disease.

Uses of cholecystography

1. The diagnosis of radio-translucent gall-stones.
2. The evaluation of gall bladder function and the diagnosis of chronic cholecystitis.
3. The differentiation of calcified opacities or other masses in the right upper quadrant of the abdomen.
4. Intra-mural lesions of the gall bladder are shown as small fixed radiolucent zones, unaffected by posture, in a well-visualized gall bladder best seen after cholecystokinin.
5. Small fixed filling defects in a well-concentrating gall bladder are usually due to cholesterol deposits [15].
6. Adenomyomatosis is shown as small outpouches, particularly fundal, in a gall bladder which is concentrating the medium extremely well.
7. Rokitansky–Aschoff sinuses are shown as a dotted second contour around the gall bladder.
8. A large gall bladder may be seen after vagotomy or in diabetes [5].

INTRAVENOUS CHOLANGIOGRAPHY

The contrast is concentrated by the liver so that the cystic, hepatic and common bile ducts are regularly demonstrated before the gall bladder

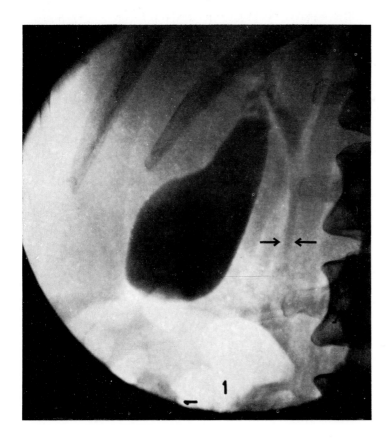

Fig. 60. Intravenous cholangiography. The common bile duct is indicated by the arrows.

becomes opaque (fig. 60). Intravenous cholangio-graphy is more costly and time consuming than the oral technique. It is indicated to visualize the bile ducts after cholecystectomy or when gall bladder and ducts are not seen with the oral methods.

Intravenous cholangiography is performed in the non-fasting state 2–3 hours after breakfast. 50 ml Ioglycamide (biligram forte) are injected intravenously in 10% glucose over 30–60 minutes. Toxic reactions [1] are more common than with oral cholecystography and include nausea, vomit-ing and hypotension. Renal failure can develop especially in those with underlying renal or hepatic disease. Dehydration should be avoided. Wal-denström's macroglobulinaemia is an absolute contraindication.

Films are exposed 15, 30 and 45 minutes later. Tomography is done after the 45 minute film. The gall bladder may be shown after 24 hours.

Intravenous cholangiography is not so satisfac-tory as the oral method in showing stones. A dilated duct, however, is always pathological and never simply follows cholecystectomy [31].

Infusion cholangiography should not be per-formed if serum bilirubin concentration exceeds 4 mg/100 ml. It may be very helpful in mild chole-stasis, for instance in primary biliary cirrhosis.

Isotopic cholangiography (see Chapter 5).

ENDOSCOPIC RETROGRADE CHOLANGIO-PANCREATOGRAPHY (ERCP) [6, 10, 33]

The ampulla of Vater can be visualized and the common bile duct or pancreatic duct cannulated and contrast material injected (fig. 61). The tech-nique demands an experienced team. The patient must be under observation for 24 hours after the procedure which is done under light sedation (atropine and diazepam) and local (never general) anaesthesia. Duodenal ileus is maintained by intermittent intravenous hyoscine N-butylbromide (Buscopan) or glucagon. The fibrescope, usually an Olympus JFB2 duodenoscope, is passed. The papillary region is easily reached. The stomach

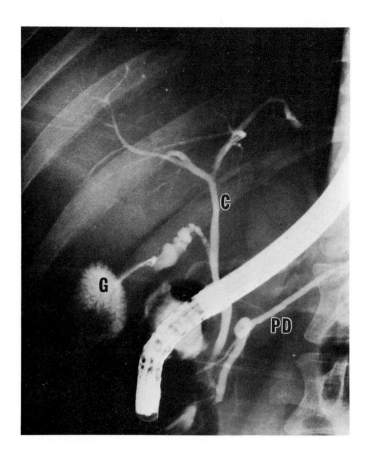

Fig. 61. ERCP, normal appearances. PD = pancreatic duct; G = gall bladder; C = common bile duct.

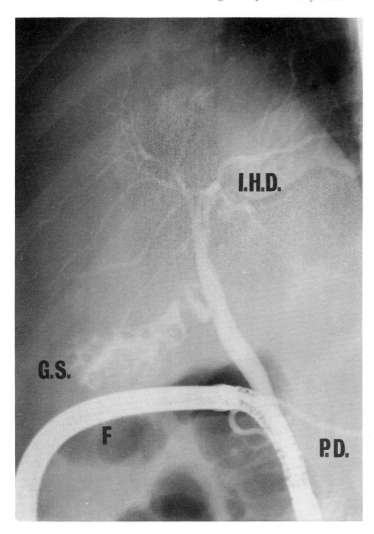

Fig. 62. ERCP in a patient with primary biliary cirrhosis and deep cholestatic jaundice in whom intravenous cholangiography had failed to show bile ducts. The main bile ducts are patent. The gall bladder contains many gall-stones. F = fibrescope; PD = pancreatic duct; GS = gall-stone; IHD = intra-hepatic ducts.

and duodenum having been surveyed, biopsy and cytology specimens and photographs are taken as necessary. The papilla is identified and any lesion in the area biopsied. The cannula is then introduced under direct vision into the papilla and bile duct and contrast (angiografin 65%) injected under fluoroscopic control. Posturing is needed to fill the intra-hepatic biliary tree, cystic and common bile ducts and the gall bladder (fig. 61). The pancreatic duct is similarly cannulated and photographed (fig. 61). Patients with suspected biliary obstruction or cholangitis are given antibiotics (gentamicin and ampicillin) before the examination and afterwards if cholestasis has been observed.

The success rate is about 80% but much depends on the experience of the operator. Other causes of failure include papillary stenosis or tumour, previous gastric surgery, duodenal diverticulum or previous ulceration.

COMPLICATIONS

Febrile reactions and septicaemias may follow ERCP in those with cholangitis [30]. Sepsis is only seen where contrast is injected into diseased and obstructed ducts. Bile leakage and haemorrhage have been seen in those with tumours. It is also possible to damage the papillary region and to perforate the duodenum.

Serum amylase levels rise considerably after ERCP, and acute pancreatitis is a complication. Suspected pancreatic pseudocyst is an absolute contraindication to ERCP.

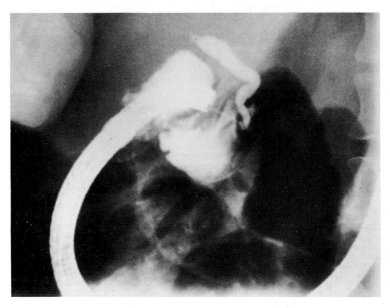

Fig. 63. ERCP showing nipple-like obstruction at
the hilum of the liver due to bile duct carcinoma.

CLINICAL INDICATIONS

ERCP adds to the speed of diagnosis of the jaundiced patient as it can be performed irrespective
of depth of icterus or state of liver function. It outlines the site of any biliary obstruction and in many
instances indicates the cause (fig. 63).

It can be used to diagnose gall bladder and common bile duct stones (fig. 64). These are outlined
more clearly than by intravenous cholangiography
and ERCP may be used after i.v. cholangiography
has failed [22].

ERCP may be performed after biliary surgery
in the investigation of benign post-cholecystectomy symptoms or to define more serious sequelae
such as residual calculi, biliary strictures and
choledocho-duodenal fistulas.

ERCP may be used to diagnose pancreatic
disease and particularly in those with coincident
hepato-biliary problems such as alcoholic pancreatitis with biliary obstruction (fig. 320).

ERCP is used in the investigation of the patient
with obscure epigastric pain. It allows visualization of stomach and duodenum as well as pancreatic and biliary ducts, all at one sitting.

THERAPEUTIC USES (see Chapter 29)

In a patient with choledocholithiasis the procedure
may be combined with section of the duodenal

papilla (*papillotomy*). This may allow the gall-
stones to pass into the duodenum. Alternatively
the stones may be extracted from the common bile
duct using a Dormia basket. As an extension of
ERCP, fine baby instruments can now be passed
through mother scopes through the papilla and
into the biliary and pancreatic ducts. Such scopes
can be used for choledochoscopy and even for oral
biliary drainage [6].

CHOLEDOCHOSCOPY [28]

This procedure allows the surgeon to see directly
into the lumen of the intra-hepatic and extra-
hepatic biliary system. The scope is introduced at
surgery into the common bile duct. The majority
of stones missed by conventional manipulation
can be seen and removed. Biliary tumours may be
diagnosed.

**PERCUTANEOUS TRANS-HEPATIC
CHOLANGIOGRAPHY** [11, 17, 21, 24]

This technique involves the direct percutaneous
injection, via a fine needle, of contrast into bile
ducts within the liver (fig. 65). The procedure is
done in the radiology department with intravenous diazepam pre-medication and under

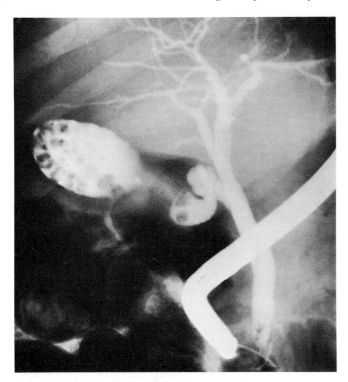

Fig. 64. ERCP showing gall-stones in gall bladder and common bile duct. The common bile duct is dilated.

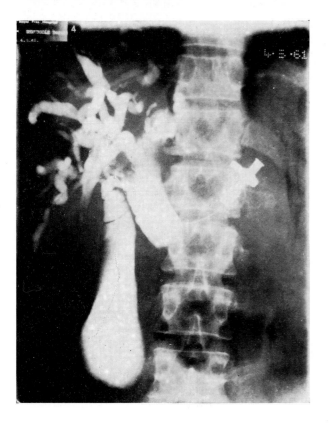

Fig. 65. Percutaneous trans-hepatic cholangiography showing grossly distended intra-hepatic bile ducts and gall bladder. The common bile duct is totally obstructed. Surgery revealed a carcinoma of the head of the pancreas.

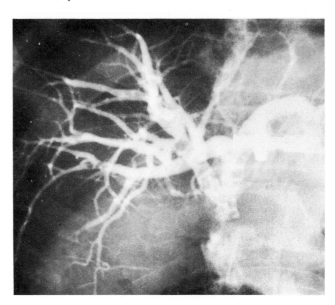

Fig. 66. Percutaneous cholangiogram showing stones in the intra-hepatic bile ducts above a stricture. Some contrast material is reaching the duodenum.

local anaesthesia. Preliminary antibiotics are given 24 hours before the procedure. The 'skinny' Chiba needle is 0.7 mm outside diameter. It does not have an outer sheath and is very flexible so that the patient is able to breathe normally with it *in situ* [21].

The patient lies supine. The needle is introduced in the seventh, eighth or ninth right intercostal space at a point of maximal dullness to percussion. It is advanced parallel to the table top as far as the spine, bisecting a sagittal line between the dome of the diaphragm and the duodenal cap identified by an air bubble. Contrast is injected continuously as the needle is withdrawn. Bile ducts are identified by centripetal flow, the contrast remaining for some time. Portal and hepatic veins are recognized by the direction of flow and rapid disappearance of contrast medium when injection is stopped. Lymphatics can be filled but usually after injection of contrast into hepatic parenchyma. Such deposits take 5–10 minutes to be cleared by the lymphatic channels. Up to six needle 'passes' are allowed before the procedure is usually abandoned. After injection of contrast material into obstructed and dilated ducts the patient is tilted upright so that the common bile duct has an opportunity to fill. Using the 'skinny' needle, the technique is relatively safe so that surgery need not inevitably follow. If dilated ducts are encountered, however, external biliary drainage using a slightly wider needle, should continue until surgery is done [9]. The bile should be cultured. The patient must be observed carefully in hospital.

The technique is easy and the success rate is at least 90% if intra-hepatic bile ducts are dilated. With undilated ducts, such as in primary biliary cirrhosis, sclerosing cholangitis or with some cases of choledocholithiasis the success rate drops to some 60% but can rise to 96% in specially skilled hands [24] and to 85% if unlimited attempts are allowed.

CLINICAL INDICATIONS

Trans-hepatic cholangiography is valuable in jaundiced, presumably cholestatic, patients where oral or intravenous cholangiography would not succeed. It is particularly useful when ultrasound has demonstrated intra-hepatic biliary dilatation and the site and possible nature of the biliary obstruction must be defined.

THERAPEUTIC USES

In a patient with cholestasis and with dilated intra-hepatic bile ducts, percutaneous cholangiography may be followed by catheterization of the bile ducts and external biliary drainage for some days [9, 19]. This allows a biliary infection to be controlled and the patient to be operated upon with normal serum bilirubin and bile acid values. This procedure may reduce operative mortality [19] and the incidence of renal complications. An endoprosthesis may be introduced through a malignant growth or a benign inoperable biliary stricture [9, 25] (figs. 67, 68).

CHOICE BETWEEN PERCUTANEOUS TRANS-HEPATIC CHOLANGIOGRAPHY OR ERCP (table 6, overleaf)

Using one or both of these procedures the biliary tree can be visualized in over 90% of patients in whom surgical cholestasis has to be excluded [10]. The choice of the first procedure depends on many factors. These include the availability of skilled operators for ERCP and of the economic resources for the maintenance of endoscopes. In general where intra-hepatic bile ducts are dilated then the percutaneous cholangiogram should be the first procedure. Post-cholecystectomy problems, the diagnosis of gall-stones and where pancreatic lesions are suspected should indicate ERCP as the first choice. Any large hospital should have both techniques available.

Operative and post-operative cholangiography [12, 13]

In the jaundiced subject, operative cholangiography is being replaced by the percutaneous trans-hepatic or endoscopic techniques. In patients with gall-stones, however, there is much to be said for routine operative cholangiography. The contrast is introduced by catheter into the cystic duct. This allows stones in the common bile duct to be diagnosed. After exploration of the common bile duct cholangiography may be performed to exclude residual calculi.

Debris may cause filling defects which are less sharply defined than those caused by gall-stones. Air bubbles may simulate gall-stones. Small stones

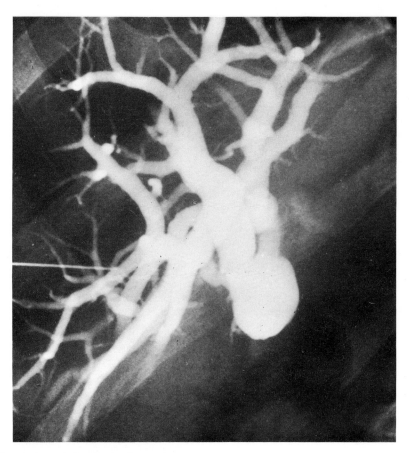

Fig. 67. Percutaneous cholangiogram in a patient with hilar stricture due to bile duct carcinoma (Dooley *et al* 1979).

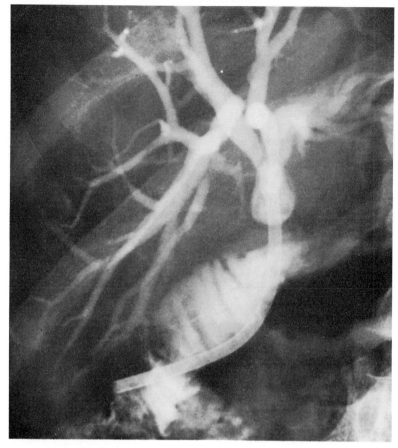

Fig. 68. The same patient as fig. 67. An
endoprosthesis is in position allowing biliary
drainage into the duodenum (Dooley *et al* 1979).

Table 6. A comparison of percutaneous trans-
hepatic (PTC) and endoscopic cholangio-
pancreatographic cholangiography (ERCP).

	PTC	ERCP
Technique	Easy	Difficult
Time taken (min.)	15	15–60
Anatomical difficulties	Few	Many
Cost	Moderate	High
Complications	5% biliary leaks	1% cholangitis
	Cholangitis	Pancreatitis Rupture duodenum
Success %		
Overall	80	80
Dilated ducts	100	80
Undilated ducts	60	80
Pancreatic ducts	0	80

may be obliterated by the contrast medium. Post-
operative cholangiography should be undertaken
routinely before final removal of a T tube draining
the biliary tree.

During the injection, biliary duct contents, including bacteria, probably regurgitate into the
blood. This is particularly marked in the presence
of biliary obstruction.

A surprising number of operative and post-
operative cholangiograms are technically unsatisfactory through failure to visualize bile ducts or
the trans-duodenal or sphincteric segment of the
ducts. Practice is necessary.

Hepatic ultrasound and scanning (see Chapter 5)

The bile ducts above an obstruction dilate and can
be visualized by ultrasound or CT scan. Isotope

scanning is less satisfactory. Ultrasound is an essential first step in the diagnosis of cholestasis.

Barium meal

A barium meal or enema may be useful in diagnosing obstructive jaundice by disclosing a primary neoplasm or revealing pressure deformities or internal fistulae. Gall-stones keep a constant relationship to the first or second part of the duodenum.

A pancreatic carcinoma may cause pressure effects on adjacent organs. Duodenography, using gas distension of the duodenum by oxygen after relaxation by local xylocaine and intravenous oxyphenonium may be very useful in demonstrating ampullary and pancreatic lesions.

Internal biliary fistulae or a lax sphincter may allow the passage of intestinal barium into the biliary tree, confirming a suspicion aroused in the plain film by the presence of gas in the biliary tract.

REFERENCES

1. ANSELL G. (1970) Adverse reactions to contrast agents: scope of problem. *Invest. Radiol.* **5**, 374.
2. ASHKIN J.R., LYON D.T., SHULL S.D. *et al* (1978) Factors affecting delivery of bile to the duodenum in man. *Gastroenterology* **74**, 560.
3. BELSITO A.A., MARTA J.B., CRAMER G.G. *et al* (1977) Measurement of biliary tract size and drainage time. *Radiology* **122**, 65.
4. BERK R.N. & CLEMETT A.R. (eds.) (1977) *Radiology of the Gallbladder and Bile Ducts.* Monographs in Clinical Radiology, vol. 12. W.B. Saunders, Philadelphia.
5. BLOOM A.A. & STACHENFELD R. (1969) Diabetic cholecystomegaly. *J. Am. med. Assoc.* **208**, 357.
6. COTTON P.B. (1977) ERCP. *Gut* **18**, 316.
7. CSENDES A., KRUSE A., FUNCH-JENSEN P. *et al* (1979) Pressure measurements in the biliary and pancreatic duct systems in controls and in patients with gallstones, previous cholecystectomy, common bile duct stones. *Gastroenterology* **77**, 1203.
8. DIETSCHY J.M. (1966) Recent developments in solute and water transport across the gall bladder epithelium. *Gastroenterology* **50**, 692.
9. DOOLEY J.S., DICK R., OLNEY J. *et al* (1979) Non-surgical treatment of biliary obstruction. *Lancet* ii, 1040.
10. ELIAS E. (1976) Progress report: cholangiography in the jaundiced patient. *Gut* **17**, 801.
11. ELIAS E., HAMLYN A.N., JAIN S. *et al* (1976) A randomised trial of percutaneous transhepatic cholangiography with the Chiba needle versus endoscopic retrograde cholangiography for bile duct visualisation in jaundice. *Gastroenterology* **71**, 439.
12. FARHA G.J. & PEARSON R.N. (1976) Transcystic duct operative cholangiography: personal experience with 500 consecutive cases. *Am. J. Surg.* **131**, 228.
13. FARIS I., THOMSON J.P., GRUNDY D.J. *et al* (1975) Operative cholangiography: a reappraisal based on a review of 400 cholangiograms. *Br. J. Surg.* **62**, 966.
14. GEENEN J.E., HOGAN W.J., DODDS W.J. *et al* (1980) Intraluminal pressure recording from the human sphincter of Oddi. *Gastroenterology* **78**, 317.
15. GRIECO R.V., BARTONE N.F. & VASILAS A. (1963) A study of fixed filling defects in the well opacified gallbladder and their evolution. *Am. J. Roentgenol.* **90**, 844.
16. JACOB H., APPELMAN R. & STEIN H.D. (1979) The radiology corner. Emphysematous cholecystitis. *Am. J. Gastroenterol.* **71**, 325.
17. JAIN S., LONG R.G., SCOTT J. *et al* (1977) Percutaneous transhepatic cholangiography using the 'Chiba' needle—80 cases. *Br. J. Radiol.* **50**, 175.
18. JAMES O.F.W., AGNEW J.E. & BOUCHIER I.A.D. (1973) Assessment of the ^{14}C-glycocholic acid breath test. *Br. med. J.* iii, 191.
19. NAKAYAMA T., IKEDA A. & OKUDA K. (1978) Percutaneous transhepatic drainage of the biliary tract: technique and results in 104 cases. *Gastroenterology* **74**, 554.
20. ODDI R. (1887) D'une disposition à sphincter spéciale de l'ouverture du canal cholédoque. *Arch. ital. Biol.* **8**, 317.
21. OKUDA K., TANIKAWA K., EMURA T. *et al* (1974) Nonsurgical, percutaneous transhepatic cholangiography—diagnostic significance in medical problems of the liver. *Am. J. dig. Dis.* **19**, 21.
22. OSNES M., GRØNSETH K., LARSEN S. *et al* (1978) Comparison of endoscopic retrograde and intravenous cholangiography in diagnosis of biliary calculi. *Lancet* ii, 230.
23. OSTROW J.D. (1969) Absorption by the gallbladder of bile salts, sulfobromophthalein and iodipamide. *J. lab. clin. Med.* **74**, 482.
24. PEREIRAS R.V. Jr, CHIPRUT R.O., GREENWALD R.A. *et al* (1977) Percutaneous transhepatic cholangiography with the 'skinny' needle. *Ann. intern. Med.* **86**, 562.
25. PEREIRAS R.V. Jr, RHEINGOLD O.J., HUTSON D. *et al* (1978) Relief of malignant obstructive jaundice by percutaneous insertion of a permanent prosthesis in the biliary tree. *Ann. intern. Med.* **89**, 589.
26. SALZMAN E., SPURCK R.P. & WATKINS D.H. (1959) X-ray diagnosis of bile duct calculi. *Gastroenterology* **37**, 587.
27. SCOTT A.J. & KHAN G.A. (1968) Biliary infection producing a blind loop syndrome. *Gut* **9**, 187.
28. SHORE J.M., BERCI G. & MORGENSTERN L. (1975) The value of biliary endoscopy. *Surg. Gynecol. Obstet.* **140**, 601.
29. SPELLMAN S.J., SHAFFER E.A. & ROSENTHALL L. (1979) Gallbladder emptying in response to cholecystokinin. *Gastroenterology* **77**, 115.
30. THURNHERR N., BRÜHLMANN W.F., KREJS G.I. *et al* (1976) Fulminant cholangitis and septicaemia after endoscopic retrograde cholangiography

(ERC) in two patients with obstructive jaundice. *Am. J. dig. Dis.* **21,** 477.

31. WAKIM K.G. & MAHOUR G.H. (1971) Pathophysiologic consequences of cholecystectomy. *Surg. Gynecol. Obstet.* **133,** 113.

32. WHEELER H.O. (1971) Concentrating function of the gallbladder. *Am. J. Med.* **51,** 588.

33. ZIMMON D.S., CHANG J. & CLEMETT A.R. (1979) Advances in the management of bile duct obstruction. *Med. Clin. N. Am.* **63,** 593.

Chapter 7
Hepato-cellular Failure

Hepato-cellular failure can complicate almost all forms of liver disease. It may follow virus hepatitis, or the cirrhoses, fatty liver of pregnancy, hepatitis due to drugs such as halothane, overdose with drugs such as acetaminophen (paracetamol), ligation of the hepatic artery near the liver, or occlusion of the hepatic veins. The syndrome does not complicate portal venous occlusion alone. Circulatory failure, with hypotension, may precipitate liver failure, especially in the cirrhotic.

It may be terminal in chronic cholestasis, such as primary biliary cirrhosis or surgical cholestatic jaundice associated with malignant replacement of liver tissue or acute cholangitis. It should be diagnosed cautiously in a patient suffering from acute biliary obstruction, and certainly not until other possible complications have been excluded.

It might be questioned whether so many different conditions should be included under one heading. Although the clinical features may differ, the overall picture and treatment are similar, irrespective of the aetiology. Acute hepato-cellular failure (fulminant hepatic necrosis) poses special problems and will be considered as a whole in Chapter 9. Hepatic encephalopathy and ascites are discussed in Chapters 8 and 10.

There is no constant hepatic pathology and in particular necrosis is not always seen. The syndrome is therefore a functional rather than an anatomical one. It comprises some or all of the following features:

General failure of health.
Jaundice.
Circulatory changes and cyanosis.
Fever.
Neurological changes (hepatic encephalopathy) (Chapters 8, 9).
Ascites (Chapter 10).
Changes in nitrogen metabolism.
Skin and endocrine changes.
Disordered blood coagulation (Chapter 4).

General failure of health

The most conspicuous feature is weakness and easy fatiguability. Loss of flesh can be related to difficulty in synthesizing tissue proteins. Anorexia and poor dietary habits add to the malnutrition.

Jaundice

Jaundice is largely due to failure of the liver cells to metabolize bilirubin, so it is some guide to the severity of liver cell failure.

In acute failure, due to such causes as virus hepatitis, jaundice parallels the extent of liver cell damage. This is not so evident in the chronic failure of cirrhosis, where jaundice may be absent or mild. This is due to the balance achieved between hepatic necrosis and regeneration. When present it represents active hepato-cellular disease and indicates a bad prognosis. Diminished erythrocyte survival adds a haemolytic component to the jaundice.

CIRCULATORY AND PULMONARY CHANGES

HYPERKINETIC CIRCULATION

This is associated with all forms of hepato-cellular failure. It is shown by flushed extremities, bounding pulses and capillary pulsations. Peripheral blood flow is increased and this is due mainly to increased skin blood flow [13, 14]. Splenic flow is increased [4]. Renal blood flow, and particularly renal cortical perfusion, is reduced [9]. Cardiac output is raised [10, 15] and this is evidenced by tachycardia, an active precordial impulse and frequently an ejection systolic murmur (figs. 69, 70). These circulatory changes only rarely result in heart failure [1].

The blood pressure is low and, in the terminal few days, further reduces kidney function. At this stage the impaired liver blood flow contributes to hepatic failure and the fall in cerebral blood flow adds to the mental changes [6]. Such hypotension is ominous and attempts at elevation by raising circulatory volume by blood transfusion or by such drugs as noradrenaline are of only temporary benefit [4] (fig. 109).

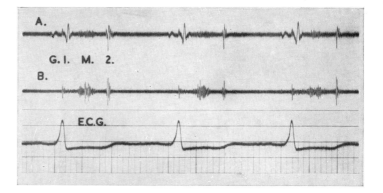

Fig. 69. Cirrhosis. Phonocardiogram at apex (A) and base (B) show ejection-type systolic murmur (M) and an auricular sound (presystolic gallop) (G) (Murray *et al* 1958).

Liver cell failure is the major factor in causation. Although commoner in patients with an extensive portal–collateral circulation, this is of secondary importance for the cardiac output is raised in fulminant virus hepatitis without major collaterals and is normal in patients with extra-hepatic portal venous obstruction and a large collateral circulation [15]. However, following porta-caval shunt, the hyperdynamic circulation may become even more gross and this is a bad prognostic sign [5].

Vasomotor tone is decreased as shown by reduced vasoconstriction in response to mental exercise, the Valsalva manœuvre and tilting from horizontal to vertical (fig. 71) [12, 13]. The circulation resembles that found in systemic arteriovenous fistulae. It seems possible that large numbers of normally present, but functionally inactive,

arteriovenous anastomoses have opened under the influence of a vasodilator substance. The diseased liver might produce such a vasodilator or fail to metabolize one formed elsewhere. False neuromuscular transmitters of gut origin have been invoked as the cause; this has not been proven (fig. 87).

PULMONARY CHANGES AND CYANOSIS

About a third of patients with decompensated cirrhosis have reduced arterial oxygen saturation and are sometimes cyanosed [16]. This is probably due to intrapulmonary shunting through microscopic arteriovenous fistulae. Injection studies of the pulmonary artery in cirrhotic patients have shown a marked arterial dilatation in fine peripheral

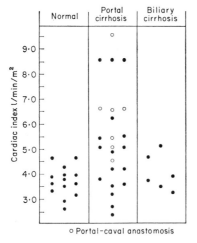

Fig. 70. The cardiac output is raised in many patients with hepatic cirrhosis but within normal limits in biliary cirrhosis. Mean normal cardiac index is $3.68 \pm 0.60 \, l/min.^{-1}/m^{-2}$. Mean in hepatic cirrhosis is $5.36 \pm 1.98 \, l/min.^{-1}/m^{-2}$ (Murray *et al* 1958).

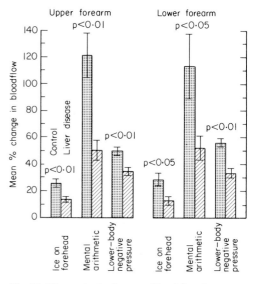

Fig. 71. Change in the forearm blood flow in response to autonomic stimuli in control subjects and patients with liver disease (Lunzer *et al* 1975).

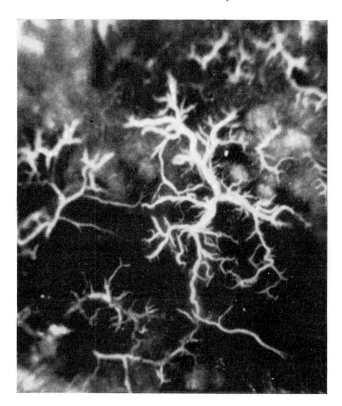

Fig. 72. Cirrhosis. Macroscopic
appearances of the pleura
showing dilated pleural vessels
resembling a spider naevus
(Berthelot *et al* 1966).

branches of the pulmonary artery both within the respiratory parts of the lung and on the pleura where spider naevi are sometimes seen (fig. 72) [2]. Rarely actual pulmonary arteriovenous shunts have been demonstrated [8, 11, 18] (fig. 73). Cardiac catheterization studies in one cyanosed patient with cirrhosis showed a right-to-left shunt with an arterial oxygen saturation of 91% falling to 68% on exercise [8]. In another, the right-to-left shunt was estimated at 42% of the cardiac output [7]. Such pulmonary arteriovenous anastomoses have been confirmed by pulmonary angiography [7].

Reduction of diffusing capacity is present without a restrictive ventilatory defect [21]. This is likely to be due to dilatation of small pulmonary blood vessels, a complication both of advanced cirrhosis and fulminant hepatic failure [2, 22, 24]. A reduction in transfer factor is a consistent finding, perhaps related to thickening of the walls of the small veins and capillaries by a layer of collagen [22]. In chronic hepatitis, radiological mottling has been related to interstitial pulmonary fibrosis [23] but, in fact, this is an excessively rare finding at autopsy.

Lung perfusion studies by scanning or radionuclide methods show dilated pulmonary capillaries and/or arteriovenous communications [25].

The pulmonary vasodilatation is associated with a low pulmonary vascular resistance. The pulmonary resistance fails to respond to hypoxia [3]. This also leads to failure of the lung to match perfusion with ventilation [17].

Functioning porto-pulmonary anastomoses have been demonstrated [19]. It is, however, theoretically impossible for such shunts to produce marked arterial oxygen desaturation owing to the high oxygen content of portal venous blood. Moreover, the flow through these channels in life is probably small.

The oxyhaemoglobin dissociation curve is shifted to the right, making transfer of oxygen to the tissues more difficult [26]. This is not of sufficient magnitude to account for the cyanosis.

Finger clubbing is a frequent but not constant association of the cyanosis and increased cardiac index [20]. Cyanosis is often seen without clubbing.

Other mechanisms for the cyanosis include the raised diaphragm and basal collapse associated

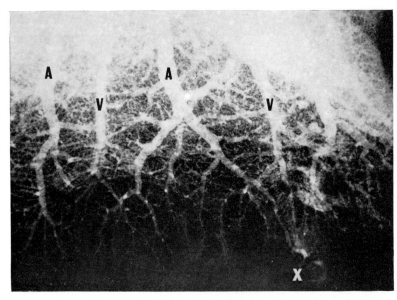

Fig. 73. Arteriogram from a patient with cirrhosis showing a slice of the basal region of the left lung. Arteries (A) and veins (V) alternate: X is the site of the arteriovenous shunting, into which a large arterial branch can be directly traced. The injection medium was barium suspension (Berthelot *et al* 1966).

with tense ascites and the chronic lung disease of the heavy-smoking alcoholic.

The most profound cyanosis and clubbing are associated with chronic active hepatitis and long-standing cirrhosis. Improvement in liver function is associated both with lessening of the cyanosis and the nodularity seen on the chest radiograph [20].

The pulmonary changes of hepato-cellular failure may thus be summed up as pulmonary vasodilatation with pulmonary arteriovenous shunting combined with ventilation–perfusion inequality.

REFERENCES

1. ABELMANN W.H., KOWALSKI H.J. & MCNEELY W.F. (1955) The hemodynamic response to exercise in patients with Laennec's cirrhosis. *J. clin. Invest.* **34,** 690.
2. BERTHELOT P., WALKER J.G., SHERLOCK S. *et al* (1966) Arterial changes in the lungs in cirrhosis of the liver—lung spider nevi. *New Engl. J. Med.* **274,** 291.
3. DAOUD F.S., REEVES J.T. & SCHAEFER J.W. (1972) Failure of hypoxic pulmonary vasoconstriction in patients with liver cirrhosis. *J. clin. Invest.* **51,** 1076.
4. GITLIN N., GRAHAME G.R., KREEL L. *et al* (1970) Splenic blood flow and resistance in patients with

cirrhosis before and after portacaval anastomoses. *Gastroenterology* **59,** 208.
5. GREENSPAN M. & DEL GUERCIO L.R.M. (1968) Cardiorespiratory determinants of survival in cirrhotic patients requiring surgery for portal hypertension. *Am. J. Surg.* **115,** 43.
6. HECKER R. & SHERLOCK S. (1956) Electrolyte and circulatory changes in terminal liver failure. *Lancet* ii, 1211.
7. HUTCHISON D.C.S., SAPRU R.P., SUMERLING M.D. *et al* (1968) Cirrhosis, cyanosis and polycythaemia: multiple pulmonary arteriovenous anastomoses. *Am. J. Med.* **45,** 139.
8. KARLISH A.J., MARSHALL R., REID L. *et al* (1967) Cyanosis with hepatic cirrhosis: a case with pulmonary arterio-venous shunting. *Thorax* **22,** 555.
9. KEW M.C., VARMA R.R., WILLIAMS H.S. *et al* (1971) Renal and intrarenal blood-flow in cirrhosis of the liver. *Lancet* ii, 504.
10. KOWALSKI H.J. & ABELMANN W.H. (1953) The cardiac output at rest in Laennec's cirrhosis. *J. clin. Invest.* **32,** 1025.
11. KRAVATH R.E., SCARPELLI E.M. & BERNSTEIN J. (1971) Hepatogenic cyanosis: arteriovenous shunts in chronic active hepatitis. *J. Pediat.* **78,** 238.
12. LUNZER M.R., MANGHANI K.K., NEWMAN S.P. *et al* (1975) Impaired cardiovascular responsiveness in liver disease. *Lancet* ii, 382.
13. LUNZER M.R., NEWMAN S.P. & SHERLOCK S. (1973) Skeletal muscle blood flow and neurovascular reactivity in liver disease. *Gut* **14,** 354.
14. MARTINI G.A. & HAGEMANN J.E. (1956) Über Fingernagelveränderungen bei Lebercirrhose als

Folge veränderter peripherer Durchblutung. *Klin. Wschr.* **34**, 25.

15. MURRAY J.F., DAWSON A.M. & SHERLOCK S. (1958) Circulatory changes in chronic liver disease. *Am. J. Med.* **24**, 358.
16. RODMAN T., SOBEL M. & CLOSE H.P. (1960) Arterial oxygen unsaturation and the ventilation-perfusion defect of Laennec's cirrhosis. *New Engl. J. Med.* **263**, 73.
17. RUFF F., HUGHES J.M.B., STANLEY N. *et al* (1971) Regional lung function in patients with hepatic cirrhosis. *J. clin. Invest.* **50**, 2403.
18. RYDELL R. & HOFFBAUER F.W. (1956) Multiple pulmonary arteriovenous fistulas in juvenile cirrhosis. *Am. J. Med.* **21**, 450.
19. SHALDON S., CAESAR J., CHIANDUSSI L. *et al* (1961) The demonstration of porta-pulmonary anastomoses in portal cirrhosis with the use of radioactive krypton (Kr^{85}). *New Engl. J. Med.* **265**, 410.
20. STANLEY N.N. & WOODGATE D.J. (1971) The circulation, the lung, and finger clubbing in hepatic cirrhosis. *Br. Heart J.* **33**, 469.
21. STANLEY N.N. & WOODGATE D.J. (1972) Mottled chest radiograph and gas transfer defect in chronic liver disease. *Thorax* **27**, 315.
22. STANLEY N.N., WILLIAMS A.J., DEWAR C.A. *et al* (1977) Hypoxia and hydrothoraces in a case of liver cirrhoses: correlation of physiological, radiographic, scintigraphic and pathological findings. *Thorax* **32**, 457.
23. TURNER-WARWICK M. (1968) Fibrosing alveolitis and chronic liver disease. *Q.J. Med.* **37**, 133.
24. WILLIAMS A., TREWBY P., WILLIAMS R. *et al* (1979) Structural alterations to the pulmonary circulation in fulminant hepatic failure. *Thorax* **34**, 447.
25. WOLFE J.D., TASHKIN D.P., HOLLY F.E. *et al* (1977) Hypoxemia of cirrhosis. Detection of abnormal small pulmonary vascular channels by a quantitative radionuclide method. *Am. J. Med.* **63**, 746.
26. ZIMMON D.S. (1967) Oxyhemoglobin dissociation in patients with hepatic encephalopathy. *Gastroenterology* **52**, 647.

FEVER AND SEPTICAEMIA

About a third of patients with active, advanced cirrhosis show a continuous low-grade fever which rarely exceeds 38 °C [7]. The pyrexia is unaffected by antibiotics or by altering the protein content of the diet. It seems to be attributable to the liver disease alone. It is frequent in alcoholics.

Intercurrent infections, often with coliform organisms, are frequent. The human liver is bacteriologically sterile [3] and the portal venous blood only rarely contains organisms [5]. Such organisms could, however, reach the general circulation either by passing through a faulty hepatic filter or through portal–systemic collaterals [1]. Patients with cirrhosis have been shown to develop Gram-negative bacteraemia in this way.

Positive blood cultures were found in 6.4% of cirrhotic patients (both biliary and non-biliary) [4]. The mortality of those with hepato-cellular disease was 59% and the organisms were frequently Gram-positive. This compared with 29% of those with predominantly biliary disease in which infection was often with Gram-negative organisms. Septicaemia is frequent in terminal hepato-cellular failure. Clinical features may be atypical with inconspicuous fever, no rigors and only slight leucocytosis. Spontaneous bacterial peritonitis may be a complication [2] and also bacterial endocarditis [6]. These patients have often been receiving previous corticosteroid or neomycin therapy.

REFERENCES

1. CAROLI J. & PLATTEBORSE R. (1958) Septicémie porto-cave. Cirrhosis du foir et septicémie à colibacille. *Sem. Hôp. Paris* **34**, 472.
2. CONN H.O. (1976) Spontaneous bacterial peritonitis. Multiple revisitations. *Gastroenterology* **70**, 455.
3. FROM P. & ALLI J.H. (1956) Bacteriologic study of human liver in one-hundred-one cases. *Gastroenterology* **31**, 33.
4. JONES E.A., CROWLEY N. & SHERLOCK S. (1967) Bacteraemia in association with hepato-cellular and hepatobiliary disease. *Postgrad. med. J.* **43**, suppl. 7–11.
5. ORLOFF M.J., PESKIN G.W. & ELLIS H.L. (1958) A bacteriologic study of human portal blood: implications regarding hepatic ischemia in man. *Ann. Surg.* **148**, 738.
6. SNYDER N., ATTERBURY C.E., PINTO CORREIA J. (1977) Increased concurrence of cirrhosis and bacterial endocarditis. *Gastroenterology* **73**, 1107.
7. TISDALE W.A. & KLATSKIN G. (1960) The fever of Laennec's cirrhosis. *Yale J. biol. Med.* **33**, 94.

FETOR HEPATICUS

This is a sweetish, slightly faecal smell of the breath which has been likened to that of a freshly opened corpse or mice. It occurs in patients with severe hepato-cellular disease and also in those with an extensive collateral circulation. It is presumably of intestinal origin, for it becomes less intense after defaecation or when the gut flora is changed by wide-spectrum antibiotics. Methyl mercaptan has been found in the urine of a patient with hepatic coma who exhibited fetor hepaticus [1]. This substance can be exhaled in the breath and might be derived from methionine, the normal demethylating processes being inhibited by liver damage.

In patients with acute liver disease, fetor hepaticus, particularly if so extreme that it pervades the room, is a bad omen and often precedes coma. It is very frequent in patients with an extensive portal collateral circulation, when it is not such a grave sign. Fetor may be a useful diagnostic sign in patients seen for the first time in coma.

REFERENCE

1. CHALLENGER F. & WALSHE J.M. (1955) Fœtor hepaticus. *Lancet* i, 1239.

CHANGES IN NITROGEN METABOLISM

Ammonia metabolism (Chapter 8). The failing liver is unable to convert ammonia to urea.

Urea production is impaired, but the reserve powers of synthesis are so great that the blood urea concentration in hepato-cellular failure is usually normal. Low values may be found in fulminant hepatitis. Maximal rate of urea synthesis is a good measure of hepato-cellular function, but is too complicated for routine use [3].

Amino acid metabolism. An almost constant excess is present in the urine [4]. In both acute and chronic liver disease a common pattern of plasma amino acids is found. The aromatic amino acids, tyrosine and phenylalanine, are raised together with methionine. The concentration of the three branched chain amino acids, valine, isoleucine and leucine, is reduced [2]. This results in a lowering of the ratio of branched chain to aromatic amino acids and this is irrespective of the presence or absence of hepatic encephalopathy [1] (fig. 21).

Serum albumin level falls in proportion to the degree of hepato-cellular failure and its duration. The protein is absorbed and retained, but is not used for serum protein manufacture. The low serum protein values may also reflect an increased plasma volume.

Plasma prothrombin is also a protein and falls with the serum protein levels. The consequent prolonged prothrombin time is not restored to normal by vitamin K therapy. Other proteins concerned in blood clotting may be deficient (fig. 29). In terminal liver failure the bleeding diathesis may be so profound that the patient is exsanguinated by such simple procedures as a paracentesis abdominis.

REFERENCES

1. MORGAN M.Y., MILSOM J.P. & SHERLOCK S. (1978) Plasma ratio of valine, leucine and isoleucine to phenylalanine and tyrosine in liver disease. *Gut* **19**, 1068.
2. MORGAN M.Y., MILSOM, J.P. & SHERLOCK S. (1981) Plasma amino acid patterns in liver disease. *Gut*, in press.
3. RUDMAN D., DI FULCO T.J., GALAMBOS J.T. *et al* (1973) Maximal rates of excretion and synthesis of urea in normal and cirrhotic subjects. *J. clin. Invest.* **53**, 2241.
4. WALSHE J.M. (1953) Disturbances of amino-acid metabolism following liver injury. *Q.J. Med.* **22**, 483.

SKIN CHANGES

An older Miss Muffett
Decided to rough it
And lived upon whisky and gin.
Red hands and a spider
Developed outside her—
Such are the wages of sin. [3]

Vascular spiders [3, 17]

Synonyms: arterial spider, spider telangiectasis, spider angioma

Arterial spiders are found in the vascular territory of the superior vena cava and very rarely below a line joining the nipples. Common sites are the necklace area, the face, forearms and dorsum of the hand (see fig. 74 in colour section). They are rarely found in the mucous membrane of the nose, mouth and pharynx. They fade after death.

An arterial spider is so called because it consists of a central arteriole, radiating from which are numerous small vessels resembling a spider's legs (fig. 75). It ranges in size from a pinhead to 0.5 cm in diameter. When sufficiently large it can be seen or felt to pulsate, and this effect is enhanced by pressing on it with a glass slide. Pressure on the central prominence with a pin causes blanching of the whole lesion, as would be expected from an arterial lesion.

Arterial spiders may disappear with improving hepatic function, whereas the appearance of fresh spiders is suggestive of progression of liver damage. The spider may also disappear if the blood pressure falls due to shock or haemorrhage. Spiders can bleed profusely.

In association with vascular spiders, and having

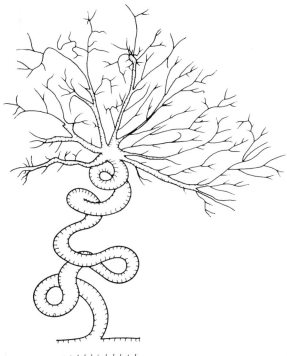

Fig. 75. Schematic diagram of an arterial spider (Bean 1953).

a similar distribution, numerous small vessels may be scattered in random fashion through the skin, usually on the upper arms. These resemble the silk threads in United States dollar bills and the condition is called *paper money skin*.

A further association is the appearance of *white spots* on arms and buttocks on cooling the skin [17]. Examination with a lens shows that the centre of each spot represents the beginnings of a spider.

Vascular spiders are most frequently associated with cirrhosis, especially of the alcoholic. They may appear transiently with viral hepatitis. Rarely they are found in normal persons, especially children. During pregnancy, they appear between the second and fifth months, disappearing within two months of delivery. A few spiders should not be sufficient to diagnose liver disease, but many new ones, with increasing size of old ones, arouse suspicion.

DIFFERENTIAL DIAGNOSIS

Hereditary haemorrhagic telangiectasia. The lesions are usually on the upper body. Mucosal ones are common inside the nose, on the tongue, lips, palate, in the pharynx, oesophagus and stomach. The nail beds, palmar surfaces and fingers are frequently involved. Visceral angiography usually shows lesions elsewhere.

The telangiectasis is punctiform, flat or a little elevated, with sharp margins. It is connected with a single vessel, or with several, which makes it resemble the arterial spider. Pulsation is difficult to demonstrate.

The lesion is a thinning of the telangiectatic vessel, but the veins show muscular hypertrophy [18].

Telangiectasia may be associated with cirrhosis. Calcinosis, Raynaud's phenomena, sclerodactyly and telangiectasia (*CRST syndrome*) may be found in patients with primary biliary cirrhosis.

Campbell de Morgan's spots are very common, increasing in size and number with age. They are bright red, flat or slightly elevated and occur especially on the front of the chest and the abdomen.

The venous star is found with elevation of venous pressure. It usually overlies the main tributary to a vein of large size. It is 2–3 cm in diameter and is not obliterated by pressure; the blood flow is from the periphery to the central collecting vein (opposite to that of the arterial spider). Venous stars are seen on the dorsum of the foot, legs, back and on the lower border of the ribs.

Palmar erythema (liver palms) (see fig. 76 in colour section)

The hands are warm and the palms bright red in colour, especially the hypothenar and thenar eminences and pulps of the fingers. Islets of erythema may be found at the bases of the fingers. The soles of the feet may be similarly affected. The mottling blanches on pressure and the colour rapidly returns. When a glass slide is pressed on the palm it flushes synchronously with the pulse rate. The patient may complain of throbbing, tingling palms.

Palmar erythema is not so frequently seen in cirrhosis as are vascular spiders. Although both may be present, they may appear independently, making it difficult to define a common aetiology. Many normal people have *familial* palmar flushing, unassociated with liver disease.

A similar appearance may be seen in prolonged rheumatoid arthritis and in pregnancy, with chronic febrile diseases, with chronic leukaemia and with thyrotoxicosis.

White nails

White nails, due to opacity of the nail bed, were found in 82 of 100 patients with cirrhosis and occasionally in certain other conditions [23] (fig. 77). A pink zone is seen at the tip of the nail and in a severe example the lunula cannot be distinguished. The lesions are bilateral, thumb and index being especially involved.

Mechanism of the skin changes

The selective distribution of vascular spiders is not understood. Exposure of upper parts of the body to the elements may damage the skin so that it becomes susceptible to the development of spiders when the appropriate internal stimulus exists [17]. Children may develop the lesion on the knees and one nudist with cirrhosis is said to be covered with vascular spiders. The number of arterial spiders does not correlate with the hyperdynamic circulation, although when the cardiac output is very high the spiders pulsate particularly vigorously.

The vascular spiders and palmar erythema have been traditionally attributed to oestrogen excess. They are also seen in pregnancy when circulating oestrogens are increased. Oestrogens have an enlarging, dilating effect on the spiral arterioles of the endometrium, and such a mechanism may

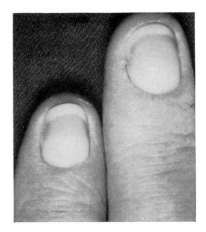

Fig. 77. White nails in a patient with hepatic cirrhosis.

explain the closely similar cutaneous spiders [3]. Oestrogens have induced cutaneous spiders in man [3] although this is not usual when such therapy is given for prostatic carcinoma. The liver certainly inactivates oestrogens. Higher plasma oestradiol levels are found in patients with vascular spiders than in those without [2]. However, spider naevi and palmar erythema appear and disappear irrespective of changes in plasma oestradiol.

The aetiology of the other skin lesions remains unknown.

ENDOCRINE CHANGES

Endocrine changes may be found in association with chronic hepato-cellular failure (cirrhosis). They are more common in cirrhosis of the alcoholic and if the patient is in the active, reproductive phase of life. In the male, the changes are towards feminization, and in the female towards masculinization or gonadal atrophy. Very few studies have been made in females.

Hypogonadism

Diminished libido and potency are frequent in men with active cirrhosis [16] and a large number are sterile. Patients with well-compensated disease may have large families. The testes are soft and small [16]. Seminal fluid is abnormal in some.

Secondary sexual hair is lost and men shave less often. Prostatic hypertrophy has a lower incidence in men with cirrhosis [4]. Incidence of metaplasia of the prostatic glandular and ductal epithelium is increased.

In the female, gonadal changes are not conspicuous for the patients are usually post-menopausal and any breast or uterine atrophy is of little significance. In younger patients, libido is lowered and the patient is usually infertile; menstruation is erratic, diminished or absent but rarely excessive. The breasts usually atrophy, although an occasional patient develops cystic hyperplasia. The uterus is atrophic.

MECHANISMS

Plasma testosterone is reduced in cirrhotic men due to reduced production of testosterone by the testes [9]. Furthermore, 15% of the testosterone produced in these men is derived not from the testes but from peripheral conversion of circulating androstenedione [9].

There is an even greater fall in the non-protein bound (biologically active) fraction of plasma testosterone caused by increased concentrations of sex hormone binding globulin (SHBG) in cirrhotic men.

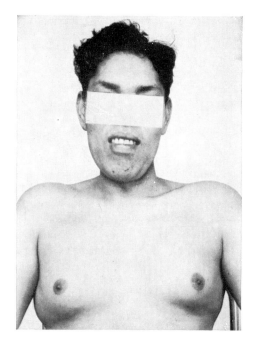

Fig. 78. Gynaecomastia in a patient with Laennec's cirrhosis. Note also scanty body hair.

Feminization

Gynaecomastia, sometimes unilateral, occasionally complicates cirrhosis usually in alcoholics (fig. 78), but also in young men with chronic active hepatitis. The breasts may be tender. It is caused by hyperplasia of the glandular elements [4].

Spironolactone therapy is the commonest cause of gynaecomastia in cirrhotic patients.

Other signs include female body habitus and a female escutcheon. The changes of feminization are particularly common in alcoholics.

MECHANISM

Despite improved biochemical techniques for measuring sex hormones in blood this remains unclear [2, 11, 15].

The three principal unconjugated oestrogens (oestrone, oestradiol and oestriol) are found in the plasma of normal men. They are produced by the testes and adrenals and also from peripheral conversion of major circulating androgens. Oestradiol is the most biologically potent oestrogen. It is bound to SHBG and to albumin. The biologically active unbound form has been reported as marginally raised in patients with cirrhosis [2]. The total

is only minimally raised. Levels of oestrone—the precursor of oestradiol but only weakly feminizing—and oestriol, which is also biologically relatively inactive, are increased in cirrhotic patients (the level of plasma oestradiol correlates only slightly with gynaecomastia [2]).

The peripheral conversion of androgens to oestrogens may be increased in cirrhosis. Feminization could be related to changes in the androgen/oestrogen ratio. Testosterone enanthate has been given therapeutically [14]. This raises the plasma testosterone and also increases oestrogen due to greater conversion from testosterone to oestrone and oestradiol. The testosterone : oestrogen ratio does in fact increase, but whether this will be beneficial is uncertain.

Oestrogen binding sites increase in the liver after castration and it is possible that the hyperoestrogenism is secondary to testicular atrophy. There is no evidence of changes in the metabolism of biologically potent oestrogens in patients with chronic liver disease. There is also no clear evidence of increased circulating potent oestrogens. Feminization remains unexplained.

Primary liver cancer occasionally presents with feminization [13]. Serum oestrone levels are high and can return to normal when the tumour is removed. The tumour can be shown to function as trophoblastic tissue.

Relation to alcoholism

Feminization is more frequent with alcoholic cirrhosis than with other types and may be related more to the effect of alcohol than to the liver disease. Acute administration of alcohol to normal men increases hepatic metabolism of testosterone [8]. Chronic administration raises SHBG, so reducing the free fraction of plasma testosterone [11]. Acutely alcohol also raises plasma gonadotrophins. A direct toxic effect of alcohol on the testes is also likely. Malnutrition, which is so frequent in alcoholics, inhibits pituitary gonadotrophic function with subsequent testicular atrophy.

Hypothalamic–pituitary function

Plasma gonadotrophins are usually normal although a minority of cirrhotic patients have high values. These normal levels in spite of testicular failure suggest either a primary testicular defect or a failure of the pituitary–hypothalamus to raise plasma gonadotrophin values.

Clomiphene, which interrupts the normal steroidal feedback inhibition of gonadotrophin secretion, secondarily stimulates the testis and enhances testicular function. In a patient with alcoholic cirrhosis, clomiphene caused a transient increase in plasma testosterone but with little effect on sexual potency [2, 5]. Bromocriptine may have similar properties and with fewer side-effects.

Prolactin cells are increased in the pituitary of cirrhotic males [12]. Serum prolactin levels are occasionally raised. This might be a response to circulating oestrogens or a direct effect of alcohol [19]. The values do not correlate with aetiology, with severity of the liver disease or with gynaecomastia.

Metabolism of hormones [1]

A reduced rate of hormonal metabolism might be related to a decrease in hepatic blood flow, to shunting of blood through or around the liver or to an increase in plasma protein binding globulin (SHBG) which would reduce the free diffusable fraction of circulating hormone.

Steroid hormones are made more polar by conjugation in the liver. Derivatives of oestrogens, cortisol and testosterone are conjugated as a glucuronide or sulphate and so excreted in the bile or urine. There seems to be little difficulty in the process even in the presence of hepato-cellular disease. The conjugated hormones excreted in the bile undergo an entero-hepatic circulation. In cholestasis the biliary excretion of oestrogens and especially of polar conjugates is greatly reduced. There are changes in the urinary pattern of excretion. Any failure of hormone metabolism results in a rise in blood hormone levels. This alters the normal homeostatic balance between secretion rates of hormones and their utilization. These feedback mechanisms between plasma hormone levels and hormone secretion prevent any but temporary rises in circulating levels. This may explain some of the difficulty in relating plasma hormone levels to clinical features.

Testosterone is converted to a more potent metabolite—dihydrotestosterone. It is degraded in the liver and conjugated for urinary excretion as 17-oxysteroids [22].

Oestrogens are metabolized and conjugated for excretion in urine or bile.

Cortisol is degraded primarily in the liver by a ring reduction to tetrahydrocortisone and subsequently conjugated with glucuronic acid [20] (fig. 79).

Prednisone is converted to prednisolone [21].

The liver extracts aldosterone from the blood and converts it to tetrahydroaldosterone [6].

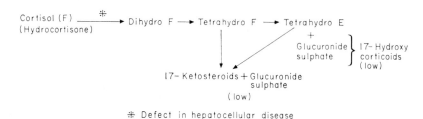

Fig. 79. The metabolism of cortisol by the liver. In hepato-cellular disease there is difficulty in reducing the 4–3 ketonic group but not in conjugation. Urinary 17-ketosteroids and 17-hydroxycorticoids are therefore reduced.

REFERENCES

1. ADLERCREUTZ H. (1974) Hepatic metabolism of estrogens in health and disease. *New Engl. J. Med.* **290**, 1081.
2. BAKER H.W.G., BURGER H.G., DE KRETSER D.M. *et al* (1976) A study of the endocrine manifestations of hepatic cirrhosis. *Q.J. Med.* **45**, 145.
3. BEAN W.B. (1959) *Vascular Spiders and Related Lesions of the Skin*. Blackwell Scientific Publications, Oxford.
4. BENNETT H.S., BAGGENSTOSS A.H. & BUTT H.R. (1950) The testis, breast and prostate of men who die of cirrhosis of the liver. *Am. J. clin. Path.* **20**, 814.
5. BJORK J.T., VARMA R.R. & BORKOWF H.I. (1977) Clomiphene citrate therapy in a patient with Laennec's cirrhosis. *Gastroenterology* **72**, 1308.
6. COPPAGE W.S. Jr, ISLAND D.P., COONER A.E. *et al* (1962) The metabolism of aldosterone in normal subjects and in patients with hepatic cirrhosis. *J. clin. Invest.* **41**, 1672.
7. GALVÃO-TELES A., ANDERSON D.C., BURKE C.W. *et al* (1973) Biologically active androgens and oestradiol in men with chronic liver disease. *Lancet* i, 173.
8. GORDON G.G., ALTMAN K., SOUTHREN A.L. *et al* (1976) Effect of alcohol (ethanol) administration on sex-hormone metabolism in normal men. *New Engl. J. Med.* **295**, 793.
9. GORDON G.G., OLIVO J., RAFII F. *et al* (1975) Conversion of androgens to estrogens in cirrhosis of the liver. *J. clin. Endocrin. Metab.* **40**, 1018.
10. GORDON G.G., VITTEK J., HO R. *et al* (1979) Effect of chronic alcohol use on hepatic testosterone 5α-A-ring reductase in the baboon and in the human being. *Gastroenterology* **77**, 110.
11. GREEN J.R.B. (1977) Mechanism of hypogonadism in cirrhotic males. *Gut* **18**, 843.
12. JUNG Y. & RUSSFIELD A.B. (1972) Prolactin cells in the hypophysis of cirrhotic patients. *Arch. Path.* **94**, 265.
13. KEW M.C., KIRSCHNER M.A., ABRAHAMS G.E. *et al* (1977) Mechanism of feminisation in primary liver cancer. *New Engl. J. Med.* **296**, 1084.
14. KLEY H.K., STROHMEYER G. & KRÜSKEMPER H.L. (1979) Effect of testosterone application on hormone concentrations of androgens and estrogens in male patients with cirrhosis of the liver. *Gastroenterology* **76**, 235.
15. LESTER R., EAGON P.K. & VAN THEIL D.H. (1979) Feminization of the alcoholic: the estrogen/testosterone ratio (E/T). *Gastroenterology* **76**, 415.
16. LLOYD C.W. & WILLIAMS R.H. (1948) Endocrine changes associated with Laennec's cirrhosis of the liver. *Am. J. Med.* **4**, 315.
17. MARTINI G.A. (1955) Über Gefässveränderungen der Haut bei Leberkranken. *Z. klin. Med.* **15**, 470.
18. MARTINI G.A. & STRAUBESAND J. (1953) Zur Morphologie der Gefässspinnen. ('vascular spider') in der Haut Leberkranker. *Virchows Arch.* **324**, 147.
19. MORGAN M.Y., JAKOBOVITS A.W., GOPE M.B.R. *et al* (1978) Serum prolactin in liver disease and its relationship to gynaecomastia. *Gut* **19**, 170.
20. PETERSON R.E. (1960) Adrenocortical steroid metabolism and adrenal cortical function in liver disease. *J. clin. Invest.* **39**, 320.
21. POWELL L.W. & AXELSEN E. (1972) Corticosteroids in liver disease: studies on the biological conversion of prednisone to prednisolone and plasma protein binding. *Gut* **13**, 690.
22. SOUTHREN A.L., GORDON G.G., OLIVO J. *et al* (1973) Androgen metabolism in cirrhosis of the liver. *Metabolism* **22**, 695.
23. TERRY R. (1954) White nails in hepatic cirrhosis. *Lancet* i, 757.

GENERAL TREATMENT

Results are at the same time depressing and encouraging. Once the liver is chronically damaged, as in cirrhosis, it will never regain normal structure. Much can be achieved by symptomatic measures. The liver cells retain such an enormous regenerative capacity that, even though liver structure may not return to normal, functional compensation may be attained.

Precipitating factors

Any factor depressing hepato-cellular function may throw the patient with a hitherto compensated liver disease into failure. Gastro-intestinal haemorrhage or the fall in blood pressure following surgical operation may necessitate blood transfusion. An acute infection must be dealt with along general lines and by antibiotics. If failure has followed an alcoholic episode, the patient is denied alcohol. Diuretic-induced electrolyte disturbances must be corrected.

General measures

Bed rest reduces the functional demands on the liver. In the acute case, it is advisable; in the subacute and chronic bed rest is continued while improvement is maintained. If, after four weeks' bed rest, the condition remains static, the patient should be allowed moderate activity.

Diet. A high protein diet may be of particular value in the alcoholic. In most cirrhotic patients 80–100 g protein and 2500 calories suffice. Fat need not be restricted within the caloric total. Folic acid may be deficient. Meals must be attractively presented—the patient with hepato-cellular failure has a fickle appetite, but if he can be persuaded to eat well clinical improvement will follow.

Diet is more important in the alcoholic who has been depriving himself of food than in the non-alcoholic who has usually been eating well.

Dietary supplements. Methionine, choline and amino acid supplements do not increase the rate of recovery. Very high methionine and cystine levels are found in the plasma in severe hepatitis and cirrhosis. There is no deficiency but rather difficulty in utilization.

Alcohol. Patients with acute hepato-cellular failure should abstain from all alcohol for six months to one year after recovery. If alcoholism can be terminated the patient should, if possible, become a total and lifelong abstainer. If the chronic liver disease is non-alcoholic, one glass of wine or of beer daily will not be harmful.

Anaemia. The haemoglobin level must be kept above 10 g/100 ml if necessary by transfusion. The anaemia may remit only when liver function improves.

Corticoid hormones. Prednisolone and ACTH do not affect the basic cirrhotic process. They have complications including an increased risk of serious infection.

Sedatives (p. 104). Morphine is very likely to pre-cipitate coma. Paraldehyde may also precipitate coma and should be avoided.

Barbiturates vary in their mode of excretion. The long-acting, short-chain barbiturates such as barbitone or phenobarbitone are excreted largely by the kidney and small doses are reasonably well tolerated by the patient with cirrhosis. The short-acting, long-chain barbiturates such as pentobarbitone and the thiobarbitones such as pentothal are metabolized largely by the liver and should be avoided. If a barbiturate is used, the initial dose must be small.

Chlordiazepoxide (Librium) may lead to over-sedation in patients with liver disease [1]. The deposition of oxazepam is normal and this may be the drug of choice in cirrhosis [2].

REFERENCES

1. ROBERTS R.K., WILKINSON G.R., BRANCH R.A. *et al* (1978) Effect of age and parenchymal liver disease on the deposition and elimination of chlordiazepoxide (Librium). *Gastroenterology* **75,** 479.
2. SHULL H.J., WILKINSON G.R., JOHNSON R. *et al* (1976) Normal deposition of oxazepam in acute viral hepatitis and cirrhosis. *Ann. intern. Med.* **84,** 420.

Chapter 8
Hepatic Encephalopathy

The relationship of the liver to mental function has been recognized from earliest times. The Babylonians (*circa* 2000 B.C.) attributed powers of augury and divination to the liver, designating it by the term also used for 'soul' or 'mood'. In the medicine of ancient China (Neiching 1000 B.C.) the liver was regarded as the storer of blood containing the soul. Hippocrates (460–370 B.C.) described a patient with hepatitis who 'barked like a dog, could not be held and said things which could not be comprehended'. Frerichs, the father of modern hepatology, described the terminal mental changes in patients with liver disease [14].

'Cases have occurred to me in which individuals who for a long period have suffered from cirrhosis of the liver have suddenly presented a series of morbid symptoms which are foreign to that disease. They have become unconscious, and have been afterwards seized with noisy delirium, from which they passed into deep coma and in this state have died.'

It is now recognized that a neuropsychiatric syndrome of the same basic pattern may complicate liver disease of almost all types. It can culminate in coma and death.

The syndrome of hepatic encephalopathy is difficult to synthesize into an entity. A spectrum of syndromes exists (table 7). In acute (fulminant) hepatic failure the syndrome is not simply an encephalopathy but a virtual hepatectomy (Chapter 9); mortality is very high. The encephalopathy of cirrhosis has portal–systemic shunting as a component but hepato-cellular damage is also important; various precipitating factors play a part. Chronic neuropsychiatric states exist, usually in those with chronic portal–systemic shunting, and these may be associated with irreversible brain damage. In these cases the hepato-cellular disease is relatively mild.

CLINICAL FEATURES [1, 9, 46]

The picture is complex and affects all parts of the brain. The disorder is an organic mental reaction associated with a neurological disturbance. Variability is a marked feature, particularly in the more chronic forms. The features differ in acuteness and in symptomatology, depending on the nature and intensity of aetiological and precipitating factors. Children show a particularly acute reaction, often with mania.

Disturbed consciousness with disorder of sleep is usual. Hypersomnia appears early and progresses to inversion of the sleep rhythm. Reduction of spontaneous movement, a fixed stare, apathy and

Table 7. Factors in hepatic encephalopathy.

Type of encephalopathy	% survival	Aetiological factors
Chronic portal–systemic encephalopathy	100	Portal–systemic shunting Dietary protein intake Intestinal bacteria
Cirrhosis with precipitant	70–80	Diuresis Haemorrhage Paracentesis Diarrhoea and vomiting Surgery Alcoholic excess Sedatives Infections
Acute liver failure	20	Viral hepatitis Alcoholic hepatitis Drug reactions and overdose

slowness and brevity of response are early signs. Further deterioration results in reaction only to intense or noxious stimuli. Coma at first resembles normal sleep, but progresses to complete unresponsiveness. Deterioration may be arrested at any level. Rapid changes in the level of consciousness are accompanied by delirium.

Personality changes are most conspicuous with chronic liver disease. These include childishness, irritability and loss of concern for family. Even in remission the patient may present similar personality features suggesting frontal lobe involvement. They are usually co-operative, pleasant people with an ease in social relationships and frequently a jocular, euphoric mood.

Intellectual deterioration varies from slight impairment of organic mental function to gross confusion. Focal defects appearing in a setting of clear consciousness relate to disturbances in visual spatial gnosis. These are most easily elicited as constructional apraxia, shown by inability to reproduce simple designs with blocks or matches (fig. 80). The *Reitan trail-making test* (fig. 81) may be used serially to assess progress [5, 58]. Psychometric tests may show intellectual impairment when clinical investigations are normal [36, 37]. Writing is oblivious of rulings and a daily writing chart is a good check of progress (fig. 80). Failure to distinguish objects of similar size, shape, function and position leads to symptoms

such as micturating and defaecating in inappropriate places. Insight into such anomalies of behaviour is frequently preserved.

Speech is slow and slurred and the voice is monotonous. In deep stupor dysphasia becomes marked and is always combined with perseveration.

The most characteristic neurological abnormality is the 'flapping' tremor ('*asterixis*'). This is due to impaired inflow of joint and other afferent information to the brain-stem reticular formation resulting in lapses in posture. It is demonstrated with the patient's arms outstretched and fingers separated or by hyper-extending the wrists with the forearm fixed (fig. 82). The rapid flexion–extension movements at the metacarpophalangeal and wrist joints are often accompanied by lateral movements of the digits. Sometimes arms, neck, jaws, protruded tongue, retracted mouth and tightly closed eyelids are involved and the gait is rendered ataxic. Absent at rest, mitigated by intentional movement and maximum on sustained posture, the tremor is usually bilateral, although not bilaterally synchronous, and one side may be affected more than the other. In coma the tremor disappears. It can occasionally be appreciated by gentle elevation of a limb or by the patient gripping the physician's hand. A 'flapping' tremor is not specific for hepatic pre-coma. It can also be observed in uraemia [47], in respiratory failure and

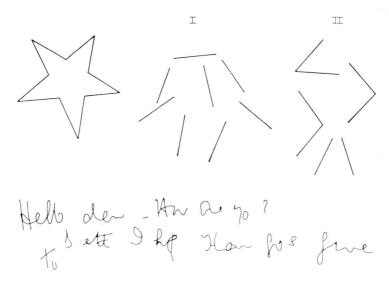

Fig. 80. Focal disorders in chronic portal–systemic encephalopathy elicited in patients with full consciousness and minimal intellectual defect, in the absence of gross tremor or visual disorder.

Above Constructional apraxia. *Below* Writing difficulty. 'Hello dear. How are you? Better I hope. –That goes for me too.' (Davidson & Summerskill 1956.)

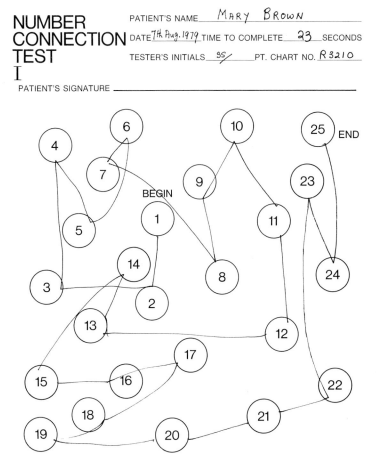

NUMBER CONNECTION TEST I

PATIENT'S NAME _MARY BROWN_

DATE _7th Aug. 1979_ TIME TO COMPLETE _23_ SECONDS

TESTER'S INITIALS _SS_ PT. CHART NO. _R 3210_

PATIENT'S SIGNATURE _____

Fig. 81. The Reitan number correction test.

in severe heart failure. Deep tendon reflexes are usually exaggerated although patients during coma become flaccid and lose their reflexes. Increased muscle tone is present at some stage and rigidity usually persists through passive flexion and extension. Sustained ankle clonus is often associated with rigidity. The plantar responses are usually flexor becoming extensor in deep stupor or coma. Hyperventilation and hyperpyrexia may be terminal. The diffuse nature of the cerebral disturbance is further shown by excessive appetite, muscle twitchings, grasping and sucking reflexes, and disorders of vision.

The clinical course is very fluctuant, and frequent observation of the patient is necessary. A rough clinical grading should be used, for example:

Grade 1. Confused. Altered mood or behaviour. Psychometric defects.
Grade 2. Drowsy. Inappropriate behaviour.

Grade 3. Stuporous but speaking and obeying simple commands. Inarticulate speech. Marked confusion.
Grade 4. Coma.
Grade 5. A very severe grade with deep coma and no response to painful stimuli.

Cerebro-spinal fluid

This is usually clear and under normal pressure. Patients in hepatic coma may show an increased CSF protein concentration, but the cell count is normal. Glutamic acid and also glutamine may be increased.

Electroencephalogram [30]

There is a slowing of the frequency from the normal alpha range of 8–13 cps right down to the delta range of below 4 cps (fig. 83). This is best graded

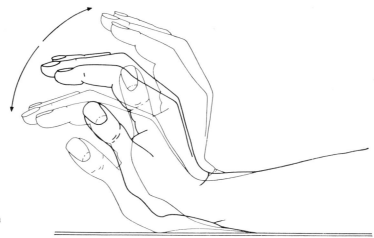

Fig. 82. 'Flapping' tremor elicited by attempted dorsiflexion of the wrist with the forearm fixed.

using frequency analysis. Alerting stimuli, such as opening the eyes, fail to reduce the background rhythmic activity. The change commences in the frontal or central region and progresses posteriorly.

This technique is useful for diagnosis and to assess the results of treatment (fig. 94). Borderline changes may be clarified by exacerbations produced by high protein feeding.

In very chronic cases with permanent neuronal damage the tracing may be slow or rapid and flat. Such changes may be 'fixed' and unaltered by diet.

EEG changes occur very early even before

psychological or biochemical disturbances. They are non-specific, being found also in conditions such as uraemia, CO_2 retention, vitamin B_{12} deficiency or hypoglycaemia. These changes, however, in a conscious patient with liver disease are virtually diagnostic.

NEUROPATHOLOGICAL CHANGES [1, 51]

Grossly the brain may be normal. About half, usually the younger patients dying with prolonged,

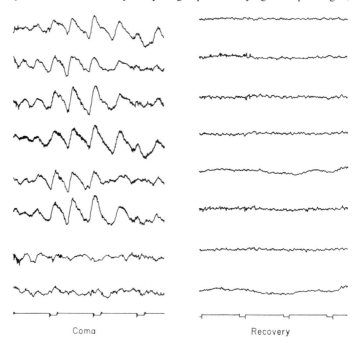

Fig. 83. Hepatic cirrhosis with encephalopathy. During coma the EEG tracing shows large bilaterally synchronous slow waves maximal in the frontal and central regions. After recovery (only two days later) a normal alpha rhythm is seen.

Coma   Recovery

deep coma, show cerebral oedema [53] (see fig. 84 in colour section); the pathogenesis is unknown. In some, positive pressure ventilation may contribute.

Microscopically, the characteristic changes are increase in number and enlargement of the astrocytes. The commonest is the Alzheimer type 2 change. The Alzheimer type 1 change is rarer. The changes can be studied experimentally in rats or chimpanzees [50] after porta-caval anastomosis. The change is diffusely found in the grey matter of cerebrum and cerebellum and in the putamen and globus pallidus. The nerve cells show relatively minor alterations. This combination, and the extent, seem virtually specific for liver disease. The changes bear a rough relationship to the duration and severity of coma and develop within a few days.

Early astrocyte changes are probably reversible. In a very longstanding case the structural changes are irreversible and unresponsive to treatment of the liver disease. The cortex is thinned; neurones and fibres are lost. The deep layers of cortex may show laminar necrosis. The cerebellum and basal ganglia are also involved. Demyelination in the pyramidal tracts is associated with spastic paraplegia.

Mechanisms [8, 16, 59]

The essentially reversible nature of the cerebral disturbance, at least in the early stages, and the diffuse involvement suggest that the change is a metabolic one. Research has proceeded to determine firstly the nature of the toxic metabolite(s), secondly the route by which it reaches the brain, and thirdly other possible disturbances of cerebral metabolism which might develop in the presence of a failing liver [43].

THE CONCEPT OF PORTAL–SYSTEMIC ENCEPHALOPATHY

Every patient presenting the features of hepatic pre-coma or coma has a circulatory pathway through which portal blood may enter the systemic veins and reach the brain without being metabolized by the liver [46].

In patients with poor hepato-cellular function, such as acute hepatitis, the shunt is through the liver itself. The damaged cells are unable to metabolize the contents of the portal venous blood completely so that they pass unaltered into the hepatic veins (fig. 85).

In patients with more chronic forms of liver disease, such as cirrhosis, the portal blood bypasses the liver through large natural 'collaterals'. The portal–hepatic vein anastomoses, developing around the nodules in a cirrhotic liver, may also act as internal shunts. The picture is a common complication of porta-caval anastomosis (p. 170). The condition is analogous to the neuro-psychiatric disturbance developing in the dog with an Eck fistula if it is given meat.

Encephalopathy is unusual if liver function is adequate. In hepatic schistosomiasis where the collateral circulation is great and liver function adequate, coma is rare [55]. If shunting is sufficiently great, however, encephalopathy may develop in the absence of obvious liver disease, for instance in extra-hepatic portal hypertension.

Patients going into hepatic coma are suffering from cerebral intoxication by intestinal contents which have not been metabolized by the liver (*portal–systemic encephalopathy*) [46]. The nature of the cerebral intoxicant is nitrogenous. A picture indistinguishable from impending hepatic coma can be induced in some patients with cirrhosis by the oral administration of a high-protein diet, ammonium chloride, urea, or methionine [31, 33, 46].

INTESTINAL BACTERIA

Symptoms can often be relieved by oral antibiotics. The intoxicant therefore seems to be produced by intestinal bacteria acting on the nitrogenous content of the intestine, and especially on protein. Other measures which diminish the colonic flora, for instance colonic exclusion or purgation, may also be effective. Moreover, urea-splitting bacteria and the small intestinal flora generally are increased in patients with liver disease [24].

AMMONIA TOXICITY

Ammonia has been the most widely investigated toxic substance. The syndrome may be reproduced in some patients by ammonium salts given orally or intravenously and arterial ammonium levels may be high in patients in hepatic coma. Ammonium can be derived from the nitrogenous contents of the intestine by bacterial action. It is present in high concentration in portal blood and

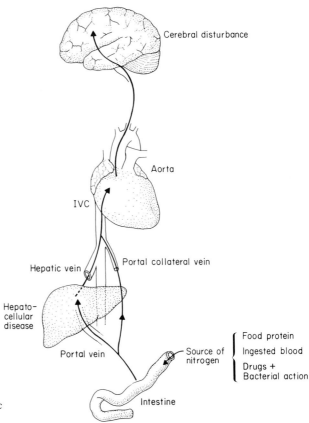

Cerebral disturbance

Aorta

IVC

Portal collateral vein

Hepatic vein

Hepato-
cellular
disease

Portal vein

Source of
nitrogen

{ Food protein
  Ingested blood
  Drugs +
  Bacterial action

Intestine

Fig. 85. The mechanism of portal–systemic
encephalopathy (Sherlock *et al* 1954).

is metabolized by the liver to urea [56]. The failing
liver cell may also be unable to metabolize
ammonium formed by the kidney [42] and, in the
terminal stages of hepatic coma, by the peripheral
tissues and brain [49]. Gastric urease is another
source of ammonia.

Theoretically ammonium intoxication could interfere with cerebral metabolism. This could be by
two mechanisms: increased glutamine synthesis
and reductive amination of ketoglutarate (fig. 86)
[2]. The increase in glutamine in the cerebrospinal
fluid in hepatic coma suggests that combination of
ammonium with glutamic acid is increased.

Combination of ammonium with α-ketoglu-
tarate to form glutamic acid removes an important
link in the Krebs' citric acid cycle. The brain depends for most of its activity on aerobic glycolysis
and this cycle. Experimentally, ammonia can
depress cerebral blood flow and glucose metabolism. Ammonia also has a direct effect on the
neuronal membrane. Diversion of α-ketoglutarate
to glutamate and glutamine would reduce the
energy available for oxidative cell metabolism (fig.

86). The diminished oxygen consumption of the
brain in hepatic coma and the increased blood and
cerebrospinal fluid pyruvic acid concentrations
[10] would support this hypothesis.

There are, however, points that suggest hepatic
coma and ammonium intoxication cannot be
equated. The brain in hepatic coma does not
always remove ammonium from the blood but may
in fact occasionally add to it, the jugular vein concentration exceeding that in an artery. Germfree animals with porta-caval shunts can develop
classic encephalopathy [27].

When ammonium citrate was used to induce a
high blood ammonia in patients with liver disease
the EEG changed in only one of 19 patients
although the arterial and venous ammonia levels
were often high [4]. The raised blood ammonium
level in hepatic coma may well be more a non-specific indicator of disturbed brain metabolism than
the toxic causative factor.

Unfortunately, there is no clear evidence asso-
ciating the amounts of ammonia in the *brain* and
the mental state.

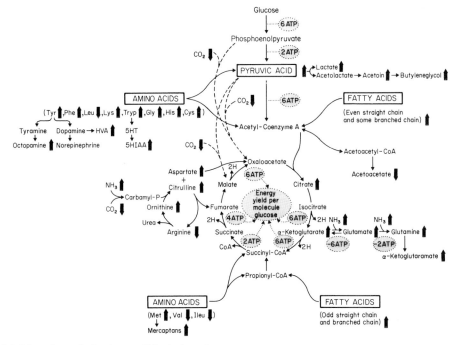

Fig. 86. Map of metabolic abnormalities in hepatic coma. Vertical heavy arrows indicate abnormalities that have been observed in blood (Zieve 1974).

Blood ammonia levels. Estimations are time consuming and must be performed immediately. The upper limit of normal is $0.8–1\,\mu g/ml$ blood.

Levels usually correlate with severity, but 10% of values are in the normal range regardless of the depth of coma [32]. Estimations in terminal hepatic coma show wide fluctuations. Some patients, particularly after porta-caval anastomosis, may seem normal with raised blood ammonium levels. Levels rise after gastro-intestinal bleeding. The level does not relate to prognosis. Blood ammonium values are not necessary for routine use.

CSF glutamine is a sensitive index of portal–systemic encephalopathy.

OTHER NITROGENOUS SUBSTANCES

Pharmacologically active amines can be formed by intestinal bacteria acting on protein and are present in portal blood. They are difficult to estimate in biological fluids.

Methionine precipitates hepatic coma without rises in blood ammonia levels [31]. Tetracycline is preventative. This effect might be related to mercaptans which are derived by bacterial metabolism

of methionine and are extremely toxic. They are usually removed by the liver. Raised blood mercaptan levels are found in portal–systemic encephalopathy but not in all patients [23].

Tryptophan is increased in the brain in experimental hepatic coma. This is metabolized to serotonin and has profound effects on the central nervous system. Increased tryptophan is found in the CSF of patients with hepatic coma. This is related to an increase in free plasma tryptophan levels [28].

Survival of the perfused brain of dogs depends on substances released by the liver. Infusion of the nucleosides, cytidine and uridine, corrected the faulty cerebral metabolism in hepatectomized animals, but these nucleosides were ineffective therapeutically in man [41]. Nevertheless it is possible that absence of a protective substance, manufactured by the healthy liver, is important, particularly in the acute coma of fulminant liver failure.

FALSE NEUROCHEMICAL TRANSMITTERS
(fig. 87)

Intestinal bacterial decarboxylation results not only in ammonia but also in hydroxyphenylamines such as beta phenylethanolamine and octopamine,

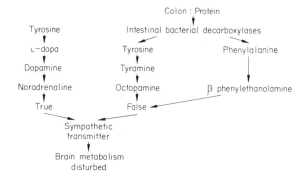

Fig. 87. The role of false sympathetic
neurotransmitters in the disturbed cerebral
metabolism in liver disease.

which is formed from tyramine. The true sympathetic neurochemical transmitters are noradrenaline
and dopamine. The bacterial products may act as
false transmitters interfering with the production
and balance of the true transmitters and so dis-
turbing neurotransmission at the synapses of the
brain [12]. The clinical features of portal–systemic
encephalopathy include akinesia, rigidity and
tremor. These are also seen in parkinsonism where
dopamine depletion in the striatum and basal
ganglia is proven.

Tyramine is known to interfere with the formation of dopamine and adrenaline and contributes
to the production of octopamine. These amines are
normally metabolized by the liver but could reach

the systemic circulation in the presence of liver
disease or a large portal collateral circulation.
Serum and urinary octopamine levels are increased in hepatic encephalopathy (fig. 88) [22].
However, intraventricular infusion of enormous
quantities of octopamine with resulting depression
of brain dopamine and noradrenaline failed to
cause coma in normal rats [59].

AMINO ACIDS [38]

Neurotransmitter synthesis is controlled by the
brain concentration of the precursor amino acids
(fig. 89).

Aromatic and branched chain amino acids compete for entry at the blood–brain barrier which is
probably disrupted in portal–systemic encephalopathy[19]. Aromatic amino acids, tyrosine, phenylalanine and tryptophan, are increased in liver
disease, perhaps due to failure of hepatic deamination. The branched chain amino acids, valine, leucine and isoleucine, are decreased perhaps due to
increased catabolism by skeletal muscle and kidney secondary to the hyperinsulinism of chronic
liver disease.

A reduced ratio between valine plus leucine plus
isoleucine and phenylalanine and tyrosine has
been related to the development of portal–systemic encephalopathy [48]. However, in a large
group of cirrhotic patients the ratio was reduced
both in those with and without encephalopathy
(fig. 90) [26].

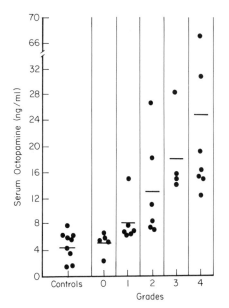

Fig. 88. Serum octopamine levels correlate with the
degree of hepatic encephalopathy. As the degree of
encephalopathy increases, so does the level of serum
octopamine (Manghani *et al* 1975).

OTHER METABOLIC ABNORMALITIES

These patients are often alkalotic. This may result
from toxic stimulation of the respiratory centre by
ammonium, from administration of alkalis such as
citrate in transfusions or with potassium supplements, or from hypokalaemia.

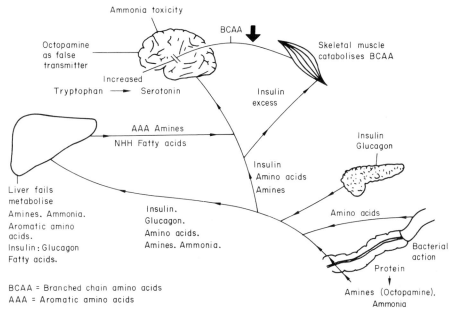

BCAA = Branched chain amino acids
AAA = Aromatic amino acids

Fig. 89. The factors concerned in hepatic encephalopathy. Important concepts illustrated are:
1 Failure of hepatic cellular function.
2 Portal–systemic bypassing.
3 Failure to metabolize insulin and glucagon coming from the pancreas.

4 Increase in false neurochemical transmitters arising from the colon.
5 Amino acid imbalance.
6 Increased change from tryptophan to serotonin in the brain.

The transfer of ionized ammonia across cell membranes and hence into the brain increases in the presence of extracellular alkalosis [54]. Alkalosis, therefore, increases ammonium toxicity and so might exacerbate the neurological state.

Hypoxia increases cerebral sensitivity to ammonia. The stimulation of the respiratory centre results in increase in depth and rate of respiration. Hypocapnia follows and this reduces cerebral blood flow. The increase in the blood organic acids (lactate and pyruvate) is correlated with the reduction in CO_2 tension.

Any potent diuretic can precipitate hepatic coma. This may be related to hypokalaemia [34] with increased ammonium output into the renal vein [42] and to readier penetration of ammonium ion through the blood–brain barrier in the presence of alkalosis [54]. In addition to hypokalaemia, other electrolyte disturbances or a profound diuresis seem to initiate encephalopathy [44].

CHANGES IN CARBOHYDRATE METABOLISM

The hepatectomized dog dies in hypoglycaemic coma. Hypoglycaemic episodes are rare in chronic

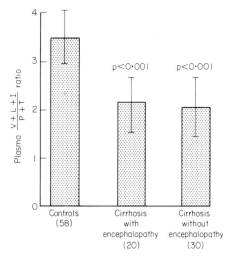

Fig. 90. The plasma $\dfrac{V+L+I}{P+T}$ ratio in control subjects and in patients with cirrhosis with and without hepatic encephalopathy. $\bar{I}$ = mean ratio $\pm$ s.d.; p = student's t test. V = valine, L = leucine, I = isoleucine, P = phenyl alanine, T = tyrosine (Morgan et al 1978).

liver disease but may complicate fulminant hepatitis (Chapter 9).

α-Ketoglutaric and pyruvic acids are transported from the periphery to the metabolic pool in the liver, and blood levels increase as the neurological state deteriorates [10]. These probably reflect severe liver damage rather than encephalopathy *per se*. The fall in blood ketones also reflects severity of hepatic dysfunction. There is progressive impairment of intermediate carbohydrate metabolism as the liver fails.

FATTY-ACID METABOLISM

Increases in short-chain fatty acids have been found in hepatic coma. These will depress mid-brain reticular activity systems in animals. The EEG appearances are very similar to those of impending hepatic coma. Long-chain fatty acids are also increased. Fatty acids seem to inhibit the detoxification of ammonia [59]. The fatty acids might act synergistically with ammonia in producing coma. However, a direct association of encephalopathy with fatty acids, either long- or short-chain, has not been established [57].

Conclusions (fig. 91)

The brain of the patient with liver disease seems unduly sensitive to insults that would be without effect in the normal. A small dose of morphine (8 mg) will induce EEG changes in a patient who has experienced pre-coma but not in one who has not [17]. A similar sensitivity is shown to electrolyte imbalance. Indeed, whether cause or effect, cerebral metabolism is undoubtedly abnormal in liver disease. In the chronic case, actual structural changes in the brain can be demonstrated and the EEG is fixed and abnormal and unresponsive to changes in dietary protein or to neomycin.

Such factors as infection, hypotension or anoxia act both on liver and brain. Multiple factors may operate; for instance the addition of protein to the diet will increase and the giving of neomycin will decrease the EEG response to morphine in susceptible cirrhotic subjects.

The picture of hepatic pre-coma and coma is non-specific. The organic psychosis, the 'flapping' tremor, the EEG changes and the raised blood ammonium values may be encountered, in whole or in part, in other disturbances such as uraemia, or respiratory failure. There is no sure laboratory method of diagnosis, and recognition depends on clinical acumen with the association of other features of liver disease such as fetor hepaticus, jaundice or ascites. The syndrome is not *only* due to the passage of toxic substances of intestinal origin to the brain. Many other metabolic events occur when the liver fails. The causes of this complex clinical picture are in most part unknown [59].

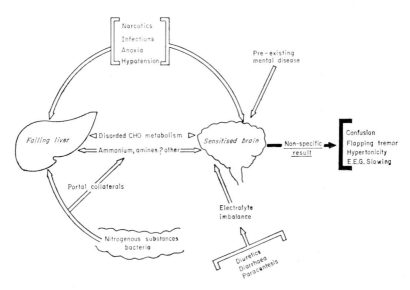

Fig. 91. The pathogenesis of a hepatic coma. Many factors affecting hepatic or cerebral function, or both, can lead to the picture of hepatic pre-coma in a patient with liver disease. The brain in such subjects may be particularly sensitive to these factors (Sherlock 1961).

No one cause has been found. Interactions between various factors are likely. Moreover some events, such as depression of cerebral oxygen and glucose metabolism, may be, in part, effects of the coma rather than primary.

Clinical associations

The syndrome is most frequently associated with *virus hepatitis* (Chapter 15) and *cirrhosis*. Fetor hepaticus is usually present.

Hepatic cirrhosis

ACUTE TYPE

The syndrome may appear spontaneously, without a precipitant, usually in a deeply jaundiced patient with ascites and in the terminal stages. Precipitating factors act by depressing liver cell or cerebral function, increasing nitrogenous material in the intestine, or raising the portal collateral flow.

The commonest precipitant is a brisk response to a potent *diuretic*. *Paracentesis abdominis* may also precipitate coma; the mechanism is uncertain. Electrolyte imbalance following removal of large quantities of electrolytes and water, changes in hepatic circulation and hypotension may contribute. Other causes of fluid and electrolyte depletion, such as *diarrhoea* or *vomiting*, may be precipitants.

Gastro-intestinal haemorrhage, usually from oesophageal varices, is another common precipitant. Coma is precipitated by the large protein meal (as blood) in addition to the depression in hepato-cellular function due to anaemia and reduction in liver blood flow.

Surgical procedures are tolerated extremely poorly. Hepatic function is depressed by the blood loss, anaesthesia and 'shock', and coma may follow.

Acute alcoholism precipitates coma both by depressing cerebral function and by the associated acute alcoholic hepatitis. *Morphia* [17] and *barbiturates* depress cerebral function and have a prolonged action when hepatic detoxication is delayed.

Infections, especially with bacteraemia and including 'spontaneous' bacterial peritonitis, may be the precipitant.

Coma may occasionally be initiated by a large *protein meal* or severe *constipation*.

CHRONIC TYPE

The portal–systemic collateral circulation is particularly extensive. This may consist simply of the myriad of small anastomotic vessels developing in the cirrhotic patient or, more often, one major collateral channel, such as the umbilical vein or inferior mesenteric vein, predominates. The construction of a surgical porta-caval anastomosis is often followed by chronic neuropsychiatric symptoms.

Fluctuations are related to dietary protein and diagnosis can be confirmed by noting the effect clinically and on the EEG of a precipitant such as a high-protein diet or by demonstrating improvement by protein withdrawal. Clinical and biochemical evidence of liver disease may be equivocal or absent, and the neuropsychiatric disorder may dominate the picture.

The intermittent neuropsychiatric disturbance may continue for as long as six years [49] and the diagnosis is very liable to fall between the stools of the various specialist interests. The psychiatrist is interested in the non-specific organic reaction and may not consider underlying liver disease. The neurologist focuses attention on the neurological features, while the hepatologist, recognizing the cirrhosis, fails to elicit the neurological signs or assumes that the patient is just 'odd' or an alcoholic. The patient may be seen for the first time in coma or in remission, adding to the diagnostic difficulty.

The acute psychiatric states often present shortly (two weeks to eight months) after porta-caval anastomosis as a paranoid-schizophrenic picture or as hypomania [35]. 'Classical' portal–systemic encephalopathy, with EEG slowing, is usually present in addition. Formal psychiatric treatment may be required in addition to that of the hepatic encephalopathy.

More persistent neuropsychiatric syndromes are probably related to organic changes in the central nervous system, not only in the brain but also in the spinal cord [51]. Twelve patients have been reported with progressive *paraplegia* commencing insidiously in those with a large portal–systemic collateral circulation [39, 40, 51]. The encephalopathy is not severe. The spinal cord shows demyelination. The paraplegia is progressive and the usual treatment for portal–systemic encephalopathy is ineffective.

Chronic cerebellar and *basal ganglia signs* with parkinsonism, the tremor being unaffected by intention, may develop after some years of chronic hepatic encephalopathy [35, 51]. Permanent cerebral damage is presumably present for treatment has little effect on the tremor. *Focal cerebral symptoms*, epileptic attacks and dementia have also been noted [35].

These persistent neuropsychiatric changes are presumably due to some unknown central nervous system poison which passes through a large portal–systemic shunt in the presence of liver disease.

Differential diagnosis

A *low sodium state* can develop in cirrhotic patients on a restricted sodium diet and having diuretics and abdominal paracenteses. This is shown by apathy, headache, nausea and hypotension. The diagnosis is confirmed by finding low serum sodium levels with a rise in blood urea concentration. The condition may be combined with impending hepatic coma.

Acute alcoholism [9] provides a particularly difficult problem especially as the two syndromes may co-exist (see table 55). Many symptoms attributed to alcoholism may be due to portal–systemic encephalopathy. Delirium tremens is distinguished by the continuous motor and autonomic overactivity, total insomnia, terrifying hallucinations and a finer, more rapid tremor. The patient is flushed, agitated, inattentive and perfunctory in his replies. Tremor, absent at rest, becomes coarse and irregular on activity. Profound anorexia, often with retching and vomiting, is common.

Portal–systemic encephalopathy in an alcoholic has similar features to that in the non-alcoholic except for the frequent absence of rigidity, hyperreflexia and ankle clonus due to concomitant peripheral neuritis. An EEG is helpful, as is the observation of a favourable response to dietary protein withdrawal and neomycin.

Wernicke's encephalopathy is common with profound malnutrition and with alcoholism.

Hepato-lenticular degeneration (*Wilson's disease*) is found in young people, often with a family history. The symptoms do not fluctuate, the tremor is choreo-athetoid rather than 'flapping', the Kayser–Fleischer corneal ring is seen and disturbances in copper metabolism can usually be demonstrated.

Latent *functional psychoses* such as depression or paranoia are frequently released by impending hepatic coma. The type of reaction is related to the previous personality, and to intensification of personality traits. The psychiatric importance of the syndrome is emphasized by such patients often being admitted to mental hospitals. Conversely a chronic psychiatric state in patients with known liver disease may not be related to the liver dysfunction. In such patients investigations are designed to demonstrate the chronic syndrome and in particular a large collateral circulation by splenic venography. Clinical and EEG changes induced by high and low protein feeding may also be useful.

Prognosis

Prognosis depends on the extent of liver cell failure. The chronic group with relatively good liver function but with an extensive collateral circulation combined with increased intestinal nitrogen have the best prognosis, and the acute hepatitis group the worst. In cirrhosis, the outlook is poor if the patient has ascites, jaundice and a low serum-albumin level—all indicative of liver failure. If treatment is begun early in the pre-comatose state, the chances of success are increased. The prognosis is better if the precipitant can be treated, for instance infection, diuretic overdose or haemorrhage.

Assessment of therapy is made difficult by fluctuations in the clinical course. The value of any new method can only be assessed after large numbers of patients have been treated on controlled regimes with recovery (defined as ability to be discharged from hospital) as the sole criterion for success. Results in patients with chronic encephalopathy (largely related to portal–systemic shunting), with recovery as the rule, must be separated from acute hepato-cellular failure in which recovery is rare.

TREATMENT OF HEPATIC PRE-COMA AND COMA

Hepatic coma is of multiple causation, and the factors acting in the particular patient must be defined and treated (table 8). The major ones are toxic nitrogenous substances formed in the intestine by bacterial action on proteins [45].

DIET

All dietary protein is stopped. At least 1600 calories are supplied daily as glucose drinks or as

Table 8. Treatment of hepatic pre-coma and coma.

Acute

1 Identify precipitating factor, e.g. haemorrhage, infection, alcoholism, electrolyte imbalance, sedatives, large protein meal
2 Empty bowels of nitrogen-containing materials
   (a) Stop nitrogen-containing drugs, e.g. ammonium chloride, urea
   (b) Enema and magnesium sulphate purge
3 Protein-free diet
   Raise dietary protein slowly with recovery
4 Antibiotic
   Neomycin 1 g 4 times a day by mouth for 1 week
5 Maintain calorie, fluid and electrolyte balance
6 Stop diuretics, check serum electrolyte levels

Chronic

1 Avoid nitrogen-containing drugs
2 Protein, largely vegetarian intake, at limit of tolerance (about 50 g daily)
3 Ensure at least one free bowel movement daily
4 Lactulose 10–30 ml three times a day
5 If symptoms worsen then adopt a regime for acute neurological complications
6 Consider trial of bromocriptine

20% glucose through a gastric drip. Twenty per cent or 40% dextrose is given via antecubital or femoral vein into the innominate vein or vena cava.

During recovery protein is added in 20 g increments on alternate days. The protein is divided between four meals. Any relapse is treated by a return to the former regime. In patients with an acute episode of coma, a normal protein intake is soon achieved. In the chronic group, permanent protein restriction is needed to control mental symptoms [49]; the limits of tolerance are usually 40–60 g per day. Protein derived from vegetables may be tolerated better than animal protein [15]. Vegetable protein is less ammoniagenic and contains smaller amounts of methionine and aromatic amino acids.

An exacerbation of symptoms is treated by rest and abstention from protein.

In the acute cases a few days' to a few weeks' deprivation of protein does not prove harmful and, even in the chronic group in whom dietary protein has to be restricted for many months, clinical protein malnutrition is not seen [45]. The risk of temporary depletion is preferable to the hazards of nitrogen toxicity. This measure, however, is indicated only in the patients showing signs of coma. Other patients with liver disease may benefit by high protein feeding particularly if alcoholic or if ascites is forming.

ANTIBIOTICS

Tetracyclines are effective for short periods. Neomycin, given orally, is very effective in decreasing gastro-intestinal ammonium formation [24]. Little is absorbed from the gut although blood levels have been detected. Impaired hearing or deafness follow its long-term use [18]. However, it remains the most satisfactory antibiotic for the treatment of acute short-term coma [11]. In the acute case 4–6 g are given daily in divided doses. The EEG improves, blood ammonium levels fall and fetor hepaticus goes. Clinical improvement is difficult to correlate with the changes in faecal flora [11].

LACTULOSE [3] (fig. 92)

The human intestinal mucosa does not produce a lactulase to split this synthetic disaccharide. When given by mouth the bulk reaches the caecum where it is broken down by bacteria to lactic acid and small amounts of acetic acid. The faecal pH drops. The growth of lactose-fermenting organisms is favoured and organisms such as bacteroides, which are ammonia formers, are suppressed. Lactulose is therefore of benefit in chronic hepatic encephalopathy. Neuropsychiatric symptoms are relieved and blood ammonia falls [5, 7, 8]. However, the improvement precedes changes in bacterial flora and is effective in those receiving neomycin who have no lactobacilli in their stools. An alternative mode of action could be related to increased faecal acidity. This would reduce the ionization of ammonium (NH_4) (unabsorbed) to ammonia (NH_3) (absorbed) and so the ammonium excreted in the faeces. NH_3 may also be attracted from the blood into the colon and then excreted. Amines and other toxic nitrogenous compounds would be similarly excreted. However, faecal ammonia is not increased by lactulose, making this view unlikely [52].

The mechanism of action of lactulose in hepatic encephalopathy is still uncertain [6]. It may provide a carbohydrate source to facilitate ammonia utilization by gut bacteria [52].

The aim is to produce acid stools without diarrhoea. The dose is 10–30 ml three times a day and is adjusted to produce two semi-solid stools daily. Lactulose is non-toxic and should certainly be tried in the chronic case. It should not be given in acute hepatic coma where nitrogenous intoxication is best controlled by neomycin.

Lactulose therapy

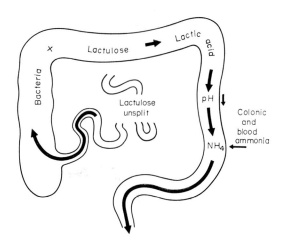

Fig. 92. Lactulose reaches the colon unsplit. It
is then converted by bacteria to organic acids
and an acid stool test results. This may also
affect the ionization of ammonia in the colon
and reduce its absorption.

Purgation. Relapses with increasing coma may
follow constipation, and remissions are associated
with free bowel action. In the chronic group, drastic purgation can result in some improvement
clinically and in the EEG. The value of enemata
and routine purgation with magnesium sulphate
in patients with hepatic coma must be emphasized.
Lactulose or lactulose enemas may be used. All
enemas must be neutral or acid to reduce
ammonium absorption.

OTHER PRECIPITATING FACTORS

Patients in impending coma are extremely sensitive to sedatives and whenever possible these are
avoided. If an overdose is suspected, the appropriate antagonist should be given. If the patient is uncontrollable and some sedation is necessary, half
the usual dose of barbitone or oxazepam is given;
morphine and paraldehyde are absolutely contraindicated. An antihistaminic such as phenergan
may be useful. Diazepoxide is valuable in the
alcoholic with impending hepatic coma. Drugs
known to induce hepatic coma such as amino acids
and diuretics are disallowed.

Potassium deficiency can be treated by liberal
administration of fruit juices or by effervescent or
slow release potassium chloride. If it is urgent,
0.1% potassium chloride may be incorporated in
an infusion.

The possibility of delirium tremens should not
tempt the clinician to give alcohol to an alcoholic
patient in impending hepatic coma. Delirium

tremens may be treated by diazepoxide or
heminevrin.

LEVODOPA AND BROMOCRIPTINE

If portal–systemic encephalopathy is related to a
defect in dopaminergic neurotransmission then re-
plenishment of cerebral dopamines should be
beneficial. Dopamine does not pass the blood–
brain barrier, but its precursor, levodopa, does
and can cause temporary arousal in acute hepatic
encephalopathy [20]. It is sometimes of benefit in
the chronic case [20]. However, only a few patients
benefit. Nausea and psychiatric disturbances are
side-effects [20].

Bromocriptine is a specific dopamine receptor
agonist with a prolonged action. In a dose of up
to 15 mg daily it causes clinical, psychometric and
electroencephalographic improvement in patients
with chronic portal–systémic encephalopathy [25].
Cerebral blood flow, oxygen and glucose consumption increase. Bromocriptine treatment
should be considered in the rare patient with
chronic portal–systemic encephalopathy resistant
to dietary protein restriction and lactulose.

AMINO ACIDS AND KETO ACIDS

Infusions of high concentrations of branched
chain and low levels of aromatic amino acids with
high arginine concentrations have been used [13].
The treatment has been uncontrolled. Keto-
analogues of essential amino acids are also said to
be beneficial but are not readily available [21].

TEMPORARY HEPATIC SUPPORT

Complicated methods of temporary hepatic support are not, in general, applicable to hepatic coma in the cirrhotic. Such a patient is either terminal or can be expected to come out of coma without them. They are discussed under acute hepatic failure (Chapter 9).

HEPATIC HOMOTRANSPLANTATION

This may be the ultimate answer to the problem of chronic hepatic encephalopathy. One such patient with a history of three years showed marked improvement lasting nine months following transplantation [29]. At the present time, however, the problems of liver transplantation have not been solved.

REFERENCES

1. ADAMS R.D. & FOLEY J.M. (1953) The neurological disorder associated with liver disease. *Res. Publ. Assn. Res. nerv. ment. Dis.* **32**, 198.
2. BESSMAN S.P. & BESSMAN A.N. (1955) The cerebral and peripheral uptake of ammonia in liver disease with an hypothesis for the mechanism of hepatic coma. *J. clin. Invest.* **34**, 622.
3. BIRCHER J., HAEMMERLI U.P., SCOLLO-LAVIZZARI G. *et al* (1971) Treatment of chronic portal–systemic encephalopathy with lactulose. *Am. J. Med.* **51**, 148.
4. COHN R. & CASTELL D.O. (1966) The effect of acute hyperammonemia on the electroencephalogram. *J. Lab. clin. Med.* **68**, 195.
5. CONN H.O. (1977) Trailmaking and Reitan-connection tests in the assessment of mental state in portal systemic encephalopathy. *Am. J. dig. Dis.* **22**, 541.
6. CONN H.O. (1978) Lactulose: a drug in search of a modus operandi. *Gastroenterology* **74**, 624.
7. CONN H.O., LEEVY C.M., VLAHCEVIC Z.R. *et al* (1977) Comparison of lactulose and neomycin in the treatment of chronic portal–systemic encephalopathy. *Gastroenterology* **72**, 573.
8. CONN H.O. & LIEBERTHALL M.M. (1979) *The Hepatic Coma Syndromes and Lactulose*. Williams and Wilkins, Baltimore.
9. DAVIDSON E.A. & SUMMERSKILL W.H.J. (1956) Psychiatric aspects of liver disease. *Postgrad. med. J.* **32**, 487.
10. DAWSON A.M., DE GROOTE J., ROSENTHAL W.A. *et al* (1957) Blood pyruvic-acid and alpha-keto glutaric-acid levels in liver disease and hepatic coma. *Lancet* i, 392.
11. DAWSON A.M., MCLAREN J. & SHERLOCK S. (1957) Neomycin in the treatment of hepatic coma. *Lancet* ii, 1263.
12. FISCHER J.E. & BALDESSARINI R.J. (1971) False neurotransmitters and hepatic failure. *Lancet* ii, 75.
13. FISCHER J.E., ROSEN H.M., EBEID A.M. *et al* (1976) The effect of normalisation of plasma amino acids on hepatic encephalopathy in man. *Surgery* **80**, 77.
14. FRERICHS F.T. (1860) *A Clinical Treatise on Diseases of the Liver*, vol. I, p. 241. Translated by C. MURCHISON. New Sydenham Society, London.
15. GREENBERGER N.J., CARLEY J., SCHENKER S. *et al* (1977) Effect of vegetable and animal protein diets in chronic hepatic encephalopathy. *Am. J. dig. Dis.* **22**, 845.
16. HOYUMPA A.M., DESMOND P.V., AVANT G.R. *et al* (1979) Hepatic encephalopathy. *Gastroenterology* **76**, 184.
17. LAIDLAW J., READ A.E. & SHERLOCK S. (1961) Morphine tolerance in hepatic cirrhosis. *Gastroenterology* **40**, 389.
18. LAST P.M. & SHERLOCK S. (1959) Systemic absorption of orally administered neomycin in liver disease. *New Engl. J. Med.* **262**, 385.
19. LIVINGSTONE A.S., POTVIN M., GORESKY C.A. *et al* (1977) Changes in the blood–brain barrier in hepatic coma after hepatectomy in the rat. *Gastroenterology* **73**, 697.
20. LUNZER M., JAMES I.M., WEINMAN J. *et al* (1974) Treatment of chronic hepatic encephalopathy with levodopa. *Gut* **15**, 555.
21. MADDREY W.C., WEBER F.L., COULTER A.W. *et al* (1976) Effects of keto analogues of essential amino acids in portal–systemic encephalopathy. *Gastroenterology* **71**, 190.
22. MANGHANI K.K., LUNZER M.R., BILLING B.H. *et al* (1975) Urinary and serum octopamine in patients with portal–systemic encephalopathy. *Lancet* ii, 943.
23. MCLAIN C.J., ZIEVE L., DOIZAKI W.M. *et al* (1980) Blood methanethiol in alcoholic liver disease with and without hepatic encephalopathy. *Gut* **21**, 318.
24. MARTINI G.A., PHEAR E.A., RUEBNER B. *et al* (1957) The bacterial content of the small intestine in normal and cirrhotic subjects: relation to methionine toxicity. *Clin. Sci.* **16**, 35.
25. MORGAN M.Y., JAKOBOVITS A.M., LENNOX R. *et al* (1980) Successful use of bromocriptine in the treatment of chronic hepatic encephalopathy. *Gastroenterology* **78**, 663.
26. MORGAN M.Y., MILSOM J.P. & SHERLOCK S. (1978) Plasma ratio of valine, leucine and isoleucine to phenylalanine and tyrosine in liver disease. *Gut* **19**, 1068.
27. NANCE F.C. & KLINE D.G. (1971) Eck's fistula encephalopathy in germfree dogs. *Ann. Surg.* **174**, 856.
28. ONO J., HUTSON D.G., DOMBRO R.S. *et al* (1978) Tryptophan and hepatic coma. *Gastroenterology* **74**, 196.
29. PARKES J.D., MURRAY-LYON I.M. & WILLIAMS R. (1970) Neuropsychiatric and electro-encephalographic changes after transplantation of the liver. *Q.J. Med.* **39**, 515.
30. PARSONS-SMITH B.G., SUMMERSKILL W.H.J., DAWSON A.M. *et al* (1957) The electroencephalograph in hepatic coma. *Lancet* ii, 867.
31. PHEAR E.A., RUEBNER B., SHERLOCK S. *et al* (1955) Methionine toxicity in liver disease and its prevention by chlortetracycline. *Clin. Sci.* **15**, 93.

32. PHEAR E.A., SHERLOCK S. & SUMMERSKILL W.H.J. (1955) Blood ammonium levels in liver disease and 'hepatic coma'. *Lancet* i, 836.

33. PHILLIPS G.B., SCHWARTZ R., GABUZDA G.J. Jr *et al* (1952) The syndrome of impending hepatic coma in patients with cirrhosis of the liver given certain nitrogenous substances. *New Engl. J. Med.* **247**, 239.

34. READ A.E., LAIDLAW J., HASLAM R.M. *et al* (1959) Neuropsychiatric complications following chlorothiazide therapy in patients with hepatic cirrhosis; possible relation to hypokalaemia. *Clin. Sci.* **18**, 409.

35. READ A.E., SHERLOCK S., LAIDLAW J. *et al* (1967) The neuropsychiatric syndromes associated with chronic liver disease and an extensive portal-systemic collateral circulation. *Q.J. Med.* **36**, 135.

36. REHNSTRÖM S., SIMERT G., HANSSON J.A. *et al* (1977) Chronic hepatic encephalopathy, a psychometrical study. *Scand. J. Gastroent.* **12**, 305.

37. RIKKERS L., JENKO P., RUDMAN D. *et al* (1978) Subclinical hepatic encephalopathy: detection, prevalence and relationship to nitrogen metabolism. *Gastroenterology* **75**, 462.

38. ROSEN H.M., YOSHIMURA N., HODGMAN J.M. *et al* (1977) Plasma amino acid patterns in hepatic encephalopathy of differing etiology. *Gastroenterology* **72**, 483.

39. SCHÜTZ R.-M., BRUNNER L., SANRADIT M. *et al* (1965) Myelopathie bei Lebercirrhose. *Acta hepato-splenol. (Stuttg.)* **12**, 361.

40. SCOBIE B.A. & SUMMERSKILL W.H.J. (1964) Permanent paraplegia with cirrhosis. *Arch. intern. Med.* **113**, 805.

41. SHAFER W.H. & ISSELBACHER K.J. (1961) Uridine metabolism in chronic liver disease. *Gastroenterology* **40**, 782.

42. SHEAR L. & GABUZDA G.J. (1970) Potassium deficiency and endogenous ammonium overload from kidney. *Am. J. clin. Nutr.* **23**, 614.

43. SHERLOCK S. (1961) Hepatic coma. *Gastroenterology* **41**, 1.

44. SHERLOCK S., SENEWIRATNE B., SCOTT A. *et al* (1966) Complications of diuretic therapy in hepatic cirrhosis. *Lancet* i, 1049.

45. SHERLOCK S., SUMMERSKILL W.H.J. & DAWSON A.M. (1956) The treatment and prognosis of hepatic coma. *Lancet* ii, 689.

46. SHERLOCK S., SUMMERSKILL W.H.J., WHITE L.P. *et al* (1954) Portal–systemic encephalopathy. Neurological complications of liver disease. *Lancet* ii, 453.

47. SMYTHE C.M. & BAROODY N.B. (1957) Hepatic type 'flapping tremor' occurring in patients without hepatic disease. *J. Am. med. Assoc.* **165**, 31.

48. SOETERS P.B. & FISCHER J.E. (1976) Insulin, glucagon, amino acid imbalance and hepatic encephalopathy. *Lancet* ii, 880.

49. SUMMERSKILL W.H.J., DAVIDSON E.A., SHERLOCK S. *et al* (1956) The neuropsychiatric syndrome associated with hepatic cirrhosis and an extensive portal circulation. *Q.J. Med.* **25**, 245.

50. TAYLOR P., SCHOENE W.C., REID W.A. Jr *et al* (1979) Quantitative changes in astrocytes after porta-caval shunting. *Arch. Path.* **103**, 82.

51. VICTOR M., ADAMS R.D. & COLE M. (1965) The acquired (non-Wilsonian) type of chronic hepato-cerebral degeneration. *Medicine (Baltimore)* **44**, 345.

52. VINCE A., KILLINGLEY M. & WRONG O.M. (1978) Effect of lactulose on ammonia production in a faecal incubation system. *Gastroenterology* **74**, 544.

53. WARE A.J., D'AGOSTINO A.N. & COMBES B. (1971) Cerebral edema: a major complication of massive hepatic necrosis. *Gastroenterology* **61**, 877.

54. WARREN K.S., IBER F.L., DÖLLE W. *et al* (1960) The effect of alterations in blood pH on the distribution of ammonia from blood to cerebrospinal fluid in patients in hepatic coma. *J. Lab. clin. Med.* **56**, 687.

55. WARREN K.S. & REBOUÇAS G. (1964) Blood ammonia during bleeding from esophageal varices in patients with hepatosplenic schistosomiasis. *New Engl. J. Med.* **271**, 921.

56. WHITE L.P., PHEAR E.A., SUMMERSKILL W.H.J. *et al* (1955) Ammonium tolerance in liver disease. Observations based on catheterization of the hepatic veins. *J. clin. Invest.* **34**, 158.

57. WILCOX H.G., DUNN G.D. & SCHENKER S. (1978) Plasma long chain fatty acids and esterified lipids in cirrhosis and hepatic encephalopathy. *Am. J. med. Sci.* **276**, 293.

58. ZEEGEN R., DRINKWATER J.E. & DAWSON A.M. (1970) Method for measuring cerebral dysfunction in patients with liver disease. *Br. med. J.* ii, 633.

59. ZIEVE L. (1979) Hepatic encephalopathy: summary of present knowledge with an elaboration on recent developments. In *Progress in Liver Disease*, eds H. Popper & F. Schaffner, vol. 6. Grune and Stratton, New York.

Chapter 9
Acute (Fulminant) Hepatic Failure

This is defined as a clinical syndrome resulting from massive necrosis of liver cells, or sudden and severe impairment of liver function. There should be no evidence of preceding liver disease and, in the case of viral hepatitis, the syndrome should have developed within eight weeks of the onset of symptoms.

The problem is not only that of hepatic encephalopathy. Virtual hepatectomy does not lead only to portal–systemic bypassing of nitrogenous products coming from the gastro-intestinal tract—although these play a part.

The prognosis is much worse than that of chronic liver failure, but the hepatic lesion is potentially reversible, and survivors usually recover completely. This makes intensive care and temporary hepatic support vitally important.

Causes [3, 32, 34] (table 9)

The most frequent cause is acute virus hepatitis of both A [30] and B types. Non-A, non-B hepatitis can also become fulminant [42]. Drug reactions comprise the next group. These include sensitivity reactions to halothane, to monoamine oxidase inhibitors such as iproniazid and phenelzine, and to anti-tuberculous drugs, especially isoniazid.

Carbon tetrachloride poisoning usually causes

Table 9. Fulminant hepatic failure 1969–1979 (grade 3 or more). Royal Free Hospital, London.

Viral hepatitis		92
type A or non-A, non-B	57	
type B	35	
Drugs		74
Halothane	28	
MAO	9	
Anti-TB	12	
Acetaminophen (paracetamol)	25	
Fatty liver, pregnancy		6
	—	—
	166	172

Survival (grade 4) 24%

more kidney damage than hepatic damage. Acetaminophen (paracetamol) self-poisoning has a high mortality from acute hepatic necrosis [9]. Acute alcoholic hepatitis can present with a picture of fulminant liver failure.

Mushroom poisoning is common in France [3] and in areas where unusual fungi are gathered and eaten.

Fatty liver of pregnancy is often unrecognized but is a cause of acute liver failure in the last stages of pregnancy (Chapter 24).

Surgical shock with or without Gram-negative septicaemia must also be considered.

Prognosis and causes of death (table 10)

The survival of a patient with fulminant hepatitis reaching grade 4 or 5 coma is of the order of 12–20% [3, 34]. The variability reflects the number of patients in each series: the smaller the series the better the prognosis is likely to be, for the good result is likely to be reported. The depth of coma reached is important. If only grade 2 is reached then 66% survival is expected. Early recognition is all important.

Table 10. Fulminant hepatic failure. Royal Free Hospital, London.

		No.	% survival
Age	> 30	25	9
	< 30	35	40
Sex	Male	25	13
	Female	35	26

Advanced age and the coexistence of other diseases worsen the prognosis. The outlook is best in children and most spectacular recoveries have been in this group. Women tend to do worse than men. With increasing duration of coma the chances of recovery become less. If recovery follows a course of less than four weeks, clinical normality can ultimately be expected. The prognosis depends on the capacity of the liver to regenerate

[7]. Those who survive do not develop cirrhosis [22].

If any precipitant can be identified, particularly the administration of sedatives and tranquillizers, the prognosis is better. The patient improves as the sedative is eliminated.

Decerebrate rigidity, with loss of the oculo-vestibular reflex [16], and respiratory failure are particularly ominous features.

Bleeding precludes liver biopsy. Hepatic histology, obtained as soon as is possible, in those that recover or immediately *post mortem* has shown that the extent of parenchymal necrosis and interlobular confluent necrosis is critical in determining outcome [12]. No single histological feature, however, allows certain prediction [15].

The causes of death are bleeding, respiratory and circulatory failure, cerebral oedema, renal failure, infection, hypoglycaemia and pancreatitis.

Clinical picture

The neuropsychiatric picture is of stimulation of the reticular system of the brain followed by terminal depression of brain-stem function.

One of the earliest signs is change in personality. The patient may show anti-social behaviour or character disturbance. Nightmares, headaches and dizziness are other inaugural, non-specific symptoms. Delirium, mania and fits indicate stimulation of the reticular system. Unco-operative behaviour often continues while consciousness is clouded. The delirium is of the noisy, restless variety and attacks of screaming are spontaneous or induced by slight stimuli. Violent behaviour is common. 'Flapping' tremor may be transient and overlooked. Fetor hepaticus is usually present.

In the later stages the picture is that of decerebrate rigidity [11, 21] with spasticity, extension and hyperpronation of the arms, extension of the legs and plantar flexor responses. Fits may occur. The plantar responses remain flexor until very late. Dysconjugate eye movements and skew positions of the eyes may be seen. Pupillary reflexes usually persist until very late. Respiratory and circulatory failure with hypotension, cardiac arrhythmias and respiratory arrest are other indications of depressed brain-stem function.

In the early stages jaundice bears little relation to the neuropsychiatric changes which may even develop before jaundice. Later jaundice is deep. Liver size is usually small.

The clinician must be alert to liver damage due to acetaminophen (paracetamol) which may present after a period of 2–3 days of apparent clinical recovery.

DISTINCTION FROM CHRONIC LIVER DISEASE (table 11)

A note should be made of any history of liver disease, duration of symptoms, the presence of a hard liver, marked splenomegaly and vascular spiders on the skin. A problem arises in the alcoholic where recent heavy drinking adds acute hepatitis to underlying chronic liver disease. In these circumstances the liver is large. Potential

Table 11. Fulminant hepatic failure: distinction between acute and acute-on-chronic types.

	Acute	Acute-on-chronic
History	Short	Long
Nutrition	Good	Poor
Liver	±	+ Hard
Spleen	±	+
Spiders	0	+ +

Table 12. Investigations of acute hepato-cellular failure.

Essential
Electroencephalogram, electrocardiogram, X-ray of chest and abdomen, fluid intake and output

Biochemical
Store 8 ml serum for later use. Blood glucose (urgent), serum bilirubin, aspartate transaminase, albumin, globulin, immunoglobulins
Serum urea, sodium, potassium, bicarbonate, chloride, calcium, phosphate, alkaline phosphatase
Serum amylase

Haematology
Haemoglobin, platelets, WBC, prothrombin, blood group

Microbiology
Hepatitis B antigen and antibody
Hepatitis A (IgM) antibody
Blood culture aerobic and anaerobic. Sputum, urine, stool (culture and microscopy)
Store serum for virological studies

Additional (not always necessary)
Blood alcohol or other drug level
Cerebrospinal fluid cells, protein and culture
Urine electrolyte concentration
Plasma fibrin split products, euglobulin lysis time
Hepatic scintiscan

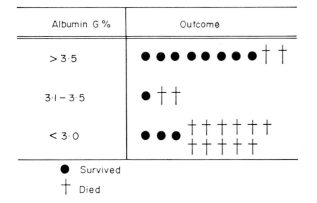

Albumin G %	Outcome
> 3·5	● ● ● ● ● ● ● ● † †
3·1 – 3·5	● † †
< 3·0	● ● ● † † † † † † † † † † †

● Survived
† Died

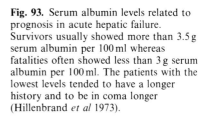

Fig. 93. Serum albumin levels related to prognosis in acute hepatic failure. Survivors usually showed more than 3.5 g serum albumin per 100 ml whereas fatalities often showed less than 3 g serum albumin per 100 ml. The patients with the lowest levels tended to have a longer history and to be in coma longer (Hillenbrand *et al* 1973).

irreversibility of acute alcoholic hepatitis merits more supportive effort in these patients than could be given to the usual end-stage cirrhosis where the liver would not be expected to regenerate.

LIVER FUNCTION TESTS

Serum bilirubin level is measured as a base line and to check progress.

Serum aspartate transaminase is measured initially but is of little prognostic value. Levels tend to fall as the patient's condition worsens.

Serum albumin is usually initially normal, but later a low albumin reflects a poor prognosis (fig. 93). In the recovery stage infusions of salt-poor albumin may hasten liver regeneration. Serum α-fetoprotein falls, rising with regeneration [6]. The C_3 component of complement falls progressively.

CEREBRO-SPINAL FLUID

Unless the diagnosis is in doubt a lumbar puncture is not necessary. Cerebro-spinal fluid glutamine levels are usually increased.

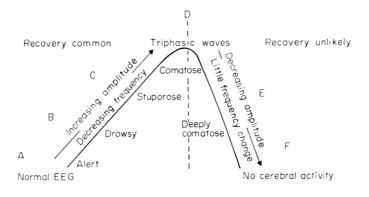

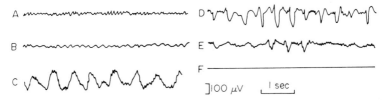

Fig. 94. Evolution of the EEG in liver failure. The progression from grade A to D is marked by increasing amplitude, decreasing frequency and increasing drowsiness. At D, triphasic waves appear and the interrupted line indicates the limit beyond which recovery is unlikely. From E to F amplitude decreases with little frequency change and at F there is no cerebral activity (Kennedy *et al* 1973).

ELECTROENCEPHALOGRAM (fig. 94)

This should be performed as often as possible. It may be used to assess the clinical state and to determine prognosis [23]. Normally the EEG correlates well with the clinical state although early on it may be more severe than the clinical picture suggests and later may be abnormal for some weeks although the patient's level of consciousness is normal.

Stage A is normal and the patient is alert. From stage B to D the EEG shows increasing amplitude while frequency decreases. The patient passes from drowsiness to coma. At stage D triphasic waves appear. These carry a poor prognosis. They are never seen in patients under the age of 20 years and are uncommon under 30. In the younger patient stage D abnormality is shown as high voltage, diffuse, slow activity. Beyond this stage recovery is unlikely. The amplitude decreases and the frequency does not change. Finally at stage F there is absence of rhythmic activity.

MANAGEMENT (table 13)

Improvement in survival of patients with fulminant hepatitis in deep coma has come from attention to the details of good supportive care combined with better knowledge of the most important functions lost when the liver cell fails. These patients are rare and should, if at all possible, be treated in a special unit experienced in their management. The recommendations below apply to grade 4 or 5 coma and must be modified for the lower grades. Their early institution may prevent a less serious grade passing to a worse one.

GENERAL

The usual measures for the unconscious patient are adopted. The patient is barrier nursed, attendants wearing gloves, gowns and masks. They should be educated concerning personal hygiene.

Because of the risk of fluid overload the patient should preferably be nursed in a bed that can be weighed. They should be placed on fluid intake and output balance.

A large bore catheter is introduced via the right arm into the right atrium. This is used for manometry, blood sampling and for feeding. Arterial sampling should not be performed because of the risk of continued bleeding from the puncture site.

Table 13. Management of acute hepato-cellular failure with coma.

Problem	Treatment
Portal–systemic encephalopathy	No protein by mouth Neomycin 1 g orally four times a day Magnesium sulphate enema, then twice daily bowel washouts using 1% dextrose No sedation
Hypoglycaemia	100 ml 50% glucose if blood glucose falls below 100 mg Up to 3 litres 10% glucose per .24 hours 120–200 mEq KCl daily (if normal urine output)
Hypocalcaemia	10 ml 10% calcium gluconate i.v. daily
Renal failure	i.v. salt-poor albumin Dialysis
Respiratory failure	Intubation (*not* tracheostomy) Ventilator Oxygen
Infection	No inguinal i.v. catheters No routine antibiotics Specific antibiotics if organism isolated
Bleeding	No arterial puncture Cimetidine intravenously

A nasogastric tube is passed. Because of the risk of mucosal erosion the stomach should not be actively aspirated but kept empty by gravity drainage.

All comatose patients should have an indwelling urinary catheter.

CLINICAL

The grade of coma (p. 93) must be charted two-hourly.

Temperature, pulse and blood pressure should be recorded at least hourly and preferably continuously. In the later stages hypothermia may be due to brain-stem involvement.

Liver size is determined daily by percussion and the lower margin marked on the abdominal wall (fig. 95).

HEPATIC ENCEPHALOPATHY AND CEREBRAL OEDEMA

In contrast to the coma of cirrhotic patients, portal–systemic encephalopathy is of minor importance in patients with fulminant hepatitis. Blood ammonium (and presumably amine) levels

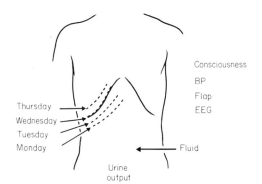

Fig. 95. Clinical daily check in patients with fulminant hepatic failure.

are increased but do not correlate with the depth of coma or with the prognosis. Such estimates are not necessary for management. The routine treatment for acute portal–systemic encephalopathy is, however, given (table 8).

Sedation must be avoided if at all possible. If the patient is uncontrollable by physical means a small dose of diazoxide, an antihistaminic or barbitone soluble may be given. All are liable to increase depth of coma.

Cerebral oedema is present at autopsy in 32% (see fig. 84 in colour section) [15]. It is marked clinically by fixed dilated pupils and respiratory arrest. Papilloedema is rare. Experimentally, pigs with acute liver necrosis show a progressive rise in intracranial pressure [19]. Treatment with mannitol or corticosteroids is unavailing.

AMINO ACIDS

Amino-aciduria is a feature of massive hepatic necrosis [39] and urinary tyrosine and leucine crystals are classical associations of 'acute yellow atrophy'. An increase in amino acids can also be seen in the plasma [32] involving methionine, glutamate and aspartate, phenyl alanine and tyrosine. Levels of leucine and isoleucine are normal or low. The significance of these findings is uncertain but might be related to the theory that 'false neurochemical transmitters' play a role in hepatic coma (fig. 87). Methionine, tyrosine and phenyl alanine are important in neuromuscular transmission. Infusion of branched-chain amino acids has been recommended but is not of proven value. Levodopa is of no permanent value in acute hepatic coma although temporary arousal sometimes follows its use [14].

HYPOGLYCAEMIA AND LACTIC ACIDOSIS

Frank hypoglycaemia is rare in fulminant hepatitis but can occur, especially in children [20]. It may be persistent and intractable [33]. Plasma insulin levels are high. Hypoglycaemia can cause sudden death in these patients and is one aspect of the condition which can be treated satisfactorily.

If it is necessary to move a patient from one centre to another a 20% glucose infusion should be given during the journey.

On arrival the blood glucose is estimated by a quick procedure such as 'dextrostix'. Fifty millilitres 50% glucose is given orally or intravenously if the blood glucose level is less than 100 mg/ 100 ml. Subsequently dextrostix are used every hour and 50% glucose is again given if the blood glucose level is 90 mg/100 ml or less.

Ten per cent glucose is given continuously, up to 3 litres daily with added potassium chloride. Ascorbic acid 500 mg is given daily in the infusion.

Lactic acidosis is due to failure of hepatic gluconeogenesis and increased anaerobic metabolism.

ELECTROLYTES

Serum sodium levels tend to be low, falling markedly in the terminal stages. Persistent hyponatraemia reflects impending cell death. It should not be corrected with hypertonic sodium chloride unless there is clear evidence of a profound loss of sodium from the body.

Serum potassium tends to fall related to urinary losses, poor intake and high glucose feeding. A metabolic alkalosis follows and this potentiates ammonium toxicity. Potassium chloride supplements must be given both orally and intravenously. If urinary output is normal at least 120 mEq daily are needed. Later renal failure leads to hyperkalaemia.

Serum calcium values tend to be low and may reflect pancreatitis [28] and hypoalbuminaemia. Ten millilitres 10% calcium gluconate daily are added to the intravenous infusion and another 10 ml for every unit of citrated blood transfused.

RENAL FAILURE

In the early stages blood urea levels may be reduced due to failure of Krebs' cycle enzymes in the liver. Later azotaemia is progressive. Many factors contribute and include jaundice, infection, endotoxaemia and haemorrhage—especially gastro-intestinal. Most important, however, is the reduced renal cortical perfusion associated with hepatic failure [17] (fig. 105). Forty-three per cent of patients develop renal failure [41].

If hyperkalaemia reaches dangerous levels peritoneal or haemo-dialysis should be performed.

RESPIRATORY AND CIRCULATORY FAILURE

Early stimulation of medullary vital centres causes over-breathing, but later, depression of brain-stem function leads to respiratory arrest. Aspiration of gastric contents and haemorrhage into the lungs with infection add to the problems.

The respiratory alkalosis with low $PaCO_2$ seems to be in some way beneficial, for coma increases if carbon dioxide is given [29]. Metabolic alkalosis is added due to hypokalaemia, continuous gastric aspiration, and accumulation of basic compounds in the circulation.

An airway or endotracheal tube and a mechanical respirator should be employed at the first sign of an impaired 'gag' reflex. Tracheostomy is not advisable. Hypoxaemia may be related to intrapulmonary shunting and to pulmonary oedema [36]. Oxygen by mask should be given routinely to the unconscious patient.

Until terminally, the circulation is hyperdynamic and the cardiac output increased. Later, depression of brain-stem function leads to circulatory failure [40]. Bradycardia is ominous, and finally there is cardiac arrest. Arrhythmias and circulatory failure are frequent, especially with acetaminophen overdose.

An electrocardiograph should be taken and cardiac monitoring performed if possible.

Volume depletion should be guarded against as it enhances circulatory failure.

BLEEDING (fig. 29) (Chapter 4)

Bleeding is a frequent cause of death. It is shown by spontaneous bruising, bleeding from mucous membranes, from the gastro-intestinal tract and into the brain. The patient often dies bleeding from everywhere and in spite of all therapeutic efforts. Portal hypertension may contribute [24].

Local trauma is avoided. Arterial punctures are not performed, the stomach is not aspirated, corticosteroids are not given.

Although it will not completely correct the bleeding tendency vitamin K_1 10 mg is given daily, intravenously.

Thrombotest	Outcome
> 25 %	● ●
21 – 25 %	●
16 – 20%	●
11–15 %	● ● † † † †
5–10%	● ● ● † † † †
<5%	† † † † †

● Survived
† Died

Fig. 96. Thrombotest before intramuscular vitamin K_1 related to outcome. Patients with less than 10% thrombotest usually died (Hillenbrand *et al* 1974).

The prothrombin index is an excellent prognostic guide. If the thrombotest after vitamin K_1 therapy is less than 20% the outlook is ominous; if less than 10% death is the rule (figs 96, 97) [18]. Defects in clotting factors are repaired by fresh frozen plasma, fresh blood and platelets (pp. 37–40). Intravascular coagulation should be diagnosed only if the euglobulin lysis time is prolonged, fibrin split products are found in the blood and there is thrombocytopenia. Intravenous heparin treatment is rarely justified [18, 37].

Thrombotest	Outcome
> 25%	● ●
21 – 25%	● †
16 – 20%	● ● † † †
11 – 15%	● † † † †
5 – 10%	● ● ● † † † †
<5%	†

● Survived
† Died

Fig. 97. Thrombotest after intramuscular vitamin K_1 related to outcome. Despite the severe hepatocellular failure many patients improved their thrombotest after treatment, but prognosis was still very poor in those with less than 20% (Hillenbrand *et al* 1974).

Gastric erosions are frequent, and prophylactic cimetidine should be given intravenously in full dosage [26].

INFECTION

Tests for hepatitis B antigen are performed urgently. Positivity emphasizes the need for more stringent measures to avoid spread of infection.

Infection is frequent particularly in relation to the respiratory tract, bladder catheterization and intravenous therapy. It is often Gram-negative and is an important contributory cause of death.

Potential pathogens were isolated from the inguinal area in 85% of patients with acute hepatic failure and this part should be avoided for intravenous catheterization.

Routine antibiotics should not be given for these favour skin colonization with potential pathogens. Appropriate antibiotics are given only when clear evidence of infection exists.

A blood culture is performed and repeated particularly while intravenous therapy is being given and the patient is comatose. Septicaemia is often clinically latent. Sputum, urine and stools should also be examined bacteriologically. All catheter tips are cut off and put into culture media.

CORTICOSTEROID THERAPY

The use of corticosteroids is not based on sound evidence. Controlled trials have failed to show benefit for large doses of corticosteroids in fulminant hepatic failure; they may even be of negative value [38]. This therapy is not being used at the present time. The complications include infections, gastric erosions and pancreatitis, and these outweigh any possible benefits.

ACUTE PANCREATITIS [2, 28]

Acute haemorrhagic and necrotic pancreatitis is frequent in patients dying with fulminant massive hepatic failure [28]. It is difficult to recognize in the comatose patient but rarely it may be the cause of death. Serum amylase levels are raised in about a third of patients and these should be repeated frequently. Aetiological factors include 'duodenitis' found with fulminant hepatitis, haemorrhage into and around the pancreas, the causative virus, corticosteroid therapy and shock. Preven-

tion includes the avoidance of corticosteroid therapy and keeping the stomach empty.

ARTIFICIAL HEPATIC SUPPORT

Review of current data reveals no controlled evidence that any therapy now in use for patients with acute hepatic necrosis in coma is of value in salvaging life [4, 5, 31]. Supportive measures are of value. Many procedures lead to the patient waking up, but only temporarily. Such measures must be considered [19]. They apply only to patients with potentially reversible acute hepato-cellular failure. They cannot be considered for temporary resuscitation of an otherwise moribund cirrhotic patient, who would succumb within the next few months. Eventually they may have a wider application in hepatic transplantation.

The aim is to remove toxic metabolites and to keep the patient alive until his own liver can function satisfactorily. Results therefore depend on the capacity of the liver to regenerate. The factors controlling this process remain unknown. This enigma therefore is unsolved.

Exchange blood [20] *or plasma* [25] *transfusion* removes protein-bound, non-dialysable, toxic substances from the blood, or possibly adds essential substances made by the normal liver. Consciousness is often regained, but the overall mortality is unaffected [20]. This treatment cannot be recommended.

Cross-circulation from a donor may not be ethically justifiable [8]. The treatment and benefit are only short-term.

The baboon has also been used [1], but this is clearly not generally applicable.

Extra-corporeal liver perfusion using pig [13], bovine [10] or cadaver [1] liver has had more success, but has now been largely abandoned.

Charcoal haemoperfusion. The difficulty is in defining the relevant toxic metabolites, which seem to be both water-soluble and protein-bound. Charcoal removes water-soluble substances, but has problems in biocompatibility [19]. No increase in survival has been reported.

Rhone–Poulenc haemodialysis system has a highly permeable polyacrylonitrile membrane which removes middle-rate substances (up to molecular weight 5000). Significant improvements in consciousness may follow its use, but percentage survival does not improve [27, 35]. The use of resins which will remove protein-bound toxins is in the preliminary stages.

REFERENCES

1. ABOUNA G.M., COOK J.S., FISHER L. McA. *et al* (1972) Treatment of acute hepatic coma by *ex vivo* baboon and human liver perfusions. *Surgery* **71**, 537.
2. ACHORD J.L. (1968) Acute pancreatitis with infectious hepatitis. *JAMA* **205**, 129.
3. BENHAMOU J-P., RUEFF B. & SICOT C. (1972) Severe hepatic failure: a critical study of current therapy. In *Liver and Drugs*, eds. F. Orlandi & A.M. Jezequel, p. 213. Academic Press, New York.
4. BERK P.D. (1978) Artificial liver: a baby delivered prematurely. *Gastroenterology* **74**, 789.
5. BERK P.D. & POPPER H. (1978) Fulminant hepatic failure. *Am. J. Gastroenterol.* **69**, 349.
6. BLOOMER J.R., WALDMANN T.A., McINTIRE R. *et al* (1977) Serum alpha-fetoprotein in patients with massive hepatic necrosis. *Gastroenterology* **72**, 479.
7. BUCHER N.L.R. & MALT R.A. (1971) *Regeneration of Liver and Kidney*. Little Brown, Boston.
8. BURNELL J.M., DAWBORN J.K., EPSTEIN R.B. *et al* (1967) Acute hepatic coma, treated by cross-circulation or exchange transfusion. *N. Engl. J. Med.* **276**, 935.
9. CLARK R., THOMPSON R.P.H., BORIRAKCHANYA-VAT V. *et al* (1973) Hepatic damage and death from overdose of paracetamol. *Lancet* i, 66.
10. CONDON R.E., BOMBECK C.T. & STEIGMANN F. (1970) Heterologous bovine liver perfusion therapy of acute hepatic failure. *Am. J. Surg.* **119**, 147.
11. CONOMY J.P. & SWASH M. (1968) Reversible decerebrate and decorticate postures in hepatic coma. *N. Engl. J. Med.* **278**, 876.
12. DESMET V.J., DE GROOTE J. & VAN DAMME B. (1972) Hepatocellular failure: A study of 17 patients treated with exchange transfusion. *Hum. Pathol.* **3**, 167.
13. EISEMAN B. (1967) Hepatic perfusion. *Colston Papers: Liver Diseases*. Butterworth Scientific Publications, 279. Butterworth, London.
14. FISCHER J.E. & BALDESSARINI R.J. (1971) False neurotransmitters and hepatic failure. *Lancet* ii, 75.
15. GAZZARD B.G., PORTMANN B., MURRAY-LION I.M. *et al* (1975) Causes of death in fulminant hepatic failure and relationship to quantitative histological assessment of parenchymal damage. *Q. J. Med.* **44**, 615.
16. HANID M.A., SILK D.B.A. & WILLIAMS R. (1978) Prognostic value of the vestibular reflex in fulminant hepatic failure. *Br. med. J.* i, 1029.
17. HECKER R. & SHERLOCK S. (1956) Electrolyte and circulatory changes in terminal liver failure. *Lancet* ii, 1121.
18. HILLENBRAND P., PARBHOO S.P., JEDRYCHOWSKI A. *et al* (1974) Significance of intravascular coagulation and fibrinolysis in acute hepatic failure. *Gut* **15**, 83.
19. JENKINS P.J. & WILLIAMS R. (1980) Fulminant viral hepatitis. *Clin. Gastroenterol.* **9**, 171.
20. JONES E.A., CLAIN D., CLINK H.M. *et al* (1967) Hepatic coma due to acute hepatic necrosis treated by exchange blood transfusion. *Lancet* ii, 169.
21. JUNEJA I. & YOVIC A. (1972) Hepatic decerebration. *Neurology* **22**, 537.
22. KARVOUNTZIS G.G., REDEKER A.G. & PETERS R. (1974) Long-term follow-up studies on patients surviving fulminant viral hepatitis. *Gastroenterology* **67**, 870.
23. KENNEDY J., PARBHOO S.P., MACGILLIVRAY B. *et al* (1973) Effect of extra-corporeal liver perfusion on the electro-encephalogram of patients in coma due to acute liver failure. *Q. J. Med.* **42**, 549.
24. LEBREC D., NOUEL O., BERNAU J. *et al* (1980) Portal hypertension in fulminant viral hepatitis. *Gut* **21**, 962.
25. LEPORE M.J. & MARTEL A.J. (1970) Plasmapheresis with plasma exchange in hepatic coma. *Ann. intern. Med.* **72**, 165.
26. MACDOUGALL B.R.D., BAILEY R.J. & WILLIAMS R. (1977) H_2 receptor antagonists and antacids in the prevention of acute gastrointestinal haemorrhage in fulminant hepatic failure. *Lancet* i, 617.
27. OPOLON P., DENIS P. & DARNIS F. (1978) Assistance extra-corporelle par hémofiltration continue au cours des hépatites graves. *Nouv. Presse Med.*, **7**, 2473.
28. PARBHOO S.P., WELCH J. & SHERLOCK S. (1973) Acute pancreatitis in patients with fulminant hepatic failure. *Gut* **14**, 428.
29. POSNER J.B. & PLUM F. (1960) The toxic effects of carbon dioxide and acetazolamide in hepatic encephalopathy. *J. clin. Invest.* **39**, 1246.
30. RAKELA J., REDEKER A.G., EDWARDS V.M. *et al* (1978) Hepatitis A virus infection in fulminant hepatitis and chronic active hepatitis. *Gastroenterology* **74**, 879.
31. RITT D.J., WHELAN G., WERNER D.J. *et al* (1969) Acute hepatic necrosis with stupor or coma. *Medicine (Baltimore)* **48**, 151.
32. ROSEN A.M., YOSHIMURA N., HODGMAN J.M. *et al* (1977) Plasma amino acid patterns in hepatic encephalopathy of differing etiology. *Gastroenterology* **72**, 483.
33. SAMSON R.I., TREY C., TIMME A.H. *et al* (1967) Fulminating hepatitis, recurrent hypoglycemia and hemorrhage. *Gastroenterology* **53**, 291.
34. SHERLOCK S. & PARBHOO S.P. (1971) The management of acute hepatic failure. *Postgrad. med. J.* **47**, 493.
35. SILK D.B.A., HANID M.A., TREWBY P.N. *et al* (1977) Treatment of fulminant hepatic failure by polyacrylonitrile-membrane haemodialysis. *Lancet* ii, 1.
36. TREWBY P.N. & WILLIAMS R. (1978) Incidence and pathophysiology of pulmonary edema in fulminant hepatic failure. *Gastroenterology* **74**, 859.
37. TUCKER J.S., WOOLF I.L., BOYES E.B. *et al* (1973) Coagulation studies in acute hepatic failure. *Gut* **14**, 418.
38. TYGSTRUP N. & JUHL E. *et al* (1979) Randomised trial of steroid therapy in acute liver failure. Report from the European Association for the Study of the Liver (EASL). In press.
39. WALSHE J.M. (1951) Observations on the sympto-

matology and pathogenesis of hepatic coma. *Q. J. Med.* **20,** 421.

40. WESTON M.J., TALBOT I.C., HOWORTH P.J.N. *et al* (1976) Frequency of arrhythmias and other cardiac abnormalities in fulminant hepatic failure. *Br. heart J.* **38,** 1179.

41. WILKINSON S.P., ARROYO V.A., MOODIE H. *et al* (1976) Abnormalities of sodium excretion and other disorders of renal function in fulminant hepatic failure. *Gut* **17,** 501.

42. WYKE R.J., THORNTON A., PORTMANN B. *et al* (1979) Transmission of non-A, non-B hepatitis to chimpanzees by factor IX concentrates in patients with chronic liver disease. *Lancet* i, 520.

Chapter 10
Ascites

MECHANISMS OF ASCITES FORMATION

Starling (1896) [39] suggested that the interchange of fluid between the blood and the tissue spaces is controlled by the balance between the capillary blood pressure, forcing fluid into the tissue spaces, and the osmotic pressure of the plasma proteins, retaining fluid in the vascular compartment (fig. 98).

Plasma colloid osmotic pressure − ascitic colloid osmotic pressure

= portal capillary pressure − intra-abdominal hydrostatic pressure.

There are thus two important factors in the formation of ascites: the plasma colloid osmotic pressure and the portal venous pressure (figs. 98, 99).

In cirrhosis, albumin synthesis is decreased [41] and plasma albumin and colloid osmotic pressure

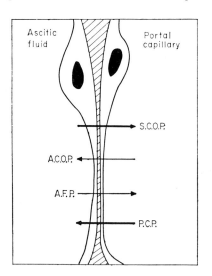

Fig. 98. The ascitic fluid is separated from the capillary lumen by the peritoneal membrane and the portal capillary wall. The forces keeping fluid in the capillaries are the colloid osmotic pressure of the serum (SCOP) and the hydrostatic pressure of the ascitic fluid (AFP). The forces tending to form ascites are the portal capillary pressure (PCP) and the colloid osmotic pressure of the ascitic fluid (ACOP). In a steady state these forces should balance.

are reduced [11]. This pressure in many instances provides an accurate discriminant between patients with cirrhosis and ascites and those without [11].

Portal venous pressure cannot be quantitatively related to ascites. For instance, portal hypertension due to cirrhosis may exist with or without ascites. Experimental obstruction to the portal vein is not sufficient to produce ascites unless, at the same time, the animal is rendered hypoproteinaemic by plasmapheresis [7]. Similarly, if a patient with extra-hepatic portal hypertension suffers a gastro-intestinal haemorrhage or if for any other reason the plasma protein level falls, then ascites will develop [44]. As the plasma proteins recover, the ascites disappears even though the portal hypertension remains. The portal hypertension serves to localize the fluid retention in the peritoneal cavity rather than in the peripheral tissues.

Plasma–ascites interchange

Fluid exchange between the ascitic and vascular compartments is mainly through the visceral peritoneum; the role of lymphatics will be considered later. Once formed, ascitic fluid can exchange with blood through an enormous capillary bed under the visceral peritoneum.

The visceral peritoneum is not a simple, semipermeable membrane as in the Starling equilibrium. It plays a vital, dynamic role, sometimes actively facilitating transfer of fluid into the ascites and sometimes retarding it. The mechanism by which patients with ascites may attain a steady state is not known.

Ascites is continuously circulating, about half entering and leaving the peritoneal cavity every hour, there being a rapid transit in both directions [6]. The constituents of the fluid are in dynamic equilibrium with those of the plasma.

The role of hepatic lymph

Ascites can be produced in the dog by obstruction to hepatic venous outflow by constricting the in-

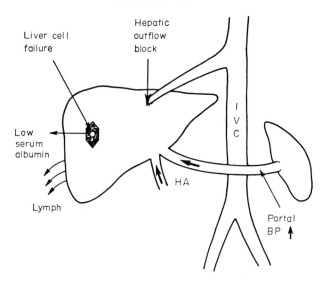

Ascites in cirrhosis

Liver cell failure

Hepatic outflow block

Low serum albumin

I V C

H A

Lymph

Portal BP ↑

Fig. 99. Important factors for ascites production are liver cell failure leading to a low serum albumin level, portal venous obstruction (pre-sinusoidal, sinusoidal and post-sinusoidal) and hepatic outflow block with over-production of hepatic lymph.

ferior vena cava above the entry of the hepatic veins [7]. Hepatic lymph production increases and this extravasates into the peritoneal cavity. In cirrhosis the obstruction to hepatic blood flow is partly post-sinusoidal, presumably secondary to pressure of regenerating nodules on hepatic veins. In severe alcoholic liver disease there may be actual lesions of the central hepatic veins (*sclerosing hyaline necrosis*). Some of the hepatic lymph undoubtedly enters the ascitic fluid, particularly when the transport capacity of the hepatic lymph system is exceeded [48]. The numbers of subcapsular and hilar lymphatics are increased in patients with ascites [1]. Ascites disappears if hepatic outflow block is relieved by side-to-side porta-caval shunt [45]. Enormous ascites can rarely follow the end-to-side procedure.

Increased lymph production does not explain the development of ascites in patients with extrahepatic portal obstruction who become hypoproteinaemic. Moreover, ascites usually clears after end-to-side porta-caval shunt which certainly does not relieve the hepatic 'outflow block'.

Renal changes (fig. 100)

Sodium retention [17]

Cirrhotic patients with ascites retain sodium avidly, urinary sodium excretion being usually less than 5 mEq daily. Serum sodium levels are somewhat reduced. This does not reflect sodium de-

ficiency for, because of a greatly expanded extracellular sodium space, the actual total body stores of sodium are increased.

As ascites develops there is progressive diminution of the effective intravascular volume. This acts as a signal for the renal tubules to retain sodium, 99.5% of the filtered load being re-absorbed. Diminished perfusion of the kidney stimulates the juxta-glomerular system to produce renin which leads to aldosterone release by the adrenal cortex. The plasma renin levels are increased in cirrhosis

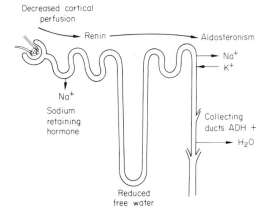

Decreased cortical perfusion

Renin

Aldosteronism

Na⁺
K⁺

Na⁺

Sodium retaining hormone

Collecting ducts ADH +

H₂O

Reduced free water

Fig. 100. Renal changes in ascites. Decreased renal cortical perfusion leads to renin release with aldosterone excess. Reduced extracellular fluid volume leads to release of sodium-retaining hormone and sodium reabsorption. 'Free' water clearance is reduced. ADH plays a minor role.

[36] and the juxta-glomerular apparatus is hypertrophied. Increased proximal tubular sodium re-absorption is probably more important. The hormone concerned is unidentified but is presumably produced in response to a change in extracellular fluid volume. It has been called natriuretic hormone or third factor [16].

An alternative 'forward' theory propounds that inappropriate renal sodium retention with expansion of the plasma volume is the primary event in ascites formation [30]. As the portal blood pressure is high and the serum colloid osmotic pressure is low, the excess fluid is localized to the peritoneal cavity. This theory seems unlikely as volume expansion seems to improve rather than impair urinary sodium and water clearance.

Prostaglandin E2 increases renal blood flow and sodium excretion. Rises in cirrhotic patients might represent an attempt to improve renal blood flow and sodium excretion [8, 49].

Plasma prekallikrein levels are reduced in liver disease and these might be related to changes in intrarenal blood flow and sodium handling [46].

Water excretion is defective because proximal tubular re-absorption of sodium is so great that none passes to the distal 'loop' site to allow 'free' water to be generated. It can be treated by giving an osmotic diuretic which flushes sodium distally and so allows free water to be generated.

Serum potassium is normal or slightly depressed, but the body's exchangeable potassium is decreased [6, 9]. This is not only due to excessive loss of the ion from secondary aldosteronism but to failure of the cells to maintain their potassium content (cellular depletion). Reduction in total muscle mass is contributory. Diarrhoea is a factor in alcoholics.

Renal function

A normal renal circulation and glomerular filtration rate are necessary for sodium excretion. In

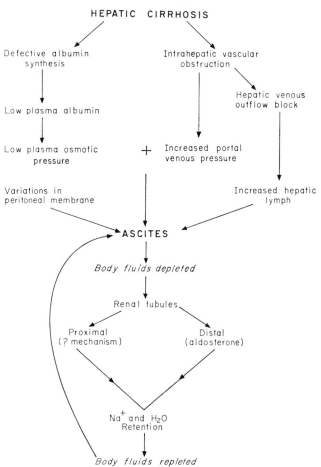

Fig. 101. The possible mechanisms of ascites formation in cirrhosis.

patients with cirrhosis these may be depressed by intensive diuretic therapy, by complicating renal disease, by increased abdominal pressure of tense ascites on the renal veins, by altered distribution of intrarenal flow [25], or chronic liver failure with hypotension [23].

Summary (figs. 99, 101)

The two most important factors in the development of ascites are failure of the liver to synthesize albumin and hence a lowered plasma osmotic pressure, and portal venous hypertension. More fluid enters the peritoneal cavity than leaves it and ascites develops. This results in depletion of the effective intravascular volume which causes the renal tubules to retain sodium and water. The distal effect is presumably mainly through aldosterone; the mechanism of the proximal tubular sodium retention is uncertain.

By these various methods sodium and water are retained, body fluids are again replete, more ascites is formed, and the whole cycle starts again.

An active role of the peritoneal capillary membrane in controlling the passage of fluid is possible.

The increase in intra-sinusoidal pressure found in cirrhosis and hepatic venous obstruction may stimulate hepatic lymph formation and add to the ascites.

CLINICAL FEATURES

ONSET

Ascites may appear suddenly or develop insidiously over the course of months with accompanying flatulent abdominal distension.

Ascites may develop suddenly when hepatocellular function is reduced, for instance by haemorrhage, 'shock', infection or an alcoholic debauch. This might be related to the fall in serum albumin values and/or to increased aldosterone production. Increased portal venous pressure due to thrombosis of the portal vein may precipitate ascites in a patient with a low serum albumin level.

The insidious onset proclaims a worse prognosis, possibly because it is not associated with any rectifiable factor. There is gradually increasing abdominal distension and the patient may present with dyspnoea.

EXAMINATION

The patient is sallow and dehydrated. Sweating is diminished. Muscle wasting is profound. The thin limbs with the protuberant belly lead to the description of the patient as a 'spider man'.

The abdomen is distended not only with fluid but also by air in the dilated intestines. The fullness is particularly conspicuous in the flanks. The umbilicus is everted and the distance between the symphysis pubis and umbilicus seems diminished.

The increased intra-abdominal pressure favours the protrusion of hernias in the umbilical (fig. 117), femoral or inguinal regions or through old abdominal incisions. Scrotal oedema is frequent.

Distended abdominal wall veins may represent portal–systemic collateral channels which radiate from the umbilicus and persist after control of the ascites (figs. 114, 115). Inferior vena caval collaterals result from a secondary, functional block of the inferior vena cava due to pressure of the peritoneal fluid. They commonly run from the groin to the costal margin or flanks and disappear when the ascites is controlled and intra-abdominal pressure is reduced. Abdominal striae may develop.

Dullness on percussion in the flanks is the earliest sign and can be detected when about 2 litres are present. The distribution of the dullness differs from that due to enlargement of the bladder, to an ovarian tumour or a pregnant uterus when the flanks are resonant to percussion. With tense ascites, it is difficult to palpate the abdominal viscera, but with moderate amounts of fluid the liver or spleen may be balloted.

A fluid thrill means much free fluid; it is a very late sign of fluid under tension.

Secondary effects

A *pleural effusion* is found in about 6% of cirrhotics and in 67% of these it is right-sided. It is due to defects in the diaphragm allowing ascites to pass into the pleural cavity. This can be shown by introducing ^{131}I albumin or air into the ascites and examining the pleural fluid afterwards [29].

The pleural fluid is in equilibrium with the ascites and control depends on medical control of the ascites. Thoracentesis is followed by rapid filling up of the pleural space by ascitic fluid. Occasionally recurrent pleural effusions demand obliteration of the pleural space [18].

The lung bases may be dull to percussion due to elevation of the diaphragm.

Oedema usually follows the ascites and is related to hypoproteinaemia. A functional inferior vena caval block due to pressure of the abdominal fluid is an additional factor.

The *cardiac apex beat* is displaced up and out, by the raised diaphragm.

The *neck veins* are distended. This is secondary to the increase in right auricular pressure and in-trapleural pressure which follows tense ascites and a raised diaphragm. A persisting increase in jugu-lar venous pressure after ascites is controlled implies a cardiac cause for the fluid retention.

Ascitic fluid and paracentesis abdominis

Diagnostic paracentesis (of about 50 ml) is always performed, however obvious the cause of the ascites. *Therapeutic* paracentesis is very rarely necessary unless the patient is in severe discomfort. Complications, including bowel perforation and haemorrhage, can develop after paracentesis in patients with cirrhosis. Special care must, there-fore, be taken [31].

Protein concentration rarely exceeds 1–2 g/100 ml. Higher values suggest infection. Obstruc-tion to the hepatic veins (Budd–Chiari syndrome) is usually, but not always, associated with a very high ascitic fluid protein. Pancreatic ascites is also found with a high ascitic protein value. *Electrolyte concentrations* are those of other extracellular fluids.

Fluid appears clear, green, straw-coloured or bile-stained. The volume is variable and up to 70 litres have been recorded. A blood-stained fluid in-dicates malignant disease or a recent paracentesis or invasive investigation, such as splenic veno-graphy or trans-hepatic cholangiography or veno-graphy.

The *volume* of the ascitic fluid can be approxi-mately estimated by a dilution method [2], but this is not usually necessary.

The *rate of accumulation of fluid* is variable and depends on the dietary intake of sodium and the ability of the kidney to excrete it. Rate of fluid re-absorption is limited to 700–900 ml daily.

The *pressure* exerted by the ascitic fluid rarely exceeds 10 mmHg above the right atrium. At high pressures discomfort makes paracentesis obliga-tory. Vasovagal fainting may follow too rapid release of ascites.

A *low sodium state* may follow paracentesis, especially if the patient has been on a restricted sodium intake. Approximately 1000 mEq of sodium are lost in every 7 litres of ascites. This is rapidly replenished from the blood and the serum sodium level falls. Water may be retained in excess of sodium. The patient collapses with weakness, abdominal distension, cramps, falling blood pressure, a low serum sodium and a raised blood urea level [32]. This syndrome is treated by 200 ml hypertonic (5%) sodium chloride intravenously.

Hepatic coma may be precipitated.

Peritonitis, bacteriology and leucocyte (WBC) counts

Infection of the ascitic fluid is very common. This may be 'spontaneous' or follow a previous para-centesis. The spontaneous type develops in about 8% of cirrhotic patients with ascites [14]. It is parti-cularly frequent if the cirrhosis is severely decom-pensated. In these instances the infection is usually part of a septicaemia [13]. Intra-arterial vasopres-sin therapy for upper gastro-intestinal haemor-rhage can predispose to peritonitis [4]. The arterial vasoconstriction presumably allows transmural migration of enteric organisms from the lumen of the bowel into the ascites-filled peritoneal cavity.

The ascitic fluid possesses humoral anti-microbial activity for Gram-negative organisms [20]. This seems to be complement-mediated and the alternate pathway may be particularly impor-tant. Susceptibility for Gram-negative spon-taneous bacterial peritonitis may be related to low C_3' concentrations in ascitic fluid in cirrhosis resulting in the lack of bactericidal activity. Absence of humoral antimicrobial activity against Gram-positive organisms may in part explain their relative prevalence in spontaneous bacterial peritonitis.

Spontaneous bacterial peritonitis should be sus-pected if the patient with known cirrhosis under-goes a sudden deterioration, particularly with encephalopathy. Pyrexia, local abdominal pain and tenderness and systemic leucocytosis may be noted. These features, however, are by no means constant and the diagnosis is made on the index of suspicion with examination of the ascitic fluid. This shows a WBC count exceeding 500 per mm^3 of which 75–100% are polymorphs [5]. Although the values are not conclusive evidence of bacterial peritonitis, they are sufficiently alarming to merit antibiotic therapy.

The infecting organisms are usually Gram-nega-tive coliforms or streptococci. The infection may be mixed. Other organisms described include meningococci [3], campylobacter fetus [40], a micro-aerophilic Gram-negative bacillus, and organisms of the pasteurella group [22]. Anaerobic bacteria are conspicuous by their near absence. In many instances, opportunist organisms are identified, often in patients with cirrhosis on corticosteroid therapy. The patient can present without any localizing or systemic evidences of peritonitis. The infection represents invasion of a pre-existing transudate, often by chance organisms. Centrifuged deposits of ascitic fluid are therefore stained by Gram's method and the fluid cultured.

Tuberculous peritonitis should be suspected particularly in the severely malnourished alcoholic. The patient is usually pyrexial. The cell count in the ascitic fluid is usually mononuclear. The deposit must always be stained for tubercle bacilli and suitable cultures set up.

Cytology of ascitic fluid is of little value. The normal endothelial cells in the peritoneum resemble malignant cells, so leading to an over-diagnosis of cancer.

Urine

The urine volume is diminished, deeply pigmented and of high osmolarity.

The daily urinary output of sodium is greatly reduced, usually less than 5 mEq and in a severe case less than 1 mEq.

Radiological features

Plain X-ray of the abdomen shows a diffuse 'ground-glass' appearance. Distended loops of bowel simulate intestinal obstruction. Ultrasound shows an echo-free space round the liver and can be used to demonstrate quite small amounts of fluid.

Differential diagnosis

Malignant ascites. There may be symptoms and localizing signs due to primary tumour. After paracentesis, the liver may be enlarged and nodular. The peritoneal fluid may be characteristic.

Tuberculous ascites. Abdominal distension is rarely great. After paracentesis lumps of matted omentum can be palpated. The ascitic fluid is of high protein content, usually with many lymphocytes and sometimes polymorphs. Tubercle bacilli may be cultured.

Constrictive pericarditis. Diagnostic points in-clude the very high jugular venous pressure, the paradoxical pulse, the radiological demonstration of a calcified pericardium and the characteristic electrocardiogram.

Hepatic venous obstruction (Budd–Chiari syndrome) must be considered, especially if the protein content of the ascitic fluid is high.

Ovarian tumour is suggested by resonance in the flanks. The maximum bulge is antero-posterior and the maximum girth is below the umbilicus.

Pancreatic ascites. This is rarely gross. It develops as a complication of acute pancreatitis. The amylase content of the ascitic fluid is very high.

TREATMENT

Indications

The availability of so many potent diuretics and of the patient with obvious ascites who will respond to them may seem a challenge to the physician. Therapy is positive and the results are apparent to one and all. The initial gratitude of the patient and his family may be overwhelming. Nevertheless, although the initial response may be excellent, the ultimate result can be a patient in renal failure or hepatic encephalopathy, 'dry and demented rather than wet and wise'. Indications for therapy must always be clear cut and caution must always be the working rule in deciding therapy.

The mere presence of ascites does not merit active treatment. Indications include:

Uncertain diagnosis. Control of ascites may allow such procedures as better abdominal examination, needle biopsy or splenic or trans-hepatic venography to be performed.

Gross ascites, i.e. it is so gross that it is causing abdominal pain and/or dyspnoea.

Tense ascites so that an umbilical hernia has ulcerated and is near to rupture. This complication has a very high mortality. The patient may develop shock and pass into renal failure.

Cosmetic reasons are only relative.

Management

Unless the ascites is very slight the patient will have to be admitted to hospital for diagnosis, general assessment and treatment. The control of ascites in patients with cirrhosis is more difficult than in other forms of fluid retention for diuretic therapy is liable to be followed by electrolyte disturbances, encephalopathy and renal failure.

The patient is confined to bed. Restriction of physical activity reduces metabolites which have to be handled by the liver. Renal perfusion increases in recumbency. He is weighed daily at the same time. Urine volume is measured. Urinary electrolyte determinations are helpful but are costly and not essential. Urine volume and body weight provide a satisfactory guide to progress. Abdominal girth is unreliable for gaseous distension is common. Serum electrolytes are measured twice weekly while in hospital.

The cirrhotic patient who is accumulating ascites on an unrestricted sodium intake excretes less than 10 mEq (0.2 g) sodium daily in the urine. Extra-renal loss is about 0.5 g. Sodium taken in excess of 0.75 g will result in ascites, every gram retaining 200 ml fluid. If the ascites is to be absorbed the daily intake of sodium must be restricted to less than 22 mEq (0.5 g) daily and even to less than 10 mEq daily. Fluid intake is restricted to one litre daily.

Diet: general remarks

1. Food to be cooked without added salt. No salt on table. Use salt substitute.
2. Use *salt-free* bread, crispbread, crackers or matzos and *salt-free* butter or margarine—as much as you like.
3. Seasonings such as lemon juice, orange peel, onion, vinegar, garlic, salt-free ketchup and mayonnaise, pepper, mustard, sage, parsley, thyme, marjoram, bay leaves, cloves or low-salt yeast extract, help to make salt-free foods more palatable.
4. **Omit** anything containing baking powder or baking soda. This includes pastry, biscuits, cake, self-raising flour and ordinary bread.
5. **Omit** pickles, olives, ham, bacon, corned beef, tongue, oyster, shell-fish, canned fish and meat, chutney, salad cream, meat and fish paste, bottled sauces, sausages, kippers and all cheese and ice cream.
6. **Omit** dry cereals, except shredded wheat, puffed wheat or sugar puffs. **Omit** salted canned foods. Regular canned fruit may be used in place of fresh fruit.
7. Meat or poultry, rabbit, tripe, sweetbreads or fish—4 oz (100 g) daily and one egg. Egg may be used as substitute for 2 oz (50 g) meat.

8. Do not use more than 10 oz ($\frac{1}{2}$ pint, $\frac{1}{4}$ litre) of milk daily. Heavy (double) cream is allowed.
9. Boiled rice (without salt) is permissible.
10. Eat fresh and home cooked fruit and vegetables of all kinds.
11. No candy, pastilles or milk chocolate.

Most protein-containing foods, such as meat, eggs and dairy produce, have a high sodium content and, to maintain a good protein intake, a low-sodium protein supplement should be taken, e.g. Casilan, Edosol or Lanolac. Salt-free bread and butter is used and all cooking is done without added salt. Many low-sodium foods are now available including soups, ketchups and crackers. It is possible to give a diet containing 1500–2000 calories, 70 g protein and only 22 mEq sodium (table 14). The patient should be virtually vegetarian.

Failure to adhere to a low-sodium diet is the usual reason for ascites to be termed 'resistant' or 'refractory'. In a severe case, even combinations of the newer diuretics in huge doses will not compensate for a high dietary sodium intake.

The patient may respond rapidly to this regime

Table 14. Specimen salt-free diet.

Calories 2000–2200. Protein 70 g (approx)
Sodium 380–450 mg (18–20 mEq)

Breakfast
Shredded wheat with cream and sugar or stewed fruit
2 oz (60 g) salt-free bread or Matzos or salt-free Ryvita, unsalted butter, marmalade or jelly or honey
1 egg or 2 oz white fish
Tea or coffee with milk from allowance

Lunch
2 oz meat or poultry or 3 oz white fish
Potatoes
Green vegetables or salad
Fresh or stewed fruit

Tea
2 oz salt-free bread or Matzos
Unsalted butter, jam, honey or tomato
Tea or coffee with milk from allowance

Supper
Grapefruit or salt-free soup
Meat, fish or poultry as for lunch
Potatoes
Green vegetables or salad
Fresh or stewed fruit or jelly made with fruit juice and gelatine
Heavy cream
Coffee or tea with milk from allowance

without the need for diuretics. Such easy responders are liable to be those:

—with ascites and oedema presenting for the first time—'virgin' ascites;
—with a 24-hour urine sodium excretion of more than 10 mEq;
—with a normal glomerular filtration rate (creatinine clearance);
—with underlying reversible liver disease such as fatty liver of the alcoholic;
—in whom the ascites has developed acutely in response to a treatable complication such as infection or bleeding;
—with ascites following excessive sodium intake, such as in sodium-containing antacids or purgatives, or spa waters with a high sodium content.

Diuretics

These should be given only if the weight loss is less than 2 lb (1 kg) after four days on the dietetic and fluid restriction regime alone. The dose and frequency of administration must be calculated for each individual patient. Too rapid diuresis must be followed by stopping the diuretic; too slow by increasing the dose or frequency.

Therapy is aimed at blocking all the renal sodium-conserving mechanisms. Diuretics can be divided into two main groups (table 15, fig. 102). The first group comprises the thiazides, frusemide, bumetamide, piretamide and ethacrynic acid. These are powerful natriuretic agents, but also powerful kaliuretics. Potassium chloride supplements are always necessary when these diuretics are given alone to cirrhotic patients.

The second group comprises spironolactone (an aldosterone antagonist), amiloride and triamterene. These are weakly natriuretic but conserve potassium. When they are combined with a group

Table 15. Diuretics for ascites.

Urine loss			
Group 1			
Na^{++}	K^{++}		Thiazides
			Frusemide
			Ethacrynic acid
			Bumetamide
			Piretamide
Group 2			
Na^+	K^-		Spironolactone
			Triamterene
			Amiloride

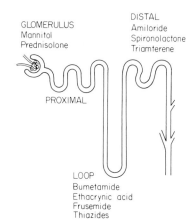

Fig. 102. The site of action of diuretics.

I diuretic, the potassium chloride supplements are reduced and may even become unnecessary. In general it is advisable to start with one of these diuretics and then add a first group diuretic as required (figs 103, 104).

The choice of a diuretic from the first group depends on effectiveness, length of action, incidence of complications and cost. The longer acting diuretics, such as the thiazides and ethacrynic acid, have disadvantages in patients with liver disease because the action may continue when electrolyte disturbances have already developed. The patient may thus continue to lose urinary potassium and become more alkalotic even after stopping the diuretic. Frusemide or bumetamide are the drugs of choice. The best second group diuretic is amiloride but, if unobtainable, spironolactone may be used. It has the disadvantage of causing gynaecomastia in cirrhotic males. Satisfactory control is usual and failures are in those with very poor hepato-cellular function who are usually dead within six months of starting therapy (table 16). In such refractory patients diuretics have eventually had to be withdrawn because of intractable uraemia, hypotension or encephalopathy.

Complications are avoided by treating the ascites slowly [15] and allowing at least two weeks in hospital. From time to time diuretics need to be stopped for a few days. The rate of ascitic fluid re-absorption is limited to 700–900 ml a day. If a diuresis of some 3 litres is induced much of the fluid must have come from non-ascitic extracellular fluids including oedema fluid and the intravenous compartment. This is safe as long as oedema persists, but if the diuresis continues and exceeds the limits of ascites absorption in the

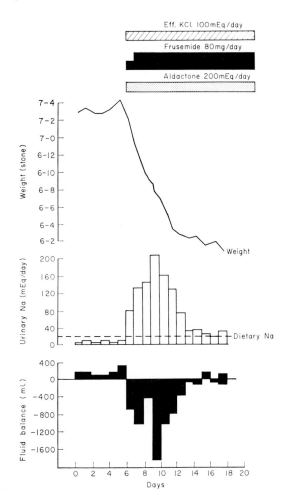

Fig. 103. Before treatment this patient with hepatic cirrhosis and ascites excreted less than 10 mEq sodium daily in the urine and was in positive fluid balance. He was treated with frusemide 80 mg and aldactone 200 mg a day with extra potassium chloride 100 mEq a day. A marked natriuresis ensued. Fluid balance became negative and body weight dropped 15 lb (33 kg) in two weeks.

absence of oedema, then the plasma volume would fall. Renal perfusion is reduced and the stage is set for the development of functional renal failure (hepato-renal syndrome).

The general management of ascites using diuretics is shown in table 17.

In a few patients, on discharge from hospital, diuretics are no longer required. In the majority, however, the diuretic and dietetic regime has to be continued according to the individual needs.

COMPLICATIONS (table 18)

Encephalopathy

This follows any profound diuresis (table 18). The mechanism is uncertain. It is usually thought to be associated with hypokalaemia [35]. There is an overall correlation with any form of electrolyte

imbalance in patients with cirrhosis and perhaps most closely with hypochloraemic alkalosis.

Encephalopathy should be recognized early by daily examination for confusion and 'flapping' tremor. The diuretic is then stopped, serum electrolyte levels are checked, dietary protein is withdrawn and a purge given.

Electrolyte disturbances

These are frequent [38]. The development of a profound serum electrolyte abnormality with azotaemia indicates a very poor prognosis. This probably reflects the severity of the underlying liver disease. Large doses of potent diuretics in seriously ill patients with cirrhosis and ascites may induce a diuresis, but the terminal, hyponatraemic azotaemic state ('hepato-renal syndrome') may be accelerated.

Hypokalaemia reflects not only diuretic effect but also secondary hyperaldosteronism. Its incidence is reduced by adding a potassium-sparing diuretic (table 15). The serum potassium level is an inaccurate but simple estimate of body potassium, particularly so in liver disease. Levels of less than 3.1 mEq/l indicate severe potassium depletion.

Such levels necessitate stopping the diuretic and giving potassium *chloride* supplements.

Hyponatraemia reflects urinary excretion of sodium in excess of water in patients on a greatly restricted sodium intake. In the particularly ill terminal patient it may also indicate the passage of sodium into the cells. When combined with

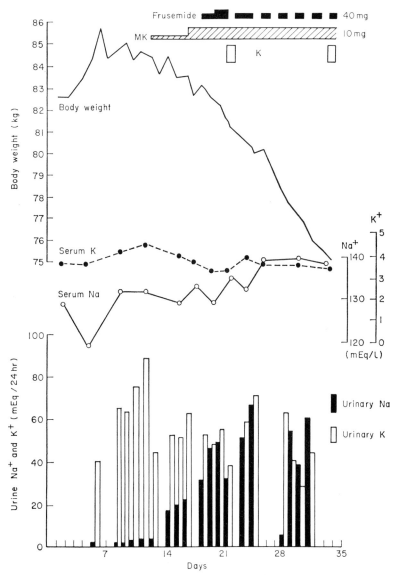

Fig. 104. Hepatic cirrhosis with ascites. Before treatment the urinary sodium was less than 5 mEq and potassium greater than 60 mEq per 24 hours, reflecting marked secondary hyperaldosteronism. The patient was first treated with amiloride (MK), 5–10 mg a day. When this was combined with frusemide 40–80 mg every other day a profound natriuresis ensued but urinary potassium did not increase. Body weight fell 9 kg in three weeks. Potassium supplements (K) were given on only two occasions. The serum potassium level did not fall below 3.5 mEq/l.

Table 16. Dietetic and diuretic control of ascites.

No. patients	Controlled
157	148 (94%)
Failures all dead in 6 months	

Table 17. General management of ascites.

1 Bed rest. 22 mEq Na diet. Restrict fluids to 1
   litre daily.
   Check serum (if possible urinary) electrolytes.
   Weigh daily. Measure urinary volume.
   Add KCl 100 mEq daily.

2 After four days if weight loss less than 1 kg start
   spironolactone 100 mg or amiloride 10 mg daily.
   Reduce KCl to 50 mEq daily.

3 After one more day check serum electrolytes.
   Add frusemide 80 mg or bumetamide 1 mg daily
   as required.

4 After four more days check serum electrolytes. If
   weight loss less than 2 kg, amiloride 10 mg twice
   daily or spironolactone 200 mg daily.

5 If necessary increase frusemide to 120 mg daily.
   Stop diuretic drugs if pre-coma ('flap'),
   hypokalaemia, azotaemia or alkalosis or weight
   loss more than 0.5 kg daily.

other electrolyte abnormalities it indicates a particularly bad prognosis and has similar significance to the terminal hyponatraemic state [23]. It is treated by stopping the diuretic and restricting fluid intake to 500 ml or even less per day. Alternatively, mannitol (2 litres 10% intravenously) will act as an osmotic diuretic and increase free water clearance. Prednisolone has the same result for it increases the glomerular filtration rate and reduces tubular re-absorption of water. Unfortunately, fulminant infections often complicate use of prednisolone in these patients.

The clinician may be tempted to give sodium supplements. In fact body stores of sodium and water are excessive and giving more sodium will only lead to gain in weight and pulmonary oedema. It is therefore contraindicated.

Hypochloraemic alkalosis complicates treatment with potent diuretics such as frusemide and ethacrynic acid given alone. It is due to urinary sodium and chloride loss with normal tubular re-absorption of bicarbonate. Hypokalaemia is not a necessary accompaniment. This complication can be repaired only by chloride replacement.

Hyperchloraemic acidosis can complicate spironolactone therapy in alcoholic cirrhosis [21].

Azotaemia in cirrhotic patients reflects altered renal circulation rather than any lesion of the parenchyma [25] (fig. 105). A brisk diuresis results in contraction of the extracellular fluid volume and accentuates this tendency. The greater the potency of the diuretic, the greater the azotaemia. When azotaemia is part of a profound electrolyte disturbance the prognosis is poor. Many of these patients will progress to the terminal picture of renal failure.

Follow-up advice

On discharge from hospital the patient should adhere to the strict low sodium diet as far as possible. He should purchase bathroom scales and weigh himself daily, naked. A daily record should be kept and brought to the physician at each attendance.

Diuretics should be continued. The dose depends on the severity of the liver disease. A usual routine is 100–200 mg spironolactone or 10–20 mg amiloride daily with frusemide 40–80 mg every

Table 18. Diuretics in cirrhosis—percentage of complications.

	No.	Hepatic encephalopathy	Serum†		
			K	Na	Urea
Chlorothiazide	31	22	55	40	22
+K sparer*	39	28	16	49	31
Frusemide	17	26	64	43	43
+K sparer*	24	4	16	40	40

* Spironolactone or amiloride.
† Serum potassium level < 3.1 mEq/l, serum sodium level < 130 mEq/l, blood urea level > 40 mg/dl.

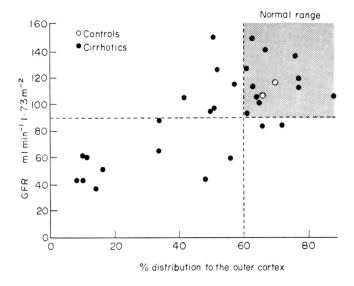

Fig. 105. Distribution of renal blood flow measured by injection of ^{133}xenon into the renal artery and external counting. Cirrhotic patients tend to have reduced distribution of renal blood to the outer cortex and this may be present with a normal creatinine clearance (GFR) (Kew *et al* 1971).

other day. Potassium chloride supplements, about 50 mEq potassium daily, are given. Serum electrolytes, blood urea nitrogen and liver function tests are monitored every four weeks. As liver function improves it may become possible to stop first the frusemide and then the spironolactone or amiloride. Finally the low sodium diet is relaxed, first to 'no added salt' and then to a normal diet.

'REFRACTORY' ASCITES

The majority of patients will respond to the dietary diuretic regime (table 17). Failures indicate either failure to comply or such severe liver failure that the patient is terminal. In some patients, however, ascites is gross and diuretics have to be pushed to extreme doses in an attempt to produce a diuresis. In such refractory patients there is particular danger of depletion of the intravascular compartment and the development of the hepato-renal syndrome. In these resistant cases alternative therapy must be considered. Large paracenteses are contraindicated because of the loss of albumin with the fluid and the temporary effect. The infusion of dextran, salt-poor albumin or ascitic fluid itself expands the plasma volume and may initiate diuresis, albeit temporarily.

Porta-caval anastomosis

Side-to-side porta-caval shunt decompresses splanchnic veins and relieves the hepatic venous outflow block (fig. 153).

Ascites implies defective hepato-cellular function. The mortality of porta-caval anastomoses when performed for ascites is very high, even 35.2% [45]. Hypoalbuminaemia persists post-operatively. When the portal pressure falls, fluid no longer localizes in the abdomen but peripheral oedema develops instead. Post-operatively, neuro-psychiatric complications of varying degree are extremely frequent in these patients.

Ascites ultrafiltration and reinfusion (fig. 106) [33, 34, 42]

The automated ultrafiltration apparatus (Rhodiascit) removes ascitic fluid via a peritoneal dialysis catheter and passes it over an ultrafilter which selects molecules of less than 50000. The concentrate, which contains two to four times as much protein as the ascitic fluid, is returned to the patient intravenously. Up to 13 litres of ascites can be removed in 24 hours. Weight loss is greater than would be accounted for by the volume of fluid ultrafiltered because urine flow increases during and after the procedure (fig. 107). The patient is more responsive to diuretics. High-protein ascitic fluids clog the membrane and the technique is unsuitable for malignant ascites. Infection of the fluid is also a contraindication. The procedure is costly, but this must be weighed against the price of a longer stay in hospital. Transient pyrexia, pulmonary oedema and intraperitoneal haemorrhage are complications. Central venous pressure rises in almost all instances so that the infusion rate must

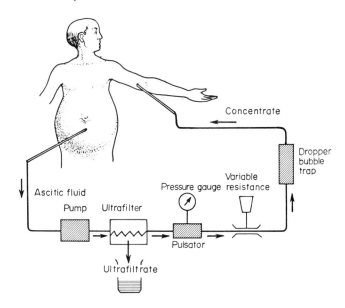

Fig. 106. The concentration–reinfusion technique for removal of ascitic fluid (Parbhoo *et al* 1974).

be monitored else fluid overload may lead to heart failure and precipitate variceal haemorrhage.

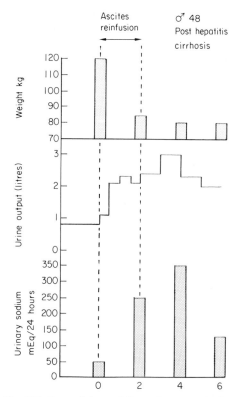

Fig. 107. Successful use of the ascites concentration–reinfusion technique. In two days, body weight fell 36 kg. Urine output increased and urinary sodium output rose.

LeVeen shunt

This peritoneal–venous shunt system gives more continuous treatment over many months [27]. The peritoneal cavity is drained by a long perforated plastic tube that reaches into the pelvis. This connects with a special pressure-sensitive valve lying extraperitoneally and deep through the abdominal muscles. This again connects with a silicone rubber tube which passes subcutaneously from the abdominal wound towards the neck and so into the internal jugular vein. The end of the tube is left in position in the superior vena cava. The operation is performed under antibiotic cover with local anaesthesia although occasionally a light general anaesthetic is necessary. As the diaphragm descends during inspiration the intraperitoneal fluid pressure rises whereas that in the intrathoracic superior vena cava falls. This results in a pressure differential of about 5 cm H_2O. Respiration provides the force which opens the valve and propels the fluid into the superior vena cava. The venous tube remains patent only when its interior contains ascitic fluid. The specially designed pressure-sensitive valve totally prevents entry of blood into the venous tubing.

Well over 300 treated patients have been reported. Ten of 22 patients treated after 1973 survived at least 12 months [27]. The technique may be particularly useful in the Budd–Chiari syndrome. The shunt has been used to manage the hepato-renal syndrome [43]. Complications include fever, leakage of peritoneal fluid, blocked shunt, infections both subcutaneous and systemic, and bacterial endocarditis. Disseminated intravascular coagulation always occurs and occasionally may be severe and fatal. Complications are numerous and severe in those who have severe underlying hepato-cellular failure. The patient with well compensated cirrhosis and ascites as a major problem may do exceedingly well with improved nutrition, rise in serum albumin levels, increased urinary flow and continued control of ascites.

With the modern diuretic and dietetic regimes, such an operation as the LeVeen shunt should rarely be necessary. It may be useful in those who cannot co-operate with diet and diuretics, the alcoholic who insists on imbibing, and those coming from countries where medical services are insufficient to manage the diet and diuretic regime.

Prognosis

Despite modern dietetic and diuretic measures the prognosis is always grave after ascites develops in a patient with cirrhosis. It is better if the ascites has accumulated rapidly, especially if there is a well defined precipitating factor such as gastrointestinal haemorrhage.

Even with adequate treatment, a patient with cirrhosis developing ascites has only a 40% chance of being alive two years later. Much depends on the major factor in the aetiology of the fluid retention. If liver cell failure, evidenced by jaundice and hepatic encephalopathy, is severe, the prognosis is poor. If the major factor is a particularly high portal pressure, the patient may respond well to treatment.

Ascites cannot be divorced from the underlying liver disease that caused it and, although it may be controlled, the patient is still liable to die from another complication such as haemorrhage, hepatic coma or primary liver cancer. It is questioned whether control of ascites *per se* increases life span. It certainly makes the patient more comfortable.

FUNCTIONAL RENAL FAILURE ('HEPATO-RENAL SYNDROME') [23, 24, 37, 47]

Renal failure in patients with hepato-cellular failure may be due to primary kidney disease or acute tubular necrosis due to haemorrhage or in-

Table 19. Diagnosis of hepato-renal syndrome.

Chronic liver disease with ascites
Slow onset azotaemia (plasma creatinine > 1.5 mg/dl)
Tubular function good
  Urine to plasma osmolarity ratio > 1.0
  Urine to plasma creatinine ratio > 30
  Urine sodium concentration < 10 mEq/dl
No sustained benefit by expansion of intravascular spaces

fection. However, in most instances the uraemia and oliguria arise either spontaneously or in response to changes in blood volume or shifts of fluid within body compartments. The histology of the kidney is virtually normal and the failure is a functional one. Such kidneys have even been successfully transplanted when they functioned normally [26]. Conversely apparently moribund patients with this syndrome have returned to normal kidney function after liver transplantation.

The syndrome is marked by renal failure with normal tubular function in a patient with chronic liver disease (table 19).

The renal failure is often initiated by reduction in the intravascular volume due to over-vigorous diuretic therapy, paracentesis or diarrhoea. It may develop without a precipitant. The classical features of uraemia are usually absent. The syndrome is particularly common in patients with end-stage alcoholic cirrhosis. The prognosis is extremely grave.

In the mildest pre-azotaemic stage, renal dysfunction is shown by failure to excrete a water load, reduction in urinary sodium excretion and hyponatraemia. Hepatic dysfunction is usually severe and ascites is usual.

The more advanced stages are characterized by progressive azotaemia usually with hepatic failure and ascites difficult to control. The patient complains of anorexia, weakness and fatigue. The blood urea concentration is raised. Hyponatraemia is invariable. Sodium is avidly re-absorbed by the renal tubules and urine osmolarity is increased. Fluid accumulates in spite of a normal urinary volume, dietary sodium restriction and diuretic therapy. In the later stages nausea, vomiting and thirst are added. The patient is drowsy. The picture may be indistinguishable from that of hepatic encephalopathy.

The serum urea and creatinine levels rise progressively. The serum sodium is usually less than 120 mEq/l. Urinalysis is virtually normal. Urinary sodium excretion is very low. Ascites is refractory.

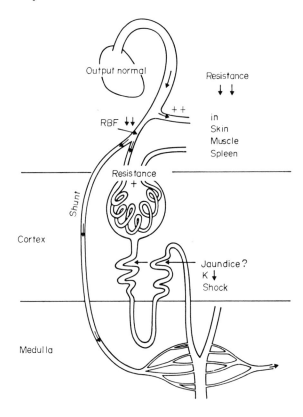

Fig. 108. Factors contributing to renal failure in cirrhosis ('hepato-renal syndrome').

Terminally, coma deepens, blood pressure drops and urine volume falls even more. The terminal stages last from a few days to more than six weeks [37].

It may be difficult to distinguish hepatic from renal failure although the patients die with biochemical azotaemia rather than the full clinical picture of kidney failure [24]. Death is due to liver failure; survival depends on the reversibility of the *liver* disease.

Mechanisms

Renal failure is related to a reduction of effective renal circulation (see fig. 105) [28]. Cardiac output is normal or even increased but is distributed to skin, splanchnic area, spleen and brain so that renal plasma flow is reduced. Changes in intrarenal circulation are of great importance. An increased pre-glomerular vascular resistance leads to reduced glomerular filtration rate and plasma renin rises. Blood flow is thus diverted away from the renal cortex [25] (see fig. 108). This change in intrarenal distribution of blood flow can be shown even in well-compensated cirrhotic patients. It

may explain their susceptibility to develop oliguric renal failure after haemorrhage not sufficiently large to reduce the blood pressure or after minor shifts of fluid within body compartments, such as with abdominal paracentesis [25] or diuretic therapy. Reduced effective plasma volume may be a factor. Volume expansion may increase renal blood flow and institute a diuresis, but the response is not maintained and variceal haemorrhage may be precipitated. Endotoxaemia may be an important contributory factor [12].

Treatment

The syndrome is prevented by avoiding diuretic overdose, by treating ascites slowly and by early recognition of any complication such as electrolyte imbalance, haemorrhage or infection. The conservative management is that of renal and hepatic failure whatever the cause. Hepatic failure holds the key to the problem and must be treated. Conservative measures include restriction of fluids, sodium, potassium and protein, and withdrawal of potentially nephrotoxic drugs such as neomycin. Blood cultures should be taken and any septicaemia treated appropriately. Mannitol is useless and may lead to intracellular acidosis. High doses of frusemide are unavailing and are hepatotoxic. Renal dialysis does not improve survival and may precipitate gastro-intestinal haemorrhage and shock.

The renal cortical circulatory failure has been related to the action of false neuro-transmitter amines of intestinal origin [19]. This has led to the administration of such drugs as L-dopa or metara-minol; they have not been successful. Introduction of a peritoneo-jugular (LeVeen) shunt has resulted in improved renal function in ascitic patients with refractory ascites [43]. However, this technique in patients with the hepato-renal syndrome and advanced liver failure is not recommended as disseminated intravascular coagulation and death are usually precipitated.

Terminal hyponatraemia [23] is in part dilutional (over-hydration), in part due to over-administration of diuretics and in part to redistribution of sodium, a raised proportion occurring in the intracellular compartments. It should not be treated

with intravenous hypertonic sodium chloride as pulmonary oedema will develop and death will be accelerated.

The final combination of azotaemia, hyponatraemia and hypotension is terminal and quite unresponsive to all forms of therapy.

REFERENCES

1. BAGGENSTOSS A.H. & CAIN J.C. (1957) The hepatic hilar lymphatics of man. *N. Engl. J. Med.* **256**, 531.
2. BAKER L., PUESTOW R.C., KRUGER S. *et al* (1952) Estimation of ascitic fluid volumes. *J. lab. clin. Med.* **39**, 30.
3. BAR-MEIR S., CHOJKIER M., GROSZMANN R.J. *et al* (1978) Spontaneous meningococcal peritonitis. A report of two cases. *Am. J. dig. Dis.* **23**, 119.
4. BAR-MEIR S. & CONN H.O. (1976) Spontaneous bacterial peritonitis reduced by intra-arterial vasopressin therapy. *Gastroenterology* **70**, 418.
5. BAR-MEIR S., LERNER E. & CONN H.O. (1979) Analysis of ascitic fluid in cirrhosis. *Dig. Dis. Sci.* **24**, 136.
6. BIRKENFELD L.W., LEIBMAN J., O'MEARA M.P. *et*

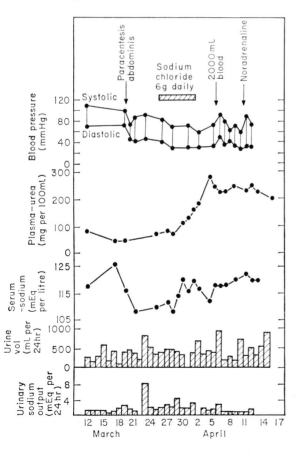

Fig. 109. Terminal sub-acute virus hepatitis. Note the low blood pressure which was only temporarily increased by blood transfusion and noradrenaline. Serum sodium values and urinary sodium excretion were profoundly depressed and were uninfluenced by oral sodium chloride. Blood urea rose progressively in the last two weeks (Hecker & Sherlock 1956).

al (1958) Total exchangeable sodium, total exchangeable potassium, and total body water in edematous patients with cirrhosis of the liver and congestive heart failure. *J. clin. Invest.* **37**, 687.

7. BOLTON C. (1914) The pathological changes in the liver resulting from passive venous congestion experimentally produced. *J. Path. Bact.* **19**, 258.

8. BOYER T.D., ZIA P. & REYNOLDS T.B. (1979) Effect of indomethacin and prostaglandin A1 on renal function and plasma renin activity in alcoholic liver disease. *Gastroenterology* **77**, 215.

9. CASEY T.H., SUMMERSKILL W.H.J. & ORVIS A.L. (1965) Body and serum potassium in liver disease. I. Relationship to hepatic function and associated factors. *Gastroenterology* **48**, 198.

10. CHART J.J., GORDON E.S., HELMER P. *et al* (1956) Metabolism of salt-retaining hormone by surviving liver slices. *J. clin. Invest.* **35**, 254.

11. CHERRICK G.R., KERR D.N.S., READ A.E. *et al* (1960) Colloid osmotic pressure and hydrostatic pressure relationships in the formation of ascites in hepatic cirrhosis. *Clin. Sci.* **19**, 361.

12. CLEMENTE C., BOSCH J., RODÉS J. *et al* (1977) Functional renal failure and haemorrhagic gastritis associated with endotoxaemia in cirrhosis. *Gut* **18**, 556.

13. CONN H.O. (1964) Spontaneous peritonitis and bacteremia in Laennec's cirrhosis caused by enteric organisms. *Ann. intern. Med.* **60**, 1964.

14. CONN H.O. (1976) Spontaneous bacterial peritonitis. Multiple revisitations. *Gastroenterology* **70**, 455.

15. CONN H.O. (1977) Diuresis of ascites: fraught with or free from hazard. *Gastroenterology* **73**, 619.

16. DE WARDENER H.E. (1977) Natriuretic hormone. *Clin Sci. mol. Med.* **53**, 1.

17. EPSTEIN M. (1979) Deranged sodium homeostasis in cirrhosis. *Gastroenterology* **76**, 622.

18. FALCHUK K.R., JACOBY I., COLUCCI W.S. *et al* (1977) Tetracycline-induced pleural symphysis for recurrent hydrothorax complicating cirrhosis. *Gastroenterology* **72**, 319.

19. FISCHER J.E. & JAMES J.H. (1972) Treatment of hepatic coma and hepatorenal syndrome: mechanism of action of L-dopa and Aramine. *Am. J. Surg.* **123**, 222.

20. FROMKES J.J., THOMAS F.B., MEKHJIAN H.S. *et al* (1977) Antimicrobial activity of human ascitic fluid. *Gastroenterology* **73**, 668.

21. GABOW P.A., MOORE S. & SCHRIER R.W. (1979) Spironolactone-induced hyperchloremic acidosis in cirrhosis. *Ann. intern. Med.* **90**, 338.

22. GERDING D.N., KHAN M.Y., EWING J.W. *et al* (1976) *Pasturella multocida* peritonitis in hepatic cirrhosis with ascites. *Gastroenterology* **70**, 413.

23. HECKER R. & SHERLOCK S. (1956) Electrolyte and circulatory changes in terminal liver failure. *Lancet* ii, 1121.

24. KEW M. (1972) Renal changes in cirrhosis. *Gut* **13**, 748.

25. KEW M.C., BRUNT P.W., VARMA R.R. *et al* (1971) Renal and intrarenal blood-flow in cirrhosis of the liver. *Lancet* ii, 504.

26. KOPPEL M.H., COBURN J.W., MIMS M.M. *et al* (1969) Transplantation of cadaveric kidneys from patients with hepatorenal syndrome. *N. Engl. J. Med.* **280**, 1367.

27. LEVEEN H.H., WAPNICK S., GROSBERG S. *et al* (1976) Further experience with peritoneo-venous shunt for ascites. *Ann. Surg.* **184**, 574.

28. LIEBERMAN F.L. (1970) Functional renal failure in cirrhosis. *Gastroenterology* **58**, 108.

29. LIEBERMAN F.L., HIDEMURA R., PETERS R.L. *et al* (1966) Pathogenesis and treatment of hydrothorax complicating cirrhosis with ascites. *Ann. intern. Med.* **64**, 341.

30. LIEBERMAN F.L., ITO S. & REYNOLDS T.B. (1969) Effective plasma volume in cirrhosis with ascites. Evidence that a decreased value does not account for renal sodium retention, a spontaneous reduction in glomerular filtration rate (GFR), and a fall in GFR during drug-induced diuresis. *J. clin. Invest.* **48**, 975.

31. MALLORY A. & SCHAEFER J.W. (1978) Complications of diagnostic paracentesis in patients with liver disease. *JAMA* **239**, 628.

32. MARTINI G.A. & RAUSCH-STROOMANN J.G. (1959) Das hyponatriämiesyndrom nach kochsalzfreier Kost, erzwungener Diurese und/oder Ascitesponktion bei chronischer Leberinsuffizienz. *Klin. Wschr.* **37**, 835.

33. MOULT P.J.A., PARBHOO S.P. & SHERLOCK S. (1975) Clinical experience with the Rhone-Poulenc ascites reinfusion apparatus. *Postgrad. med. J.* **51**, 574.

34. PARBHOO S.P., AJDUKIEWICZ A. & SHERLOCK S. (1974) Treatment of ascites by continuous ultra-filtration and reinfusion of protein concentrate. *Lancet* i, 949.

35. READ A.E., LAIDLAW J., HASLAM R.M. *et al* (1959) Neuropsychiatric complications following chlorothiazide therapy in patients with hepatic cirrhosis: possible relation to hypokalaemia. *Clin. Sci.* **18**, 409.

36. ROSOFF L. Jr, ZIA P., REYNOLDS T. *et al* (1975) Studies of renin and aldosterone in cirrhotic patients with ascites. *Gastroenterology* **69**, 698.

37. SHEAR L., HALL P.W. III & GABUZDA G.J. (1965) Renal failure in patients with cirrhosis of the liver. II. Factors influencing maximal urinary flow rate. *Am. J. Med.* **39**, 199.

38. SHERLOCK S., SENEWIRATNE B., SCOTT A. *et al* (1966) Complications of diuretic therapy in hepatic cirrhosis. *Lancet* i, 1049.

39. STARLING E.H. (1896) On the absorption of fluids from the connective tissue spaces. *J. Physiol. (Lond.)* **19**, 312.

40. TARGAN S.R., CHOW A.W. & GUZE L.B. (1976) Spontaneous peritonitis of cirrhosis due to *Campylobacter fetus*. *Gastroenterology* **71**, 311.

41. TAVILL A.S., CRAIGIE A. & ROSENOER V.M. (1968) The measurement of the synthetic rate of albumin in man. *Clin. Sci.* **34**, 1.

42. VILLENEUVE J.P., THOUT C., MARLEAU D. *et al* (1977) Treatment of resistant ascites by continuous infiltration–reinfusion of ascitic fluid. *Can. med. Assoc. J.* **117**, 1296.

43. WAPNICK S., GROSBERG S., KINNEY M. *et al* (1978) Renal failure in ascites secondary to hepatic, renal and pancreatic disease. *Arch. Surg.* **113**, 581.

44. WEBB L. & SHERLOCK S. (1979) Extra-hepatic portal venous destruction. *Q. J. Med.* **48,** 627.

45. WELCH H.F., WELCH C.S. & CARTER J.H. (1964) Prognosis after surgical treatment of ascites: results of side-to-side shunt in 40 patients. *Surgery* **56,** 75.

46. WONG P.Y., COLMAN R.W., TALAMO R.C. *et al* (1972) Kallikrein–bradykinin system in chronic alcoholic liver disease. *Ann. intern. Med.* **77,** 205.

47. WONG P.Y., McCOY G.C., SPIELBERG A. *et al* (1979) The hepatorenal syndrome. *Gastroenterology* **77,** 1326.

48. ZIMMON D.S., ORATZ M., KESSLER R. *et al* (1969) Albumin to ascites: demonstration of a direct pathway bypassing the systemic circulation. *J. clin. Invest.* **48,** 2074.

49. ZIPSER R., HOEFS J., SPECKART P. *et al* (1977) Prostaglandins: a critical modulator of renin release, blood pressure and renal function in liver disease. *Clin. Res.* **25,** 151A.

Chapter 11
The Portal Venous System and Portal Hypertension

The portal system includes all veins which carry blood from the abdominal part of the alimentary tract, the spleen, pancreas and gall bladder. The portal vein enters the liver at the porta hepatis in two main branches, one to each lobe; it is without valves in its larger channels [30].

The *portal vein* is formed by the union of the superior mesenteric vein and the splenic vein just posterior to the head of the pancreas at about the level of the second lumbar vertebra. It extends slightly to the right of the midline for a distance of 5.5–8 cm to the porta hepatis. The portal vein has a segmental, intra-hepatic distribution.

The *superior mesenteric vein* is formed by tributaries from the small intestine, colon and head of the pancreas, and irregularly from the stomach via the right gastro-epiploic vein.

The *splenic veins* (5–15 channels) originate at the splenic hilum and join near the tail of the pancreas with the short gastric vessels to form the main splenic vein. This proceeds in a transverse direction in the body and head of the pancreas, lying below and in front of the artery. It receives numerous tributaries from the head of the pancreas, and the left gastro-epiploic vein enters it near the spleen. The *inferior mesenteric vein* bringing blood from the left part of the colon and rectum usually enters its medial third. Occasionally, however, it enters the junction of superior mesenteric and splenic veins.

Portal blood flow in man is about 1000–1200 ml/min.

Portal oxygen content. The fasting arterioportal oxygen difference is only 1.9 volumes per cent (range 0.4–3.3 volumes per cent) [120] and the portal vein contributes 40 ml/min or 72% of the total oxygen supply to the liver.

During digestion, the arterioportal venous oxygen difference increases due to increased intestinal utilization [120]. The portal vein is therefore an undependable source of oxygen, supplying least during digestion when hepatic activity is greatest.

Stream-lines in the portal vein. There is no consistent pattern of hepatic distribution of portal inflow. Using portal venography and radio-isotopic

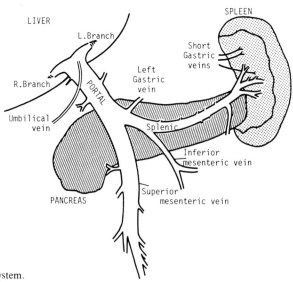

Fig. 110. The anatomy of the portal venous system.

methods, some workers have shown stream-lining [40] while others have not [45]. Scinti-photospleno-portography, injecting only 1 ml ^{99m}Tc into the spleen with gamma scanning over the liver, has shown that sometimes splenic blood goes to the left and sometimes to the right lobe [58]. Crossing-over of the blood stream can occur in the human portal vein. Flow is probably stream-lined rather than turbulent.

Hepatotrophic factors in the portal vein may determine hepato-cellular regeneration [92].

Portal pressure. In normal man this is about 7 mmHg.

Collateral circulation

When the portal circulation is obstructed, whether it be within or outside the liver, a remarkable collateral circulation develops to carry portal blood into the systemic veins (fig. 111).

Intra-hepatic obstruction (cirrhosis)

Normally 100% of the portal vein blood flow can be recovered from the hepatic veins whereas in cirrhosis only 13% is obtained [67]. The remainder enters collateral channels which form four main groups.

Group I: Where protective epithelium adjoins absorptive epithelium:

(*a*) At the cardia of the stomach, where the left gastric (coronary) vein and short gastric veins of the portal system anastomose with the intercostal, diaphragmo-oesophageal and azygos minor veins of the caval system. Deviation of blood into these channels leads to varicosities in the submucous layer of the lower end of the oesophagus and upper part of the stomach.

(*b*) At the anus the superior haemorrhoidal vein of the portal system anastomoses with the middle and inferior haemorrhoidal veins of the caval system. Deviation of blood into these channels may lead to haemorrhoids.

Group II: In the falciform ligament through the para-umbilical veins, relics of the umbilical circulation of the foetus (fig. 112).

Group III: Where the abdominal organs are in contact with retroperitoneal tissues or adherent to the abdominal wall. These collaterals include veins from the liver to the diaphragm, veins in the lieno-renal ligament and omentum, lumbar veins and veins developing in the scars of previous laparotomies.

Group IV: Portal venous blood is carried to the left renal vein (fig. 127). This may be through blood entering directly from the splenic vein or via diaphragmatic, pancreatic, left adrenal or gastric veins.

Blood from the left gastric, short gastric, retro-peritoneal and venous systems of the abdominal wall ultimately reaches the superior vena cava via the azygos or hemiazygos systems. A small volume enters the inferior vena cava. Collaterals running to the pulmonary veins have also been described.

Extra-hepatic obstruction

Additional collaterals are found, for blood is trying to bypass an extra-hepatic block and so return *towards* the liver. These enter the portal vein in the porta hepatis beyond the block. They include the veins at the hilum; venae comitantes of the portal vein and hepatic artery; veins in the suspensory ligaments of the liver; diaphragmatic and omental veins. The larger oesophageal, gastric, rectal, spleno-renal and lumbar collaterals may also be prominent, especially if the block is extensive, when return of blood through the vena cava is necessary.

Effects

When the liver cell is cut off from portal blood by the development of the collateral circulation it depends more and more on blood from the hepatic artery. Hepatic function is impaired, perhaps by deprivation of the hepatotrophic factors and other factors carried in the portal vein. The liver as a whole atrophies. Collaterals usually imply portal hypertension, although occasionally if the collateral circulation is very extensive, portal pressure may fall (fig. 117). Conversely, portal hypertension of short duration can exist without a demonstrable collateral circulation.

The diversion of portal blood into the collateral may be so great that in a splenic venogram the portal vein seems to be empty.

The large portal–systemic shunt may lead to chronic portal–systemic encephalopathy, septi-caemias due to intestinal organisms and there may be other circulatory and metabolic effects.

Pathology of portal hypertension

Collateral venous circulation is disappointingly insignificant at autopsy. This is particularly true of oesophageal varices which collapse.

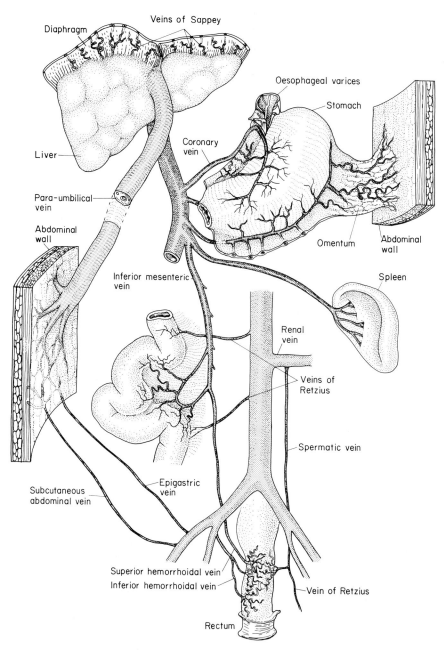

Fig. 111. The sites of the portal–systemic collateral circulation in cirrhosis of the liver (McIndoe 1928).

The spleen is enlarged with a thickened capsule. The consistency is tough and the surface oozes dark blood (*fibrocongestive splenomegaly*). Malpighian bodies are inconspicuous. Histologically [68] (fig. 113) dilated sinusoids show thickening of the reticulin in their walls. Histiocytes proliferate in the sinusoids with occasional erythrophagocytosis. Periarterial haemorrhages may progress to siderotic, fibrotic nodules.

Splenic and portal vessels. The splenic artery and portal vein are enlarged and tortuous and may be aneurysmal. The portal and splenic vein may

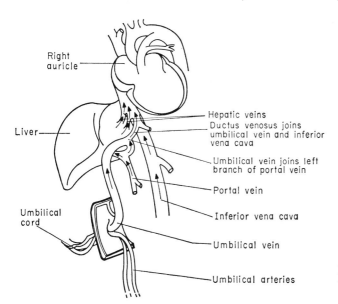

Right auricle

Liver

Umbilical cord

Hepatic veins

Ductus venosus joins umbilical vein and inferior vena cava

Umbilical vein joins left branch of portal vein

Portal vein

Inferior vena cava

Umbilical vein

Umbilical arteries

Fig. 112. The hepatic circulation at the time of birth.

show endothelial haemorrhages, mural thrombi and intimal plaques [51] and may calcify (fig. 118). Such veins may be unsuitable for successful portal–systemic shunts.

The intra-splenic venous and especially the arterial volume are increased and in 50% of cirrhotics small, deeply placed arterial aneurysms are seen [72].

Hepatic changes depend on the cause of the portal hypertension.

The height of the portal venous pressure correlates poorly with the apparent degree of cirrhosis

and in particular of fibrosis. There is a much better correlation with the degree of nodular regeneration.

CLINICAL FEATURES OF PORTAL HYPERTENSION

HISTORY AND GENERAL EXAMINATION

Hepatic cirrhosis is the commonest cause of portal venous hypertension. Any possible aetiological factor such as alcoholism or past hepatitis should

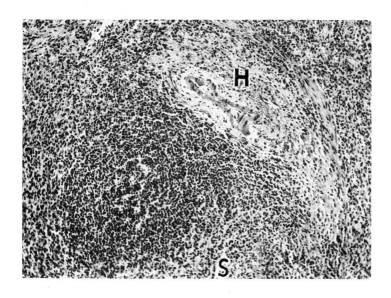

Fig. 113. The spleen in portal hypertension. The sinusoids (S) are congested and the sinusoidal wall is thickened. A haemorrhage (H) lies adjacent to an arteriole of a Malpighian corpuscle. H & E, × 70.

Table 20. Investigation of a patient with suspected portal hypertension.

History

Relative to cirrhosis or chronic hepatitis (table 51)
Gastro-intestinal bleedings: number, dates, amounts, symptoms, treatment
Results of previous barium series examinations and endoscopies
P/H: Alcoholism, jaundice, intra-abdominal, neonatal or other sepsis, oral contraceptives, myeloproliferative disorder

Examination

Signs of hepato-cellular failure
Abdominal wall veins:
    Site
    Direction of blood flow
Splenomegaly
Liver size and consistency
Ascites
Oedema of legs

Rectal examination

Barium swallow and meal

Endoscopy of oesophagus, stomach and duodenum

Additional investigations

Plain film abdomen for liver and spleen size
Aspiration liver biopsy
Transplenic portal venography
Intra-splenic pressure
Hepatic vein catheterization
Selective splanchnic arteriography
Hepatic scintiscanning, ultrasound or CT scan

---

be considered. Past abdominal inflammation, especially in the neonatal period, is particularly important in the aetiology of extra-hepatic portal block. Some oral contraceptives conduce to portal and hepatic venous thrombosis.

Haematemesis is the commonest presentation. The number and severity of previous haemorrhages should be noted together with their immediate effects, whether there was associated confusion or coma and whether blood transfusion was required. Melaena, without haematemesis, may result from bleeding varices. The absence of dyspepsia and epigastric tenderness and a previously normal barium meal help to exclude haemorrhage from peptic ulcer.

The stigmata of cirrhosis include jaundice, vascular spiders and palmar erythema. Anaemia and the prodromata of coma should be noted.

ABDOMINAL WALL VEINS

In intra-hepatic portal hypertension, some blood from the left branch of the portal vein may be deviated via para-umbilical veins to the umbilicus, whence it reaches veins of the caval system (fig. 114). In extra-hepatic portal obstruction, dilated veins may appear in the left flank.

Distribution and direction. A number of prominent collateral veins radiating from the umbilicus is termed *caput Medusae*. This is rare and usually only one or two veins, frequently epigastric, are seen (figs. 114, 115). The blood flow is away from the umbilicus, whereas in inferior vena caval obstruction the collateral venous channels carry blood upwards to reach the superior vena caval system (fig. 114). Tense ascites may lead to functional obstruction of the inferior vena cava and cause difficulty in interpretation.

Abdominal veins can be visualized by *infra-red photography* (fig. 116).

Murmurs [12]. A venous hum may be heard, usually in the region of the xiphoid process or umbilicus, occasionally radiating to the praecordium, sternum or over the liver [85]. A thrill, detectable by light pressure, may be felt at the site of the maximum intensity. The sound may be accentuated during systole, in inspiration or in the erect or sitting positions. It is due to blood rushing through a large umbilical or para-umbilical channel in the falciform ligament from the left branch of the portal vein to the superior epigastric, internal mammary or inferior epigastric veins in the abdominal wall. A venous hum may also occasionally be heard over other large collaterals such as the inferior mesenteric vein or after a successful or even unsuccessful porta-caval anastomosis. An arterial systolic murmur usually indicates primary liver cancer or alcoholic hepatitis.

The association of dilated abdominal wall veins and a loud abdominal venous murmur at the umbilicus is termed the *Cruveilhier–Baumgarten* syndrome [7, 25]. This was originally believed to be due to congenital failure of obliteration of the umbilical vein with subsequent hepatic atrophy. In fact, it is usually due to cirrhosis with a congenitally patent umbilical vein.

The para-xiphoid umbilical hum and *caput Medusae* indicate the presence of portal obstruction beyond the origin of the umbilical veins from the left branch of the portal vein. They therefore indicate intra-hepatic portal venous hypertension (cirrhosis).

Distinction of portal from caval collaterals. Substances taken by mouth are absorbed from the intestine into the abdominal vein. After oral glucose, the abdominal, portal collateral blood has a glu-

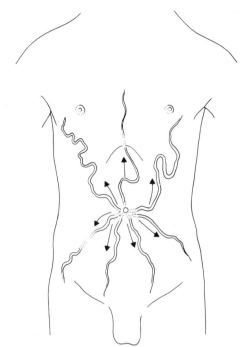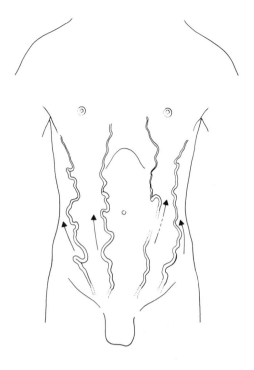

Fig. 114. Distribution and direction of blood flow in anterior abdominal wall veins in portal venous obstruction (left) and in inferior vena caval obstruction (right) (Sherlock 1950).

cose concentration higher than that in antecubital venous blood, since it reflects the portal venous glucose level [115].

SPLEEN

The spleen enlarges progressively. The edge is firm. Size bears little relation to the portal pressure. It is larger in young people and in macronodular rather than micronodular cirrhosis.

An enlarged spleen is the single most important diagnostic sign of portal hypertension. If the spleen cannot be felt or is not enlarged radiologically, the diagnosis of portal hypertension is questionable.

The peripheral blood shows a pancytopenia associated with an enlarged spleen whatever the cause (*secondary 'hypersplenism'*). This is related more to the reticulo-endothelial hyperplasia than to the hypertension and is unaffected by lowering the pressure by porta-caval anastomosis.

LIVER

A small liver may be as significant as a large one, and the size should be evaluated by careful percus-

sion. Liver size correlates poorly with the height of the portal venous pressure, although high pressures are more often found with the small, contracted, fibrotic organ.

Liver consistency, tenderness or nodularity should be recorded. A soft liver suggests extrahepatic portal venous obstruction. A firm liver supports cirrhosis.

ASCITES

This is rarely due to the portal hypertension alone although a particularly high pressure may be a major factor. The portal hypertension raises the capillary filtration pressure, increases the quantity of ascitic fluid and determines its localization to the peritoneal cavity. Ascites in cirrhosis always indicates liver cell failure in addition to portal hypertension.

HAEMORRHOIDS

Dilated rectal veins should be a common accompaniment of portal hypertension. The relationship is difficult to establish as haemorrhoids are so frequent anyway. In the cirrhotic, bleeding can be profuse.

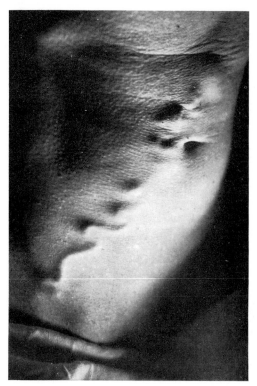

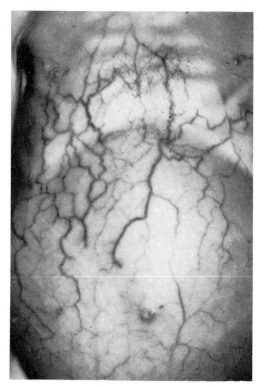

Fig. 115. Anterior abdominal wall vein in patient with cirrhosis of the liver (Sherlock & Walshe 1946).

Fig. 116. Infra-red photograph of a patient with cirrhosis and ascites. The portal collateral circulation is demonstrated. Note the everted umbilicus.

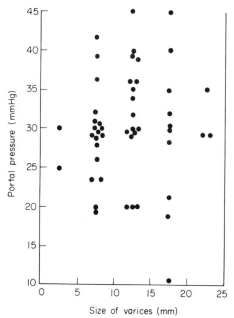

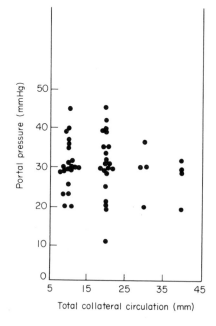

Fig. 117. Relationship between portal pressure measured during trans-hepatic portography and extent of variceal and non-variceal collateral circulation.

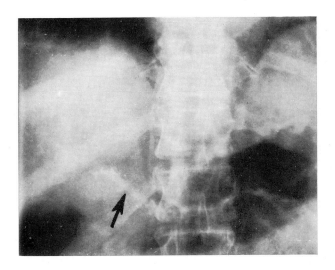

Fig. 118. Plain X-ray of the abdomen. Calcification is seen in the line of the splenic and portal vein (Smallwood & Davidson 1968).

PLAIN X-RAY OF THE ABDOMEN

This is useful to delineate liver and spleen shape and size. Rarely, a calcified portal vein may be shown [118] (fig. 118).

Branching, linear, gas-shadows in the portal vein radicles, especially near the periphery of the liver and due to gas-forming organisms, may rarely be seen in adults with intestinal infarction or infants with enterocolitis [38]. Portal gas may be associated with disseminated intravascular coagulation and heparin may be of value [117].

RADIOLOGY OF THE MEDIASTINUM

Tomography of the azygos vein may show enlargement [32] (fig. 119). This is not surprising for

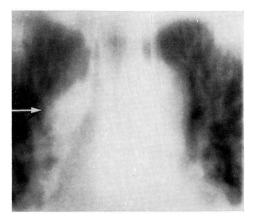

Fig. 119. Tomography of the mediastinum of a patient with large portal–systemic collaterals shows enlargement of the azygos vein (marked with arrow).

the bulk of the collateral flow enters the azygos system.

A widened left paravertebral shadow may be due to lateral displacement of the pleural reflection between aorta and vertebral column by a dilated hemiazygos vein [32].

Massively dilated **para-oesophageal collaterals** may be seen on the plain chest radiograph as a retrocardiac posterior mediastinal mass [79].

OESOPHAGEAL AND GASTRIC VARICES

Oesophageal varices lie in the submucous and subepithelial layer along the whole length of the oesophagus. They are usually permanent although fluctuating in size.

Oesophageal varices may occur transiently in patients with virus hepatitis, and in cirrhosis they have also been noted to disappear [9]. This may be related to alcoholic patients stopping drinking or to the development of a large collateral circulation elsewhere.

The mechanism of formation is uncertain. A possible hypothesis is that, with inspiration, portal pressure rises whereas the oesophageal venous pressure falls. Blood tends to flow from the portal veins into the oesophageal veins which become varicose because of their poor sub-mucosal support.

Radiology. Barium swallow is performed using both thick and thin emulsions and taking care that the oesophagus is not overfilled. Multiple films in both erect and supine positions are necessary to obtain good definition of the mucosal pattern. The films should be taken while the oesophagus is

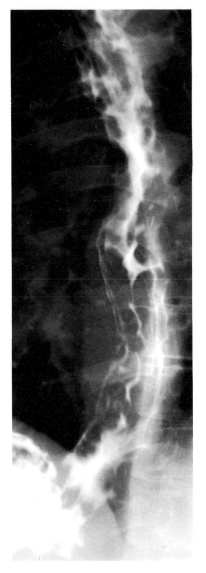

Fig. 120. Barium swallow X-ray shows a dilated oesophagus. The margin is irregular. There are multiple filling defects representing oesophageal varices.

relaxed following simple inspiration. Cinefluorography may increase the recognition rate.

Normal mucosa shows long, thin, evenly spaced lines. These are disturbed by the varices, which show as filling defects in the regular contour of the oesophagus. They are most often seen in the lower third but may spread upwards so that the entire oesophagus is involved. Widening and finally gross dilatation are helpful signs.

Oesophageal varices are nearly always accom-

panied by gastric varices which pass through the cardia, line the fundus in a worm-like fashion and may be difficult to distinguish from mucosal folds. Examination in the prone position is particularly helpful for a double contrast is obtained with the fundal air bubble. Occasionally gastric varices show as a lobulated mass in the gastric fundus simulating a carcinoma [3]. Splenic venography is useful in differentiation. Very rarely, barium meal shows lobulated filling defects in the duodenal bulb and duodenal sweep [53], representing duodenal and antral varices. Similarly, barium enema may show colonic varices [116]. These are confirmed by angiography.

Endoscopy. Oesophageal varices show as blue, rounded projections under the mucosa and occasionally may bulge out into the lumen, looking very much like internal haemorrhoids [88]. Gastric and duodenal varices may also be visualized.

Radiology versus endoscopy. It is difficult to find a standard of reference between radiologists and endoscopists. Varices are not well shown at autopsy and portal venography shows not only sub-mucosal channels but also para-oesophageal ones which are of little clinical significance. Barium swallow revealed varices in 66 of 77 patients in whom collaterals were shown by splenic venography [127]. On the whole fibroscopy seems the more reliable method although a permanent record of the varices is not usually available.

Visualizing the portal venous system (table 21) [113]

OPERATIVE INJECTION OF CONTRAST
MATERIAL DIRECTLY INTO PORTAL VEIN
OR ONE OF ITS TRIBUTARIES

This method has the obvious disadvantage of necessitating surgery. Filling of the portal system can be so great that interpretation of anatomy is difficult.

PERCUTANEOUS TRANS-SPLENIC PORTAL
VENOGRAPHY

Contrast material, injected into the pulp of the spleen, is absorbed into the portal blood stream with sufficient rapidity to outline the splenic and portal veins [4, 127].

Table 21. Methods of visualizing the portal vein.

Method	Scanning	Splenic venography	Splanchnic arteriography
Definition of			
portal vein	+	+++	++
splenic vein	±	+++	±
collaterals	±	+++	+
hepatic artery	0	0	+++
Estimation of portal pressure	No	Yes	No
Quantity contrast	None	100 ml	300–600 ml
Technical skill	Great	Minimal	Great
Complications	None	Intraperitoneal haemorrhage	Femoral arterial haemorrhage, renal failure

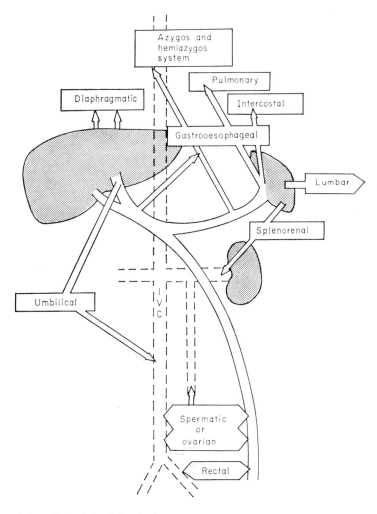

Fig. 121. The sites of the collateral circulation in the presence of intra-hepatic portal vein obstruction.

In adults local anaesthesia is used, but children require general anaesthesia. A fine plastic tube (0.75 mm outside diameter), fitted with a stilette, is inserted at the point of maximum splenic dullness in the mid-axillary line, usually in the 8th or 9th intercostal space with its tip directed at an angle of 45° to the transverse plane. When the spleen is reached a resistance is felt and thereafter the patient is asked to take shallow breaths or, if under general anaesthesia, apnoea is induced. After penetrating 2 cm into the spleen, the stilette is removed and blood can be seen to drip from the tubing. The swing of the needle with respiration is not in any way impeded. During any manipulation the patient holds his breath.

The intra-splenic pressure is measured and 100 ml contrast injected under considerable pressure. For children, 40–60 ml is used. The use of a fine needle or plastic tubing which can move freely within the spleen considerably increases the safety of the procedure.

Deep jaundice is a contraindication even if the prothrombin time is normal, for intra-peritoneal haemorrhage has followed simple intra-splenic puncture in such patients [127].

The prothrombin time should be normal, and the platelet count should exceed 100 000 per mm³.

If a venogram is indicated in a patient with ascites, the fluid should be removed before the investigation.

Serious complications are rare, provided a careful technique is employed. It is important to use a fine needle and to be sure that respiration ceases while it is inserted deeply into the splenic pulp. Trans-splenic portal venograms have been performed in more than 1000 patients without fatality.

The only serious complication is haemorrhage. Bleeding usually ceases and, although blood transfusion may be necessary, splenectomy is indicated only if it does not stop. Haemorrhage may be delayed for five days after the puncture. When the spleen is examined later, at autopsy or operation, it shows either no change, a small haematoma or a depressed scar [5].

Extra-splenic injection of contrast material causes pain both local and referred to the left shoulder.

Venographic appearances

When the portal circulation is *normal*, the material reaches the liver within 2–3 seconds, the splenic and portal veins are filled but no other vessels are outlined (fig. 122). A filling defect is frequently observed at the point of junction of splenic and superior mesenteric veins. The size and direction of the splenic and portal veins are very variable. The intra-hepatic branches of the portal vein show a gradual branching and reduction in calibre. Later the liver becomes opaque due to sinusoidal filling. The hepatic veins may very rarely be seen in the later films. Leakage of contrast medium outlines the spleen, giving some indication of its size and shape.

In *cirrhosis* the venogram varies widely. It may be completely normal or may show filling of large numbers of collateral vessels with gross distortion of the intra-hepatic pattern ('tree in winter' appearance) (fig. 123). Failure to find an abnormality in the intra-hepatic portal branches does not exclude the presence of cirrhosis.

In *extra-hepatic portal* or *splenic vein obstruction* large numbers of vessels run from the spleen and

Fig. 122. Normal portal venogram obtained by percutaneous splenic puncture. All the dye injected into the spleen passes through the splenic and portal vein into the liver. S = pool of dye in spleen; SP = splenic vein; PV = portal vein; L.Br.PV = left branch of right portal vein; I.H.P. = intra-hepatic pattern.

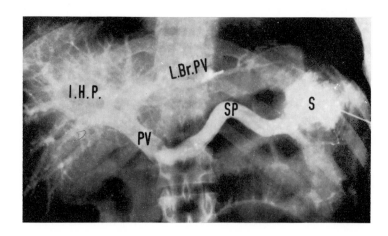

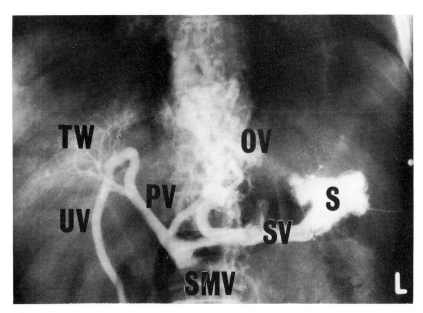

Fig. 123. Splenic venogram from a patient with cirrhosis of the liver. The gastro-oesophageal collateral circulation can be seen and the intra-hepatic portal vascular tree is distorted ('tree in winter' appearance). S = splenic pulp; SV = splenic vein; SMV = superior mesenteric vein; PV = portal vein; OV = oesophageal vein; UV = umbilical vein; TW = 'tree in winter' appearance.

splenic vein to the diaphragm, thoracic cage and abdominal wall. Intra-hepatic branches are not usually seen, although if the portal vein block is localized, paraportal vessels may short-circuit the lesion and produce a delayed but definite filling of the vein beyond.

Difficulties in interpretation. The splenic venogram may not reveal the true state of the portal circulation if inadequate material is injected into the spleen or too few films are taken. With a very large collateral circulation, the dye may enter collaterals and not fill the portal vein (fig. 127). Retrograde flow in the portal vein may contribute.

This 'empty' portal vein is seen in about 6% of examinations although the portal vein is infact patent [15].

Indications [127]

The method is most useful in the clinical management of *gastro-intestinal haemorrhage* and in suspected portal hypertension. If a technically satisfactory splenic venogram fails to show oesophageal collaterals, bleeding from varices is unlikely.

A venogram is essential before surgical procedures involving the portal system.

Splenic venography is a useful method in deter-

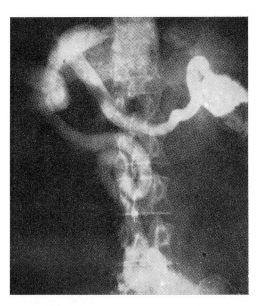

Fig. 124. Portal venogram of a patient with cirrhosis. A very large amount of contrast medium is diverted in a large umbilical vein, which is filled from the left branch of the portal vein and passes towards the iliac veins. Later films showed filling of the inferior vena cava. This patient had a normal portal venous pressure. She presented with a chronic dementia. Abdominal wall veins were not seen and there was no venous hum (Summerskill *et al* 1956).

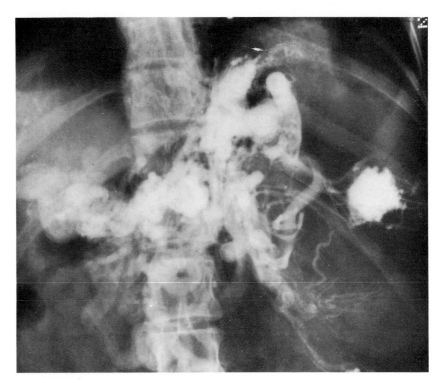

Fig. 125. Splenic venogram showing extra-hepatic
portal venous obstruction. The portal and splenic
veins are replaced by many small veins.

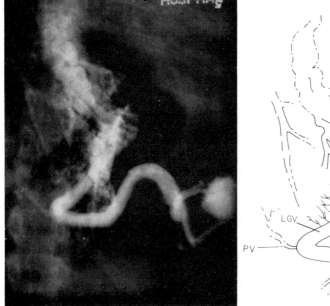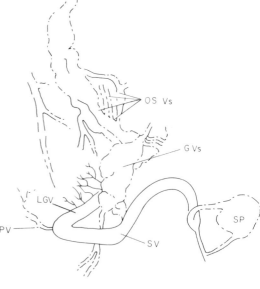

Fig. 126. Female patient with portal cirrhosis. The
bulk of the contrast medium is diverted through the
gastric and oesophageal veins and only a trickle
enters the portal vein. The portal vein was patent.

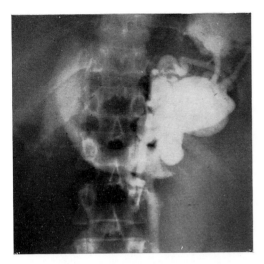

Fig. 127. Patient with Laennec's cirrhosis and a non-filled portal vein. The dye is diverted via spleno-renal collaterals to the inferior vena cava. This patient had a normal portal venous pressure (Turner *et al* 1957).

mining the patency of a portal-caval anastomosis (figs. 154, 155).

Splenomegaly, especially in childhood, may be due to a symptomless cirrhosis or portal vein anomaly. This can be elucidated by splenic venography.

Chronic neuropsychiatric disorders. The demonstration of a large portal collateral circulation is compatible with the diagnosis of chronic portal–systemic encephalopathy (fig. 124). Its absence excludes it.

The technique is occasionally of value in demonstrating a *filling defect* in the portal vein or in the liver due to a space-occupying lesion such as a pancreatic tumour or a liver abscess or cancer.

SCINTI-PHOTOSPLENOPORTOGRAPHY [59]

Serial scans, using a gamma camera, are made after injection of ^{133}Xe or ^{99m}TcO$_4$ into the spleen. Flow patterns can be defined and particularly

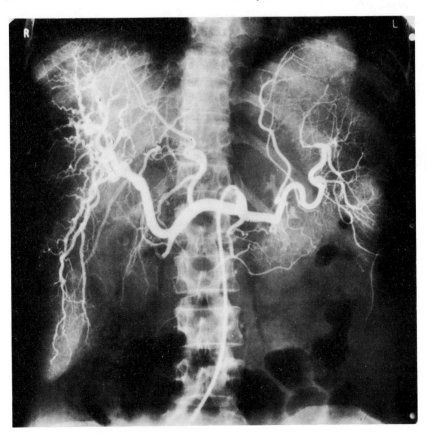

Fig. 128. Selective coeliac angiogram shows intrahepatic arterial pattern. A Reidel's lobe is shown.

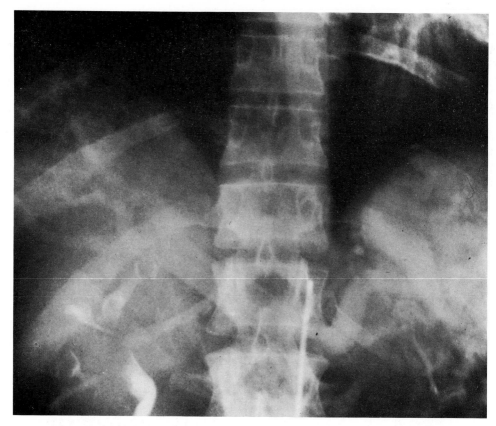

Fig. 129. Venous phase of selective coeliac
angiogram shows a patent portal and splenic vein.

whether the flow in the portal vein is centrifugal
or centripetal. Collateral flow can be shown.

It may be diagnosed by splenic or trans-hepatic
portography.

Collaterals may form at unusual sites leading to
ileal, colonic or rectal haemorrhage [49].

SELECTIVE VISCERAL ANGIOGRAPHY

The coeliac axis is catheterized via the femoral
artery with a pre-formed opaque catheter and the
injection of a bolus of radio-opaque contrast
material is injected [50, 129]. The portion of contrast material that flows into the splenic artery
returns through the splenic and portal veins and
produces a splenic and portal venogram of variable quality. Similarly, a bolus of contrast material
introduced into the superior mesenteric artery
returns through the superior mesenteric and portal
veins, which can be seen in radiographs exposed
at the appropriate intervals (figs. 128, 129). The
portal vascular bed is not seen so clearly as with
splenic venography.

Because splenic venous blood may be diverted
into large gastro-oesophageal collaterals a splenic
venogram may occasionally show a non-filled
portal vein, even though the vein is patent. In such
cases, a mesenteric angiogram shows whether or
not the main portal vein is, in fact, occluded.

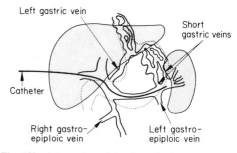

Fig. 130. A trans-hepatic catheter is shown
advanced in the splenic hilum. Major variceal supply
veins (left gastric and short gastric veins) are shown.
Gastro-epiploic veins may occasionally also feed
gastro-oesophageal varices (Scott *et al* 1976).

Visceral angiography has the additional advantage that the hepatic arterial system can be seen, so allowing space-filling lesions in the liver to be identified. A tumour circulation may help to diagnose primary liver cancer or other tumours. Knowledge of splanchnic and hepatic arterial anatomy is useful if surgery is contemplated. Haemangiomas and arteriovenous aneurysms may be identified. A disadvantage is that the portal venous pressure cannot be measured.

Large quantities of contrast material are necessary and these may precipitate renal failure, particularly in those with a tendency to the hepatorenal syndrome [106].

UMBILICAL VEIN CATHETERIZATION

The umbilical vein of the adult can be re-opened, and catheterized, so allowing access to the left branch of the portal vein and hence to the portal–venous system [62, 102]. The technique is not easy and the failure rate high. The procedure fails if there has been previous upper abdominal surgery.

TRANS-HEPATIC PORTOGRAPHY [119]

This technique gives excellent visualization of the portal and splenic veins and the portal–systemic collateral circulation. It is, however, technically difficult and carries a greater risk than the other procedures. It is usually performed as a preliminary to trans-hepatic obliteration of varices (figs. 130–133).

SCANNING PROCEDURES

These have the advantage of being rapid, non-invasive and safe. The relatively inexpensive grey

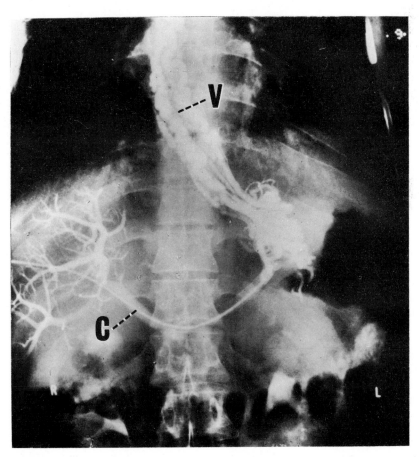

Fig. 131. Trans-hepatic portogram shows cannula passed through liver and portal vein into the left gastric vein. Contrast material has been injected and massive oesophageal varices filled. C = cannula, V = varices.

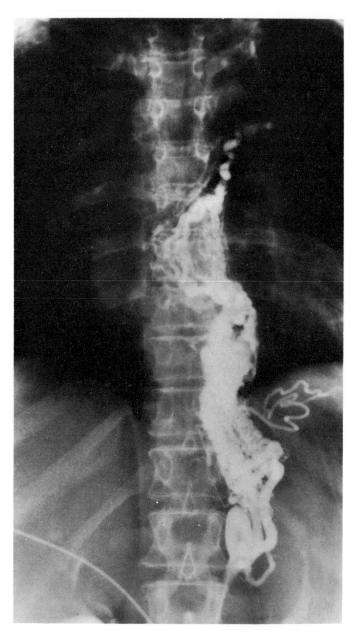

Fig. 132. The left gastric vein has been successfully catheterized.

scale ultrasound may be used to visualize the portal vein at the hilum of the liver [136] (figs. 134, 135). A normal portal vein is easily seen, while an incomplete or recanalising vein is irregular and reduced in diameter, and a thrombosed vein is not detected. The more costly CT scanner allows better definition of the portal vein. With either technique the visualization of the whole portal venous tree is not as good as with techniques such as splenic venography or splanchnic arterio-graphy. The collateral circulation is not well shown and pressure measurements are not possible (table 21).

Portal venous pressure

In any patient with portal hypertension the actual height of the portal venous pressure must be recorded.

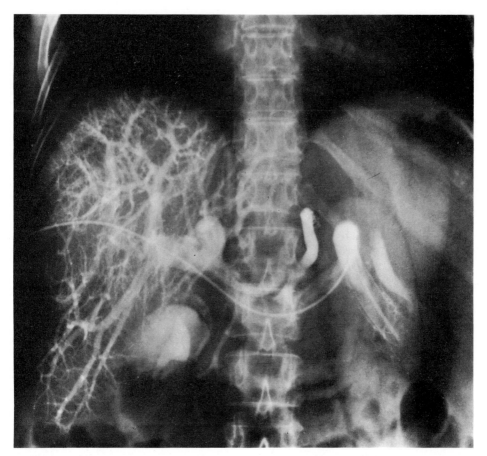

Fig. 133. After successful sclerosis the trans-hepatic portogram shows obliteration of the gastro-oesophageal collateral circulation.

Intrasplenic puncture

This is the most convenient technique [5].

Operative

These measurements are unreliable, as they are affected by the anaesthetic, blood loss, position of the patient, and duration of the operation.

Umbilical vein catheterization

This procedure allows the pressure in the left branch of the portal vein to be recorded [62, 102].

Trans-hepatic [119]

This is an excellent technique for measuring portal pressure, but the invasive nature of the procedure

and the technical skill required negate its general use.

Wedged hepatic venous pressure [89, 102, 128]

The pressure recorded through a catheter introduced into an hepatic venous radicle until it will go no further is termed the *wedged hepatic venous pressure* (fig. 136). The catheter now prevents blood from flowing through the hepatic vein radical. The pressure measured represents that at the next point of free communication with the hepatic circulation, which is the sinusoid. The pressure is therefore the sinusoidal venous pressure. The catheter is properly wedged if it shows buckling in the right atrium, if the pressure tracing shows regular oscillations related to transmission of hepatic arterial pressure and, finally, if a small amount of contrast material injected along

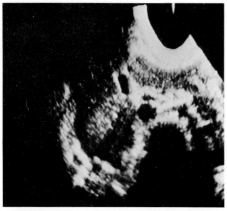

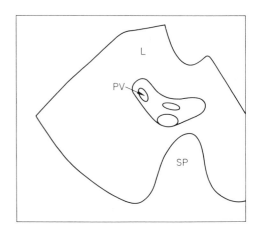

Fig. 134. Grey-scale ultrasound scan through porta hepatis showing a normal portal vein. PV=portal vein; L=liver; SP=spine (Webb *et al* 1977).

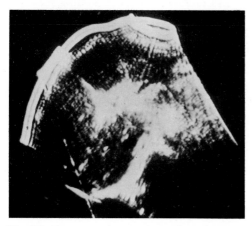

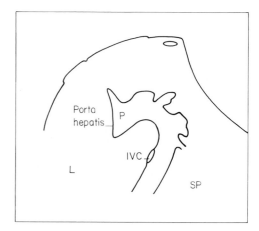

Fig. 135. Transverse ultrasound scan through porta hepatis showing a thrombosed portal vein with surrounding scar tissue. P=portal vein collaterals; L=liver; SP=spine; IVC=inferior vena cava (Webb *et al* 1977).

it is seen radiologically to pass against the predominant flow into the sinusoidal bed. Measurements are then taken with the catheter withdrawn about 5 cm to the *free position*. The standard of reference is the pressure in the inferior vena cava, measured before or after entering the liver. The technique is relatively easy. It is safe and can be performed in patients with a bleeding tendency. It also allows the sinusoidal pressure to be measured in the splenectomized.

The normal wedged hepatic vein pressure is 5–6 mmHg and values of about 20 mmHg are found in patients with portal hypertension, such as cirrhosis.

A balloon catheter may be used [46]. This allows

wedging from the femoral approach and repeated measurements in a larger segment of liver.

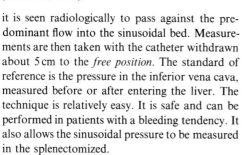

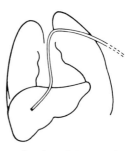

Fig. 136. The estimation of the portal venous pressure by hepatic vein catheterization.

ESTIMATION OF HEPATIC BLOOD FLOW

Constant infusion method

Hepatic blood flow may be measured by a constant infusion of the dye bromsulphalein (BSP) and catheterization of the hepatic vein [14].

The formula for calculating flow, by the Fick principle, is as follows:

$$EHBF = \frac{\text{rate of dye removal}}{\text{arterial–hepatic vein dye difference}} \times \frac{1}{\text{Hct}}$$

EHBF = estimated hepatic blood flow. Hct = haematocrit.

If arterial level constant:

rate of infusion = rate of hepatic removal

e.g.

$$Q = 5 \text{ mg/min.}$$
$$A = 1.94 \text{ mg/100 ml plasma}$$
$$H = 1.34 \text{ mg/100 ml plasma}$$

$$EHPF = \frac{5 \times 100}{0.6} = \frac{500}{0.6} = 834 \text{ ml/min.}$$

If haematocrit = 45%

$$\text{Hepatic blood flow (EHBF)} = \frac{834 \times 100}{(100 - 45)} = 1520 \text{ ml/min.}$$

This method depends on the dye being removed only by the liver at a steady rate, shown by maintenance of constant arterial levels, and on the absence of significant entero-hepatic circulation.

BSP may be replaced by indocyanine green (IG) [17] which has the advantage of being removed only by the liver, and entero-hepatic circulation is minimal. It is not conjugated. Plasma arterial levels are steadier in those with borderline hepatic function. Calculated hepatic flow is lower than for BSP and this is especially so in the cirrhotic.

This method has been used to show a fall in hepatic blood flow in recumbency, fainting [8], heart failure and cirrhosis, and exercise. Fever increases flow and it is unaltered in such high cardiac output states as thyrotoxicosis and pregnancy.

Plasma disappearance method

Hepatic blood flow can be measured after an intravenous injection of indocyanine green, followed by analysis of the disappearance curve in a peripheral artery and hepatic vein [28].

$$EHBF = K \times \frac{\text{blood volume}}{E}$$

where

K = fraction retained plasma dye disappearing per minute

$$= \frac{0.693}{t_{\frac{1}{2}}}$$

E = percentage extraction by liver

$$= \frac{\text{arterial–hepatic venous conc.}}{\text{arterial conc.}} \times 100$$

If the extraction of a substance is 100%, i.e. the substance is completely removed in one passage through the liver, then hepatic blood flow could be measured from the peripheral–arterial disappearance curve. A heat-denatured albumin colloidal complex tagged with ^{131}I (^{131}CAI) has minimal extra-hepatic removal and 94% extraction by the liver in man [108]. In normal subjects hepatic blood flow can be determined from the peripheral clearance, without hepatic vein catheterization, by the formula:

$$EHBF = K \times \text{blood volume}$$

where

K = fraction retained plasma colloid disappearing per minute

$$= \frac{0.693}{t_{\frac{1}{2}}}$$

and assuming 100% extraction of colloid by liver.

In patients with cirrhosis up to 20% of the blood perfusing the liver may not go through normal channels [108] and hepatic extraction is reduced. This must be measured by hepatic vein catheterization to obtain estimates of flow in patients with liver disease. Galactose has been used in similar fashion.

Electromagnetic flow meters

Flows in exposed vessels may be measured directly using the square-wave electromagnetic flow meter [94]. This enables flow in portal vein and hepatic artery to be measured separately.

Estimation of portal–systemic collateral flow

This is a difficult problem. The fraction of portal–systemic shunting may be computed by direct injection of isotope into splenic or mesenteric vein and measurement of the area of an isotope dilution curve recorded in the hepatic vein [16, 47].

Trans-hepatic catheterization allows injection of isotopically-labelled materials into splenic or portal vein [86]. Subsequent differential counting over liver and lungs allows calculations of intra- and extra-hepatic shunts. The intra-hepatic shunt indices vary from 1 to 78.4% and the extra-hepatic shunt indices range from 0 to 50%. These values correlate closely with the size of collaterals opacified by portography.

Experimental portal venous occlusion and hypertension

Survival following acute occlusion depends on the development of an adequate collateral circulation. In the rabbit, cat or dog this does not develop and death supervenes rapidly. In the monkey or man, the collateral circulation is adequate and survival is usual [21].

Acute occlusion of one branch of the portal vein is not fatal. The liver cells of the ischaemic lobe atrophy, but bile ducts, Kupffer cells and connective tissues survive. The unaffected lobe hypertrophies.

Experimentally, portal hypertension can be produced by occluding the portal vein with cellophane, injecting silica into the portal vein, infecting mice with schistosomiasis or by any experimental type of cirrhosis. An extensive collateral circulation develops, the spleen enlarges but ascites does not form.

CLASSIFICATION OF PORTAL HYPERTENSION [112]

Portal hypertension usually follows obstruction to the portal blood flow anywhere along its course. Intra-splenic pressure reflects pressure in the splenic vein. The trans-hepatic route can be used to measure pressure in the main portal vein [119]. The wedged hepatic venous pressure represents sinusoidal pressure. Splenic or portal venography or visceral angiography show the site of obstruction and the nature of the collateral circulation. Liver biopsy helps in localization and diagnosis of the cause of obstruction. Using a selection of these techniques, portal hypertension can be classified into two groups, presinusoidal (extra-hepatic or intra-hepatic) and a big general group of intra-hepatic causes (fig. 137, table 22) [113]. This distinction is a practical one. The pre-sinusoidal forms, which include obstruction to the sinusoids by Kupffer and other cellular proliferation, are associated with relatively normal hepato-cellular function. Consequently, if patients with this type suffer a haemorrhage from oesophageal varices, liver failure is rarely a consequence. In contrast, the intra-hepatic types are associated with hepato-cellular disease. Patients with this type suffering haemorrhage frequently go into liver failure.

EXTRA-HEPATIC PORTAL VENOUS OBSTRUCTION [135]

This causes extra-hepatic presinusoidal portal hypertension. The obstruction may be at any point

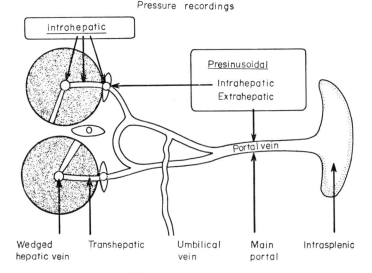

Pressure recordings

Fig. 137. Portal hypertension can be classified into two main groups: pre-sinusoidal and intra-hepatic. The pre-sinusoidal is further divided into extra-hepatic, where the obstruction is in the main portal vein and pre-sinusoidal, where the obstruction is usually in the portal tracts. Pressure recordings allow the anatomical site of the obstruction to be located.

Table 22. Classification of portal hypertension.

	Pressure		Type	Example
	Intra-splenic	Wedged hepatic vein		
Presinusoidal	Raised	Normal	Extra-hepatic	Block portal or splenic vein
				Increased splenic flow
			Intra-hepatic	Schistosomiasis
				Congenital fibrosis
				Portal zone infiltrations
Intra-hepatic	Raised	Raised		Cirrhosis
				Veno-occlusive disease
				Block hepatic vein

in the course of the portal vein. The *venae comitantes* enlarge in an attempt to deliver portal blood to the liver, so assuming a leash-like cavernous appearance [127]. The portal vein, represented by a fibrous strand, is recognized with difficulty in the multitude of small vessels. This cavernous change follows any block in the main vein.

AETIOLOGY

Infections, whether septicaemic or intra-abdominal, are the commonest causes. Umbilical infection with or without catheterization of the umbilical vein may be responsible in neonates [125]. The infection spreads along the umbilical vein to the left portal vein and hence to the main portal vein (fig. 138). Acute appendicitis and peritonitis are causative in older children.

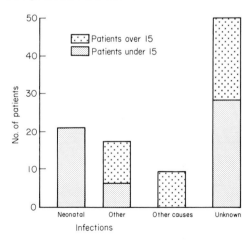

Fig. 138. Aetiology of portal vein occlusion in 97 patients over and under 15 years old (Webb & Sherlock 1979).

In later life, biliary tract surgery may be responsible.

Thrombosis may follow abdominal trauma [69]. It may complicate pregnancy or extreme dehydration.

Congenital anomalies of the portal vein, anywhere along the line of the right and left vitelline veins, from which the portal vein develops, may be responsible. The association with congenital defects, such as cardiovascular anomalies and choledochal cyst, would support this possibility [84, 135].

Splenic arteriovenous fistulae can cause portal hypertension and have been diagnosed by arteriography [57, 121]. *Hepatic arterial–portal venous aneurysms*, congenital or traumatic, are being increasingly diagnosed by hepatic angiography [36].

Thrombosis, presumably secondary to a slow circulation, is a rare complication of *cirrhosis*. The apparent non-filling of the portal vein in a splenic venogram is often related to diversion of portal blood into an enormous collateral circulation (figs. 126, 127); the vein is, in fact, patent. When the portal vein becomes occluded in the patient with cirrhosis it is usually due to invasion by a primary carcinoma (fig. 388).

Malignant growths in pancreas, stomach, colon, or adjacent lymph glands, acute pancreatitis, chronic pancreatitis [65] or pancreatic pseudocysts [126] may involve the portal vein.

The portal vein may block in patients with *blood diseases* complicated by increased clotting such as polycythaemia, myelofibrosis and thrombotic thrombocythaemia. It may complicate the use of oral contraceptives.

Occlusion may follow an unsuccessful porta-caval anastomosis or splenectomy, especially if the platelet count is normal preoperatively.

CLINICAL FEATURES

Patients present with the features of portal hyper-tension, usually haemorrhage or splenomegaly. If blood replacement is adequate, recovery usually ensues in a matter of days. There are no stigmata of cirrhosis, jaundice is absent and bleeding does not precipitate hepatic coma. Respiratory infec-tions or salicylate ingestion often precede a haemorrhage.

Before a bleeding episode, the patients, often children, may present with splenomegaly and pan-cytopenia. This may be symptomless and so dis-covered incidentally. In those of neonatal origin, the first bleed is at about the age of four (fig. 139). The frequency of bleeds increases between 10 and 15 years and decreases after puberty.

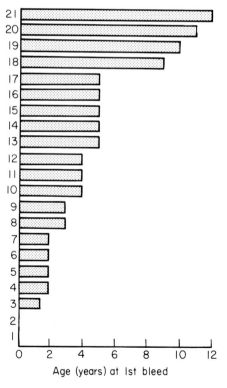

Fig. 139. Portal vein occlusion in neonates. Age at time of first haemorrhage in 21 patients in whom the portal vein block occurred in the neonatal period (Webb & Sherlock 1979).

PROGNOSIS

The shunting of portal blood away from liver cells eventually impairs liver function [126]. As age advances, signs of liver failure may develop. These include ascites and encephalopathy. These results may represent an acceleration of the normal effect of age on hepatic function. Ascites and encepha-lopathy may also be precipitated by acute portal vein thrombosis or by haemorrhage.

Pregnancies are usually well tolerated although occasionally bleeding may occur, particularly dur-ing labour [135]. Infertility may result from blocked tubes secondary to the intra-abdominal sepsis which led to the portal vein thrombosis.

The prognosis is relatively good. In one series, 24 of 97 patients died, 19 of haemorrhage [135]. The mean time between presentation and death was ten years; 60 survived more than ten years. The prognosis is better in children than adults. Predic-tion of the frequency of haemorrhage is impossible and there is no common pattern.

TREATMENT

Children should certainly survive haemorrhage from varices with proper management, including blood transfusion. Care must be taken always to give compatible blood and to preserve peripheral veins. Aspirin ingestion should be avoided. Upper respiratory infections should be treated seriously as they seem to precipitate haemorrhage.

Vasopressin infusions may be needed and occa-sionally the Sengstaken tube.

Definitive surgery for reduction of portal pressure is usually impossible as there are no suit-able veins for a shunt. Even apparently normal-looking veins seen on venography turn out to be in poor condition, presumably related to extension of the original thrombotic process. In children, veins are very small and difficult to anastomose. Myriads of collateral channels add to the technical difficulties.

Results for all forms of surgery are very unsatis-factory (table 23). Splenectomy is the least success-ful and has the highest complication rate. Meso-caval shunt is the preferred technique, but there are difficulties in finding suitable veins. Portal dis-connections such as oesophageal transection, gas-tric transection and gastrectomy are of limited long-term value. Surgery is indicated only rarely, when conservative therapy has failed. However, when the patient is exsanguinating, despite mas-

Table 23. Haemorrhage due to portal vein occlusion (Webb & Sherlock 1979).

Operation	No.	Re-bled		Operative deaths (within one month of surgery)
		no.	mean time (years)	
Splenectomy	19	18	1.9	1
Splenorenal shunt	20	14	3.2	0
Meso- and porta-caval shunt	16	12	2.1	1
Transections and disconnections	52	44	2.7	4

sive blood transfusion, then an oesophageal transection may have to be performed. Post-operative complications are common.

Mild pancreatic hypofunction may be present and pancreatic supplements may be useful [137] (fig. 140).

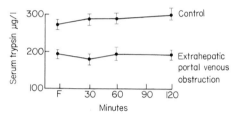

Fig. 140. Patients with extra-hepatic portal venous obstruction show lower fasting serum trypsin values and respond less well to a Lundh meal than control subjects (Webb *et al* 1980).

Intra-hepatic presinusoidal portal hypertension (fig. 141)

In schistosomiasis, the portal hypertension results from the ova causing a reaction in the minute portal–venous radicals [2].

In congenital hepatic fibrosis the portal hypertension is probably due to a deficiency of terminal branches of the portal vein in the fibrotic portal zones [61].

The portal hypertension sometimes complicating the myelo-proliferative diseases results from infiltration of the portal zones with haemopoietic tissue. Portal hypertension has been reported with myelosclerosis, myeloid leukaemia and Hodgkin's disease. Wedged hepatic venous pressure is normal while intrasplenic pressure is increased [104, 111]. Increased hepatic flow is presumably related to the enlarged spleen.

In systemic mastocytosis, portal hypertension is related to increased intra-hepatic resistance secondary to mast cell infiltration. Increased splenic flow, perhaps with splenic arteriovenous shunting and with histamine release, may contribute [48].

In primary biliary cirrhosis, portal hypertension may be a presenting feature long before the development of the nodular regeneration characteristic of cirrhosis (p. 229). The mechanism is uncertain, although portal zone lesions and narrowing of the sinusoids because of cellular infiltration have been incriminated. The portal hypertension of sarcoidosis may be similar [130].

The intra-hepatic portal venous radicals and sinusoidal cells may be injured by toxic factors. Portal hypertension complicates the treatment of psoriasis with inorganic arsenic [78]. The arsenic

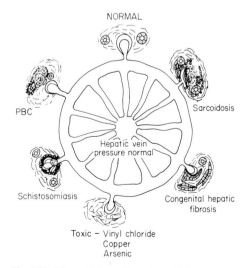

Fig. 141. The aetiology of presinusoidal intra-hepatic portal hypertension.

may be directly injurious to the intra-hepatic portal veins, causing fibrosis and sclerosis.

The non-cirrhotic portal fibrosis found in India has been related to arsenic taken in drinking water, in unorthodox medicines, and in opium obtained illegally [27].

Liver disease in vineyard sprayers in Portugal may be related to exposure to sprays containing copper [90]. Angio-sarcoma may be a complication.

Exposure to the vapour of the polymer of vinyl chloride leads to sclerosis of portal venules in the portal zones, with a development of portal hypertension and angiosarcoma [11].

Portal hypertension secondary to peri-sinu-soidal fibrosis may develop in recipients of renal transplants and be related to prolonged administration of 6-mercaptopurine and azathioprine [83].

Congenital intra-hepatic shunting

A three-year-old child has been described with portal hypertension due to an hepatic artery ductus venosus fistula [74].

An adult with portal–systemic encephalopathy had congenital intra-hepatic shunts between the portal and hepatic veins [95]. Portal hypertension was not present.

'Idiopathic' (primary) portal hypertension (fig. 142)

Patients with portal hypertension are described with no obvious obstruction to the portal venous system. These patients often have very large spleens. Malaria is one cause (*tropical splenomegaly*). Increased splenic flow *per se* is invoked as a cause of portal hypertension but is not a major factor [42]. Impaired distensibility of the liver as a whole, in the face of increased splenic blood flow may also be concerned.

In addition, intra-hepatic resistance is usually increased indicating some obstruction to portal flow. Splenic venography shows secondary and subsequent branches of the portal vein to be narrowed [138]. Liver histology in most instances of so-called 'idiopathic' portal hypertension shows sclerosis and sometimes obliteration of the intra-hepatic portal venous bed [13]. Such changes seem to be secondary to any form of portal hypertension. They may also represent a reaction to some chemical or plant toxin not hitherto identified.

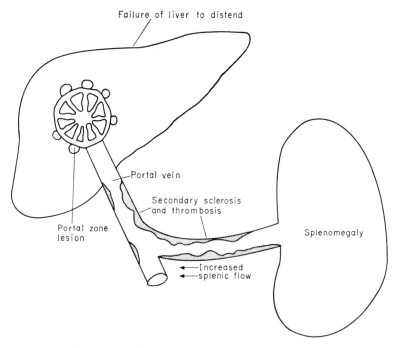

Fig. 142. Factors concerned in so-called idiopathic 'primary' portal hypertension.

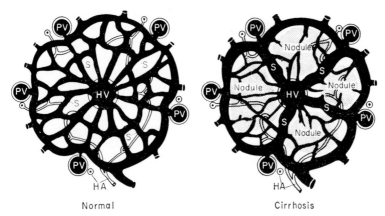

Normal   Cirrhosis

Fig. 143. Cirrhosis of the liver. The formation of portal venous (PV), hepatic venous (HV) anastomoses or internal Eck fistulae at the site of

pre-existing sinusoids (S). Note that the regeneration nodules are supplied by the hepatic artery (HA) (after Elias 1952).

Idiopathic portal hypertension has not been established as an entity.

Intra-hepatic portal hypertension

CIRRHOSIS

All forms of cirrhosis lead to intra-hepatic portal hypertension. The mechanism is complex. The portal vascular bed is distorted and diminished and the portal blood flow is mechanically obstructed [67]. Some of the portal venous blood is diverted into collateral venous channels and some bypasses the liver cells and is shunted directly into the hepatic venous radicles in the

fibrous septa. These portal–hepatic anastomoses develop from pre-existing sinusoids enclosed in the septa [93] (fig. 143). The hepatic vein is displaced further and further outwards until it lies in a fibrous septum linked with the portal venous radicle by the original sinusoid. The regenerating nodules become divorced from their portal blood supply and are nourished by the hepatic artery. About one-third of the total blood flow perfusing the cirrhotic liver may bypass sinusoids, and hence functioning liver tissue, through these channels [108].

The hepatic venous radicles and the sinusoids are readily compressed by the nodules [60] (fig. 151). The portal venous radicles, being supported

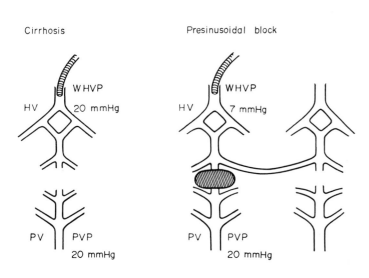

Cirrhosis   Presinusoidal block

Fig. 144. In patients with cirrhosis the wedged hepatic venous pressure (20 mmHg) is equal to the pressure in the main portal vein (20 mmHg) (measured via umbilical vein). Resistance to flow extends from the central hepatic vein, through the sinusoids to the portal vein. In pre-sinusoidal portal hypertension normal anastomoses exist between small vascular units and prevent the blocking catheter from producing a large area of stasis. Wedged hepatic venous pressure (7 mmHg) is therefore less than the pressure in the main portal vein (20 mmHg) (Reynolds *et al* 1970).

by connective tissue in the portal tract, withstand the pressure. This has led to the concept of hepatic venous outflow block as a major factor in the aetiology of portal hypertension in cirrhosis. It was supported by the observation that the pressure in the main portal (or intra-splenic) vein exceeded the wedged hepatic vein and the obstruction was therefore assumed to be in the sinusoidal bed. However, the wedged hepatic venous pressure and the main portal venous pressure were found to be virtually identical in cirrhosis [102, 128]. The stasis therefore extends to the portal inflow vessels (fig. 144). The concept of simple, post-sinusoidal portal hypertension in cirrhosis has been abandoned. The obstruction is now believed to be at all levels from portal zones through the sinusoids to the hepatic venous outflow.

The hepatic artery provides the liver with a small volume of blood at a high pressure. The portal vein provides the liver with a large volume of blood at a low pressure. These two systems are equilibrated in the sinusoids. The hepatic artery delivers blood directly into the sinusoids and so raises the intra-sinusoidal pressure. Even in the normal subject the height of the portal venous pressure may depend on the hepatic aterial pressure. In the cirrhotic liver more direct arterioportal shunting has been suspected [29]. Micro-angiographic studies show arterioles entering the venous channels surrounding the nodules instead of the sinusoids [20]. A pathway between hepatic arterial and portal venous branches certainly exists in the cirrhotic liver for retrograde flow can be shown in the portal vein.

NON-CIRRHOTIC NODULES

Various nodular conditions of the liver lead to portal hypertension but without a cirrhosis being present. They are difficult to diagnose, usually being confused with cirrhosis or with 'idiopathic'

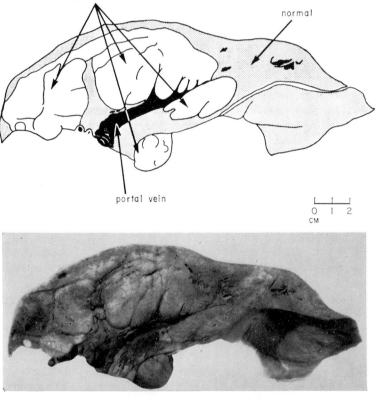

Fig. 145. Partial nodular transformation of the liver. Cross-section of liver through the porta hepatis, in which nodules can be seen obstructing the portal vein. The rest of the liver appears normal (Sherlock *et al* 1960).

portal hypertension. A 'normal' needle liver biopsy does not exclude the diagnosis.

In Felty's syndrome, nodules may be found not outlined by fibrous tissue. The hepatic venous radicle shows a reversed position being found at the periphery of the nodule with compressed columns of hepatocytes [10, 100].

Nodular regenerative hyperplasia has also been associated with monoclonal gammopathy and hyperviscosity syndromes [105, 133].

In these nodular conditions shunt therapy for the treatment of bleeding oesophageal varices should be well tolerated as hepato-cellular function is good.

Partial nodular transformation [114]

This is a very rare disease. The peri-hilar region is replaced by nodules. The periphery of the liver is normal or atrophic (fig. 145). Portal hypertension results from obstruction to hepatic blood flow by the nodules. Liver cell function remains good. Fibrosis is inconspicuous, diagnosis is difficult, confirmation often awaits autopsy. The cause is unknown.

Veno-occlusive disease

This phlebitis of minute hepatic venous radicles leads to post-sinusoidal intra-hepatic portal hypertension (Chapter 12).

Hepatic venous obstruction (Budd–Chiari syndrome)

This may be due to obstruction of the main hepatic veins or to a rise in hepatic venous pressure resulting from constrictive pericarditis or congestive heart failure (Chapter 12).

BLEEDING OESOPHAGEAL VARICES

Mechanism of rupture

This is unclear. The height of the portal blood pressure is important [87]. Gastro-oesophageal reflux is not contributory [35]. Gastric acidity is low and microscopically no oesophagitis has been found [87]. Haemorrhage, however, often follows the use of anti-inflammatory drugs. In children, the bleeding may follow an upper respiratory infection [135].

Diagnosis of bleeding

The *clinical features* are those of gastro-intestinal bleeding with the added picture of portal hypertension.

Bleeding may be a slow ooze with melaena, rather than a sudden haematemesis. The intestines may be full of blood before the haemorrhage is recognized and bleeding is liable to continue for days.

Bleeding varices in cirrhosis have injurious effects on the liver cells. These may be due to anaemia, diminishing hepatic oxygen supply, or to increased metabolic demands resulting from the protein catabolism following haemorrhage. The fall in blood pressure diminishes hepatic arterial flow, on which the regenerating liver nodules depend, and necrosis may ensue. The increased nitrogen absorption from the intestines often leads to hepatic coma (Chapter 8). Deteriorating liver cell function may precipitate jaundice or ascites.

Gastro-oesophageal bleeding in patients with cirrhosis may not be from oesophageal varices. Non-variceal bleeding is particularly frequent in alcoholic patients in whom duodenal ulcers, gastric erosions [37] and the Mallory–Weiss syndrome are frequent.

Fibroscopy will usually visualize the bleeding area if performed within eight hours of the haemorrhage. Patients with severe hepatic failure and stress-induced erosions are particularly important to diagnose.

Serum biochemical tests are not helpful in making the distinction between bleeding varix and bleeding ulcer.

Normal intrasplenic pressure excludes bleeding varix; a raised one confirms portal hypertension

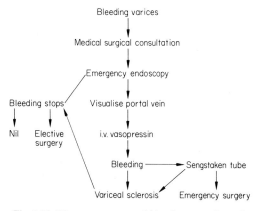

Fig. 146. The management of bleeding oesophageal varices.

but does not mean that the bleeding is variceal. Control of bleeding by inflation of the Sengstaken tube suggests an oesophageal varix.

Splenic venography, performed as an emergency, may be useful in showing an oesophageal collateral circulation.

Serial angiography can also be used to exclude arterial bleeding and to visualize the portal vein.

A wedged hepatic venous pressure 25 mm above that in the inferior vena cava supports variceal bleeding.

Prognosis

In cirrhosis, the prognosis of bleeding oesophageal varices is determined by the severity of the underlying hepato-cellular disease. The ominous triad of jaundice, ascites and encephalopathy is associated with an 80% mortality. Child classified prognosis into three risk grades: A, B and C [21]. This grading is based on nutritional status, ascites, encephalopathy, serum bilirubin and albumin levels and the prothrombin index. The one-year survival in good-risk (Child A and B) patients is about 70% and in bad-risk (Child C) about 30%. Alcoholics have a worse prognosis as hepato-cellular disease is usually greater. Patients with continuing chronic active hepatitis also do poorly. Patients with primary biliary cirrhosis tolerate the haemorrhage reasonably well.

In portal vein obstruction without cirrhosis liver failure after haemorrhage is mild and unusual. The prognosis is therefore better. It is determined by availability of peripheral veins and of adequate compatible blood for transfusion.

General measures

The patient should be hospitalized however small the haemorrhage. Bleeding is likely to continue and observation must be close. If possible, the patient should be managed by an intensive care team. A physician and a surgeon must be together in the picture from the start and subsequent management must be a joint undertaking.

Blood transfusion is a first priority if blood volume is depleted. This may need to be massive. The mean during the first 24 hours is 4 units and the mean total for a hospital admission about 10 units. Saline infusions must be avoided. Clotting factors are liable to be deficient and if possible fresh blood or fresh packed red cells or fresh frozen plasma should be used. Platelet transfusions may be necessary. Vitamin K_1 intramuscularly should be routine.

Cimetidine is given in full dosage. Although there is no controlled evidence of its benefit in patients with severe hepatic failure, stress-induced acute mucosal ulcers are frequent [37].

Hepatic encephalopathy should be anticipated in the cirrhotic patient. Sedatives should be avoided and, if essential, a small dose of a barbiturate which is excreted mainly by the kidney, such as barbitone sodium, phenobarbitone or oxazepam, should be used.

Chlordiazepoxide or heminevrin may be useful, especially if the patient is an alcoholic and delirium tremens is a possible development. If the cause of the portal hypertension is presinusoidal and hepato-cellular function is good, hepatic encephalopathy is unlikely and sedation may be liberal.

Routine measures in the cirrhotic patient to prevent hepatic encephalopathy include dietary protein abstention, neomycin 4 g daily, gastric aspiration and enemas, preferably of lactulose or lactose 300–500 ml.

If ascites is very tense, intra-abdominal pressure may be reduced by a cautious paracentesis and the use of spironolactone or amiloride.

If the haemorrhage stops spontaneously, the patient is either treated conservatively or considered for surgery or trans-hepatic variceal sclerosis. If bleeding continues the patient is given intravenous vasopressin. The portal vein is visualized by ultrasound, splenic venography or splanchnic arteriography (table 21). Recurrence of haemorrhage indicates either emergency surgery or trans-hepatic obliteration of varices. The Sengstaken tube may be used as a preliminary to either procedure.

Vasopressin (Pitressin)

This lowers portal venous pressure by constriction of the splanchnic arteriolar bed, causing an increase in resistance to the inflow of blood to the gut [109] (fig. 146). It controls haemorrhage from oesophageal varices and does so by lowering portal venous pressure [110].

Twenty units of vasopressin in 100 ml 5% dextrose are given intravenously in 10 minutes. Mean arterial pressure rises transiently and portal pressure falls for 45–60 minutes (fig. 148). Alternatively the vasopressin may be given by continuous intravenous infusion (0.4 u/min.) for a maximum of two hours [22].

Abdominal colicky discomfort and evacuation of the bowels, together with facial pallor, are usual during the infusion. If these are absent it may be questioned whether the vasopressin is pharmacologically active. Inert material is the commonest cause of failure.

Vasopressin stimulates smooth muscle and so causes coronary vasoconstriction. A preliminary electrocardiogram should be taken before vasopressin is given and evidence of myocardial ischaemia should be a contraindication.

Cessation of haemorrhage probably results from the temporary drop in portal blood pressure, allowing haemostasis at the bleeding point. The reduction in hepatic arterial blood flow in patients with cirrhosis is undesirable.

As the gastric and mesenteric arterioles are also constricted, bleeding will be controlled not only from the oesophagus but from the stomach and duodenum. The successful use of vasopressin therefore cannot distinguish a bleeding varix from a bleeding ulcer.

Gangrene may follow subcutaneous infiltration of the vasopressin [44].

Vasopressin injections may be repeated in four hours if bleeding recurs but the efficacy drops with continued use. Vasopressin may stop the bleeding but not prolong life. This reflects underlying liver failure rather than the method of treatment. The value of vasopressin lies in its simplicity. It can

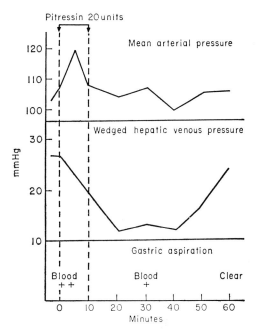

Fig. 148. Effect of 20 units of Pitressin i.v. over 10 min. on wedged hepatic venous pressure, mean arterial pressure and gastric aspirations (Shaldon & Sherlock 1960).

even be used in the home as special nursing and medical care are not essential. The short duration is obviously unsatisfactory and the side-effects are unpleasant.

Arterial vasopressin. The drug may be given by selective mesenteric arterial infusion [6]. Side-effects are similar to those of the intravenous route [22] which is easier and as effective [82].

Tryglycyl lysine vasopressin (Glypressin). This synthetic derivative of vasopressin is inactivated slowly and a single intravenous dose lasts 6–12 hours [132]. It may have fewer side-effects.

Continuous oral administration of *propranolol* in doses which reduce the heart rate by 25% lowers portal venous pressure in cirrhotic patients [64]. This is related to a reduction in cardiac output and liver blood flow—an undesirable feature of the treatment.

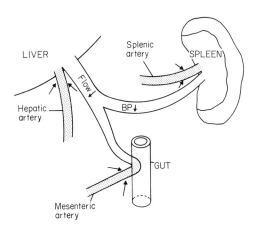

Fig. 147. The mode of action of vasopressin on the splanchnic circulation. Hepatic, splenic and mesenteric arteries are shown. Splanchnic blood flow (including hepatic blood flow) and portal venous pressure are reduced by arterial vasoconstriction (arrowed).

Sengstaken–Blakemore tube (fig. 149) [91, 96]

Oesophageal tamponade is usually done with one or other modification of the Sengstaken–Blakemore tube. The four-lumened tube has an oesophageal and a gastric balloon [91], a tube in the stomach and a fourth lumen for aspiration above

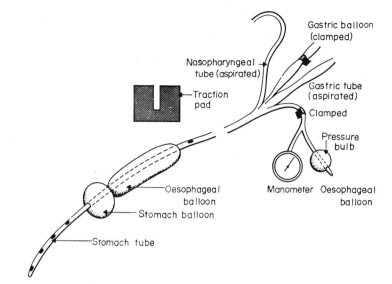

Fig. 149. Sengstaken–
Blakemore oesophageal
compression tube modified
by Pitcher (1971). Note
fourth oesophageal tube
which aspirates the
oesophagus above the
oesophageal balloon.

the oesophageal balloon. The stomach is emptied. The oesophageal tube is aspirated continuously. A *new*, tested and lubricated tube is passed through the mouth into the stomach. The gastric balloon is inflated with 250 ml air and doubly clamped. The gastric tube is aspirated continuously. The oesophageal tube is inflated to a pressure of 20–30 mmHg, slightly greater than that expected in the portal vein. Firm traction is exerted using a padded key-hole plywood retainer positioned around the tube at the angle of the mouth and held in position by adhesive tape. Too little traction means that the gastric balloon falls back into the stomach. Too much causes discomfort, with retching and also potentiates gastro-oesophageal ulceration. If necessary, the position of the tube may be checked by X-ray of the abdomen. The gastric balloon should sit well into the fundus of the stomach. The head of the bed is elevated. A trained attendant is constantly at the bedside and a pair of scissors is available to transect the tube if respiratory distress occurs. Tube traction and oesophageal balloon pressure are checked at 2–4 hour intervals. After 24 hours, traction is released, and the oesophageal balloon deflated leaving the gastric balloon inflated for a further 24 hours. If, during this period, re-bleeding occurs, the traction is re-applied and the oesophageal balloon re-inflated for another 24–28 hours or until emergency surgery is performed. Following removal, a soft diet and salt-free liquid antacids are given.

The compression tubes are very successful in controlling bleeding from oesophageal varices. They do, however, have many complications. They should not be left longer than 24 hours or ulceration will be precipitated. Their complications are numerous and include obstruction to the pharynx and asphyxia. The gastric balloon may rupture and the tube may migrate into the oeso-phagus. Ulceration of the lower oesophagus or pharynx complicates one-third of intubations par-ticularly if prolonged or repeated [96]. Aspiration of secretion into the lung with subsequent infec-tion is prevented by continuous aspiration of the naso-pharynx via the fourth tube.

The *Linton–Nachlas* tube is a single-balloon triple-lumen tube which is more effective for con-trol of gastric variceal haemorrhage but less so when the bleeding comes from the oesophagus [124].

Conclusions

The modified four-lumen Sengstaken tube is the most certain method for continued control of oesophageal bleeding over hours. Complications are frequent and are in part related to the skill and experience of the operating team [91]. It is un-pleasant for the patient. It is useful for patients who have to be transferred from one centre to another for special treatment and when vasopres-sin has failed and haemorrhage is torrential. It should not be used for much more than 24 hours.

Vasopressin is simple to give. Its action, how-ever, is short-lived. It should be the routine initial method of treating bleeding from varices. If it fails, the Sengstaken tube is the next line of management.

All these methods will be followed by the recurrence of bleeding in about the same proportion of patients. This reflects defective hepatic function and blood clotting rather than portal hypertension *per se*. The decision to introduce the Sengstaken tube repeatedly or to keep it in position for days or alternatively to give many injections of vasopressin with diminishing effect is hard to make. Emergency surgery must be considered.

Emergency surgery

This should be avoided if at all possible. Portacaval shunts, done as an emergency, have a high mortality: this was 49% in one series where the patients were alcoholics with cirrhosis and in liver failure.

If bleeding is torrential and long-term control has not been achieved by intravenous vasopressin and the Sengstaken tube, an emergency mesocaval shunt may be the most suitable procedure. Blood loss at surgery is large before the bleeding is controlled. The mortality is high in class C patients [18]. An alternative is oesophageal transection which carries a high mortality and has a high complication rate [41].

Trans-hepatic variceal sclerosis (figs. 130–133)

The main collateral venous supply of the gastro-oesophageal varices is visualized by trans-hepatic portal venography [119]. Under local anaesthesia, a catheter can be introduced into the portal vein and the dangerous variceal supply veins (left gastric and short gastric) selectively catheterized and injected with human thrombin and gel foam—so obliterating them [66, 107, 119]. The tissue adhesive, bucrylate, is an alternative sclerosant [39]. The hole in the liver is plugged with gel foam as the catheter is withdrawn. This is an excellent method of stopping variceal bleeding, particularly in those with severe liver failure. It may also be used as an elective procedure to prevent further haemorrhage. The technique allows fundal and oesophageal varices to be obliterated close to their origin. This is an advantage over oesophagoscopic injection where there is difficulty in obliterating all varices, especially those in the fundus of the stomach.

Technical failures usually occur when the supply veins to the varices are small. Complications include haemorrhage from the liver, biliary peritonitis and, possibly, portal vein thrombosis.

The duration of occlusion is uncertain. The value is as an emergency procedure in poor-risk patients.

Injection sclerotherapy

In 1939, injection sclerotherapy for the treatment of oesophageal varices was introduced [24]. At that time it did not achieve popularity, but current disenchantment with portal–systemic shunting procedures has led to its re-introduction. Veins are injected through a rigid oesophagoscope, necessitating general anaesthesia [122, 123]. If a flexible instrument is used a special rigid tube is included which fits over the endoscope. General anaesthesia is not necessary. Aspiration of blood, however, is not easy. The injection is made into the vein rather than beneath the mucosa. Ethanolamine oleate or sodium morrhuate are the usual sclerosants.

Injection is difficult if the patient is actually bleeding, and control of haemorrhage must be achieved before injection by such methods as the Sengstaken tube.

In one series, bleeding was controlled in 93% of 117 patients. The total 'admission' mortality was 18–25% [123].

Sclerotherapy has also been used long-term, the veins being injected about every two months [122]. Episodes of bleeding are reduced.

The technique is not easy. General anaesthesia is usually required. Complications include bleeding from varices at the time of puncture, retrosternal pain lasting 12–24 hours, narrowing of the lower end of the oesophagus, mediastinitis and disturbed motility of the oesophagus. Recanalization and development of fresh varices are obvious long-term problems. Gastric (fundal) varices are not injected.

Oesophageal transection

This is used as a 'last ditch' procedure in patients with intractable variceal bleeding, particularly with portal vein thrombosis [41]. The operation requires considerable technical skill, a thoracico-abdominal approach, and carries a high mortality.

A modification uses the *SPTU universal stapling gun* [56] used for the stapling of rectal and oesophageal anastomoses. The patient is stabilized, perhaps using the Sengstaken tube. The oesophagus is mobilized and the nozzle of the gun advanced into the lower oesophagus. A flange of four-thickness oesophageal wall is introduced between two sections of gun and the gap is reduced to 2.5 mm. The transection is completed by pulling the trigger when simultaneously the gun resects a full thickness section of oesophageal wall. Reanastomosis of the oesophagus is done using 12 staples. Complications include anastomotic leaks, mild dysphagia and, later, heartburn. Later bleeding follows the development of new collaterals around the transection. This may be a useful emergency method for controlling oesophageal bleeding in those fit for general anaesthesia.

SURGICAL PORTAL–SYSTEMIC SHUNTS

The aim is to reduce portal venous pressure, maintain total hepatic and, particularly, portal blood flow and, above all, not have a high incidence of complicating hepatic encephalopathy. There is no currently available procedure that fulfils all these criteria satisfactorily. Hepatic reserve determines survival. Hepato-cellular function deteriorates after shunting [101]. In animals this corresponds to a reduction in liver function of 50% of liver mass after end-to-side porta-caval shunt [63].

SELECTION OF PATIENTS

There should have been at least one haemorrhage, usually of sufficient severity to merit transfusion, from proven oesophago-gastric varices [139]. Varices must be demonstrated by fibroscopy or barium studies. Portal hypertension must be established by pressure measurements. The portal vein, shown by splenic venography or by selective splanchnic angiography, must be suitable for the shunt. Prophylactic shunts do not prolong life [23, 54, 55].

General condition must be good and age preferably less than 50 years. After 40 years, survival is reduced and encephalopathy is twice as common [52].

Hepato-cellular function must be adequate. Serum bilirubin levels should be less than 2.5 mg/100 ml in non-biliary cases. Serum albumin should exceed 3 g/100 ml. Ascites should not be present at the time of operation, but recent transient ascites, perhaps after haemorrhage, does not reduce survival. Even the mildest episode of pre-operative encephalopathy, perhaps after a major haemorrhage, should contraindicate porta-caval anastomosis for severe post-operative encephalopathy is sure to develop in these patients. The EEG should be normal.

The liver disease should be static or only slowly progressive. The overall five-year survival for elective end-to-side porta-caval anastomosis for cirrhotic patients is 55%. This is reduced in chronic active hepatitis, where hepatocellular necrosis continues, and increased in primary biliary cirrhosis where liver function is good. In the alcoholic the prognosis lies between the two and much depends on whether the patient abstains from alcohol post-operatively.

The patient must be in the best possible condition and haemoglobin should be at least 12 g/dl. Oral neomycin, 4 g daily, is started the day before operation and continued for four days. Dietary protein must be reduced pre-operatively and none given for three days after the operation. Morphine should be avoided and intravenous barbiturates given only in small doses. Halothane (fluothane) is a suitable anaesthetic.

Porta-caval anastomosis (fig. 150)

In 1877 Eck [34] first performed a porta-caval shunt in dogs and this remains the most effective way of reducing portal hypertension.

The portal vein is joined to the inferior vena cava either end-to-side with ligation of the portal vein (fig. 152) or side-to-side, maintaining its continuity (fig. 153). The portal blood pressure falls, hepatic venous pressure falls and hepatic arterial flow increases. There is decompression of the splanchnic venous bed and the portal–systemic collateral circulation disappears.

When an end-to-side porta-caval shunt is performed the ratio of the portal pressure to total blood flow is unchanged (fig. 152). In other words, the hepatic blood flow falls to the same extent as the portal pressure so that the sinusoidal resistance is unchanged and the intra-hepatic obstruction is not relieved.

If the side-to-side porta-caval shunt is made, hepatic arterial blood can, and often does, pass in a retrograde fashion in the portal vein to the inferior vena cava [80, 99] (fig. 153). This retrograde-flowing blood may contribute somewhat to hepatic function although some hepatic arterial blood flow is undoubtedly lost [81]. The post-sinu-

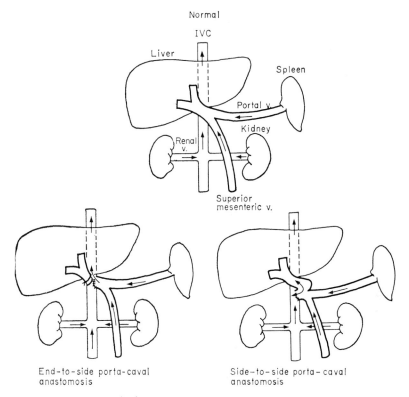

Fig. 150. The types of portal–systemic shunt operation performed for the relief of portal hypertension.

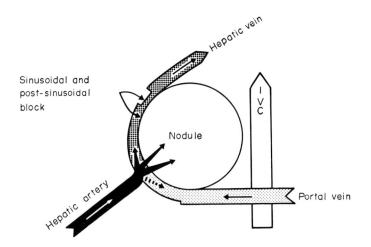

Fig. 151. The circulation in hepatic cirrhosis. A nodule obstructs the sinusoids and hepatic veins. The nodule is supplied mainly by the hepatic artery.

soidal block, which may be important in ascites formation, is relieved.

The end-to-side shunt probably gives a greater fall in portal venous pressure than does the side-to-side procedure, of the order of 10 mmHg.

Technically, it is easier to perform. The stoma is larger, kinking and tension are absent and there is smooth unidirectional blood flow. The side-to-side shunt is more difficult to perform. It does, however, allow vascular decompression and relief

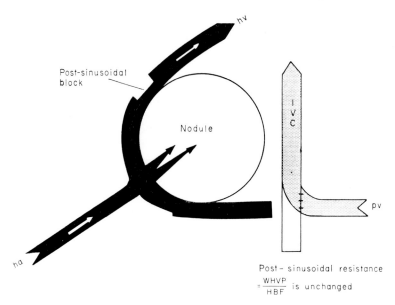

Fig. 152. End-to-side porta-caval shunt. The liver is now supplied entirely by the hepatic artery. The wedged hepatic venous pressure (WHVP) falls in proportion to the hepatic blood flow (HBF) so that the post-sinusoidal resistance is unchanged and the intra-hepatic block is not relieved.

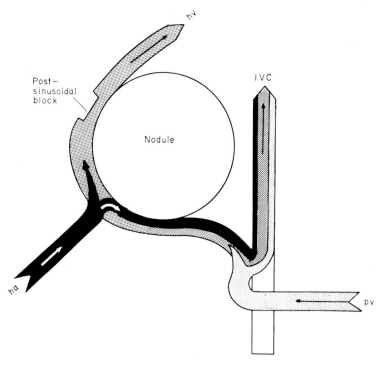

Fig. 153. Side-to-side porta-caval shunt. Continuity between the main portal vein and the liver is maintained so that retrograde flow in the portal vein is possible. The intra-hepatic block is relieved.

of hepatic outflow block. If this is particularly severe, ascites may be made worse by end-to-side shunt. Clinical comparison of the two methods showed no major differences [99] The higher incidence of severe encephalopathy after the side-to-side procedure (50% compared with 28%) [99] makes it the less desirable one.

RESULTS OF PORTA-CAVAL ANASTOMOSIS

Operative mortality depends on selection of patients with good hepato-cellular function. The good-risk patients have an operative mortality of 6–12% [52, 131] and a five-year survival of 65–70%. For poor-risk patients the mortality is 50%.

Shunt closure is often due to operating on a partially thrombosed, thickened or calcified portal vein and is often fatal [52]. Hepatic failure is the usual cause of death. Later fibrotic closure of the shunt is unusual.

Survival. The traditional end-to-side porta-caval shunt certainly prevents bleeding from gastro-oesophageal varices and probably increases survival.

General effects of a patent anastomosis. There is no further gastro-intestinal bleeding from varices [19].

Abdominal wall collateral veins disappear. Diminution in *spleen* size can be detected clinically within three months of the operation. *Oesophagoscopy* shows collapsed veins. Barium swallow and endoscopy show disappearance of *oesophageal varices* within six months to one year of the operation. *Spleno-portal venography* or superior mesenteric angiography shows passage of the contrast material from the portal vein directly into the inferior vena cava; collateral channels are not filled (figs. 154, 155).

Hepatic blood flow is reduced [98]. The oxygen supply to the liver cells is maintained as far as possible by better extraction of oxygen, the arterial–hepatic vein oxygen difference increasing. Splenic blood flow increases [42].

Intra-splenic pressure falls; a subsequent rise in pressure means that the anastomosis is blocked. Portal pressure falls.

After end-to-side porta-caval anastomosis the wedged (sinusoidal) hepatic venous pressure

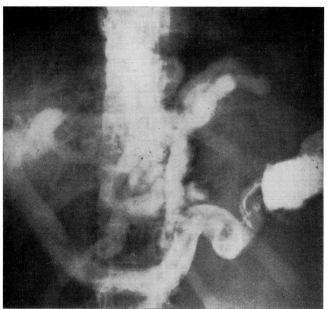

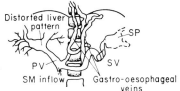

Fig. 154. Girl with post-hepatitis cirrhosis. Pre-operative splenic venography shows extensive collateral circulation via gastro-oesophageal veins.

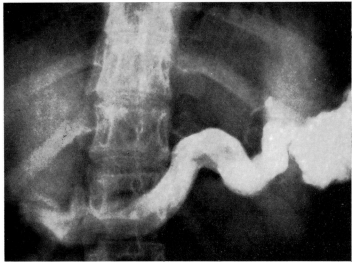

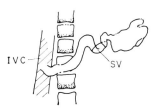

Fig. 155. Same patient as in fig. 154 after porta-caval anastomosis. The collaterals are no longer filled but the vena cava is well seen (Turner *et al* 1957).

falls with hepatic blood flow; the ratio, i.e. sinusoidal resistance, is unchanged indicating that intra-hepatic portal–venous hypertension has not been relieved (fig. 152). After side-to-side anastomosis the portal vein can, if necessary, become the outflow tract of the liver (fig. 153).

Hepatic function deteriorates slowly. This is in part due to the natural history of the chronic liver disease. It is also related to the loss of portal venous flow to the liver. It may be less where portal flow has already, pre-operatively, been deviated into collaterals and the fraction of hepatic arterial flow has increased. This may be shown on a splenic venogram by poor portal filling of the main portal vein [15] (fig. 126).

Jaundice, after shunt, reflects deterioration of hepatic function and also increased load of bilirubin due to haemolysis of transfused blood. In addition, unconjugated hyperbilirubinaemia is due to increased blood destruction after porta-caval anastomosis [26]. The mechanism is unknown.

Oedema of the ankles develops or increases in most patients with cirrhosis. Pressure in the inferior vena cava does not increase. The oedema is presumably part of the general fluid retention of cirrhosis. The portal venous pressure has been reduced but the serum albumin level remains low. Fluid therefore localizes in dependent parts rather than in the peritoneal cavity. Increased cardiac output with failure may contribute to the oedema [43].

Neuropsychiatric changes. These may be only transient in the post-operative period when liver cell function is depressed. Chronic changes, however, can also be anticipated [97]. The incidence depends on the assiduity with which the clinician searches for them and with which they are investigated.

The incidence is 20–40%. The incidence is less with end-to-side (28%) than side-to-side (50%) shunt [98] for hepatic perfusion with arterial blood is better. It is also less following a spleno-renal than porta-caval anastomosis, suggesting that the size of the shunt is important.

Progressive deterioration of hepatic function may be the major factor in determining the development of encephalopathy. This deterioration is proportional to the reduction in hepatic blood flow.

Patients whose liver disease progresses will be more likely to develop encephalopathy (table 24). Encephalopathy is greatest in conditions such as

Table 24. Post-shunt encephalopathy. Late post-operative, severe, chronic portal–systemic encephalopathy in 50 survivors with patent shunts (Hourigan *et al* 1971).

Aetiology	No. of cases	Patients with encephalopathy no.	Patients with encephalopathy %
Cryptogenic cirrhosis	28	11	39
Alcoholic cirrhosis	9	5	56
Biliary cirrhosis	4	0	0
Chronic active hepatitis with cirrhosis	5	3	60
Portal vein block	1	0	0
Schistosomal cirrhosis	1	0	0
Haemochromatosis	1	0	0
Sarcoidosis	1	0	0
Total	50	19	38

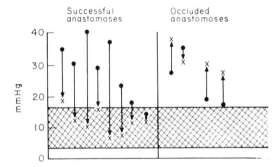

Fig. 156. Effect of end-to-side porta-caval anastomosis on intrasplenic pressure. ● = Pre-operative, *X* = post-operative. The normal range is cross-hatched (Turner *et al* 1957).

chronic active hepatitis where progression of the liver disease is more rapid [52]. The best candidates are those with excellent hepato-cellular function such as congenital hepatic fibrosis or with a blocked portal vein at the hilum of the liver.

Symptoms are commoner in older patients, perhaps due to changes in the ageing brain, so that it becomes less capable of meeting alterations in its environment.

The personality deterioration seen to a greater or lesser degree in about a third of patients is a major post-operative complication (Chapter 8).

Myelopathy, with paraplegia, has developed soon after porta-caval anastomosis. Autopsy shows pyramidal tract demyelination. Chronic parkinsonian–cerebellar syndromes may be seen (Chapter 18).

Haemosiderosis (Chapter 20).

Meso-caval shunt

The superior mesenteric vein is anastomosed side-to-side with the inferior vena cava using a

dacron graft [33 [18] (fig. 157). Hospital deaths are 9% for good-risk and 58% for poor-risk patients [18]. The early encephalopathy rate is 9% [18]. This shunt is particularly applicable to the poor-risk patient. It is technically easy. The portal vein remains patent but the blood flow through it is un-

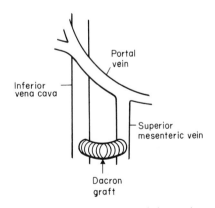

Fig. 157. The Drapanas mesocaval shunt using a dacron graft.

certain. Shunt occlusion is a complication and this is followed by re-bleeding [31].

Selective 'distal' spleno-renal shunt (fig. 158)

This aims to divide veins feeding the dangerous oesophago-gastric collaterals while allowing drainage of portal blood through short gastric spleen and splenic veins through a spleno-renal shunt to the inferior vena cava. Portal blood flow is maintained [134].

In a controlled, prospective trial, when the distal spleno-renal shunt was compared with non-selective shunts, usually meso-caval, the operative mortality was similar [103]. After four years only

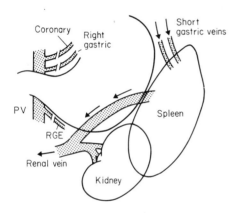

Fig. 158. The distal spleno-renal shunt. Veins feeding varices (coronary, right gastric, right gastro-epiploic—RGE) are ligated. A spleno-renal shunt is made, preserving the spleen; retrograde flow in the short gastric veins is possible. Portal blood flow to the liver is preserved.

12% of patients with selective shunts—compared with 52% of non-selective shunts—had experienced episodes of hepatic encephalopathy. Survival was increased, at least in non-alcoholic patients.

The technique is a difficult and time-consuming one. It does not always achieve its objective of preserving portal blood flow [71]. Ascites, which may be chylous and usually transient, may be a complication [75]. Comparison of the selective shunt with standard end-to-side porta-caval shunt or more conservative measures such as trans-hepatic sclerosis suggests little benefit for the more complicated procedure.

Portal vein arterialization procedures

Portal blood flow may be maintained if, after a porta-caval shunt, the splenic artery is ligated and anastomosed to the distal stump of the portal vein [70].

Alternatively a saphenous vein graft has been used from the right gastro-epiploic artery to the hepatic portion of the portal vein [1]. Arterial flow is maintained at or slightly below the level of normal portal flow. Follow-up results are awaited.

SUMMARY

The treatment of portal hypertension has not been solved. In the cirrhotic group very few patients have sufficiently adequate liver function to allow porta-caval anastomosis, the operation which has the greatest hope of success. The young patient with cirrhosis whose only complaint is recurrent haematemesis may achieve a spectacularly good result. Encephalopathy, however, remains a problem. Surgical procedures treat only the mechanical effects of portal vein obstruction and prognosis remains that of hepato-cellular function. Procedures are being tried which will lower portal pressure in the gastro-oesophageal region while maintaining hepatic blood flow (and hepato-cellular function). The problem of treating haemorrhage in patients with poor liver function remains unsolved.

In the group with extra-hepatic portal obstruction prognosis, even without surgery, is good provided adequate blood transfusion is given.

Medical measures such as bed rest and a good diet may be followed by a fall in portal pressure, especially in alcoholic subjects who lose fat from the liver. This makes assessment of surgical results even more difficult.

REFERENCES

1. ADAMSONS R.J., KINKHABWALA M., MOSKOWITZ H. *et al* (1972) Portacaval shunt with arterialisation of the hepatic portion of the portal vein. *Surg. Gynecol. Obstet.* **135**, 529.
2. ALVES C.A.P., ALVES A.R., ABREU W.N. *et al* (1977) Hepatic artery hypertrophy and sinusoidal hypertension in advanced schistosomiasis. *Gastroenterology* **72**, 126.
3. ANDERSON M.F. & DUNNICK N.R. (1977) Pseudo-tumor caused by gastric varices. *Am. J. dig. Dis.* **22**, 929.

4. ATKINSON M., BARNETT E., SHERLOCK S. *et al* (1955) The clinical investigation of the portal circulation with special reference to portal venography. *Q. J. Med.* **24**, 77.

5. ATKINSON M. & SHERLOCK S. (1954) Intrasplenic pressure as an index of the portal venous pressure. *Lancet* **i**, 1325.

6. BAUM S. & NUSBAUM M. (1971) The control of gastrointestinal hemorrhage by selective mesenteric arterial infusion of vasopressin. *Radiology* **98**, 497.

7. BAUMGARTEN P. VON (1907) Über völlstandiges Offenbleiben der Vena umbilicalis; zugleich ein Beitrag zur Frage des Morbus Bantii. *Arb. path. Anat. Inst. Tübingen* **6**, 93.

8. BEARN A.G., BILLING B., EDHOLM O.G. *et al* (1951) Hepatic blood flow and carbohydrate changes in man during fainting. *J. Physiol.* **115**, 442.

9. BENNETT H.D., LORENTZEN C. & BAKER L.A. (1953) Transient esophageal varices in hepatic cirrhosis. *Arch. intern. Med.* **92**, 507.

10. BLENDIS L.M., PARKINSON M.C., SHILKIN K.B. *et al* (1974) Nodular regenerative hypoplasia of the liver in Felty's syndrome. *Q. J. Med.* **43**, 25.

11. BLENDIS L.M., SMITH P.M., LAWRIE B.W. *et al* (1978) Portal hypertension in vinyl chloride monomer workers. *Gastroenterology* **75**, 206.

12. BLOOM H.J.G. (1950) Venous hums in hepatic cirrhosis. *Br. Heart J.* **12**, 343.

13. BOYER J.L., GUPTA K.P.S., BISWAS S.K. *et al* (1967) Idiopathic portal hypertension. *Ann. intern. Med.* **66**, 41.

14. BRADLEY S.E., INGELFINGER F.J., BRADLEY G.P. *et al* (1945) Estimation of hepatic blood flow in man. *J. clin. Invest.* **24**, 890.

15. BURCHELL A.R., MORENO A.H., PANKE W.F. *et al* (1965) Some limitations of splenic portography. I. Incidence, hemodynamics and surgical implications of the nonvisualized portal vein. *Ann. Surg.* **162**, 981.

16. CAESAR J., BARBER K.M., BARAONA E. *et al* (1962) The estimation of portal–systemic collateral flow in man using intrasplenic injection of radio-active indicator. *Clin. Sci.* **23**, 77.

17. CAESAR J., SHALDON S., CHIANDUSSI L. *et al* (1961) The use of indocyanine green in the measurement of hepatic blood flow and as a test of hepatic function. *Clin. Sci.* **21**, 43.

18. CAMERON J.L., ZUIDEMA G.D., SMITH G.W. *et al* (1979) Mesocaval shunts for the control of bleeding esophageal varices. *Surgery (St Louis)* **85**, 257.

19. CASTELL D.O. & CONN H.O. (1972) The determination of portacaval shunt patency: a critical review of methodology. *Medicine (Baltimore)* **51**, 315.

20. CHENDEROVITCH J. (1956) La microangioradiographie du foie et de la rate. Thèse, Faculté de Médecine de Paris.

21. CHILD C.G. III (1954) *The Hepatic Circulation and Portal Hypertension*. W.B. Saunders, Philadelphia.

22. CHOJKIER M., GROSZMANN R.J., ATTERBURY C.E. *et al* (1979) A controlled comparison of continuous intra-arterial and intravenous infusions of vasopressin in hemorrhage from esophageal varices. *Gastroenterology* **77**, 540.

23. CONN H.O., LINDENMUTH W.W., MAY C.J. *et al* (1972) Prophylactic porta-caval anastomosis—a tale of two studies. *Medicine (Baltimore)* **51**, 27.

24. CRAFOORD C. & FRENCKNER P. (1939) New surgical treatment of varicose veins of the oesophagus. *Acta Otolaryngol. Stockh.* **27**, 422.

25. CRUVEILHIER J. (1829–35) Anatomie pathologique du corps humain. Vol. 1. XVI livr. pl. vi—*Maladies du veines* J.B. Ballière, Paris.

26. DA SILVA L.C., JAMRA M.A., MASPES V. *et al* (1963) Pathogenesis of indirect reacting hyperbilirubinemia after portacaval anastomosis. *Gastroenterology* **44**, 117.

27. DATTA D.V., MITRA S.K., CHHUTTANI P.N. *et al* (1979) Chronic oral arsenic intoxication as a possible aetiological factor in idiopathic portal hypertension (non-cirrhotic portal fibrosis) in India. *Gut* **20**, 378.

28. DOBSON E.L. & JONES H.B. (1952) The behaviour of intravenously injected particulate matter; its rate of disappearance from the blood stream as a measure of liver blood flow. *Acta med. Scand.* **144**, suppl. 273.

29. DOCK W. (1942) Role of increased hepatic arterial flow in the portal hypertension of cirrhosis. *Trans. Ass. Am. Physicians* **57**, 302.

30. DOUGLASS B.E., BAGGENSTOSS A.H. & HOLLINSHEAD W.H. (1950) Variations in the portal systems of veins. *Proc. Mayo Clin.* **25**, 26.

31. DOWLING J.B. (1979) Ten years' experience with mesocaval grafts. *Surg. Gynecol. Obstet.* **149**, 518.

32. DOYLE F.H., READ A.E. & EVANS K.T. (1961) The mediastinum in portal hypertension. *Clin. Radiol.* **12**, 114.

33. DRAPANAS T. (1972) Interposition mesocaval shunt for treatment of portal hypertension. *Ann. Surg.* **176**, 435.

34. ECK N.V. (1877) On the question of ligature of the portal vein (trans. title). *Voyenno med. J. (St Petersburg)* **130**, Sect. 2, 1.

35. ECKARDT V.F. & GRACE N.D. (1979) Gastro-esophageal reflux and bleeding esophageal varices. *Gastroenterology* **76**, 39.

36. FOLEY W.J., TURCOTTE J.G., HOSKINS P.A. *et al* (1971) Intrahepatic arteriovenous fistulas between the hepatic artery and portal vein. *Ann. Surg.* **174**, 849.

37. FRANCO D., DURANDY Y., DEPORTE A. *et al* (1977) Upper gastrointestinal haemorrhage in hepatic cirrhosis: causes and relation to hepatic failure and stress. *Lancet* **i**, 218.

38. FRED H.L., MAYHALL C.G. & HARLE T.S. (1968) Hepatic portal venous gas. A review and report on six new cases. *Am. J. Med.* **44**, 557.

39. FREENY P.C. & KIDD R. (1979) Transhepatic portal venography and selective obliteration of gastroesophageal varices using isobutyl 2-cyanoacrylate (Bucrylate). *Am. J. dig. Dis.* **24**, 321.

40. GATES G.F. & DORE E.K. (1973) Streamline flow in the human portal vein. *J. nucl. Med.* **14**, 79.

41. GEORGE P., BROWN C., RIDGWAY G. *et al* (1973) Emergency oesophageal transection in uncontrolled variceal haemorrhage. *Br. J. Surg.* **60**, 635.

42. GITLIN G., GRAHAME G.R., KREEL L. *et al* (1970) Splenic blood flow and resistance in patients with

cirrhosis before and after portacaval anastomoses. *Gastroenterology* **59**, 208.

43. GORDON M.J. & DEL GUERCIO L.R.M. (1972) Late effects of portal systemic shunting procedures of cardio-respiratory dynamics in man. *Ann. Surg.* **176**, 672.

44. GREENWALD R.A., RHEINGOLD O.J., CHIPRUT R.O. *et al* (1978) Local gangrene: a complication of peripheral pitressin therapy for bleeding esophageal varices. *Gastroenterology* **74**, 744.

45. GROSZMANN R.J., KITELANSKI B. & COHN J.N. (1971) Hepatic lobar distribution of splenic and mesenteric blood flow in man. *Gastroenterology* **66**, 1047.

46. GROSZMANN R.J., GLICKMAN M., BLEI A.T. *et al* (1979) Wedged and free hepatic venous pressure measured with a balloon catheter. *Gastroenterology* **76**, 253.

47. GROSZMANN R., KOTELANSKI B., COHN J. *et al* (1972) Quantitation of porta-systemic shunting from the splenic and mesenteric beds in alcoholic liver disease. *Am. J. Med.* **53**, 715.

48. GRUNDFEST S., COOPERMAN A.M., FERGUSON R. *et al* (1980) Portal hypertension associated with systemic mastocytosis and splenomegaly. *Gastroenterology* **78**, 370.

49. HAMLYN A.N., LUNZER M.R., MORRIS J.S. *et al* (1974) Portal hypertension with varices in unusual sites. *Lancet* ii, 1531.

50. HERLINGER H. (1928) Arterioportography. *Clin. Radiol.* **29**, 255.

51. HOU P.C. & MCFADZEAN A.J.S. (1965) Thrombosis and intimal thickening in the portal system in cirrhosis of the liver. *J. Path. Bact.* **89**, 473.

52. HOURIGAN K., SHERLOCK S., GEORGE P. *et al* (1971) Elective end-to-side porta-caval shunt: results in 64 cases. *Br. med. J.* iv, 473.

53. ITZCHAK Y. & GLICKMAN M.G. (1977) Duodenal varices in extrahepatic portal obstruction. *Radiology* **124**, 619.

54. JACKSON F.C., PERRIN E.B., SMITH A.G. *et al* (1968) A clinical investigation of the portacaval shunt. II. Survival analysis of the prophylactic operation. *Am. J. Surg.* **115**, 22.

55. JACKSON F.C., PERRIN E.B., FELIX W.R. *et al* (1971) A clinical investigation of the portacaval shunt. V. Survival analysis of the therapeutic operation. *Ann. Surg.* **174**, 672.

56. JOHNSTON G.W. (1978) Simplified oesophageal transection for bleeding varices. *Br. med. J.* i, 1388.

57. JOHNSTON G.W. & GIBSON J.B. (1965) Portal hypertension resulting from splenic arteriovenous fistulae. *Gut* **6**, 500.

58. KASHIWAGI T., KAMADA T. & ABE H. (1974) Dynamic studies on the portal hemodynamics by scintiphotosplenoportography: the visualization of portal venous system using ^{99m}Tc. *Gastroenterology* **67**, 668.

59. KASHIWAGI T., KIMURA K., SUEMATSU T. *et al* (1980) Dynamic studies on portal haemodynamics by scintiphotosplenoportography: flow patterns of portal circulation. *Gut* **21**, 57.

60. KELTY R.H., BAGGENSTOSS A.H. & BUTT H.R. (1950) The relation of the regenerated liver nodule to the vascular bed in cirrhosis. *Gastroenterology* **15**, 285.

61. KERR D.N.S., HARRISON C.V., SHERLOCK S. *et al* (1961) Congenital hepatic fibrosis. *Q. J. Med.* **30**, 91.

62. KESSLER R.E., TICE D.A. & ZIMMON D.S. (1973) Value, complications and limitations of umbilical vein catheterization. *Surg. Gynecol. Obstet.* **136**, 529.

63. LAUTERBURG B.H., SAVTTER V., PREISIG R. *et al* (1976) Hepatic functional deterioration after portacaval shunt in the rat. *Gastroenterology* **71**, 221.

64. LEBREC D., NOUEL O., CORBIC M. *et al* (1980) Propranolol—a medical treatment for portal hypertension. *Lancet* ii, 180.

65. LONGSTRETH G.F., NEWCOMER A.D. & GREEN P.A. (1971) Extrahepatic portal hypertension caused by chronic pancreatitis. *Ann. intern. Med.* **75**, 903.

66. LUNDERQUIST A. & VANG J. (1974) Transhepatic catheterization and obliteration of the coronary vein in patients with portal hypertension and esophageal varices. *New Engl. J. Med.* **291**, 646.

67. MCINDOE A.H. (1928) Vascular lesions of portal cirrhosis. *Arch. Path.* **5**, 23.

68. MCMICHAEL J. (1934) The pathology of hepatolienal fibrosis. *J. Path. Bact.* **39**, 481.

69. MADDREY W.C., MALLIK K.C.B., IBER F.L. *et al* (1968) Extrahepatic obstruction of the portal venous system. *Surg. Gynecol. Obstet.* **127**, 989.

70. MAILLARD J.-N., BENHAMOU J.-P. & RUEFF B. (1970) Arterialization of the liver with portacaval shunt in the treatment of portal hypertension due to intrahepatic block. *Surgery* (*St Louis*) **67**, 883.

71. MAILLARD J.-N., FLAMANT Y.M., HAY J.M. *et al* (1979) Selectivity of the distal splenorenal shunt. *Surgery* **86**, 663.

72. MANENTI F. & WILLIAMS R. (1966) Injection of the splenic vasculature in portal hypertension. *Gut* **7**, 175.

73. MARION P. (1953) Les obstructions portales. *Sem. Hôp. Paris* **29**, 2781.

74. MARTIN L.W., BENZING G. & KAPLAN S. (1965) Congenital intrahepatic arteriovenous fistula: report of a successfully treated case. *Ann. Surg.* **161**, 209.

75. MAYWOOD B.T., GOLDSTEIN L. & BUSUTTIL R.W. (1978) Chylous ascites after a Warren shunt. *Am. J. Surg.* **135**, 700.

76. MORENO A.H., BURCHELL A.R., ROUSSELOT L.M. *et al* (1967) Portal blood flow in cirrhosis of the liver. *J. clin. Invest.* **46**, 236.

77. MORENO A.H., RUZICKA F.F., ROUSSELOT L.M. *et al* (1963) Functional hepatography. A study of the hemodynamics of the outflow tracts of the human liver by intraparenchymal deposition of contrast medium, with attempts at functional evaluation of the outflow block concept of cirrhotic ascites and the accessory outflow role of the portal vein. *Radiology* **81**, 65.

78. MORRIS J.S., SCHMID M., NEWMAN S. *et al* (1974) Arsenic and non-cirrhotic portal hypertension. *Gastroenterology* **66**, 86.

79. MOULT P.J.A., WAITE D.W. & DICK R. (1975) Posterior mediastinal venous masses in patients with portal hypertension. *Gut* **16**, 57.

80. Mulder D.G., Plested W.G. III, Hanafee W.N. *et al* (1966) Hepatic circulatory and functional alterations following side-to-side porta-caval shunt. *Surgery* **59**, 923.

81. Murray J.F. & Mulder D.G. (1961) The effects of retrograde portal venous flow following side-to-side portacaval anastomosis: a comparison with end-to-side shunts. *J. clin. Invest.* **40**, 1413.

82. Murray-Lyon I.M., Pugh R.N.H., Nunnerly H.B. *et al* (1973) Treatment of bleeding oesophageal varices by infusion of vasopressin into the superior mesenteric artery. *Gut* **14**, 59.

83. Nataf C., Feldmann G., Lebrec D. *et al* (1979) Idiopathic hypertension (perisinusoidal fibrosis) after renal transplantation. *Gut* **20**, 531.

84. Odièvre M., Pigé G. & Alagille D. (1977) Congenital abnormalities associated with extrahepatic portal hypertension. *Arch. Dis. Childh.* **52**, 383.

85. Ohkubo H., Okuda K., Takayasu K. *et al* (1978) Cruveilhier–Baumgarten syndrome presenting with precordial murmur and thrill. *Am. J. dig. Dis.* **23**, 65s.

86. Okuda K., Suzuki K., Musha H. *et al* (1977) Percutaneous transhepatic catheterisation of the portal vein for the study of portal hemodynamics and shunts. *Gastroenterology* **73**, 279.

87. Orloff M.J. & Thomas H.S. (1963) Pathogenesis of esophageal varix rupture. A study based on gross and microscopic examination of the esophagus at the time of bleeding. *Arch. Surg.* **87**, 301.

88. Palmer E.D. (1969) The vigorous diagnostic approach to upper-gastrointestinal tract hemorrhage. *J. Am. med. Assoc.* **207**, 1477.

89. Paton A., Reynolds T.B. & Sherlock S. (1953) Assessment of portal venous hypertension by catheterization of the hepatic vein. *Lancet* i, 918.

90. Pimentel J.C. & Menezes A.P. (1977) Liver disease in vineyard sprayers. *Gastroenterology* **72**, 275.

91. Pitcher J.L. (1971) Safety and effectiveness of the modified Sengstaken–Blakemore tube: a prospective study. *Gastroenterology* **61**, 291.

92. Popper H. (1974) Implications of portal hepatotrophic factors in hepatology. *Gastroenterology* **66**, 1227.

93. Popper H., Elias H. & Petty D.E. (1952) Vascular pattern of the cirrhotic liver. *Am. J. clin. Path.* **22**, 717.

94. Price J.B. Jr, Britton R.C., Peterson L.M. *et al* (1965) The validity of chronic hepatic blood flow measurements obtained by electromagnetic flow meter. *J. surg. Res.* **5**, 313.

95. Raskin N.H., Price J.B. & Fishman R.A. (1964) Portal-systemic encephalopathy due to congenital intrahepatic shunts. *New Engl. J. Med.* **270**, 225.

96. Read A.E., Dawson A.M., Kerr D.N.S. *et al* (1960) Bleeding oesophageal varices treated by oesophageal compression tube. *Br. med. J.* i, 227.

97. Read A.E., Laidlaw J. & Sherlock S. (1961) Neuropsychiatric complications of porta-caval anastomosis. *Lancet* i, 961.

98. Redeker A.G., Geller H.M. & Reynolds T.B. (1958) Hepatic wedge pressure, blood flow, vascular resistance and oxygen consumption in cirrhosis

before and after end-to-side portacaval shunt. *J. clin. Invest.* **37**, 606.

99. Redeker A.G., Kunelis C.T., Yamamoto S. *et al* (1964) Assessment of portal and hepatic hemodynamics after side-to-side portacaval shunt in patients with cirrhosis. *J. clin. Invest.* **43**, 1464.

100. Reisman T., Levi J.U., Zeppa R. *et al* (1977) Non-cirrhotic portal hypertension in Felty's syndrome. *Am. J. dig. Dis.* **22**, 145.

101. Resnick R.H. *et al* and the Boston Inter-Hospital Liver Group (1969) A controlled study of the prophylactic portacaval shunt—a final report. *Ann. intern. Med.* **70**, 675.

102. Reynolds T.B., Ito S. & Iwatsuki S. (1970) Measurement of portal pressure and its clinical application. *Am. J. Med.* **49**, 649.

103. Rikkers L.F., Rudman D., Galambos J.T. *et al* (1978) A randomised controlled trial of the distal splenorenal shunt. *Ann. Surg.* **188**, 271.

104. Rosenbaum D.L., Murphy G.W. & Swisher S.N. (1966) Hemodynamic studies of the portal circulation in myeloid metaplasia. *Am. J. Med.* **41**, 360.

105. Rougier P., Degott C., Rueff B. *et al* (1978) Nodular regenerative hyperplasia of the liver. *Gastroenterology* **75**, 169.

106. Schwartz R.D., Rubin J.E., Leeming R.W. *et al* (1978) Renal failure following major angiography. *Am. J. Med.* **65**, 31.

107. Scott J., Long R.D., Dick R. *et al* (1976) Percutaneous transhepatic obliteration of gastro-oesophageal varices. *Lancet* ii, 53.

108. Shaldon S., Chiandussi L., Guevara L. *et al* (1961) The measurement of hepatic blood flow and intrahepatic shunted blood flow by colloid heat-denatured human serum albumin labelled with I^{131}. *J. clin. Invest.* **40**, 1346.

109. Shaldon S., Dolle W., Guevara L. *et al* (1961) Effect of pitressin on the splanchnic circulation in man. *Circulation* **24**, 797.

110. Shaldon S. & Sherlock S. (1960) The use of vasopressin ('pitressin') in the control of bleeding from oesophageal varices. *Lancet* ii, 222.

111. Shaldon S. & Sherlock S. (1962) Portal hypertension in the myeloproliferative syndrome and the reticuloses. *Am. J. Med.* **32**, 758.

112. Sherlock S. (1974) Classification and functional aspects of portal hypertension. *Am. J. Surg.* **127**, 121.

113. Sherlock S. (1978) Portal circulation and portal hypertension. *Gut* **19**, 70.

114. Sherlock S., Feldman C.A., Moran B. *et al* (1966) Partial nodular transformation of the liver with portal hyoertension. *Am. J. Med.* **40**, 195.

115. Sherlock S. & Walshe V.M. (1946) The use of a portal anastomotic vein for absorption studies in man. *Clin. Sci.* **6**, 113.

116. Shin S.I., Easley G.W., Raquel J.A. *et al* (1971) Filling defect in the colon due to portal hypertension. *Am. Surg.* **37**, 413.

117. Sibbald W.J., Sweeney J.P. & Inwood M.J. (1972) Portal venous gas (PVG) as an indication for heparinization. *Am. J. Surg.* **124**, 690.

118. Smallwood R.A. & Davidson J.S. (1968) Cal-

cification in the portal system. *Gastroenterology* **54**, 265.

119. Smith-Laing G., Camilo M.E., Dick R. *et al* (1980) Percutaneous transhepatic portography in the assessment of portal hypertension. *Gastroenterology* **78**, 197.

120. Smythe C.McC., Fitzpatrick H.F. & Blakemore A.H. (1951) Studies of portal venous oxygen content in unanaesthetized man. *J. clin. Invest.* **30**, 674.

121. Stone H.H., Jordan W.D., Acker J.J. *et al* (1965) Portal arteriovenous fistulas. Review and case report. *Am. J. Surg.* **109**, 191.

122. Terblanche J., Northover J.M.A., Bornman P. *et al* (1979) A prospective controlled trial of sclerotherapy in the long term management of patients after esophageal variceal bleeding. *Surg. Gynecol. Obstet.* **148**, 323.

123. Terblanche J., Northover J.M.A., Bornman P. *et al* (1979) A prospective evaluation of injection sclerotherapy in the treatment of acute bleeding from esophageal varices. *Surgery* **85**, 239.

124. Terés J., Cecilia A., Bordas J.M. *et al* (1978) Esophageal tamponade for bleeding varices. *Gastroenterology* **75**, 566.

125. Thompson E.N. & Sherlock S. (1964) The aetiology of portal vein thrombosis with particular reference to the role of infection and exchange transfusion. *Q. J. Med.* n.s. **33**, 465.

126. Thompson E.N., Williams R. & Sherlock S. (1964) Liver function in extra-hepatic portal hypertension. *Lancet* ii, 1352.

127. Turner M.D., Sherlock S. & Steiner R.E. (1957) Intrasplenic pressure measurement and splenic venography in the clinical investigation of the portal circulation. *Am. J. Med.* **23**, 846.

128. Viallet A., Joly J.-G., Marleau D. *et al* (1970) Comparison of free portal venous pressure and wedged hepatic venous pressure in patients with cirrhosis of the liver. *Gastroenterology* **59**, 372.

129. Viamonte M. Jr, Warren W.D., Fomon J.J. *et al* (1970) Angiographic investigations in portal hypertension. *Surg. Gynecol. Obstet.* **130**, 37.

130. Vilinskas J., Joyeuse R. & Serlin O. (1970) Hepatic sarcoidosis with portal hypertension. *Am. J. Surg.* **120**, 393.

131. Voorhees A.B. Jr, Price J.B. Jr & Britton R.C. (1970) Portasystemic shunting procedures for portal hypertension. *Am. J. Surg.* **119**, 501.

132. Vosmik J., Jedlicka K., Mulder J.L. *et al* (1977) Action of the triglycyl hormonogen of vasopressin (glycopressin) in patients with liver cirrhosis and bleeding esophageal varices. *Gastroenterology* **72**, 605.

133. Wanless I.R. (1979) Failure to produce hepatic hyperplastic nodules in rats by portacaval anastomosis and testosterone. *Nature* **277**, 327.

134. Warren W.D., Fomon J.J. & Zeppa R. (1969) Further evaluation of selective decompression of varices by distal splenorenal shunt. *Ann. Surg.* **169**, 652.

135. Webb L.J. & Sherlock S. (1979) The aetiology, presentation and natural history of extrahepatic portal venous obstruction. *Q. J. Med.* **48**, 627.

136. Webb L.J., Berger L.A. & Sherlock S. (1977) Grey-scale ultrasonography of portal vein. *Lancet* ii, 675.

137. Webb L., Smith-Laing G., Lake-Bakaar G. *et al* (1980) Pancreatic hypofunction in extrahepatic portal venous obstruction. *Gut* **21**, 227.

138. Williams R., Parsonson A., Somers K. *et al* (1966) Portal hypertension in idiopathic tropical splenomegaly. *Lancet* i, 329.

139. Winkler K. (1972) Selection of patients with cirrhosis of the liver for shunt surgery. *Scand. J. Gastroenterol.* **7**, 679.

Chapter 12
The Hepatic Artery and Hepatic Veins:
the Liver in Circulatory Failure

THE HEPATIC ARTERY

The hepatic artery is a branch of the coeliac axis. It runs along the upper border of the pancreas to the first part of the duodenum where it turns upwards between the layers of the lesser omentum, lying in front of the portal vein and medial to the common bile duct. Reaching the porta hepatis it divides into right and left branches. Its branches include the right gastric artery and the gastroduodenal artery which descends behind the first part of the duodenum. Aberrant branches are common. Among the many variations, the right hepatic artery may arise from the superior mesenteric, the aorta or the right renal artery. An accessory left hepatic artery may come from the left gastric artery.

Anastomoses occur between the right and left branches, with subcapsular vessels of the liver and with the inferior phrenic artery.

Intra-hepatic anatomy. The hepatic artery enters sinusoids both at the periphery of the lobule and probably at various points towards the central vein [2]. Direct arterio-portal venous anastomoses are also possible. The hepatic artery also forms a capillary plexus around the bile ducts. The connective tissue in the portal tracts is supplied.

The *pressure in the hepatic artery* is equal to the general systemic blood pressure; that in the portal vein is much lower. These two pressures are equilibrated within the sinusoids (Chapter 11).

HEPATIC ARTERIAL FLOW

Animal experiments show that the hepatic artery provides 20–30% of the total hepatic blood flow. In man, during surgery, the hepatic artery supplies 35% of the hepatic blood flow and 50% of the liver's oxygen supply [17].

The proportion of hepatic arterial flow increases greatly in cirrhosis [8] and especially after portacaval anastomosis. It is the main blood supply to tumours. The proportion varies greatly under different conditions. A drop in systemic blood pressure from haemorrhage or other cause lowers the oxygen content of the portal vein and the liver becomes more and more dependent on the hepatic artery for oxygen [7]. The hepatic artery and the portal vein adapt the volume of blood and of oxygen that they supply to the liver according to demand [6].

CATHETERIZATION OF THE HEPATIC ARTERY

Hepatic arteriography (page 465) is being increasingly performed for diagnosis, especially of intra-hepatic tumours (page 468). Embolization via the catheter is done for treatment of hepatic carcinoid and other hepatic tumours.

Hepatic arterial chemotherapy is not often performed nowadays but can be complicated by intra-hepatic sepsis [16].

Hepatic artery occlusion

The effects of hepatic artery occlusion depend on the site and on the extent of available collateral circulation. If the division is distal to the origins of the gastric and gastroduodenal arteries the patient may die. Survivors have a collateral circulation via phrenic or subcapsular arteries or else the main hepatic artery has not been divided. Slow thrombosis is better than sudden block. Simultaneous occlusion of the portal vein is nearly always fatal.

The pathological consequence is infarction, the area involved depending on the extent of the collateral arterial circulation but rarely exceeding 8 cm in diameter [11]. The lesion has a pale centre with a surrounding, congested, haemorrhagic band. Liver cells in the infarcted area are jumbled together in irregular masses of eosinophilic granular cytoplasm without glycogen or nuclei. Subcapsular areas escape because they have an alternative, arterial blood supply.

Hepatic infarction may occur without arterial occlusion. Shock, cardiac failure [10] or diabetic ketosis [9] are the most important aetiological factors [15]. The gall bladder may also be infarcted [4].

AETIOLOGY

Occlusion of the hepatic artery is very rare [5]. Some of the causes are polyarteritis nodosa [1], embolism in patients with acute bacterial endocarditis and surgical trauma during cholecystectomy. In the last circumstance, fortunately only a branch is tied so that recovery may occur.

Hepatic arterial dissection can follow abdominal trauma [14]. It may also follow catheters introduced for arteriography or for cancer therapy.

CLINICAL FEATURES

The condition is rarely diagnosed *ante mortem* and descriptions are meagre. The patient exhibits the features of the cause, such as bacterial endocarditis, or polyarteritis nodosa, or has undergone a difficult upper abdominal operation. Sudden pain in the right upper abdomen is followed by collapse and hypotension. Right upper quadrant tenderness develops and the liver edge is tender. Jaundice deepens rapidly. There is usually fever and leucocytosis and liver function tests show hepato-cellular damage. The prothrombin time rises precipitously and haemorrhages develop. The patient passes into coma and is dead within ten days.

TREATMENT

If possible the causative lesion must be treated. Antibiotics may prevent secondary infection in the anoxic liver. The general management is that of acute hepato-cellular failure. Trauma to the artery has been treated by embolization [14].

Aneurysms of the hepatic artery

These are rare, about 200 cases having been recorded [12]. The aneurysm may complicate bacterial endocarditis [12], polyarteritis nodosa, trauma or cholelithiasis. The aneurysm may be extra- or intra-hepatic and varies from a pin point to a grapefruit.

The aneurysm may be recognized by angiography, incidentally at operation or at autopsy.

It may cause pain in the right upper abdomen with fever; jaundice is rare. Haematemesis can follow rupture into the biliary tree [3], stomach or duodenum. Diagnosis is confirmed by hepatic arteriography.

The aneurysm may be wrapped with cellophane, ligated or embolized with gelfoam [12].

Hepatic arteriovenous shunts

These are usually secondary to blunt trauma, needle liver biopsy or neoplasms, usually primary liver cancer. Multiple shunts may be part of hereditary haemorrhagic telangiectasia when they can be so extensive that congestive heart failure follows [13].

Large shunts cause a bruit in the right upper quadrant. The diagnosis is confirmed by hepatic angiography. Embolization with gelfoam is the usual treatment. Ligation is occasionally possible.

REFERENCES

1. COWEN R.E., MALLINSON C.N., THOMAS G.E. *et al* (1977) Polyarteritis of the liver: a report of two cases. *Postgrad. med. J.* **53,** 89.
2. ELIAS H. (1949) A re-examination of the structure of the mammalian liver. II. The hepatic lobule and its relation to the vascular and biliary systems. *Am. J. Anat.* **85,** 379.
3. HARLAFTIS N.N. & AKIN J.T. (1977) Hemobilia from ruptured hepatic artery aneurysm. *Am. J. Surg.* **133,** 229.
4. HENRICH W.L., HUEHNERGARTH R.J., RÖSCH J. *et al* (1975) Gall bladder and liver infarction occurring as a complication of acute bacterial endocarditis. *Gastroenterology* **68,** 1602.
5. KANTER D.M. (1965) Hepatic infarction. *Arch. intern. Med.* **115,** 479.
6. LAUTT W.W. (1977) Hepatic vasculature: a conceptual review. *Gastroenterology* **73,** 1163.
7. MCMICHAEL J. (1937) The oxygen supply of the liver. *Q. J. exp. Physiol.* **27,** 73.
8. MORENO A.H., BURCHELL A.R., ROUSSELOT L.M., *et al* (1967) Portal blood flow in cirrhosis of the liver. *J. clin. Invest.* **46,** 236.
9. NG R.C.K., SIGMUND C.J. Jr, LAGOS J.A. *et al* (1977) Hepatic infarction and diabetic ketoacidosis. *Gastroenterology* **73,** 804.
10. O'CONNOR P.J., BUHAC I. & BALINT J.A. (1976) Spontaneous hepatic artery thrombosis with infarction of the liver. *Gastroenterology* **70,** 599.
11. PARKER R.G.F. (1955) Arterial infarction of the liver in man. *J. Path. Bact.* **70,** 521.
12. PORTER L.L. III, HOUSTON M.C. & KADIR S. (1979) Mycotic aneurysm of the hepatic artery: treatment with arterial embolization. *Am. J. Med.* **67,** 697.
13. RADTKE W.E., SMITH H.C., FULTON R.E. *et al* (1978) Misdiagnosis of atrial septal defect in

patients with hereditary telangiectasia (Osler–Weber–Rendu disease) and hepatic arteriovenous fistulas. *Am. Heart J.* **95**, 235.

14. RUBIN B.E. & KATZEN B.T. (1977) Selective hepatic artery embolization to control massive hepatic hemorrhage after trauma. *Am. J. Roentgenol.* **129**, 253.

15. SEELEY T.T., BLUMENFIELD C.M., IKEDA R. *et al* (1972) Hepatic infarction. *Hum. Path.* **3**, 265.

16. TULLY J.L., LEW M.A., CONNOR M. *et al* (1969) Clostridial sepsis following hepatic arterial infusion chemotherapy. *Am. J. Med.* **67**, 707.

17. TYGSTRUP N., WINKLER K., MELLEMGAARD K. *et al* (1962) Determination of the hepatic arterial blood flow and oxygen supply in man by clamping the hepatic artery during surgery. *J. clin. Invest.* **41**, 447.

THE HEPATIC VEINS

The hepatic veins begin in the centres of the lobules as the central veins [10]. These join the sub-lobular veins and merge into larger hepatic veins, which enter the inferior vena cava while it is still partly embedded in the liver substance. The number, size, configuration and pattern of hepatic veins are very variable. Generally, there are three large veins, one draining the left lobe of the liver and the other two emerging from the right lobe. There are variable numbers of small accessory veins particularly from the caudate lobe.

In the normal liver there are no direct anastomoses between portal vein and hepatic vein which are linked only by the sinusoids. In the cirrhotic liver there are anastomoses between portal and hepatic veins so that the blood bypasses the regenerating liver cell nodules (fig. 143). These 'internal Eck fistulae' develop from pre-existing sinusoids enclosed in the fibrous septa. There is no evidence, either in the normal or cirrhotic liver, of anastomoses between the hepatic artery and the hepatic vein.

FUNCTIONS

The pressure in the free hepatic vein is approximately 6 mmHg.

The hepatic venous blood is only about 67% saturated with oxygen. The oxygen consumption of the liver (or splanchnic area) can be calculated as 47 ml per square metre body surface per minute.

Dogs have muscular hepatic veins near their caval orifices which form a sluice mechanism. The hepatic veins in man have little muscle.

The hepatic venous blood is usually sterile for the liver is a bacterial filter.

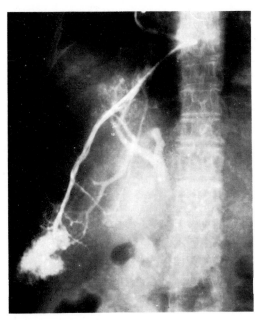
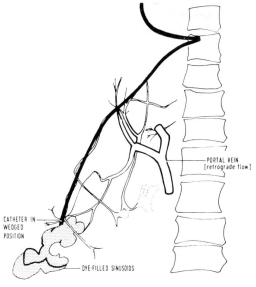

PORTAL VEIN [retrograde flow]

CATHETER IN WEDGED POSITION

DYE-FILLED SINUSOIDS

Fig. 159. Retrograde hepatic venogram in a patient with cirrhosis of the liver. The portal vein has filled by retrograde flow.

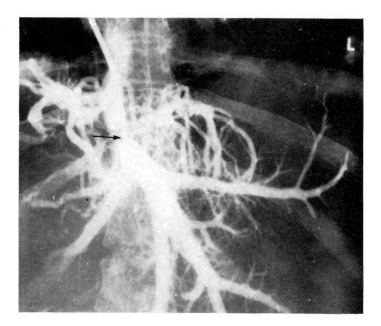

Fig. 160. Hepatic venogram obtained by hepatic vein catheterization in a patient with the Budd–Chiari syndrome. Dilated veins in the obstructed lobe have filled, the catheter having passed beyond the constriction in a main hepatic vein (marked by arrow) (Clain *et al* 1967).

Hepatic venography

Contrast material is injected into the hepatic vein through a catheter against blood flow. The medium is rapidly flushed out, but deformities and obstructions of the main hepatic vein may sometimes be demonstrated [8, 9].

Injection into the *wedged* hepatic vein radicle will result in filling of the sinusoidal area draining into the catheter and also in retrograde filling of the portal venous system in that area. The portal radicle then carries the contrast medium to other parts of the liver and so other hepatic vein branches become opacified (fig. 159). Cirrhotic nodules and tumour deposits are surrounded by portal vein–hepatic vein anastomoses and may be outlined. In cirrhosis the sinusoidal pattern is coarsened, beady and tortuous, and gnarled hepatic radicles may be seen. The extent of filling of the main portal vein may indicate the extent to which the portal vein has become the outflow tract of the liver. In the Budd–Chiari syndrome a characteristic lace-like vascular pattern may be seen [7, 30] (fig. 161).

The main hepatic veins can sometimes be visualized by a reflux of contrast material injected into the inferior vena cava while the patient performs a Valsalva manœuvre. The hepatic veins may occasionally be seen after selective coeliac or hepatic arteriography, particularly when hepatic arterial blood flow is increased [12].

Experimental hepatic venous obstruction

It is impossible to ligate all the hepatic veins individually. The usual method is to constrict the inferior vena cava by a cellophane band above the entry of the hepatic veins, and so obstruct the venous return from the liver [3].

The extent of centrizonal haemorrhage and necrosis is proportional to the degree of hepatic venous obstruction. Connective tissue proliferates round the central vein. In acute hepatic venous occlusion, the hepatic lymphatics are, at first, greatly dilated.

Ascites is the first sign of hepatic venous congestion [3]. The output of hepatic lymph through the capsule increases 10–20 times [32]. The fluid has a high protein and lymphocyte content.

Budd–Chiari (hepatic venous obstruction) syndrome [7] (fig. 162)

This condition is usually associated with the names of Budd and Chiari although Budd's description [4] omitted the features and Chiari's paper [6] was not the first to report the clinical picture. The syndrome comprises hepatomegaly, abdominal pain, ascites and hepatic histology showing centrizonal sinusoidal distension and pooling. It may arise from obstruction to hepatic veins at any site from the efferent vein of the lobule to the entry of the inferior vena cava into the right atrium (fig. 162).

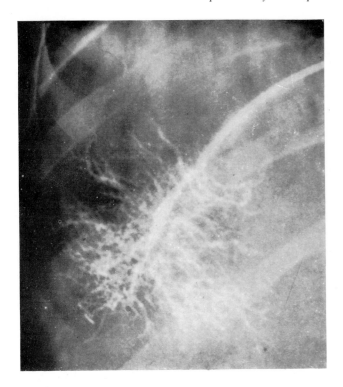

Fig. 161. Hepatic venogram in a patient with Budd–Chiari syndrome. Note lace-like spider-web pattern (Clain *et al* 1967).

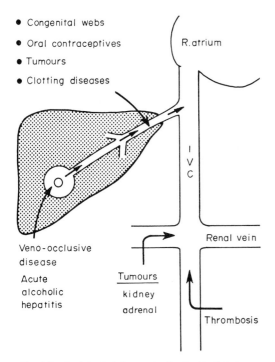

Fig. 162. Aetiological factors in the Budd–Chiari syndrome.

A similar syndrome may be produced by constrictive pericarditis or right-sided heart failure.

The Budd–Chiari syndrome is associated with clotting diseases, particularly polycythaemia, both primary and secondary [31]. It is also associated with oral contraceptives of the oestrogen–progesterone type [1, 15, 33]. It has been reported in paroxysmal nocturnal haemoglobinuria [23].

Trauma, usually of blunt abdominal type, as in automobile accidents is also an association.

Obstruction to the inferior vena cava is usually secondary to thrombosis in malignant disease, for instance an adrenal or renal carcinoma or invasion by a primary hepato-cellular cancer. Rare tumours include leiomyosarcoma of the hepatic veins [17] and metastatic testicular lesions in the right atrium [11].

Invasion of hepatic veins by masses of aspergillosis has been reported in association with leukaemia [34].

Membranous obstruction of the supra-hepatic segment of the inferior vena cava is an important condition because it is potentially curable by surgery [24]. The web varies from a thin membrane to a thick fibrotic band. The largest reported series comes from Japan [28]. The web is presumed congenital although the presentation in adults in their thirties is surprising. It could also have been acquired as a result of organized thrombosis.

The picture also follows central hepatic vein involvement in the sclerosing hyaline necrosis of alcoholics and in veno-occlusive disease (page 185).

In many instances the cause remains unknown [7, 22].

PATHOLOGICAL CHANGES

The hepatic veins show thrombosis at various points in their course from the ostia to the smaller radicles. The thrombus may have spread from an occluded inferior vena cava. Thrombus filling the veins may be purulent or may contain malignant cells, depending on the cause. In chronic cases the vein wall is thickened and there may be some recanalization of the lumen. In others it is replaced by a fibrous strand; a fibrous web may be seen.

The liver is enlarged, purplish and smooth. Venous congestion is gross and the cut surface shows an advanced 'nutmeg' change. Hepatic veins beyond the obstruction and, in the acute stage, subcapsular lymphatics, are dilated and prominent.

In the more chronic case the caudate lobe, which has separate venous drainage into the cava, is enlarged (fig. 163). The inferior vena cava as it passes posterior to the liver is compressed side-to-side by this lobe. Areas less affected by obstruction hypertrophy in nodular fashion. In such cases the spleen may be enlarged and a portal–systemic collateral circulation seen. There may be terminal thrombosis of mesenteric vessels.

Histologically, sections show centrizonal venous dilatation, sinusoidal congestion and

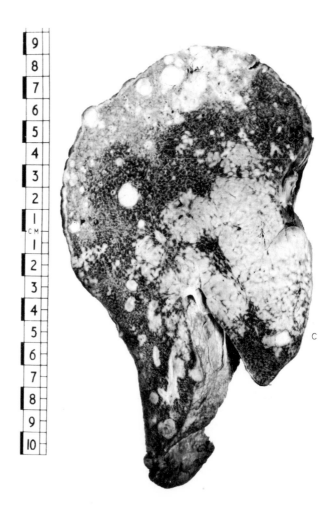

Fig. 163. Vertical section of the liver at autopsy in hepatic venous obstruction. The pale areas represent regeneration and the dark areas are congested. Note the marked hypertrophy of the caudate lobe (C).

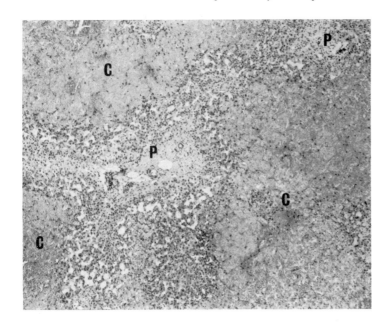

Fig. 164. Hepatic venous occlusion (Budd–Chiari syndrome). Hepatic histology shows marked centrizonal haemorrhage (C). The liver cells adjoining the portal zones (P) are spared. H & E, × 100.

haemorrhage with central necrosis of liver cells (fig. 164). Blood cells in Disse's space could represent an extra-sinusoidal circulation conducting blood toward the larger hepatic veins in an attempt to circumvent obstruction to the venous drainage in the lumen. The periportal areas are spared. The appearances are indistinguishable from those of any obstruction to the hepatic venous flow, for instance cardiac failure or constrictive pericarditis.

In the later stages centrizonal fibrosis is seen and the picture is that of a cardiac cirrhosis.

CLINICAL FEATURES

In the most *acute form* the picture is of an ill patient, often suffering from some other condition—for instance renal carcinoma, primary cancer of the liver, thrombophlebitis migrans or polycythaemia. The presentation is with abdominal pain, vomiting, liver enlargement, ascites and mild icterus. Watery diarrhoea, following mesenteric venous obstruction, is a terminal, inconstant feature. If the hepatic venous occlusion is total, delirium and coma with hepato-cellular failure and death follow rapidly.

In the more usual, *chronic form*, the patient presents with pain over an enlarged tender liver and ascites. Jaundice is mild or absent. Pressure over the liver may fail to fill the jugular vein (negative hepato-jugular reflux). As portal hypertension

increases the spleen becomes palpable. The enlarged caudate lobe, palpable in the epigastrium, may simulate a tumour.

If the inferior vena cava is blocked, oedema of the legs is gross and veins distend over the abdomen, flanks and back. Albuminuria is found.

Biochemical. Serum bilirubin rarely exceeds 2 mg/100 ml. The serum alkaline phosphatase level is raised and the serum albumin value reduced. Serum transaminase values increase and the prothrombin time is reduced. Hypoproteinaemia may be due to protein-losing enteropathy.

The protein content of the ascites should theoretically be high, but this is not always so.

Needle liver biopsy is essential. Speckled centrizonal areas can be distinguished from the pale portal ones. Histologically the picture is of centrizonal congestion. Alcoholic hepatitis or phlebitis of the hepatic veins should be noted.

Peritoneoscopy shows an enlarged purple liver.

Hepatic venography may fail or show narrow occluded hepatic veins (fig. 160). Adjacent veins show a tortuous, lace-like spider-web pattern [7] (fig. 161). This probably represents abnormal venous collaterals. The catheter cannot be advanced the usual distance along the hepatic vein and wedging occurs 2–12 cm from the diaphragm. The features of a normal wedged venogram are absent.

Inferior vena cavography both from above, via the right atrium, or below, via the femoral vein,

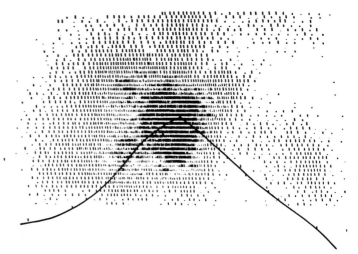

Fig. 165. Hepatic scintiscan in hepatic venous obstruction showing maximal uptake of isotope more centrally placed in the liver than normal; this represents the hypertrophied caudate lobe.

or both, establishes the patency of the inferior vena cava. The hepatic segment may show side-to-side narrowing due to distortion from the enlarged caudate lobe (fig. 166). Pressure measurements should be taken in the inferior vena cava along its length to confirm its patency and to quantitate the extent of any membranous or caudate lobe obstruction.

Splenic venography may show a collateral circulation and it is necessary to establish that the portal vein is patent.

Selective coeliac arteriography. The hepatic artery appears small for the size of the liver and the branches are of fine calibre. They appear stretched and displaced, producing the appearance of multiple space-occupying lesions simulating metastases [16]. The venous phase shows delayed emptying of the portal venous bed.

Hepatography [20] by injecting contrast material directly into the liver substance may reveal the hepatic venous block [20].

Hepatic scintiscans are abnormal with poor uptake of isotope into the areas drained by the occluded hepatic vein. The caudate lobe is relatively spared and may take up isotope normally or excessively [7, 30]. Maximal density is therefore medial to its usual position (fig. 165).

DIAGNOSIS

The condition should be suspected if a patient with a tendency to thrombosis or malignant disease in or near the liver or on oral contraceptives develops tender hepatomegaly with gross ascites. Diagnosis, prognosis and correct treatment are only possible if the block is localized, and the special

radiological and scanning techniques already described are essential.

Heart failure and constrictive pericarditis must be distinguished clinically, by fluoroscopy and by electrocardiography. Tense ascites *per se* can elevate the jugular venous pressure and displace the cardiac apex.

Cirrhosis must be distinguished and the liver biopsy is helpful. The ascitic fluid protein content is usually lower.

Portal vein thrombosis rarely leads to ascites. Jaundice is absent and the liver is not very large.

Inferior vena caval thrombosis results in distended abdominal wall veins (fig. 114) but without ascites. If the renal vein is occluded, albuminuria is gross. Hepatic venous and inferior vena caval thrombosis may, however, co-exist.

PROGNOSIS

In the acute form death in hepatic coma usually results. Thrombosis may spread to the portal and mesenteric veins with infarction of the bowel. In the more chronic and localized instances response to symptomatic therapy may allow prolongation of life for a few years [7].

Prognosis depends on the aetiology, on the extent of the occlusion and whether it can be corrected surgically.

Cases associated with clotting disease, such as polycythaemia, usually have multiple thrombosis of vessels of varying sizes. The inferior vena cava and portal vein may also be involved. Thrombosis following oral contraceptives is again usually ominous; the outlook depends on how much recanalization takes place and on the initial response to treatment.

Haemorrhage from oesophageal varices is usually terminal.

Chronic cases may survive many months or even years and up to 22 years has been recorded.

TREATMENT

Much can be achieved by controlling ascites with a low sodium diet and diuretics. Severe cases demand ever-increasing doses of combinations of potent diuretics for their control and eventually the patient is overtaken by inanition and renal failure. The less severe respond slowly and require less treatment with time. The peritoneo-jugular (LeVeen) shunt may be useful in some patients. Any cause such as polycythaemia is treated by venesection and radiophosphorus. Anticoagulants or fibrinolysin therapy are of no benefit.

Surgical correction of webs by trans-atrial membranotomy has been performed in 29 patients: 20 were successful, 6 died and 3 did not improve [14, 24]. Side-to-side porta-caval shunt may be useful if the portal vein and inferior vena cava have been proved patent [21]. The pressure in the vena cava above and below the enlarged caudate lobe must be less than the normal portal venous pressure if the shunt is to remain patent. Meso-atrial shunt may be considered if the inferior vena cava is obstructed [5].

Veno-occlusive disease (VOD)

This disease was originally described from Jamaica due to a toxic injury to the minute hepatic veins by pyrrolizidine alkaloids taken as senecio in medicinal bush teas [27]. It has since been described from Israel, Egypt and even Arizona [26]. It may be related to contamination of wheat with pyrrolizidine alkaloids [19, 29].

Toxic injury to the hepatic veins can also follow hepatic irradiation and urethane, azathioprine [18] and other chemotherapy for acute leukaemia [13]. It can develop as a graft-versus-host reaction in patients having allogenic bone-marrow transplantation [2, 25]. The central hepatic vein is also characteristically affected in acute alcoholic hepatitis (*sclerosing hyaline necrosis*).

Small hepatic veins are involved, medium-sized vessels somewhat affected and larger veins normal. The block is due to sub-endothelial oedema with

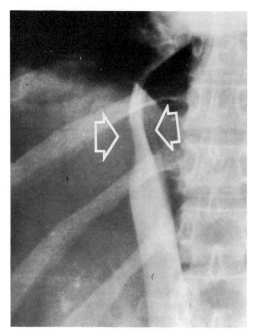

Fig. 166. Inferior venacavogram. Antero-posterior view showing side-to-side narrowing and distortion of the inferior vena cava. Extrinsic compression from the left (arrow) is due to an enlarged caudate lobe (Tavill *et al* 1975).

subsequent collagenization. Massive centrizonal congestion leads to loss of liver cells. In the subacute phase, there is persistent centrizonal fibrosis with thickened narrowed hepatic veins. The chronic stage is one of a mainly non-portal cirrhosis.

Clinical features [27]. The *acute stage* is marked by sudden painful hepatomegaly and ascites. Jaundice is inconspicuous. The patient may recover in 4–6 weeks, die of liver failure or pass into the subacute phase.

The *sub-acute stage* is characterized by firm hepatomegaly and recurrent ascites. It may follow the acute stage directly, after a few months or may appear *de novo*. The disease may subside clinically or pass into the chronic stage.

The *chronic stage* clinically resembles any other type of cirrhosis [27]. Portal hypertension is prominent. It can be suspected only from a history of an acute or sub-acute episode but can be proven by aspiration liver biopsy.

Treatment is symptomatic. Porta-caval anastomosis has been performed for relief of portal hypertension in the later stages.

Spread of disease by the hepatic veins

The hepatic veins link the portal and systemic venous systems. Malignant disease of the liver is spread by the hepatic veins to the lungs and hence to other parts. Liver abscesses can burst into the hepatic vein and metastatic abscesses may result. Parasitic disease, including amoebiasis, hydatid disease and schistosomiasis, is spread by this route. The portal–hepatic venous anastomoses developing in cirrhosis may allow intestinal organisms to cause septicaemia.

REFERENCES

1. ALPERT L.I. (1976) Veno-occlusive disease of the liver associated with oral contraceptives: case report and review of the literature. *Hum. Path.* **7**, 709.
2. BERK P.D., POPPER H., KRUEGER G.R.F. *et al* (1979) Veno-occlusive disease of the liver after allogenic bone marrow transplantation. *Ann. intern. Med.* **90**, 158.
3. BOLTON C. & BARNARD W.G. (1931) The pathological occurrences in the liver in experimental venous stagnation. *J. Path. Bact.* **34**, 701.
4. BUDD G. (1857) *On Diseases of the Liver*, 3rd edn., p. 195. Blanchard & Lea, Philadelphia.
5. CAMERON J.L. & MADDREY W.C. (1978) Mesoatrial shunt: a new treatment for the Budd–Chiari syndrome. *Ann. Surg.* **187**, 402.
6. CHIARI H. (1899) Ueber die selbständige Phlebitis obliterans der Hauptstämme der Venae hepaticae als Todesursache. *Beitr. path. Anat.* **26**, 1.
7. CLAIN D., FRESTON J., KREEL L. *et al* (1967) Clinical diagnosis of the Budd–Chiari syndrome. *Am. J. Med.* **43**, 544.
8. DOEHNER G.A. (1968) The hepatic venous system. Its normal roentgen anatomy. *Radiology* **90**, 1119.
9. DOEHNER G.A. (1968) The hepatic venous system. Its pathologic roentgen anatomy. *Radiology* **90**, 1124.
10. ELIAS H. & PETTY D. (1952) Gross anatomy of the blood vessels and ducts within the human liver. *Am. J. Anat.* **90**, 59.
11. FEINGOLD M.L., LITWAK R.L., GELLER S.S. *et al* (1971) Budd–Chiari syndrome caused by a right atrial tumor. *Arch. intern. Med.* **127**, 292.
12. GLICKMAN M.G. & HANDEL S.F. (1972) Opacification of hepatic veins during celiac and hepatic angiography. *Radiology* **103**, 565.
13. GRINER P.F., ELBADAWI A. & PACKMAN C.H. (1976) Veno-occlusive disease of the liver after chemotherapy of acute leukemia. *Ann. intern. Med.* **85**, 578.
14. HIROOKA M. & KIMURA C. (1970) Membranous obstruction of the hepatic portion of the inferior vena cava. *Arch. Surg.* **100**, 656.
15. HOYUMPA A.M. Jr, SCHIFF L. & HELFMAN E.L. (1971) Budd–Chiari syndrome in women taking oral contraceptives. *Am. J. Med.* **50**, 137.
16. HUNGERFORD G.D., HAMLYN A.N., LUNZER M.R. *et al* (1976) Pseudo-metastases in the liver: a presentation of the Budd–Chiari syndrome. *Radiology* **120**, 627.
17. MACMAHON H.E. & BALL H.G. III (1971) Leiomyosarcoma of hepatic vein and the Budd–Chiari syndrome. *Gastroenterology* **61**, 239.
18. MARUBBIO A.T. & DANIELSON B. (1975) Hepatic veno-occlusive disease in a renal transplant patient receiving azathioprine. *Gastroenterology* **69**, 739.
19. MOHABBAT O., SRIVASTAVA R.N., YOUNOS M.S. *et al* (1976) An attack of hepatic veno-occlusive disease in North-Western Afghanistan. *Lancet* ii, 269.
20. MORENO A.H., RUZICKA F.F., ROUSSELOT L.M. *et al* (1963) Functional hepatography. A study of the hemodynamics of the outflow tracts of the human liver by intraparenchymal deposition of contrast medium, with attempts at functional evaluation of the outflow block concept of cirrhotic ascites and the accessory outflow role of the portal vein. *Radiology* **81**, 65.
21. ORLOFF M.J. & JOHANSEN K.H. (1978) Treatment of the Budd–Chiari syndrome by side-to-side portacaval shunt: experimental and clinical results. *Ann. Surg.* **188**, 494.
22. PARKER R.G.F. (1959) Occlusion of the hepatic veins in man. *Medicine (Baltimore)* **38**, 369.
23. PEYTREMANN R., RHODES R.S. & HARMANN R.C. (1972) Thrombosis in paroxysmal nocturnal haemoglobinuria (PNH) with particular reference to progressive diffuse, hepatic venous thrombosis. *Ser. Haemat.* **5**, 115.
24. SCHAFFNER F., GADBOYS H.L., SAFRAN A.P. *et al* (1967) Budd–Chiari syndrome caused by a web in the inferior vena cava. *Am. J. Med.* **42**, 838.
25. SHULMAN H. M., McDONALD G.B., MATTHEWS D. *et al* (1980) An analysis of hepatic venocclusive disease and centrilobular hepatic degeneration following bone marrow transplantation. *Gastroenterology* **79**, 1178.
26. STILLMAN A.E., HUXTABLE R., CONSROE P. *et al* (1977) Hepatic veno-occlusive disease due to pyrrolizidine (Senecio poisoning in Arizona. *Gastroenterology* **73**, 349.
27. STUART K.L. & BRAS G. (1957) Veno-occlusive disease of the liver. *Q. J. Med.* n.s. **26**, 291.
28. TAKEUCHI J., TAKADA A., HASUMURA Y. *et al* (1971) Budd–Chiari syndrome associated with obstruction of the inferior vena cava. *Am. J. Med.* **51**, 11.
29. TANDON B.N., TANDON R.K., TANDON H.D. *et al* (1976) An epidemic of veno-occlusive disease of liver in Central India. *Lancet* ii, 271.
30. TAVILL A.S., WOOD E.J., KREEL L. *et al* (1975) The Budd–Chiari syndrome: correlation between hepatic scintigraphy and the clinical, radiological and pathological findings in nineteen cases of hepatic venous outflow obstruction. *Gastroenterology* **68**, 509.
31. THOMAS M. & CAROLI J. (1971) Polycythémie et syndrome de Budd–Chiari: a propos de 17 observations. *Ann. Méd. interne* **122**, 1175.

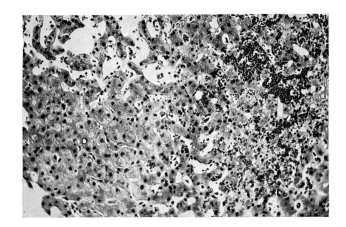

Fig. 167. Coronary thrombosis. Serum bilirubin 2.1 mg/100 ml. Liver cells have disappeared from the centre of the lobule and are replaced by frank haemorrhage. H & E, × 120 (Sherlock 1951).

32. VOLWILER W., GRINDLAY J.H. & BOLLMAN J.L. (1950) The relation of portal vein pressure to the formation of ascites—an experimental study. *Gastroenterology* **14**, 40.

33. WU S-M., SPURNY O.M. & KLOTZ A.P. (1977) Budd–Chiari syndrome after taking oral contraceptives: a case report and review of 14 reported cases. *Am. J. dig. Dis.* **22**, 623.

34. YOUNG R.C. (1969) The Budd–Chiari syndrome caused by *Aspergillus. Arch. intern. Med.* **124**, 754.

CIRCULATORY FAILURE

A rise in pressure in the right atrium is readily transmitted to the hepatic veins. Liver cells are particularly vulnerable to diminished oxygen supply so a failing heart, lowered blood pressure or reduced hepatic blood flow are reflected in impaired hepatic function.

Hepatic changes in acute heart failure and shock

Hepatic changes are particularly common in acute heart failure and in shock due to trauma, burns, haemorrhage, sepsis, peritonitis or black water fever [3, 6].

Light microscopy shows congested central areas with local haemorrhage (fig. 167). Focal necrosis with eosinophilic liver cells, hydropic change and polymorphonuclear infiltration is usually centrizonal but may appear mid-zonal if the section has been cut in a plane missing the hepatic vein. The essential reticulin structure of the liver is preserved within the necrotic zone. With recovery, particularly where the cause is trauma, mitoses may be prominent [6]. The left lobe of the liver may suffer more than the right.

MECHANISM OF THE HEPATIC CHANGES

Changes can be related to the duration of the shock: if longer than 24 hours, hepatic necrosis is almost constant; if less than 10 hours, it is unusual.

The fall in systemic blood pressure leads to a reduction in portal blood flow and the oxygen content of the blood is reduced [22]. Hepatic arterial blood flow is also reduced due to vasoconstriction following the fall in systemic blood pressure. The centrizonal cells receive blood at a lower oxygen tension than the peripheral cells and therefore more readily become anoxic and necrotic.

In man, an increased blood lactic acid and alpha amino nitrogen level has been observed in 'medical shock'. Some patients show mild icterus [9]. Jaundice has been recorded in severely traumatized patients [6]. Serum transaminase levels increase markedly and the prothrombin time rises [3, 9].

Post-operative jaundice [18]

Jaundice developing *soon* after surgery may have multiple causes [14, 18]. Increased bilirubin follows blood transfusion, particularly of stored blood. The haemoglobin in 500 ml blood contains about 250 mg of bilirubin, the normal daily production. Extravasated blood in the tissues gives an additional bilirubin load.

Impaired hepato-cellular function follows operation, anaesthetics and shock. Severe jaundice develops in approximately 2% of patients with shock resulting from major trauma [24]. Hepatic perfusion is reduced. This will be particularly evident if the patient is in incipient circulatory failure and the cardiac output is already reduced. The kidney will simultaneously suffer from reduced renal blood flow.

Halothane anaesthetics, especially if multiple, may be followed by a hepatitis-like picture. This is rare less than seven days after a first operation (Chapter 17). Other drugs used in the operative period, such as the promazines, must also be considered as the cause. Sepsis, *per se*, can produce deep jaundice which may be cholestatic.

Rarely a *cholestatic jaundice* may be noted on the first or second post-operative day. It reaches its height between the fourth and tenth day, and disappears by 14–18 days. Serum biochemical changes are variable. Sometimes, but not always, the alkaline phosphatase and transaminase levels are increased [30]. Serum bilirubin can rise to levels of 23–39 mg/100 ml. The picture simulates extra-hepatic biliary obstruction. Patients have all had an episode of shock, been transfused and suffered heart failure of recent onset. Centrizonal hepatic necrosis, however, is not conspicuous and hepatic histology shows only minor abnormalities. The mechanism of the cholestasis is uncertain. This picture must be recognized [14] and if necessary needle biopsy of the liver performed. Surgical intervention to relieve a non-existent obstruction would be disastrous.

Jaundice after cardiac surgery

Jaundice may follow major heart surgery [27]. Post-operative jaundice (serum bilirubin greater than 3 mg) was seen in 63 (8·6%) of 736 patients having open heart surgery; 58 of the 63 had acquired heart disease [29]. Jaundice was greater the more severe the valvular pathology, being particularly marked where double or triple valves were replaced.

The patient may have pre-operative centrizonal necrosis, consequent upon prolonged heart failure. Patients over 50 years old are very liable. Hypotension and shock are frequent in the operative period, further reducing hepatic blood flow. Hypothermia may contribute [17].

The lifespan of stored blood used for transfusion may be reduced by passage through the extra-corporeal circulation [2]. Mechanical prostheses may decrease the survival time of red cells [2, 19]. The bilirubin load on the liver cell is therefore increased.

The cholestatic picture following operations may also be seen. In these patients hepatic necrosis is minimal. Surprisingly, alkaline phosphatase may be normal or only slightly increased. Serum transaminases are raised [19].

Infections, drugs (including anticoagulants) and anaesthetics must also be considered.

Non-A, non-B hepatitis is now the commonest cause of post-transfusion hepatitis, particularly if commercial blood or factor IX concentrates have been used. Virus B hepatitis is rare since blood has been screened for the agent. Cytomegalo-hepatitis may develop after cardiac surgery.

The liver in congestive heart failure [10]

PATHOLOGICAL CHANGES

Hepatic autolysis is particularly rapid in the patient dying in heart failure [25, 32]. Autopsy material is therefore unreliable for the assessment of the effects of cardiac failure on the liver in life. Accurate histological data can only be obtained by aspiration liver biopsy. Haemorrhage might be anticipated from puncture of the 'congested' liver but biopsies are well tolerated [32, 33].

Macroscopic changes. The liver is usually enlarged, and purplish with rounded edges. If

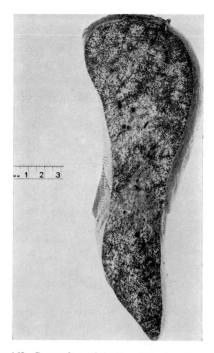

Fig. 168. Cut surface of the liver from a patient dying with congestive heart failure. Note dilated hepatic veins. Light areas corresponding to peripheral fatty zones alternate with dark areas corresponding to central zonal congestion and haemorrhage.

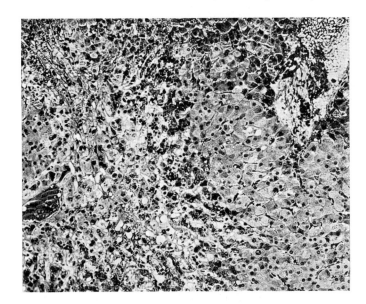

Fig. 169. Cor pulmonale. Serum bilirubin 3.4 mg/100 ml. Gross centrizonal congestion and liver cell necrosis. Pigment increase is seen in the degenerating liver cells. Liver cells at the periphery are relatively normal. H & E, × 120 (Sherlock 1951).

there is a cardiac cirrhosis, the liver may be small, but never has the same nodularity seen in other forms of cirrhosis. The cut surface (fig. 168) shows prominent hepatic veins which may be thickened. The organ drips blood. The central areas are prominent with alternation of yellow zones (fatty change) and red areas (centrizonal haemorrhage). This appearance has been likened to a nutmeg.

Histological changes. The central vein is always dilated, and the sinusoids entering it are engorged for a variable distance towards the peripheral zones (fig. 169). In severe cases, there is frank haemorrhage with focal necrosis of liver cells. The liver cells show a variety of degenerative changes in the central areas, but each portal tract is surrounded by relatively normal cells to a depth that varies inversely with the extent of the centrizonal atrophy. Surviving cells usually retain their glycogen. Biopsy sections show significant fatty change in only about a third. The absence of fat in biopsy material contrasts with the usual postmortem picture. Cellular infiltration is inconspicuous.

The centrizonal degenerating cells are often

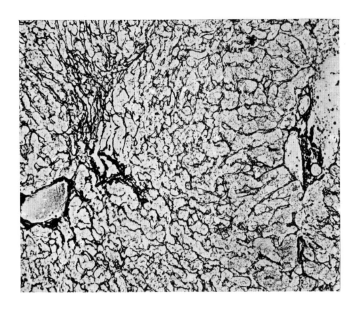

Fig. 170. Same section as in fig. 169. Reticulin stains show centrizonal condensation. H & E, × 120.

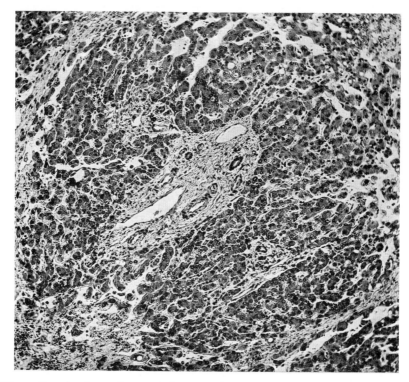

Fig. 171. Fibrous tissue bands pass from central vein to central vein. There is 'reversed lobulation' and a fully developed cardiac cirrhosis. Portal tracts show only slight fibrosis. H & E, ×90 (Sherlock 1951).

packed with brown lipochrome pigment. As they disintegrate, pigment lies free amidst cellular debris. Bile thrombi, particularly periportally, may sometimes be seen in deeply jaundiced patients.

Reticulin changes. The earliest change is centrizonal reticulin condensation following loss of liver cells. This is followed by reticulin and collagen increase and the central vein shows phlebosclerosis (fig. 170). If the heart failure continues or relapses, bridges develop between central veins [5] so that the unaffected portal zone is surrounded by a ring of fibrous tissue (reversed lobulation) (fig. 171). Later the portal tracts are involved and a complex cirrhotic picture results. Nodular regeneration is inconspicuous. A true cardiac cirrhosis is rare.

Electron microscopy [28] shows that the centrizonal cells disappear because of atrophy rather than necrosis. This atrophy may be related to extensive new fibre formation, especially in the spaces of Disse, impairing blood–liver cell exchange. Canalicular dilation and rupture may also be seen.

MECHANISM (fig. 172)

The centrizonal liver cells receive blood at a lower oxygen tension than those at the periphery. Hypoxia is known to cause both degeneration of centrizonal liver cells, dilation of sinusoids [26, 31] and slowing of bile secretion [31]. The liver attempts to compensate by increasing the oxygen extracted as the blood flows across the sinusoidal bed. The central cells (zone III of Rappaport) are the last to receive oxygen and other nutrients and therefore become necrotic. The centrizonal injury is therefore hypoxic and consequent upon a falling cardiac output. Cellular oedema and collagenosis of Disse's space may play a minor role in impairing oxygen diffusion.

The hepatic venous pressure is raised, reflecting the pressure in the right atrium, and this correlates with hepatic necrosis. However, it is doubtful

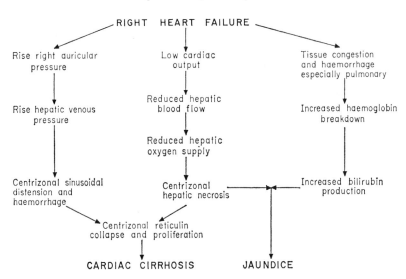

Fig. 172. Possible mechanism of production of cardiac jaundice and cardiac cirrhosis.

whether the centrizonal changes can be purely mechanical, since the rise in pressure must extend from the hepatic vein through the lobule to the portal vein.

CLINICAL FEATURES

Cardiac jaundice

Mild jaundice is common, but deeper icterus is particularly associated with mitral stenosis, especially with tricuspid incompetence. In a general hospital, cardio-respiratory disease is the commonest cause of a raised serum bilirubin level [1]. Jaundice increases with prolonged and repeated bouts of congestive failure. Occasionally, jaundice may be deep and the patient a greenish colour simulating biliary obstruction. Oedematous areas may escape, for bile pigment is attached to protein and does not enter the oedema fluid which has a low protein content [23].

Mechanisms. Jaundice is partly hepatic for the greater the extent of centrizonal necrosis the deeper the icterus [32].

Cholestasis due to bile thrombi or to pressure on bile ducts by distended veins [11] is unlikely.

Bilirubin released from infarcts, whether pulmonary, splenic or renal, or simply from pulmonary congestion, provides an overload on the anoxic liver. Patients in cardiac failure who become jaundiced with minimal hepato-cellular damage usually have clear evidence of pulmonary infarction [32]. In keeping with bilirubin overload the serum shows unconjugated bilirubinaemia and the urine and the faeces show excess of urobilinogen.

The liver

The patient may complain of right abdominal pain probably due to stretching of the nerve endings in the capsule of the enlarged liver. The firm, smooth, tender lower edge may reach the umbilicus.

A rise in right atrial pressure is readily transmitted to the hepatic veins. This is particularly so in tricuspid incompetence when the hepatic vein pressure tracing resembles that obtained from the right atrium with obliteration of the depression between the c and v waves. Palpable pulsation of liver, systolic in time, can be related to this transmission of pressure. Pre-systolic hepatic pulsation occurs in tricuspid stenosis. The expansion may be felt bimanually with one hand over the liver anteriorly and the other over the right lower ribs posteriorly. This expansibility distinguishes it from the palpable epigastric pulsation due to the aorta or an hypertrophied right ventricle. Correct timing of the pulsation is important and if necessary hepatic pulse tracings may be recorded [7].

Hepato-jugular reflux

In heart failure, pressure applied over the liver fills the large veins of the neck. The hepatic compression increases the venous return and the jugular venous pressure rises due to the inability of the failing right heart to handle the increased blood flow.

The reflux is of value for the better identification of the jugular venous pulse and to establish that venous channels between the hepatic and jugular veins are patent.

The reflux is absent if the hepatic veins are occluded or if the main mediastinal or jugular veins are blocked.

Ascites

Ascites is associated with a particularly high venous pressure, a low cardiac output and severe, centrizonal necrosis. This description applies to patients with mitral stenosis and tricuspid incompetence or constrictive pericarditis. In such patients the ascites may be out of proportion to the oedema and symptoms of congestive heart failure. The ascitic fluid may have a high protein content analogous to that observed in the Budd–Chiari syndrome.

Acute liver failure

Confusion, lethargy and coma are occasional accompaniments of heart failure and are related to cerebral anoxia. Occasionally the whole picture of impending hepatic coma may be seen [15]. This may follow not only chronic congestive but also left-sided heart failure [8].

Portal hypertension

Splenomegaly is frequent. Other features of portal hypertension are usually absent except in very severe cardiac cirrhosis associated with constrictive pericarditis. However, at autopsy, 6.7% of 74 patients with congestive heart failure showed oesophageal varices, although in only one was there evidence of bleeding [21].

Clinical recognition of cardiac cirrhosis is usually impossible [32]. It should be suspected in patients with prolonged, decompensated mitral valve disease with tricuspid incompetence or in patients with constrictive pericarditis. The incidence has fallen since both the conditions can be relieved surgically.

BIOCHEMICAL CHANGES

A rise in serum bilirubin is common. In congestive failure the level usually exceeds 1 mg/dl and in about one-third it is more than 2 mg/dl [32]. The jaundice may be deep, exceeding 5 mg/dl and even up to 26.9 mg [13]. The serum bilirubin level corresponds to the degree of heart failure.

Bromsulphalein tests parallel clinical severity, extent of hepato-cellular necrosis [12, 32] and right atrial pressure [20]. The lowered hepatic blood flow may contribute to the abnormality.

Serum alkaline phosphatase is usually normal or slightly increased. Serum albumin values may be mildly reduced and globulin raised [32]. Protein loss from the intestine may contribute.

Serum transaminases rise. They are higher in acute than chronic failure and are proportional to the degree of shock and the extent of centrizonal necrosis [16]. The association of very high values with jaundice may simulate acute viral hepatitis [4, 8].

Urine shows excess urobilinogen and faecal stercobilinogen is increased. Rarely grey stools accompany deep icterus.

PROGNOSIS

The prognosis of the liver changes is that of the underlying heart disease causing them. Cardiac jaundice, particularly if deep, is always a bad omen.

Cardiac cirrhosis *per se* does not carry a bad prognosis and if the heart failure responds to treatment, the cirrhosis can be expected to become latent.

The liver in constrictive pericarditis

The clinical picture and hepatic changes are those of the Budd–Chiari syndrome (page 180).

Cardiac cirrhosis is frequent and marked thickening of the liver capsule simulates sugar icing (*zuckergussleber*). Microscopically the picture is of cardiac cirrhosis. Portal zone fibrosis and bile duct proliferation may be prominent.

Jaundice is absent. The liver is enlarged and hard. Ascites is gross.

Diagnosis must be made from ascites due to cirrhosis or to hepatic venous obstruction. This is done by the paradoxical pulse, the venous pulse, the calcified pericardium, the electrocardiogram and by cardiac catheterization.

TREATMENT

Treatment is that of the cardiac condition. If pericardectomy is possible, prognosis as regards the liver is good although recovery may be slow. Within six months of a successful operation, liver function tests improve and the liver shrinks. The cardiac cirrhosis cannot be expected to resolve completely, but fibrous bands become narrower and avascular.

REFERENCES

1. ABBOTT R.J., CLEE M.D., CARTER N.W. *et al* (1979) A study of hyperbilirubinaemia in clinical practice. *Postgrad. med. J.* **55**, 787.
2. ANDERSON M.D., GABRIELI E. & ZIZZI J.A. (1965) Chronic hemolysis in patients with ball valve prosthesis. *J. Thorac. cardiovasc. Surg.* **50**, 510.
3. BIRGENS H.S., HENRIKSEN J., MATZEN P. *et al* (1978) The shock liver. *Acta. med. Scand.* **204**, 417.
4. BLOTH B., DE FAIRE U. & EDHAG O. (1976) Extreme elevation of transaminase levels in acute heart disease—a problem in differential diagnosis? *Acta. med. Scand.* **200**, 281.
5. BUHAC I., AGRAWAL A.B., PARK S.K. *et al* (1976) Jaundice and bridging centrilobular necrosis of liver in circulatory failure. *N. Y. State J. Med.* **76**, 678.
6. BYWATERS E.G.L. (1946) Anatomical changes in the liver after trauma. *Clin. Sci.* **6**, 19.
7. CALLEJA H.V., ROSENOW O.F. & CLARK T.E. (1961) Pulsations of the liver in heart disease. *Am. J. Med.* **30**, 202.
8. COHEN J.A. & KAPLAN M.M. (1978) Left-sided heart failure presenting as hepatitis. *Gastroenterology* **74**, 583.
9. DAVIDSON C.S., LEWIS J.H., TAGNON H.J. *et al* (1946) Medical shock; abnormal biochemical changes in patients with severe acute medical illnesses, with and without peripheral vascular failure. *N. Engl. J. Med.* **234**, 279.
10. DUNN G.D., HAYES P., BREEN K.J. *et al* (1973) The liver in congestive heart failure: a review. *Am. J. med. Sci.* **265**, 174.
11. EPPINGER H. (1937) *Die Leberkrankheiten* J. Springer, Vienna.
12. EVANS J.M., ZIMMERMAN H.J., WILMER J.G. *et al* (1952) Altered liver function of chronic congestive heart failure. *Am. J. Med.* **13**, 704.
13. GADEHOLT H. & HAUGEN J. (1964) Centrilobular hepatic necrosis in cardiac failure. One case with severe acute jaundice. *Acta. med. Scand.* **176**, 525.
14. KANTROWITZ P.A., JONES W.A., GREENBERGER N.J. *et al* (1967) Post-operative hyperbilirubinemia simulating obstructive jaundice. *N. Engl. J. Med.* **276**, 591.
15. KAYMAKCALAN H., DOURDOUREKAS D., SZANTO P.B. *et al* (1978) Congestive heart failure as cause of fulminant hepatic failure. *Am. J. Med.* **65**, 384.
16. KILLIP T. III & PAYNE M.A. (1960) High serum transaminase activity in heart disease, circulatory failure and hepatic necrosis. *Circulation* **21**, 646.
17. KINGSLEY D.P.E. (1966) Hepatic damage following profound hypothermia and extra-corporeal circulation in man. *Thorax* **21**, 91.
18. LAMONT J.T. & ISSELBACHER K.J. (1973) Current concepts: postoperative jaundice. *N. Engl. J. Med.* **288**, 305.
19. LOCKEY E., MCINTYRE N., ROSS D.N. *et al* (1967) Early jaundice after open heart surgery. *Thorax* **22**, 165.
20. LOSOWSKY M.S., IKRAM H., SNOW H.M. *et al* (1965) Liver function in advanced heart disease. *Br. heart J.* **27**, 578.
21. LUNA A., MEISTER H.P. & SZANTO P.B. (1968) Esophageal varices in the absence of cirrhosis. Incidence and characteristics of congestive heart failure and neoplasm of the liver. *Am. J. clin. Pathol.* **49**, 710.
22. MCMICHAEL J. (1937) The oxygen supply of the liver. *Q. J. exp. Physiol.* **27**, 73.
23. MEAKINS J. (1927) Distribution of jaundice in circulatory failure. *J. clin. Invest.* **4**, 135.
24. NUNES G., BLAISDELL F.W. & MARGARETTEN W. (1970) Mechanism of hepatic dysfunction following shock and trauma. *Arch. Surg.* **100**, 646.
25. POPPER H. (1948) Significance of agonal changes in the human liver. *Arch. Path.* **46**, 132.
26. REESE A.J.M. (1960) The effect of hypoxia on liver secretion studied by intra-viral fluorescence microscopy. *Br. J. exp. Pathol.* **41**, 527.
27. ROBINSON J.S., COLE F.R., GIBSON P. *et al* (1967) Jaundice following cardio-pulmonary bypass. *Thorax* **22**, 232.
28. SAFRAN A.P. & SCHAFFNER F. (1967) Chronic passive congestion of the liver in man. Electron microscopic study of cell atrophy and intralobular fibrosis. *Am. J. Pathol.* **50**, 447.
29. SANDERSON R.G., ELLISON J.H., BENSON J.A. Jr *et al* (1967) Jaundice following open heart surgery. *Ann. Surg.* **165**, 217.
30. SCHMID M., HEFTI M.L., GATTIKER R. *et al* (1965) Benign post-operative intrahepatic cholestasis. *N. Engl. J. Med.* **272**, 545.
31. SENEVIRATNE R.D. (1949) Physiological and pathological responses in the blood-vessels of the liver. *Q. J. exp. Physiol.* **35**, 77.
32. SHERLOCK S. (1951) The liver in heart failure; relation of anatomical, functional and circulatory changes. *Br. Heart J.* **13**, 273.
33. WHITE T.J., LEEVY C.M., BRUSCA A.M. *et al* (1955) The liver in congestive heart failure. *Am. Heart J.* **49**, 250.

Chapter 13
Jaundice

BILIRUBIN METABOLISM [8, 45]

Bilirubin is the end product of haem coming from haemoglobin and also from myoglobin and many respiratory enzymes including the cytochromes (fig. 173). Approximately 6 g haemoglobin are broken down daily and 30 mg bilirubin are formed. Production takes place in reticulo-endothelial cells, particularly in the liver and spleen.

The enzyme which converts haem to bilirubin is microsomal haem oxygenase which has absolute requirements for oxygen and NADPH. Cleavage of the porphyrin ring occurs selectively at the alpha methane bridge (fig. 174). The alpha bridge carbon atom is converted to carbon monoxide and the original bridge function is replaced by two oxygen atoms which are derived from molecular oxygen. The resulting linear tetrapyrrole has the structure of the IX alpha biliverdin. This is further converted to IX alpha bilirubin by an enzyme biliverdin reductase. Such a linear tetrapyrrole should be water-soluble whereas bilirubin is lipid-soluble. The lipid-solubility is explained by the structure of IX alpha bilirubin which has six intramolecular stable hydrogen bonds (fig. 175) [12]. This bonding can be broken by alcohol in the diazo (Van den Bergh) reaction converting unconjugated (indirect) bilirubin to conjugated (direct) reacting bilirubin. *In vivo* the stable hydrogen bonds are altered by esterification of the proprionic groups by glucuronic acid.

About 20% of circulating bilirubin is not formed from the haem of mature erythrocytes [7]. A very small proportion of this comes from immature erythropoietic cells in spleen and bone marrow. This component is increased in haemolytic states. The remainder is formed in the liver from haem, the cytochromes and unknown sources. This component is increased in pernicious anaemia, congenital erythropoietic porphyria and the Crigler–Najjar syndrome.

Hepatic transport of bilirubin (fig. 176)

Unconjugated bilirubin is transported in the plasma tightly bound to albumin. A very small amount is dialysable, but this can be increased by substances which compete with bilirubin for albumin binding. These include fatty acids, some drugs and antibiotics, and organic anions. All these facilitate the non-ionic diffusion of bilirubin into the liver and other tissues. This is important in the neonate where such drugs as sulphonamides and salicylates facilitate diffusion of bilirubin into brain and so increase the risk of kernicterus.

Hepatic uptake involves detachment of the albumin at the sinusoidal plasma membrane. This is carrier-mediated and shared by many organic anions including BSP, indocyanine green, and bile acids. Binding proteins, such as ligandin, may be concerned with the transport of bilirubin from the

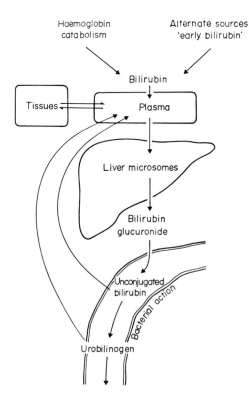

Fig. 173. The metabolism of bilirubin.

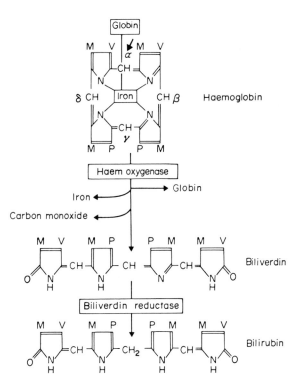

Fig. 174. The metabolism of haemoglobin to bilirubin (Billing 1972).

Fig. 175. The structure of bilirubin IXα as an involuted hydrogen-bonded structure. The propionic acid groups of pyrrole rings B and C are linked to the nitrogens of the opposite pyrrole rings (broken lines).

plasma membrane to the endoplasmic reticulum. Ligandin may also be concerned in the efflux of bilirubin from liver to plasma.

Unconjugated bilirubin is non-polar (lipid soluble). It is converted to a polar (water-soluble) compound by conjugation and this allows its excretion into the bile. This involves an enzyme of the microsomal fraction called bilirubin UDP glucuronyl transferase which converts the unconjugated bilirubin to the conjugated bilirubin monoglucuronide. The process is inducible by such drugs as phenobarbital. Reduced concentrations of the

conjugating enzyme are of importance in the neonate and in the Gilbert's and Crigler–Najjar hyperbilirubinaemias. Levels are well maintained in hepato-cellular jaundice and even increased in the cholestatic type [9].

The major bilirubin conjugate in human bile is the diglucuronide. The conversion of the monoglucuronide to the diglucuronide may take place at the liver cell surface membrane [31]. The diglucuronide is then excreted in the bile and the bilirubin presumably returns to be conjugated, but its exact fate is unknown (fig. 176).

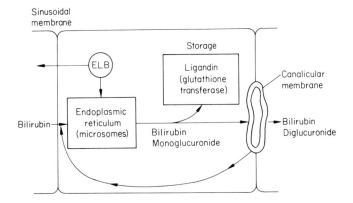

Fig. 176. The transport and conjugation of bilirubin as a monoglucuronide and diglucuronide. ELB = early labelled bilirubin.

Although conjugation as a glucuronide remains the most important mechanism, sulphate, xylose and glucose conjugation also occur to a small extent and may be increased in cholestasis.

The uptake process of bilirubin from plasma to liver cell is normally not saturated and biliary excretion of bilirubin glucuronide is the rate-limiting factor in the transport of bilirubin from plasma to bile. Secretion of the conjugated pigments probably involves a carrier-mediated active transport system which is shared by many other organic anions. Bilirubin excretion can be enhanced by taurocholate. A high proportion of the conjugated bilirubin in bile is incorporated into mixed micelles with cholesterol, phospholipids and bile salts. The role of the Golgi apparatus and of the microfilaments of the cytoskeleton in the intra-hepatic transport of conjugated bilirubin remains to be defined.

Bilirubin diglucuronide in bile is polar (water-soluble) and hence is not absorbed from the small intestine. In the colon, bacterial beta-glucuronidases hydrolyse the conjugated bilirubin, which is then reduced to urobilinogens. In the presence of bacterial cholangitis some hydrolysis of the bilirubin glucuronide is possible and unconjugated bilirubin is precipitated. This may be an important factor in the production of bilirubin gall-stones.

Urobilinogen is non-polar and is well absorbed from the small intestine, but only minimally from the colon. The little that is normally absorbed is re-excreted by the liver and kidneys (*entero-hepatic circulation*). With hepato-cellular dysfunction re-excretion by the liver is impaired and more is excreted into the urine. This accounts for the urobilinogenuria of alcoholic liver disease, pyrexia, heart failure, and the early stages of viral hepatitis.

Unconjugated bilirubin–albumin cannot cross the glomerulus and is not found in normal urine. The bilirubin–glucuronide–albumin complex on the other hand is 1% dialysable and is excreted by glomerular filtration. This unbound conjugated bilirubin is largely re-absorbed in the proximal tubules [25]. Bilirubin is therefore present in the urine in cholestatic jaundice where increases of circulating conjugated bilirubin are found.

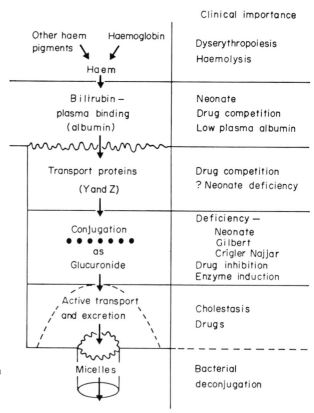

Fig. 177. The clinical importance of interference with the stages in the transport of bilirubin, from its production from haem through to its excretion in micellar form into the bile.

Distribution of jaundice in the tissues

Circulating protein-bound bilirubin finds it difficult to enter the protein-low tissue fluids. If the protein is increased, jaundice becomes more evident. A histamine wheal, with blister fluid of a high protein content, appears yellow if the serum bilirubin concentration is raised [14]. Exudates tend to be more icteric than transudates because of the greater amount of protein in them.

The cerebro-spinal fluid is more likely to be xanthochromic when meningitis is present, the classical example being Weil's disease with both jaundice and meningitis.

The basal ganglia may be bile-stained in the newborn (kernicterus). This is due to the high concentration of circulating, unconjugated, lipophilic bilirubin having an affinity for nervous tissue.

Cerebro-spinal fluid from jaundiced subjects contains a small amount of bilirubin, the level being one-tenth to one-hundredth of that found in the serum [32].

In deep jaundice, the ocular fluids are yellow, and this is considered to explain the extremely rare symptom of xanthopsia (seeing yellow).

Urine, sweat, semen and milk contain bile pigment in the deeply jaundiced patient. Bilirubin is a normal constituent of synovial fluid.

Paralysed parts and oedematous areas tend to remain uncoloured.

Bilirubin is readily bound to elastic tissue. Skin, ocular sclera and blood vessels have a high elastic tissue content, and easily become icteric. This also accounts for the disparity between the depth of skin jaundice and serum bilirubin levels during the stage of recovery.

Factors determining the depth of jaundice

Even after complete bile duct obstruction, the depth of jaundice is very variable. After an initial rapid increase, the serum bilirubin levels off after about three weeks although the obstruction persists. The jaundice deepends on both bile pigment production and the capacity for its excretion. In total bile duct obstruction the kidneys are responsible for bilirubin excretion and their powers are limited.

Rates of bilirubin production may vary in different people. Another possibility is that products other than bilirubin, which do not give the diazo reaction, are formed from haem catabolism. The intestinal mucosa may allow the passage of bilirubin, presumably unconjugated, from the blood.

In prolonged cholestasis the skin is greenish, possibly due to biliverdin, which does not give the diazo reaction for bilirubin. Other pigments may also play a part.

Conjugated bilirubin, because of its water-solubility and penetration of body fluids, produces more jaundice than unconjugated pigment. This accounts for the more intense colour of those with hepato-cellular and cholestatic rather than haemolytic jaundice.

CLASSIFICATION OF JAUNDICE
(fig. 178)

Theoretically jaundice might arise in four different ways. Firstly, there may be increased bilirubin load on the liver cell. Secondly, there may be a disturbance in uptake and transport of bilirubin within the liver cell. Thirdly, there may be defects in conjugation. Finally the defect may be in the cell membrane opposite the canaliculus for excretion into the bile. Further difficulties might be due to obstruction to the large bile channels before the bilirubin reaches the intestines. Simple classification is into three predominant types, *pre-hepatic*, *hepatic* and *cholestatic*. There is much overlap between them and particularly between the hepatic and cholestatic varieties. The differentiation nevertheless is a useful one, for the routines adopted for diagnosis, management and prognosis are completely different.

Pre-hepatic (table 27). This group is marked by an increase in total serum bilirubin levels with normal values for the serum transaminases, alkaline phosphatases and proteins. If the serum bilirubin can be fractionated then the increase may be either in the unconjugated ('indirect') component or in the conjugated ('direct') reacting one. Bilirubin cannot be detected in the urine. The cause may be haemolysis or a familial disturbance of bilirubin metabolism.

Hepatic (Chapters 15 and 17). The jaundice usually comes on rapidly and is of an orange tint. Fatigue and malaise are conspicuous. There are varying degrees of liver failure. These may be shown in a mild case as personality change and in the more severe as flapping tremor, confusion and coma. Fluid retention is shown in its mildest form by weight gain and in the more severe by oedema and ascites. The blood pressure is low. Reduced

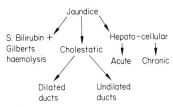

Fig. 178. Classification of jaundice.

hepatic synthesis of coagulation factors is shown by bruising in relation to venepunctures and also spontaneously. Serum biochemistry shows increases in transaminases and immunoglobulin G. Serum albumin levels are reduced in the long-standing case.

Cholestatic (Chapter 14). This is due to failure of adequate amounts of bile to reach the duodenum. The patient is relatively well, apart from the causative condition, for cholestasis *per se* is compatible with reasonably good health. Pruritus is prominent. With time the patient becomes increasingly pigmented. The serum shows increases in conjugated bilirubin, biliary alkaline phosphatase, total cholesterol and conjugated bile acids. Steatorrhoea is responsible for weight loss and malabsorption of fat-soluble vitamins A, D and K and of calcium.

DIAGNOSIS OF JAUNDICE
(tables 25, 26)

The importance of the careful history and physical examination with routine biochemical and haematological tests must be stressed. The stool should be inspected and occult blood examination performed. The urine is tested for bilirubin and urobilinogen excess. Routine radiological tests include a chest X-ray and a plain X-ray of the abdomen. The place of special tests such as ultrasonic examination, liver biopsy and cholangiography— whether percutaneous or endoscopic—will depend on the category of jaundice into which the patient has been placed.

Clinical history

Occupation of the patient should be noted; particularly any contact with rats carrying Weil's disease, or employment involving alcohol.

Place of origin (Mediterranean, African or Far East) may suggest carriage of hepatitis B antigen.

Table 25. First steps in the diagnosis of the jaundiced patient.

Clinical history and examination
Urine, stools
Serum biochemical tests
   bilirubin (conjugated and unconjugated)
   transaminase ('AST', 'SGOT')
   albumin
   quantitative immunoglobulins
   alkaline phosphatase
   total cholesterol
Haematology
   haemoglobin, WBC, platelets
Blood film
Prothrombin time (before and after i.m. vitamin K)
X-rays
   chest
   plain abdomen

Family history is important with respect to jaundice, hepatitis, anaemia, splenectomy or cholecystectomy. Positive histories are helpful in diagnosing haemolytic jaundice, congenital hyperbilirubinaemia, hepatitis and gall-stones.

Contact with jaundiced persons particularly in nurseries, camps, hospitals and schools is noted. Close contact with patients on renal units or with drug abusers is recorded. Any *injection* in the preceding six months should be recorded. 'Injections' include blood tests, drug abuse, tuberculin testing, dental treatment and tattooing as well as blood or plasma transfusions. The patient is asked about previous *drug treatment* with possible icterogenic agents. Consumption of *shell fish* and previous *travel* to areas where hepatitis is endemic should be noted.

Previous dyspepsia, fat intolerance and biliary colic suggest choledocholithiasis.

Jaundice after biliary tract surgery suggests residual calculus, traumatic stricture of the bile duct, or hepatitis. Jaundice following the removal of a malignant growth may be due to hepatic metastases. Post-operative jaundice might be related to multiple administrations of halothane.

Alcoholics usually have associated features such as anorexia, morning nausea, diarrhoea and mild pyrexia. They may complain of pain over the enlarged liver.

Progressive failure of health and weight loss favour an underlying carcinoma.

The mode of onset is extremely important. Preceding nausea, associated anorexia, in smokers— aversion to smoking, and jaundice, developing in a matter of hours and deepening rapidly, suggest

Table 26. Differential diagnosis of the common types of jaundice.

	Gall-stones in common bile duct	Carcinoma ampullary region	Acute virus hepatitis	Cholestatic drug jaundice
Antecedent history	Dyspepsia, previous attack	Nil	Contacts, injections, transfusion, or nil	Taking drug
Pain	Constant epigastric, biliary colic, or none	Constant epigastric, back, or none	Ache over liver or none	None
Pruritus	+	+	Transient	+
Rate of development of jaundice	Slow	Slow	Rapid	Rapid
Type of jaundice	Fluctuant or persistent	Usually but not always progressive	Rapid onset, slow fall with recovery	Variable, usually mild
Weight loss	Slight to moderate	Progressive	Slight	Slight
Examination				
Diathesis	Frequently female, obese	Over 40 years old	Young usually	Often female, psychotic
Depth of jaundice	Moderate	Deep	Variable	Variable, rash sometimes
Ascites	0	Rarely with metastases	If severe and prolonged	0
Liver	Enlarged, slightly tender	Enlarged, not tender	Enlarged and tender	Slightly enlarged
Palpable gall bladder	0	+ (sometimes)	0	0
Tender gall bladder area	+	0	0	0
Palpable spleen	0	Occasionally	About 20%	0
Temperature	↑	Not usually	↑ onset only	↑ onset
Laboratory investigations				
Leucocyte count	↑ or normal	↑ or normal	↓	Normal
Differential leucocytes	Polymorphs ↑	–	Lymphocytes ↑	Eosinophilia at onset
Faeces:				
colour	Intermittently pale	Acholic	Variable, light→dark	Pale
occult blood	0	+	0	0
Urine: Urobilin (ogen)	+	Absent	– Early + late	– Early + late
S. bilirubin mg/dl	Usually 3–10	Steady rise to 15–30	Varies with severity	Variable
S. alkaline phosphatase KA units/dl	> 30	> 30	< 30	> 30
S. aspartate transaminase units	< 100	< 100	> 100 (early)	< 100
S. total cholesterol mg/dl	Variable	Variable	< 300	> 300
Radiology				
Plain film abdomen	Gall-stones 10%	Hepatomegaly	Hepatomegaly, slight	Hepatomegaly, slight
Barium meal	Normal	Displacement stomach and duodenum sometimes	Normal	Normal

virus hepatitis. Cholestatic jaundice develops more slowly, often with persistent pruritus. Pyrexia with rigors suggests cholangitis associated with gall-stones or biliary stricture.

Dark urine and pale stools precede hepato-cellular or cholestatic jaundice by a few days. In haemolytic jaundice the stools are well coloured.

In hepato-cellular jaundice the patient feels ill; in cholestatic jaundice he may be inconvenienced only by the icterus, any symptoms being due to the cause of the obstruction.

Persistent mild jaundice of varying intensity suggests haemolysis. The jaundice of cirrhosis is usually mild and variable and is associated with dark stools, although patients with acute 'alcoholic hepatitis' may be deeply jaundiced and pass pale stools.

Biliary colic may be continuous for hours rather than being intermittent. Back or epigastric pain may be associated with pancreatic carcinoma.

Examination (fig. 179)

Age and sex. A parous, middle-aged, obese female

may have gall-stones. The incidence of type A hepatitis decreases as age advances but no age is exempt from type B and non-A, non-B hepatitis. The probability of cancerous biliary obstruction increases with age. Drug jaundice is very rare in childhood.

General examination. Anaemia may indicate haemolysis, cancer or cirrhosis. Gross weight loss suggests cancer. The patient with haemolytic jaundice is a mild yellow colour, with hepato-cellular jaundice is orange and with prolonged biliary obstruction is a deep greenish hue. A hunched-up position suggests pancreatic carcinoma. In alcoholics, the stigmata of cirrhosis should be noted. Sites to be examined for a primary tumour include breasts, thyroid, stomach, colon, rectum and lung. Lymphadenopathy is noted.

Mental state. Slight intellectual deterioration with minimal personality change may be extremely valuable in suggesting hepato-cellular jaundice. Fetor and 'flapping' tremor indicate impending hepatic coma.

Skin changes. Bruising may indicate a clotting

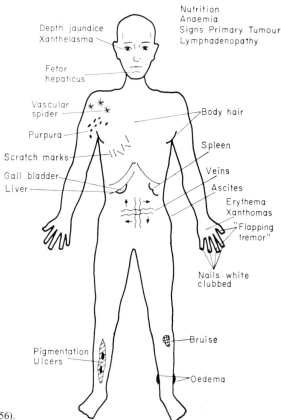

Fig. 179. Physical signs in jaundice (Sherlock 1956).

defect. Purpuric spots on forearms, axillae or shins may be related to the thrombocytopenia of cirrhosis. Other cutaneous manifestations of cirrhosis include vascular spiders, palmar erythema, white nails and loss of secondary sexual hair.

In chronic cholestasis, scratch marks, melanin pigmentation, finger clubbing, xanthomas on the eyelids, extensor surfaces and palmar creases, and hyperkeratosis may be found.

Pigmentation of the shins and ulcers may be seen in some forms of congenital haemolytic anaemia.

Malignant nodules should be sought in the skin. Multiple venous thromboses suggest carcinoma of the body of the pancreas. Ankle oedema may indicate cirrhosis, or obstruction of the inferior vena cava due to hepatic malignancy.

Abdominal examination. Dilated peri-umbilical veins indicate a portal collateral circulation and cirrhosis. Ascites may be due to cirrhosis or to malignant disease of the peritoneum. A very large nodular liver suggests cancer. A small liver may indicate severe hepatitis or cirrhosis, and its presence excludes extra-hepatic cholestasis in which the liver is enlarged and smooth. In an alcoholic, fatty change and cirrhosis may produce a uniform enlargement of the liver. The edge is tender in hepatitis, in congestive heart failure, with alcoholism, in bacterial cholangitis and occasionally in malignant disease. An arterial murmur over the liver indicates acute alcoholic hepatitis or primary liver cancer.

In choledocholithiasis the gall bladder may be tender and Murphy's sign positive. A palpable, and sometimes visibly enlarged, gall bladder suggests pancreatic cancer.

The abdomen is carefully examined for any primary tumour. A rectal examination is essential and sigmoidoscopy may be needed.

Urine and faeces. Bilirubinuria is an early sign of virus hepatitis and drug jaundice. Persistent absence of urobilinogen suggests total obstruction of the common bile duct: if it is absent for more than seven days the obstruction is probably complete and malignant. Persistent excess of urobilinogen with a negative bilirubin test supports the diagnosis of haemolytic jaundice.

The persistence of acholic stools confirms biliary obstruction. The presence of occult blood favours a diagnosis of ampullary, pancreatic or alimentary carcinoma or of portal hypertension.

The colour of the faeces must be recorded daily.

Serum biochemical tests

The serum bilirubin level confirms jaundice, indicates depth and is used to follow progress. Serum alkaline phosphatase values more than three times normal strongly suggest biliary obstruction if bone disease is absent; high values may also be found in patients with non-biliary cirrhosis. In doubtful cases the serum 5'-nucleotidase or γ-glutamyl transpeptidase level may be measured when an increase indicates hepato-biliary and not bone disease.

Serum albumin and globulin levels are little changed in jaundice of short duration. In more chronic hepato-cellular icterus the albumin is depressed and globulin increased. Electrophoretic analysis shows raised α_2- and β-globulins in cholestatic jaundice in contrast to γ-globulin elevation in hepato-cellular jaundice.

Serum transaminase increases in hepatitis compared with variable but lower levels in cholestatic jaundice.

Haematology

A low total leucocyte count with a relative lymphocytosis suggests hepato-cellular jaundice. A polymorph leucocytosis may complicate very severe virus hepatitis. Increased leucocyte counts are found with cholestatic jaundice with acute cholangitis or underlying malignant disease. If haemolysis is suspected, investigations should include reticulocyte counts, the examination of blood films, erythrocyte fragility, Coombs' test, and examination of the bone marrow.

If the prothrombin time is prolonged vitamin K_1 10 mg intramuscularly for three days leads to return to normal in cholestasis whereas patients with hepato-cellular jaundice show little change.

Radiology

A routine chest film is taken to show primary and secondary tumours and any irregularity and elevation of the right diaphragm due to an enlarged or nodular liver. A plain film of the abdomen confirms liver and spleen size; 10% of gall-stones are radio-opaque. A barium meal may show oesophageal varices and in patients with hepatomegaly the lesser curve of the stomach may be displaced and even rigid. Distortion and altered motility of the duodenum is seen in carcinoma of the head of the pancreas.

VISUALIZATION OF THE BILE DUCTS

This is indicated if the picture is cholestatic (see Chapter 14). The first technique is ultrasound or CT scanning to show whether or not the intra-hepatic bile ducts are dilated (fig. 49). This is followed by percutaneous or endoscopic cholangiography as indicated (fig. 64).

In the mildly jaundiced (total serum bilirubin less than 3 mg/100 ml) and particularly if acute, the bile ducts can sometimes be shown by intravenous cholangiography with tomography.

Percutaneous trans-hepatic cholangiography (Chapter 6) [20, 30]. This technique using the Chiba ('skinny') needle is 90% successful if intrahepatic ducts are dilated and about 60% if they are not. It carries a small risk of biliary peritonitis. External drainage [37] or surgery within four hours should usually follow puncture of dilated ducts.

Endoscopic retrograde cholangio-pancreatography (ERCP) (Chapter 6) [16] using fibreoptic endoscopes is a skilled procedure. The success rate is about 70%. Visualization of stomach, duodenum and pancreatic ducts is possible. Suspicious lesions may be biopsied.

Needle liver biopsy

Acute jaundice rarely merits liver biopsy and the technique is reserved for the patient who presents diagnostic difficulty. The method carries extra risk in the jaundiced; the Menghini technique is safest. Mere depth of jaundice is not a contraindication (table 2). Acute virus hepatitis is usually diagnosed easily. The greatest difficulty arises in the cholestatic group. However, in most instances an experienced histopathologist can distinguish appearances of intra-hepatic cholestasis, for instance due to drugs or to primary biliary cirrhosis, from the appearances of block to main bile passages. The cause of the cholestasis can be stated with much less certainty.

Peritoneoscopy

The appearance of a dark green liver with an enormous gall bladder favours extra-hepatic biliary obstruction. Tumour nodules may be seen and needle biopsy may be made under direct vision. A pale yellow-green liver suggests hepatitis and a cirrhosis is obvious. The method cannot be relied upon to distinguish extra-hepatic biliary obstruc-

tion, especially due to a carcinoma of the main hepatic ducts, from intra-hepatic cholestasis due to drugs.

If possible a permanent photographic record should be taken of the appearances. In the presence of jaundice peritoneoscopy is safer than needle biopsy but, if necessary, the two procedures may be combined.

Prednisolone test

When 30 mg prednisolone daily are given a profound fall in serum bilirubin level in five days indicates hepato-cellular jaundice. Patients with cholestasis show little change. A fall in serum bilirubin level greater than 40% strongly suggests hepatitis [49], but an equivocal one does not exclude it. This test is for the problem case usually when cholestatic viral hepatitis is suspected. It is rarely necessary.

The fate of the bilirubin disappearing from the blood after prednisolone is most obscure. The corticosteroid 'whitewash' cannot be accounted for by changes in erythrocyte survival (reflecting changes in haemoglobin catabolism), faecal or urinary urobilinogen output, or urinary bilirubin [52]. The bilirubin may take an alternative metabolic pathway.

The place of laparotomy

Jaundice is rarely a surgical emergency. If there is any doubt concerning the diagnosis, it is better to investigate further rather than to explore the bile passages of a patient with hepatic jaundice and so run the very real risk of precipitating acute liver failure. The patient rarely suffers from delay. If the diagnosis is virus hepatitis, recovery may ensue. If cirrhosis, the diagnosis should be obvious, and if cholestatic, the changes occurring in the liver are essentially reversible. Biliary cirrhosis does not develop rapidly. If the diagnosis is malignant biliary obstruction, the chances of radical removal of the tumour are so remote that they are unlikely to be affected by a few days' delay. Special investigations include liver biopsy, scanning and visualization of the bile duct by percutaneous or endoscopic cholangiography. Any laparotomy should be thorough and, if any diagnostic doubt remains, should include operative liver biopsy and direct operative or post-operative cholangiography with biopsy of any suspicious mass or enlarged nodes.

THE FAMILIAL NON-HAEMOLYTIC HYPERBILIRUBINAEMIAS (table 27)

Although the upper limit of serum bilirubin is usually taken to be 0.8 mg/100 ml, in some 5% of healthy blood donors higher values (1–3 mg/100 ml) may be found. When those suffering from haemolysis or from overt liver disease have been excluded there remain the patients with familial abnormalities of bilirubin metabolism. The commonest is Gilbert's syndrome [24]. Other syndromes can also be identified. The prognosis for all these is excellent. Accurate diagnosis, particularly from chronic liver disease, is important for it enables the patient to be reassured more convincingly. The diagnosis is based on the family history, duration, absence of stigmata of hepatocellular disease and of splenomegaly, and on the hepatic histology.

Primary 'shunt' hyperbilirubinaemia. This very rare condition is due to increased production of 'early-labelled' ('shunt') bilirubin in the bone marrow [6]. The cause is probably the premature destruction of abnormal red cell precursors (ineffective erythrocyte synthesis). The clinical picture is of compensated haemolysis. Peripheral erythrocyte destruction is normal. The condition is probably familial [3, 29].

Gilbert's syndrome

This is the commonest form of familial, unconjugated, non-haemolytic hyperbilirubinaemia. It affects some 2–5% of the population [38]. The number involved in any family is difficult to determine. The serum bilirubin may be only minimally, and inconstantly, elevated. In one study, a family history of jaundice was obtained in about 15% of patients, and in some families an incidence of 5% could be traced through successive generations [23]. In another investigation of first-degree relatives of 42 patients, unconjugated bilirubinaemia was found in 10 of 62 (16.1%) healthy parents, and 14 of 51 (27.5%) healthy siblings [40]. The distribution of serum bilirubin levels in the relatives fell into two groups. One approximated to the normal range and the other was similar to that of the patients. Gilbert's syndrome is probably inherited as an autosomal dominant. Patients are heterozygous for a single mutant gene [41].

It may be diagnosed by chance at a routine medical examination or when the blood is being examined for another reason, for instance to determine completeness of recovery from virus hepatitis. It has an excellent prognosis. Jaundice is mild and intermittent. Deepening may follow an intercurrent infection and is associated with malaise, nausea and often discomfort over the liver. These symptoms have never been explained but often lead to a mistaken diagnosis of virus hepatitis. There are no other abnormal physical signs; the spleen is not palpable.

The serum total bilirubin level rarely exceeds 3 mg/100 ml. Other biochemical tests are normal. Bilirubin is not detected in the urine. Hepatic histology is normal.

Table 27. Isolated increases in serum bilirubin.

Type	Diagnostic points
Unconjugated	
Haemolysis	Splenomegaly. Blood film. Reticulocytosis. Coombs'.
Gilbert's	Familial. S. bilirubin increases fasting and falls on phenobarbitone. Liver biopsy normal but conjugating enzyme reduced.
Crigler–Najjar	
Type 1	No conjugating enzyme in liver. No response to phenobarbitone. Usually die young with kernicterus.
Type 2	Absent or deficient conjugating enzyme in liver. Response to phenobarbitone.
Conjugated	
Dubin–Johnson	Black liver biopsy. No concentration of cholecystographic media. Secondary rise in BSP test.
Rotor	Normal liver biopsy. Cholecystography normal. BSP test normal.

Total bilirubin concentration in Gilbert's syndrome and normal subjects

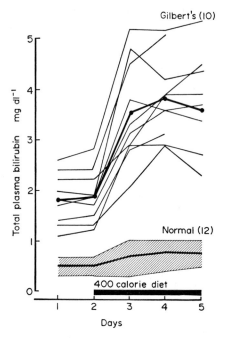

Fig. 180. Gilbert's syndrome. The serum unconjugated bilirubin level increases after a 400 calorie diet (Owens & Sherlock 1973).

The defect in bilirubin metabolism is complex. The bilirubin conjugating enzyme, UDP glucuronyl transferase, is reduced [9]. A liver cell membrane uptake defect may impair the uptake of bilirubin by the liver cell [11]. The bile contains an increased amount of bilirubin monoglucuronide over the diglucuronide, suggesting a second enzyme defect related to the conversion of monoglucuronide to diglucuronide [22]. Erythrocyte survival may be mildly reduced [41] and dyserythropoiesis may play a part [36]. The bilirubin liberated from the erythrocyte breakdown would not be sufficient to account for the jaundice [40].

Other abnormalities include a mild impairment of BSP clearance and a reduced clearance of tolbutamide, a drug which does not need conjugation. The multiplicity of abnormalities suggests that Gilbert's syndrome may not be an entity. The hyperbilirubinaemia may constitute merely the upper end of the normal range [5].

An increase in the serum unconjugated bilirubin follows a 400 calorie diet for 24 hours [21, 39] (fig. 180). This is probably due to an increase in serum

fatty acids on fasting. These compete with bilirubin for excretion by the liver cell [26]. In a doubtful case the low calorie test may be used diagnostically.

The bilirubin transferase enzyme can be enhanced by enzyme induction using phenobarbital 60 mg three times a day in the adult (fig. 181). This results in a return of the serum bilirubin level to normal [10]. Since the mild bilirubinaemia of untreated Gilbert's syndrome rarely leads to clinical icterus, few patients will gain cosmetic benefit from this treatment.

Gilbert's syndrome has a normal life expectancy. 'Sufferers' should be regarded as a normal risk for life insurance purposes.

Crigler–Najjar Type

This extreme form of familial non-haemolytic jaundice is associated with very high serum unconjugated bilirubin values [17]. Deficiency of conjugating enzyme can be demonstrated in the liver. Monoglucuronide is the major pigment fraction of bile [22]. Bilirubin tolerance is impaired but the BSP test gives normal results.

Two varieties are described [27].

In *Type I*, no bilirubin conjugating enzyme can be detected in the liver. Conjugated bilirubin is absent from the bile. Sufferers usually die with ker-

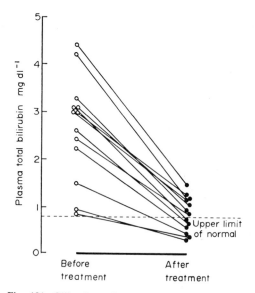

Fig. 181. Gilbert's syndrome. The effect of phenobarbital (60 mg, three times a day) on the serum bilirubin level (Black & Sherlock 1970).

nicterus in the first year of life. There is no re$ponse to phenobarbital.

In *Type II*, although the bilirubin conjugating enzyme is absent or deficient in the liver, the patients respond to phenobarbital and survive into adult life. Phototherapy (sunlight) also lowers the serum bilirubin level.

The *Gunn strain* of congenitally jaundiced rats also lacks the bilirubin glucuronyl transferase enzyme and these animals are very useful in the study of bilirubin metabolism.

Dubin–Johnson type

The Dubin–Johnson type is a chronic, benign, intermittent jaundice with conjugated hyperbilirubinaemia and bilirubinuria [18, 19, 48].

The liver, macroscopically, is greenish-black (black-liver jaundice) (figs. 182, 183). In sections the liver cells show a brown pigment which is neither iron nor bile. The pigment may be melanin, which has been found in the urine and spleen of a patient with this syndrome [51]. This seems likely since the pigment in the liver of mutant Corriedale sheep, which have a disorder similar in all respects to the Dubin–Johnson syndrome, is derived from epinephrine [4]. Electron microscopy shows the pigment in dense bodies related to lysosomes [28] (fig. 184). Lysosomal function is abnormal [46].

An unrelated virus hepatitis leads to temporary mobilization of the hepatic pigment [50].

Pruritus is absent and the serum alkaline phosphatase and bile acid levels are normal. There is difficulty in excreting both the contrast media used in intravenous cholangiography and BSP. Carriers of the abnormal gene, however, cannot be identified by simple intravenous BSP testing. In patients a more diagnostic pattern is seen in a prolonged BSP test. After an initial fall in serum level the BSP

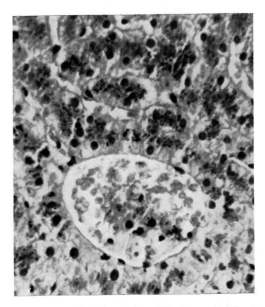

Fig. 183. Dubin–Johnson hyperbilirubinaemia. The liver cells and Kupffer cells (especially centrizonally) are packed with a dark pigment which gives the staining reactions of lipofuscin. H & E, ×275 (Sherlock 1962).

rises so that the value at 120 minutes exceeds that seen at 45 minutes [35] (fig. 185).

Total coproporphyrin excretion is slightly reduced or normal, 90% being in the form of isomer 1 [53]. The reason is unknown. There may be a relationship between canalicular excretion and porphyrin metabolism, or the two may be unrelated.

The condition may present as jaundice during pregnancy or after taking oral contraceptives, both of which reduce hepatic excretory function [15].

Study of a large family of 242 persons, some of whom had the Dubin–Johnson syndrome, suggested the inheritance was dominant with considerable invariability of expression [13]. Further study of 101 patients from Israel, however, suggested autosomal recessive inheritance.

There is no correlation between liver pigment and serum bilirubin level. Prognosis is excellent.

Rotor type

This is a similar form of chronic familial conjugated hyperbilirubinaemia. It resembles the Dubin–Johnson syndrome, the main difference

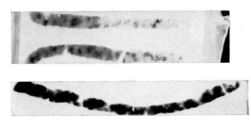

Fig. 182. Paraffin blocks of needle liver biopsies from a normal patient and (*below*) the chocolate coloured biopsy of a patient with Dubin–Johnson hyperbilirubinaemia (Sherlock 1962).

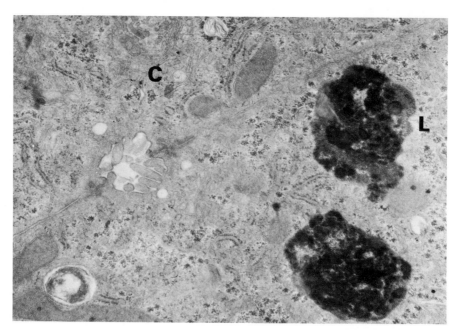

Fig. 184. Dubin–Johnson syndrome. Electron microscopy shows normal bile canaliculi with intact microvilli (C). Lysosomes (L) are enlarged, irregularly shaped and contain granular material and often membrane-bound lipid droplets.

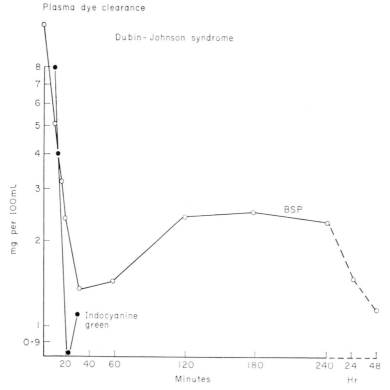

Fig. 185. Bromsulphalein tolerance test (5 mg/kg i.m.) in a patient with Dubin–Johnson syndrome. At 40 min. the BSP level has almost returned to normal. An increase is then seen at 120, 180 and 240 min. Dye can still be detected in the blood at 48 hours. The indocyanine green test is also shown and is normal at 20 min. but also has a tendency to increase at 30 min.

being the absence of brown pigment in the liver cell [44]. The condition also differs from the Dubin–Johnson type in that the gall bladder opacifies on cholecystography and there is no secondary rise in the BSP test. The abnormality causing BSP retention appears to be related to a defect in hepatic uptake rather than excretion as originally demonstrated in the Dubin–Johnson syndrome [1].

Family studies over six generations make an autosomal inheritance probable [34]. The Rotor type has an excellent prognosis.

The group of familial non-haemolytic hyperbilirubinaemias

There is much overlap between the various syndromes of congenital hyperbilirubinaemia. Patients are found in the same family with conjugated hyperbilirubinaemia but with or without pigment in the liver cells [2, 42]. Pigmented livers have been found in patients with unconjugated hyperbilirubinaemia [13, 42]. In one large family the propositi had the classic Dubin–Johnson picture, but the commonest abnormality in the family was unconjugated hyperbilirubinaemia [13]. In another family, conjugated and unconjugated hyperbilirubinaemia alternated in the same patient [43]. Such observations add to the confusion in separating the groups and in deciding the mode of inheritance.

REFERENCES

1. ABE H. & OKUDA K. (1975) Biliary excretion of conjugated sulfobromophthalein (BSP) in constitutional conjugated hyperbilirubinaemias. *Digestion* **13**, 272.
2. ARIAS I.M. (1961) Studies of chronic familial non-hemolytic jaundice with conjugated bilirubin in the serum with and without an unidentified pigment in the liver cells. *Am. J. Med.* **31**, 510.
3. ARIAS I.M. (1962) Chronic unconjugated hyperbilirubinemia (CUH) with increased production of bile pigment not derived from the hemoglobin of mature, circulating erythrocytes. *J. clin. Invest.* **41**, 1341.
4. ARIAS I.M., BERNSTEIN L., TOFFLER R. et al (1964) Black liver disease in Corriedale sheep: a new mutation affecting excretory function. *J. clin. Invest.* **43**, 1249.
5. BAILEY A., ROBINSON D. & DAWSON A.M. (1977) Does Gilbert's disease exist? *Lancet* i, 931.
6. BERK P.D. & JAVITT N.B. (1978) Hyperbilirubinemia and cholestasis. *Am. J. Med.* **64**, 311.
7. BERK P.D., BLASCHKE T.F., SCHARSCHMIDT B.F. et al (1976) A new approach to quantitation of the various sources of bilirubin in man. *J. lab. clin. Med.* **87**, 767.
8. BILLING B.H. (1978) Twenty-five years of progress in bilirubin metabolism (1952–1977). *Gut* **19**, 481.
9. BLACK M. & BILLING B.H. (1969) Hepatic bilirubin UDP-Glucuronyl transferase activity in liver disease and Gilbert's syndrome. *New Engl. J. Med.* **280**, 1266.
10. BLACK M. & SHERLOCK S. (1970) Treatment of Gilbert's syndrome with phenobarbitone. *Lancet* i, 1359.
11. BLACK M., FEVERY J., PARKER D. et al (1974) Effect of phenobarbitone on plasma (^{14}C) bilirubin clearance in patients with unconjugated hyperbilirubinaemia. *Clin. Sci. molec. Med.* **46**, 1.
12. BONNETT R., DAVIES J.E. & HURSTHOUSE M.B. (1976) Structure of bilirubin. *Nature* **262**, 326.
13. BUTT H.R., ANDERSON V.E., FOULK W.T. et al (1966) Studies of chronic idiopathic jaundice (Dubin–Johnson syndrome). II. Evaluation of a large family with the trait. *Gastroenterology* **51**, 619.
14. CAMERON J.D.S. (1943) Infective hepatitis. *Q. J. Med.* **12**, 139.
15. COHEN L., LEWIS C. & ARIAS I.M. (1972) Pregnancy, oral contraceptives, and chronic familial jaundice with predominantly conjugated hyperbilirubinemia (Dubin–Johnson syndrome). *Gastroenterology* **62**, 1182.
16. COTTON P.B. (1977) E.R.C.P. *Gut* **18**, 316.
17. CRIGLER J.F. Jr & NAJJAR V.A. (1952) Congenital familial nonhemolytic jaundice with kernicterus. *Pediatrics* **10**, 169.
18. DUBIN I.N. (1958) Chronic idiopathic jaundice. A review of fifty cases. *Am. J. Med.* **24**, 268.
19. DUBIN I.N. & JOHNSON F.B. (1954) Chronic idiopathic jaundice with unidentified pigment in the liver cells: a new clinico-pathological entity with a report of twelve cases. *Medicine (Baltimore)* **33**, 155.
20. ELIAS E. (1976) Cholangiography in the jaundiced patient. *Gut* **17**, 801.
21. FELSHER B.F., RICKARD D. & REDEKER A.G. (1970) The reciprocal relation between caloric intake and the degree of hyperbilirubinemia in Gilbert's syndrome. *New Engl. J. Med.* **283**, 170.
22. FEVERY J., BLANCKAERT N., HEIRWEGH K.P.M. et al (1977) Unconjugated bilirubin and an increased proportion of bilirubin monoconjugates in the bile of patients with Gilbert's syndrome and Crigler–Najjar disease. *J. clin. Invest.* **60**, 970.
23. FOULK W.T., BUTT H.R., OWEN C.A. Jr et al (1959) Constitutional hepatic dysfunction (Gilbert's disease): its natural history and related syndromes. *Medicine (Baltimore)* **38**, 25.
24. GILBERT A. & LEREBOULLET P. (1901) La cholémie simple familiale. *Sem. méd. Paris* **21**, 241.
25. GOLLAN J.L., DALLINGER K.J.C. & BILLING B.H. (1978) Excretion of conjugated bilirubin in the isolated perfused rat kidney. *Clin. Sci. molec. Biol.* **54**, 38.
26. GOLLAN J.L., HOLE D.R. & BILLING B.H. (1979) The role of dietary fat in the regulation of unconjugated hyperbilirubinaemia in Gunn rats. *Clin. Sci.* **57**, 327.

27. GOLLAN J.L., HUANG S.N., BILLING B. *et al* (1975) Prolonged survival in three brothers with severe type 2 Crigler–Najjar syndrome. Ultrastructural and metabolic studies. *Gastroenterology* **68**, 1543.

28. ICHIDA F. & FUNAHASHI H. (1964) Electron microscopic observations on liver cells of cases with Dubin–Johnson syndrome. *Acta hepato-splen.* **11**, 332.

29. ISRAELS L.G., SUDERMAN H.J. & RITZMANN S.E. (1959) Hyperbilirubinemia due to an alternate path of bilirubin production. *Am. J. Med.* **27**, 693.

30. JAIN S., LONG R.G., SCOTT J. *et al* (1977) Percutaneous transhepatic cholangiography using the 'Chiba' needle—800 cases. *Brit. J. Radiol.* **50**, 175.

31. JANSEN P.L.M., CHOWDHURY J.R., FISHBERG E.B. *et al* (1977) Enzymatic conversion of bilirubin monoglucuronide to diglucuronide by rat liver plasma membranes. *J. biol. Chem.* **252**, 2710.

32. KJELLIN K.G. (1971) Bilirubin compounds in the CSF. *J. neurol. Sci.* **13**, 161.

33. LEVI A.J., GATMAITAN Z. & ARIAS I.M. (1970) Deficiency of hepatic organic anion binding protein, impaired organic anion uptake by liver and 'physiologie' jaundice in newborn monkeys. *New Engl. J. Med.* **283**, 1136.

34. LIMA J.E.P., UTZ E. & ROISENBERG I. (1966) Hereditary non hemolytic conjugated hyperbilirubinemia without abnormal liver cell pigmentation. A family study. *Am. J. Med.* **40**, 628.

35. MANDEMA E., DE FRAITURE W.H., NIEWEG H.O. *et al* (1960) Familial chronic idiopathic jaundice (Dubin–Sprinz disease) with a note on bromsulphalein metabolism in this disease. *Am. J. Med.* **28**, 42.

36. METREAU J.M., YVART J., DHUMEAUX D. *et al* (1978) Role of bilirubin overproduction in revealing Gilbert's syndrome: is dyserythropoiesis an important factor? *Gut* **19**, 838.

37. NAKAYAMA T., IKEDA A. & OKUDA K. (1978) Percutaneous transhepatic drainage of the biliary tract. Technique and results in 104 cases. *Gastroenterology* **74**, 554.

38. OWENS D. & EVANS J. (1975) Population studies on Gilbert's syndrome. *J. med. Genet.* **12**, 152.

39. OWENS D. & SHERLOCK S. (1973) The diagnosis of Gilbert's syndrome: role of the reduced caloric intake test. *Br. med. J.* iii, 559.

40. POWELL L.W., BILLING B.H. & WILLIAMS H.S. (1967) An assessment of red cell survival in idiopathic unconjugated hyperbilirubinaemia (Gilbert's syndrome) by the use of radio-active diisopropylfluorophosphate and chromium. *Aust. Ann. Med.* **16**, 221.

41. POWELL L.W., HEMINGWAY E., BILLING B.H. *et al* (1967) Idiopathic unconjugated hyperbilirubinaemia (Gilbert's syndrome). A study of 42 families. *New Engl. J. Med.* **277**, 1108.

42. SAGILD U., DALBAARD O.Z. & TYGSTRUP N. (1962) Constitutional hyperbilirubinemia with unconjugated bilirubin in the serum and lipochrome-like pigment granules in the liver. *Ann. intern. Med.* **56**, 308.

43. SATLER J. (1966) Another variant of constitutional familial hepatic dysfunction with permanent jaundice and with alternating serum bilirubin relations. *Acta hepato-splen.* **13**, 38.

44. SCHIFF L., BILLING B.H. & OIKAWA Y. (1959) Familial nonhemolytic jaundice with conjugated bilirubin in the serum. A case study. *New Engl. J. Med.* **260**, 1314.

45. SCHMID R. (1978) Bilirubin metabolism: state of the art. *Gastroenterology* **74**, 1307.

46. SEYMOUR C.A., NEALE G. & PETERS T.J. (1977) Lysosomal changes in liver tissue from patient with the Dubin–Johnson–Sprinz syndrome. *Clin. Sci. molec. Med.* **52**, 241.

47. SHERLOCK S. (1962) Jaundice. *Br. med. J.* i, 1359.

48. SPRINZ H. & NELSON R.S. (1954) Persistent nonhemolytic hyperbilirubinemia associated with lipochrome-like pigment in liver cells: report of four cases. *Ann. intern. Med.* **14**, 952.

49. SUMMERSKILL W.H.J., CLOWDUS B.F. II, BOLLLMAN J.L. *et al* (1961) Clinical and experimental studies on the effect of corticotrophin and steroid drugs on bilirubinaemia. *Am. J. med. Sci.* **241**, 555.

50. VARMA R.R., GRAINGER J.M. & SCHEUER P.J. (1970) A case of the Dubin–Johnson syndrome complicated by acute hepatitis. *Gut* **11**, 817.

51. WEGMANN R., RANGIER M., ETÉVÉ J. *et al* (1960) Mélanose hépato-splénique avec ictère chronique a bilirubine directe: maladie de Dubin–Johnson? Étude clinique et biologique de la maladie. Étude histochimique et spectrographique du pigment anormal. *Sem. Hôp., Paris* **36**, 1761.

52. WILLIAMS R. & BILLING B. (1961) Action of steroid therapy in jaundice. *Lancet* ii, 392.

53. WOLKOFF A.W., WOLPERT E., PASCASIO F.N. *et al* (1976) Rotor's syndrome: a distinct inheritable pathophysiologic entity. *Am. J. Med.* **60**, 173.

Chapter 14
Cholestasis

Cholestasis is defined as failure of normal amounts of bile to reach the duodenum. The term 'obstructive jaundice' is not used, as in many instances no mechanical block can be shown in the biliary tract.

Biliary cirrhosis follows prolonged cholestasis; the time taken for its development varies from months to years. The transition is not reflected in a sudden change in the clinical picture. The term 'biliary cirrhosis' is reserved for a pathological picture. It is diagnosed when there are features of cirrhosis such as nodule formation, encephalopathy or fluid retention.

ANATOMY OF THE BILIARY SYSTEM

Conjugated bilirubin is secreted by the liver cell into the canaliculus. The biliary secretory apparatus comprises the bile canaliculus, the pericanalicular ectoplasm, lysosomes and Golgi apparatus [20] (fig. 186).

The bile canalicular membrane has enzymes, like Mg^{2+}–ATPase and Na^+–K^+–ATPase, as an integral component and some parts of the membrane such as phospholipids are released into the bile. The microvilli increase the surface area.

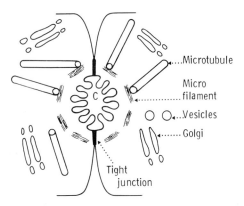

Fig. 186. The bile secretory apparatus. A diagram of the ultrastructure of the bile canaliculus (C) and peri-canalicular zone of the liver cell.

The tight junctions seal the biliary space from the blood compartment.

The pericanalicular ectoplasm contains the *cytoskeleton* of the liver cell. Microfilaments provide tone to the canalicular system. Microtubules may be concerned in the arrangement of canalicular membrane proteins and in lecithin and bile acid secretion. Pericanalicular vesicles are probably 'ferry' vesicles conveying substances from sinusoidal to canalicular zones. Lysosomes are involved in biliary excretion. The role of the Golgi apparatus in biliary secretion is unknown.

The bile canaliculi empty into ductules sometimes called cholangioles or canals of Hering (fig. 188). These are found largely in the portal zones of the liver. The ductule passes into the interlobular bile duct which is the first bile channel to be accompanied by a branch of the hepatic artery and portal vein. These are also found in the portal triad. These channels unite with one another to form septal bile ducts and so on until the two main hepatic ducts emerge from the right and left lobes of the liver at the porta hepatis.

THE SECRETION OF BILE (fig. 189)

Bile secretion is relatively independent of perfusion pressure and bile is formed by several different energy-dependent transport processes. An excellent correlation exists between bile flow and bile salt secretion. Bile salts passing into the biliary canaliculus are the most important factors promoting bile flow. This *bile salt-dependent* active secretion carries with it bile pigments, organic anions and water. The passage of the osmotically active bile salts generates water flow. The bile salts are present as micelles. Changes in micellar size influence osmotic activity and this may be the regulatory mechanism for the flow of water into the bile. The bile salts might also determine biliary flow through a solute-pump mechanism. The bile salts are steroids and could change flow by changing the function of the canalicular membrane.

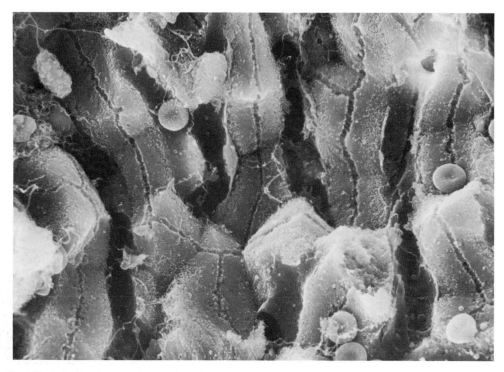

Fig. 187. Scanning electron micrograph of the
canalicular biliary system (Boyer 1975).

Bile salt-independent flow is shown by extrapola-
tion of bile salt versus bile flow data to zero bile
salt excretion when a positive intercept is shown.
This indicates that flow would continue at zero bile
salt excretion, presumably by a bile salt-independent method. In the isolated perfused rat liver a
large fraction of bile is found to be independent
of bile salt secretion [9]. This fraction may be
linked to active sodium transport. Substances such
as phenobarbital or cortisol increase bile flow
without enhancing bile salt secretion [7].

Alteration in the canalicular membrane may be
important in disease. The bile canaliculi are
limited by the plasma membranes of 2–3 adjacent
hepatocytes. Where the borders of two cells meet
is the zona occludens or tight junction which can
leak in disease states. Actin microfilaments have
an important role in cell movements and in the
maintenance of cell shape [72]. Biliary lipids (cholesterol and phospholipids) are synthesized in the
hepatocyte microsomal membranes and, in the
rat, a microtubular system transports them to the
canalicular membrane [31].

Ductular bile flow modifies canalicular flow by

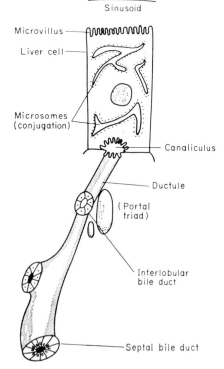

Fig. 188. The anatomy of the intra-hepatic biliary
system.

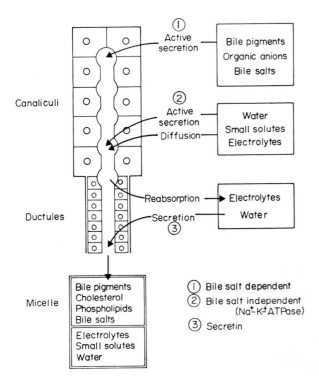

Fig. 189. Mechanisms of bile formation.

adding an inorganic electrolyte solution consisting mostly of sodium bicarbonate and sodium chloride. A limited amount of water and sodium chloride may be absorbed. Ductular flow is largely controlled by secretin. *Gall bladder contraction* is controlled by cholecystokinin. Ductular flow may serve to flush bile salts from the lower end of the common bile duct following gall bladder contraction.

In man, total bile flow is about 600 ml per 24 hours of which 225 ml is bile acid-dependent, 225 ml bile acid-independent and 150 ml ductular [71] (fig. 190).

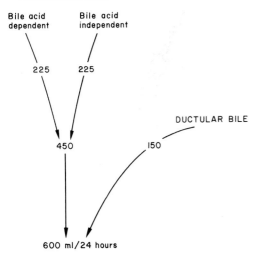

Fig. 190. Twenty-four-hour volumes of bile in man (Paumgartner 1977).

THE SYNDROME OF CHOLESTASIS

Definition. Cholestasis can result from interference with bile flow anywhere from the conjugating site in the microsomal fraction to the duodenum.

Morphologically cholestasis is defined as accumulation of bile in liver cells and biliary passages.

Clinically cholestasis is the retention in the blood of all substances normally excreted in the bile. Serum bile acid levels are increased.

Functionally [31, 34, 37] cholestasis is defined as a decrease in canalicular bile flow. There is a decreased hepatic secretion of water and/or organic anions (bilirubin–bile acid). This may be

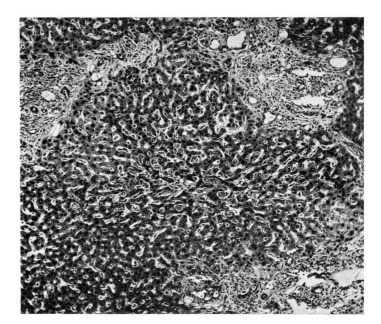

Fig. 191. Unrelieved common bile duct obstruction. Bile duct proliferation and fibrosis in the portal tracts which are becoming joined together. Bile pigment accumulations in the centrizonal areas. Hepatic lobular architecture normal. H & E, ×67.

due to failure of the pumps secreting bile or of the channels into which bile is secreted.

The bile salt-dependent pump fails if inadequate quantities of bile salts reach the canaliculus or leak from it. Failure of the entero-hepatic circulation of bile salts may contribute.

The Na^+–K^+–ATPase-mediated sodium transport (bile acid-independent) pump can also fail. This has been shown following oestrogens in rats. Decrease in canalicular Na^+–K^+–ATPase activity may be due to changes in membrane lipids. No ultrastructural modification of the canaliculus has been observed, suggesting that the cholestasis initially is due only to pump failure.

The microfilaments of the cytoskeleton may be altered. In cholestasis the layers of contractile actin microfilaments around the tight junctions between neighbouring hepatocytes are widened, reflecting a defect in the normal depolymerization of the actin/myosin microfilament. Cholestasis can be produced experimentally by agents such as phalloidin which alter microfilaments [24]. Phalloidin inhibits microfilament function, diminishes bile secretion and produces such morphological hallmarks of cholestasis as dilatation of the canalicular space and loss of microvilli. Canaliculi may become more rigid and become excessively permeable [34]. This might involve the tight junctions which are abnormal in mechanical cholestasis.

Ductular abnormalities, such as inflammation and epithelial changes, interfere with bile flow but are probably secondary rather than primary.

The primary event in extra-hepatic cholestasis is obvious, for instance a gall-stone obstructing the common bile duct. Secondary events are then initiated within the liver cell. In intra-hepatic cholestasis the primary event is particularly obscure, but again secondary changes follow within the liver cell itself. It is often impossible to differentiate the primary events from the secondary ones.

Pathology

All changes depend on duration. The liver is enlarged and green. It is swollen with a rounded edge. Nodularity develops later.

Light microscopy [11]. The hepatic changes are irrespective of cause. Accumulations of bile are seen, particularly in the centrizonal areas, the Kupffer cells and the canaliculi (fig. 191). The liver cells, especially in the centrizonal areas, show a 'feathery' degeneration, possibly due to retention of 'toxic' bile salts, with surrounding focal accumulations of mononuclear cells. Cellular necrosis, regeneration and nodular hyperplasia, however, are minimal.

With time, portal zone mononuclear cells accumulate. Portal zone fibrosis extends to meet bands from adjacent zones so that eventually the

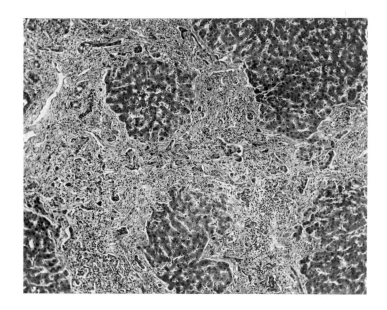

Fig. 192. Biliary cirrhosis. The normal hepatic architecture is disturbed. The wide intervening fibrous tissue bands show proliferating bile ducts and a heavy infiltration with mononuclear cells. H & E, × 63.

lobule is enclosed by a ring of connective tissue (fig. 191). In the early stages the essential relationship of hepatic vein to portal tract remains undisturbed and this distinguishes the picture from that of biliary cirrhosis.

Biliary cirrhosis follows prolonged cholestasis. The fibrous tissue bands in the portal zones widen further, coalesce and the lobules are correspondingly reduced in size. Fibrous septa from the portal zones now sub-divide the lobule joining portal and hepatic venous areas and so disturb hepatic architecture (fig. 192). Nodular regeneration of liver cells follows, although never to the same extent as in other cirrhoses. True cirrhosis rarely follows biliary obstruction. In total biliary obstruction due to cancer of the head of the pancreas death occurs before nodular regeneration has had time to develop. Biliary cirrhosis is associated with partial biliary obstruction, due for example to biliary stricture or to gall-stones. Cirrhosis defined as widespread fibrosis with nodules develops in only some 8.6% of patients dying with cholestatic jaundice [41].

In biliary cirrhosis the liver is larger and greener than in non-biliary cirrhosis. Margins of nodules are clear-cut rather than moth-eaten. Fatty change is absent and hyperplastic foci are rare.

Electron microscopy. The biliary canaliculi show constant changes irrespective of the cause. These include dilatation and oedema, blunting, distortion and sparsity of the microvilli. The Golgi apparatus shows vacuolization. Pericanali-

cular vesicles appear which contain bile and which ultimately can be identified with the feathery degeneration of liver cells seen on light microscopy. Lysosomes become more numerous. The endoplasmic reticulum is hypertrophied. These electron microscopical changes are non-specific.

Reversibility of hepatic changes

If the cholestasis can be relieved, hepatic histology shows slow regression of the portal zone fibrosis. Bile pigment is slow to disappear. Disturbed hepatic structure and function should not be a contraindication to attempts to relieve the cholestasis for the changes are potentially reversible.

Changes in other organs

The spleen is enlarged and firm due to reticuloendothelial hyperplasia and increase in mononuclear cells. Later, cirrhosis results in portal hypertension.

The intestinal contents are bulky and greasy; the more complete the cholestasis the paler the stools.

The kidneys are swollen and bile stained. Casts containing bilirubin are found in the distal convoluted tubules and collecting tubules. The casts may be heavily infiltrated with cells and the tubular epithelium is disrupted. The surrounding connective tissue may then show oedema and inflammatory infiltration. Scar formation is absent.

Clinical features

The patient develops jaundice slowly. He feels well and weight loss is slow. This is in contrast to the malaise and physical deterioration of the patient with hepato-cellular disease. Later the skin may become greenish. Skin pigmentation is due to melanin.

Pruritus in jaundice is often attributed to irritation of cutaneous sensory nerves by retained bile salts. However, even with the most sophisticated biochemical methods no association has been found between the concentration of any particular conjugated or free bile acid and the presence or absence of pruritus [69]. Moreover, in terminal liver failure, when pruritus is lost, serum bile acids may still be increased. The association of itching with cholestasis suggests that pruritus is due to some substance normally excreted in the bile. Relief by the bile salt chelating resin, cholestyramine, also suggests that bile salts are concerned. Disappearance of itching when liver cells fail indicates that the agent responsible is manufactured by the liver.

Xanthomas [1]. The planous varieties occur as xanthelasma. They are flat or slightly raised, yellow and soft. They may also be seen in the palmar creases, below the breast and on the neck (see figs. 193, 194 in colour section), chest or back. The tuberous lesions appear later, and are found on extensor surfaces, especially the wrists, elbows, knees, ankles and buttocks (fig. 195), on pressure points and in scars. The xanthomas associated with cholestatic jaundice rarely affect tendon sheaths. They may involve bone (fig. 200) or occasionally peripheral nerves [94]. Focal accumulations of xanthoma cells may be found in the liver.

The development of skin xanthomas is in proportion to the height of the total serum lipids (fig. 202). If the level is greater than 1800 mg/dl for longer than three months, then skin xanthomas become generalized. The serum cholesterol value is approximately one-fourth of the total lipid level and must be raised to over 450 mg/100 ml for longer than three months before skin xanthomas appear [57]. Skin xanthomas disappear if serum cholesterol levels fall after cholestasis is relieved or in the late stage of hepato-cellular failure.

The *liver* is usually enlarged with a firm, smooth, non-tender edge. *Splenomegaly* is unusual except in biliary cirrhosis where portal hypertension has developed or if infection is present.

Faeces

Faecal *colour* gives a good indication whether cholestasis is total, intermittent or decreasing.

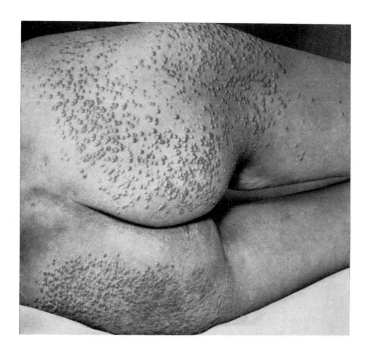

Fig. 195. Chronic obstructive jaundice. Xanthomata tuberosa affecting the buttocks.

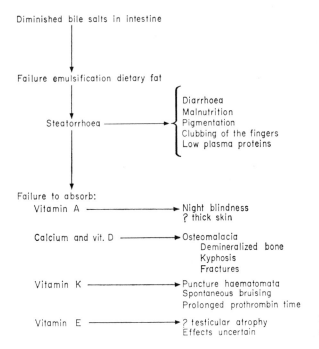

Diminished bile salts in intestine

Failure emulsification dietary fat

Steatorrhoea ⎯⎯⎯⎯⎯→ { Diarrhoea
Malnutrition
Pigmentation
Clubbing of the fingers
Low plasma proteins

Failure to absorb:
Vitamin A ⎯⎯⎯⎯→ Night blindness
? thick skin

Calcium and vit. D ⎯⎯⎯→ Osteomalacia
Demineralized bone
Kyphosis
Fractures

Vitamin K ⎯⎯⎯⎯→ Puncture haematomata
Spontaneous bruising
Prolonged prothrombin time

Vitamin E ⎯⎯⎯⎯→ ? testicular atrophy
Effects uncertain

Fig. 196. The effects of acholia in chronic cholestatic jaundice.

Bile salts, deficient in the intestine in cholestasis, are essential for the absorption of dietary fat. Steatorrhoea (fig. 196) is proportional to the depth of jaundice [5]. In cholestasis inadequate bile salts are present in small intestinal contents to achieve micellar solution of lipid [6] (fig. 197). Stools are loose, pale, bulky and offensive. Clubbing of the fingers may be associated.

Steatorrhoea results in failure of proper absorption of calcium and fat-soluble vitamins.

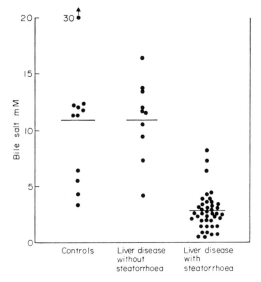

Fig. 197. Bile salt concentration of aspirated intestinal contents in patients with non-alcoholic liver disease with or without steatorrhoea (Badley *et al* 1970).

BONE CHANGES IN LIVER DISEASE [62]

Osteomalacia can complicate all forms of chronic cholestasis and also hepato-cellular disease, especially in the alcoholic. Bone pain is frequent in chronic cholestasis and occasionally in chronic active hepatitis and alcoholic liver disease [63]. Serum may show normal or low calcium and phosphate levels and calcium is reduced in the urine. Bone biopsy may reveal either osteomalacia or often osteoporosis. Bone changes cannot be predicted by serum calcium and phosphate values.

In osteomalacia the bone is weakened, osteoblasts multiply and the serum alkaline phosphatase therefore rises; in the presence of cholestasis these values may be enormous. The vertebral bodies become crushed and wedge-shaped (fig. 198) and kyphosis is gross. The thoracic cage is decalcified and pseudo-fractures are frequent. Ribbon-like areas of decalcification (Looser's zones), often symmetrical, are rarely found. The hands show rarefaction (fig. 200). The lamina dura

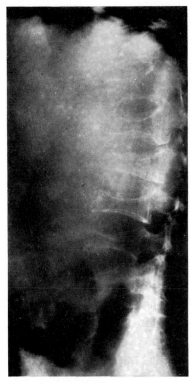

Fig. 198. Carcinoma of common hepatic duct;
jaundiced for three years. Bone biopsy showed
osteomalacia. Lumbar spine radiograph shows very
severe biconcave deformities and vertebral
compression (Atkinson *et al* 1956).

around the teeth disappear and the teeth fall out.
Bone biopsy shows wide, uncalcified, osteoid seams
surrounding the trabeculae.

Osteoporosis may also be important. It is
diagnosed by bone biopsy. It is particularly likely
in patients more than 45 years old with chronic
cholestasis or alcoholic liver disease.

Osteomalacia and osteoporosis are slow to develop and are unlikely unless the cholestasis is deep
and has lasted longer than two years. Ill-advised
prednisolone therapy hastens their progress.

Painful *osteoarthropathy* may develop in the
wrists and ankles (fig. 201) [28]. This is a non-
specific complication of chronic liver disease.

Mechanisms of bone changes. Vitamin D_2 (ergo-
calciferol) is absorbed from the gut while vitamin
D_3 (cholecalciferol) is synthesized in the skin (fig.
199). In both England and North America, the
majority of circulating vitamin D originates from
vitamin D_3 rather than vitamin D_2. Both forms
are transported in serum by vitamin D binding

globulin which is synthesized by the liver and is
usually only 2–5% saturated. 25-hydroxylation of
vitamin D takes place in the liver cell and concentrations in the serum roughly correlate with vitamin D intake. Low serum 25-(OH)D values have
been demonstrated in vitamin D untreated
patients with symptomatic primary biliary cirrhosis, alcoholic liver disease, chronic active liver
disease and large bile duct obstruction. Treatment
with vitamin D supplements usually results in normal concentrations suggesting that 25-hydroxyla-
tion is not defective. Similarly patients with primary biliary cirrhosis or cirrhosis due to chronic
active hepatitis form 1,25-dihydroxy vitamin D so
that a renal defect in dihydroxy-vitamin D metabolite synthesis seems unlikely to be present.

The main defect appears to be a lack of vitamin
D substrate. Such patients fail to go out into the
sun or to take an adequate diet. As bilirubin
absorbs light maximally at the wavelength which
is required to convert 7-dihydrocholesterol to
vitamin D, interference with the cutaneous synthesis of vitamin D_3 by bilirubin may be important
in jaundiced patients. The main problem, however, is the reduction of intraluminal bile acids
which are essential for vitamin D absorption from
the gut (fig. 203). The availability can be further
reduced by the use of cholestyramine. Malabsorption of vitamin D during its entero-hepatic circulation may be another factor.

Calcium malabsorption in chronic cholestasis
can be related to vitamin D deficiency and the
formation of unabsorbable calcium soaps in the
intestinal lumen [54]. Parenteral vitamin D_2 cor-
rects the malabsorption, but the bone disease is not
prevented.

Hyperparathyroidism is not a major problem in
patients with chronic liver disease [63].

The osteoporosis is unexplained. The degree
does not correlate with plasma albumin, hence
with the ability of liver to synthesize albumin.

FAT-SOLUBLE VITAMINS AND
COAGULATION FACTORS

Vitamin A is fat soluble and plasma levels are low.
If cholestasis is sufficiently prolonged, hepatic
reserves of the vitamin become exhausted and
failure of dark adaptation follows (night blindness).

Vitamin K and Factor VII are not absorbed and
the *prothrombin time* is prolonged. This is restored
to normal by intramuscular vitamin K_1 therapy.

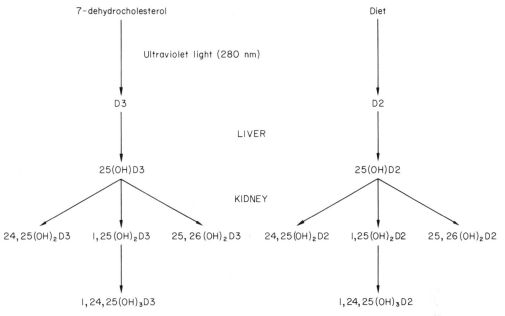

Fig. 199. Normal vitamin D metabolic pathway. Vitamin D$_3$ is formed in the skin. The 25-hydroxylation step of both D$_2$ and D$_3$ occurs in the liver; the addition of a second hydroxy group occurs predominantly in the kidney (Long & Sherlock 1979).

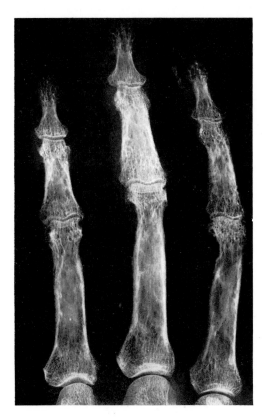

Vitamin K deficiency is shown by ready and even spontaneous bruising and by excessive bleeding with trauma.

CHANGES IN COPPER METABOLISM [52]

Approximately 80% of absorbed copper is normally excreted in the bile and lost in the faeces. In cholestasis of all types, but particularly if chronic (as in primary biliary cirrhosis), copper accumulates in the liver to levels equal to or exceeding those found in Wilson's disease [19, 88]. Pigmented corneal rings resembling the Kayser–Fleischer ring are seen rarely [33, 38].

Hepatic copper may be measured by neutron activation or demonstrated histologically on paraffin sections by rhodanine [52]. Copper-associated protein may be shown by orcine staining. These methods provide a tentative histological index of cholestasis. They are not applicable to Wilson's disease where the excess copper accumulates in a different chemical form [52].

Fig. 200. Primary biliary cirrhosis; jaundiced for five years. Many skin xanthomas. Serum cholesterol 2400 mg/dl. X-ray of digits shows gross demineralization. Erosions represent bone xanthomas.

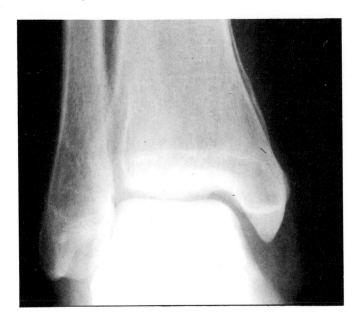

Fig. 201. Osteoarthropathy in chronic cholestasis. New sub-periosteal bone is seen at the lower end of the tibia.

HAEMATOLOGICAL CHANGES

These include reduced osmotic fragility of the erythrocytes. Target cells have been related to an accumulation of cholesterol in the red cell membrane. This increases red cell surface area and leads to target formation.

DEVELOPMENT OF PORTAL VENOUS HYPERTENSION

With increasing biliary cirrhosis and distortion of the intra-hepatic vascular system, the portal venous pressure rises. Hypertension develops more slowly than in other forms of cirrhosis. The enlarging spleen reflects portal obstruction.

DEVELOPMENT OF HEPATO-CELLULAR FAILURE

This is slow, and it is remarkable how well the liver cells function in the presence of cholestasis. After three to five years of chronic jaundice, rapidly deepening jaundice, ascites, oedema and a lowered serum albumin level indicate liver cell failure. Pruritus lessens and the bleeding tendency is not controlled by parenteral vitamin K. Hepatic encephalopathy is terminal.

Biochemistry

All the constituents of the bile show an increased level in the serum. Conjugation of biliary substances is intact but excretion defective.

The *serum ('conjugated', 'ester') bilirubin level* is raised due mainly to conjugated pigment. In unrelieved cholestasis the level rises slowly for the first three weeks and then fluctuates, always tending to increase. When the cholestasis is relieved, serum bilirubin values fall slowly to normal.

The *serum alkaline phosphatase level* is raised, usually to more than three times the upper limit of normal. Iso-enzyme studies show that the type is similar to that excreted in bile. Serum 5′-nucleotidase and γ-glutamyl transpeptidase levels are raised. The rises are due to increased synthesis or release of enzymes from liver plasma membranes.

The total *serum cholesterol* increases but not constantly. In chronic cholestasis the total serum lipids are greatly increased (fig. 202) and this involves particularly the phospholipid and total cholesterol fractions. Neutral fat is very slightly increased. In spite of the high lipid content, the serum is characteristically clear and not milky. This may be due to the surface-action effect of phospholipid, which keeps the other lipids in solution. Serum cholesterol values fall terminally.

Serum lipoproteins are increased [57], due to a rise in the low density (α_2, β) fraction. The high density lipoproteins are decreased. The increase

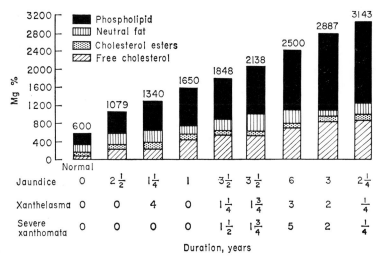

Fig. 202. Serum lipid pattern in eight patients with primary biliary cirrhosis (chronic intra-hepatic obstructive jaundice) (Ahrens & Kunkel 1949).

consists largely of an abnormal lipoprotein which has been called *lipoprotein X*. The origin is unknown but it may be an intestinal lipoprotein, normally catabolized in the liver, and accumulating as a result of hepatic dysfunction. It appears by electron microscopy as a disc-shaped particle [46]. Serum lipoprotein X is increased in both intrahepatic and extra-hepatic cholestasis [66, 86]. The lipoproteins of cholestatic jaundice differ from those found in athero-sclerosis. Atheroma is not a complication of prolonged cholestasis. Some of the lipoprotein abnormalities may be related to low lecithin-cholesterol acyltransferase (LCAT) levels [2].

Trihydroxy *bile salts* accumulate in the blood [69].

Serum albumin and globulin concentrations are normal in acute cholestasis. With the development of biliary cirrhosis the serum albumin tends to fall.

The *serum aspartate transaminase* is usually less than 100 i.u./100 ml.

Urine. Conjugated bilirubin is present. Urinary urobilinogen, which undergoes an entero-hepatic circulation, is excreted in proportion to the amount of bile reaching the duodenum.

General treatment

Cholestasis whether of intra-hepatic or extra-hepatic origin should be managed along the same general lines.

NUTRITION (table 28)

The problem is essentially that of intestinal bile salt deficiency. Calorie intake should be maintained and protein must be adequate. Neutral fat is poorly tolerated, badly absorbed and reduces calcium absorption. It should be restricted to 40 g daily. Additional fat is supplied by medium chain triglycerides (MCT) which are digested and absorbed quite well in the absence of bile salts into the portal vein as free fatty acids. They can be given as 'Portagen' (Mead–Johnson) or as MCT (coconut) oil for cooking or in salads.

In the chronic case fat soluble vitamins (A, D, K) are necessary and must be given parenterally because they are not absorbed when given by mouth.

Table 28. Management of chronic cholestasis.

Dietary fat
Low neutral fat (less than 40 g)
Add medium chain triglyceride, 40 g daily

Intramuscular vitamins
(every four weeks)   A   100 000 i.u.
                    D   100 000 i.u.
                    K_1 10 mg

Calcium
Extra defatted milk
Calcium (Sandoz) 8 tablets/day
If bone pain, calcium chloride i.v.

If there is evidence of bruising or haemorrhage associated with a prolonged prothrombin time, vitamin K_1 may be administered daily until the deficiency is corrected.

TREATMENT OF BONE CHANGES

Vitamin D_2 (100 000 units intramuscularly) should be given every four weeks to all patients with chronic cholestasis [87] (fig. 203). If possible, treatment should be monitored by measuring serum 25-(OH)D levels. Reduced levels indicate increase of the intramuscular vitamin D_2 supplements until the serum 25-(OH)D is normal. In prolonged cholestasis a maintenance oral dose of 6 g calcium gluconate or preferably effervescent calcium (Sandoz) 8 tablets daily, equivalent to 30 g calcium gluconate, should be given. The patient should be encouraged to take extra skimmed (fat-free) milk.

If the serum phosphate level is low, phosphate supplements must be given. These should be given on alternate days to calcium so that the formation of calcium phosphate complexes in the gut is prevented.

In patients with symptomatic bone disease and with osteomalacia, proven on bone biopsy, oral or parenteral 1,25-dihydroxy-D_3 appears to be the vitamin D metabolite of choice. It is biologically very active and has a short half-life. 1-alpha vitamin D_3 could also be used, but full metabolic activity would only follow hepatic 25-hydroxylation.

Severe bone pain may be controlled by intravenous calcium (15 mg calcium per kg body weight as calcium gluconate in 500 ml 5% dextrose) given over four hours daily for about seven days and repeated as necessary [4].

Osteoporosis can be crippling, but no treatment is known to reverse the process. Corticosteroids worsen the process and should be avoided.

No specific treatment is available for the periosteal reactions. Simple analgesics may be of use and, if arthropathy is present, physiotherapy may be helpful.

CHOLESTYRAMINE

Pruritus can be relieved in patients with partial biliary obstruction by intermittent, external biliary drainage [97]. This, presumably, breaks the enterohepatic circulation of bile salts. Cholestyramine (Questran) binds bile salts in the intestine, so eliminating them in the faeces (fig. 204). It will stop itching in 4–7 days in patients with partial biliary obstruction [16]. One sachet should be given before and one after breakfast so that the arrival of the drug in the duodenum coincides with gall bladder contraction. If necessary, a further dose may be taken before the mid-day and the evening meals. The maintenance dose is usually about 12 g per day. The drug causes nausea and reluctance to take it. It is particularly valuable for itching associated with primary biliary cirrhosis, biliary atresia and biliary stricture. Serum bile acid levels fall. Serum cholesterol drops and skin xanthomas diminish or disappear. Cholestyramine increases faecal fat even in normal subjects. The dose should be the smallest that controls pruritus. Hypoprothrombinaemia has developed due to failure to absorb vitamin K. This vitamin must be given by intramuscular injection.

These results suggest that bile salts are responsible for the pruritus. However, the resin might well act in some other way than by removing bile acids.

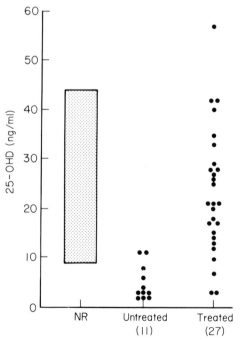

Fig. 203. Serum 25-(OH)D values in vitamin D_2-treated (100 000 iu in ethyl oleate once monthly i.m.) and untreated patients with primary biliary cirrhosis. The differences are highly significant (Skinner *et al* 1977).

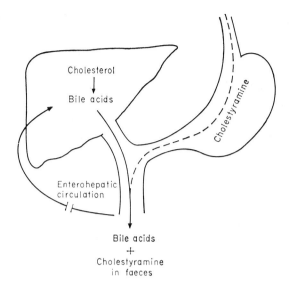

Fig. 204. Cholestyramine, a strongly basic anion exchange resin, chelates with bile salts in the intestine and the complex is excreted in the faeces. The entero-hepatic circulation is broken (Datta & Sherlock 1963).

Cholestyramine may bind other drugs having an entero-hepatic circulation, particularly digitoxin [10]. Care must be taken that the cholestyramine and other drugs are given at separate times.

Other drugs

Clofibrate (Atromid) should *not* be given to lower serum cholesterol in cholestasis as paradoxical increases occur. This could be related to increased hepatic cholesterol synthesis. Gall-stones may be precipitated [92].

Methyl testosterone, 25 mg sublingually daily, relieves itching within seven days [60]. *Norethandrolone* (Nilevar), 10 mg twice or thrice daily by mouth, is less masculinizing and better for females. Both substances greatly increase jaundice and both can themselves cause an intra-hepatic cholestasis in normal patients (Chapter 17). There are no ill effects on liver function, but these drugs should be given only for intractable, usually malignant, pruritus and in the smallest effective dose. They should be used in total biliary obstruction where cholestyramine is not effective.

Choleretics. In intra-hepatic cholestasis drugs to increase bile flow are being evaluated. They have largely been used in the neonate. Phenobarbital increases bile flow and has been used in cholestatic states but with equivocal results. Cholestyramine has also been given. It reduces serum bilirubin and may permit radiology of the biliary tree in the jaundiced.

Antibiotics may be indicated for febrile cholan-gitis but only temporary benefit is given in the presence of continued biliary obstruction.

Terminal hepato-cellular failure or *portal hypertension* are treated along the same lines.

CLASSIFICATION

The traditional classification of cholestasis is into *extra-hepatic* where there is a mechanical obstruction to the main bile ducts and *intra-hepatic* where such an obstructive lesion cannot be demonstrated and the defect is in the liver cell or in microscopic bile ducts within the liver. Practical extension of this classification has followed the development of better methods of visualizing the main bile ducts (fig. 205). Distinction is made between cholestasis where dilated bile ducts are demonstrated within the liver and cholestasis where such dilatation cannot be demonstrated. The investigation and management of the two types is very different.

The importance of a careful history with particular reference to the nature of pain or pyrexia

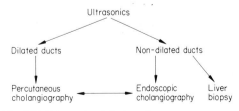

Fig. 205. Diagnosis of cholestasis.

Table 29. The differentiation of obstruction to
main bile ducts from acute intra-hepatic cholestasis.

	Cholestasis	
	Extra-hepatic	Intra-hepatic
History	Fever, pain frequent	Drugs. Onset as for hepatitis
Liver size	+ +	±
Hepatic histology		
Bile necrosis	+ (sometimes)	0
Portal zones		
Polymorphs	+	0
Eosinophils	0	Frequent
Dilated ductules	+	0
Liver cell damage	±	+
Percutaneous or endoscopic cholangiography	Block shown	No dilated bile ducts found
Ultrasound		
Intra-hepatic ducts	Dilated	Not dilated

and an accurate physical examination with routine
haematology and biochemistry must be stressed
(table 29). The stools should be inspected and
occult blood examination performed. Persistent
acholic (silver) stools and glycosuria may suggest
pancreatic malignancy. Rectal examination is
mandatory. A barium meal or enema may be
required.

If the diagnosis is not obvious by these simple
means, the next investigation is ultrasonic examination of the liver.

If dilated intra-hepatic bile ducts are seen by
ultrasound (fig. 49) percutaneous trans-hepatic
cholangiography using the 'skinny' (Chiba) needle

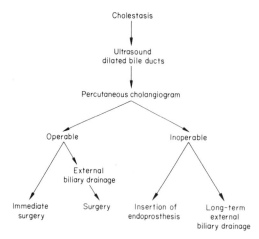

Fig. 206. Management of patient with bile duct
obstruction (Dooley *et al* 1979).

is the next investigation (fig. 61). The technique
is easy and with dilated ducts is almost always successful in visualizing the biliary tree and any
obstruction to it [25]. The procedure should be
followed by surgery within a few hours. As an
alternative procedure, the skinny needle may then
be replaced by a sheathed needle and cannula and
the bile drained externally from the dilated ducts
for hours or even days until surgery is performed
[23].

If ultrasonic scanning shows that intra-hepatic
bile ducts are undilated, cholangiography with the
skinny needle becomes more difficult. The choice
of procedure lies between endoscopic retrograde
cholangiopancreatography (ERCP) and percutaneous needle liver biopsy. The selection depends
on the circumstances in the individual patient.
ERCP is a specialist procedure requiring training
and technical expertise [14]. It has the advantage
over other forms of cholangiography in that the
stomach, duodenum and pancreatic ducts may be
visualized (fig. 61). Any suspicious lesions, for
instance at the ampulla, can be biopsied. Undilated
bile ducts can be shown.

EXTRA-HEPATIC ('SURGICAL')
CHOLESTASIS

This term implies mechanical obstruction to large
bile ducts outside the liver or within the porta
hepatis. Additional features are added to the
general picture of cholestasis.

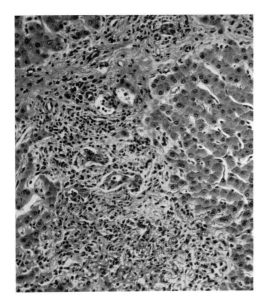

Fig. 207. Obstructive jaudice and cholangitis due to choledocholithiasis. The portal tract shows proliferating bile ducts, fibroblasts and an infiltration with polymorphonuclear and round cells. Culture of the biopsy yielded *E. coli.* H & E, × 70.

The liver is enlarged and the intra-hepatic bile ducts are widely dilated. Their contents are at first dark but later so-called *white bile* is the result of the increased pressure in the ducts which suppresses secretion of bile by the liver. White bile is free of bilirubin and bile salts and the cation composition is that of serum [26]. It is found in all forms of extra-hepatic cholestasis. Infection of the bile above the obstruction leads to *cholangitis*; the ducts contain pus and may be surrounded by small abscesses.

Hepatic histology

Bile ducts multiply in the portal zones. They are elongated and tortuous, have a wide lumen and are lined by high cuboidal epithelium (fig. 207). If infection of the bile above the obstruction has resulted in ascending cholangitis, culture of an hepatic biopsy may yield the causative organism and histology shows accumulations of polymorphonuclear leucocytes related to bile ducts (fig. 207). The sinusoids contain numerous polymorphs.

Bile is toxic and focal necrosis of liver cells, with little surrounding cellularity, is seen early in the mid-zones and later portally. Portal necroses con-

tain bile and are called *bile lakes* (fig. 208). They represent ruptured interlobular bile ducts. They are not seen in intra-hepatic cholestasis.

The hepatic changes develop very rapidly. Cholestasis is seen within 36 hours. Bile duct proliferation is early; portal fibrosis develops later. After about two weeks, duration cannot be related to the extent of hepatic change.

The distinction of *secondary biliary* from other forms of cirrhosis is difficult. In biliary cirrhosis of extra-hepatic origin, bile duct proliferation is more conspicuous; the fibrous bands are more heavily infiltrated with polymorphs. Cholestasis is greater, reflecting the deeper jaundice.

Bile is normally secreted at a pressure of about 15–25 cm H_2O. A rise to about 35 cm results in suppression of bile flow and so in jaundice.

Clinical features

There are additional features to those of general cholestasis. *Pain* varies in type. A fixed right upper quadrant ache is probably due to stretching of the capsule of the liver. The pain of gall bladder disease may be present. Finally, cholestasis of malignant origin may be associated with pain due to the primary tumour.

Fever may indicate ascending cholangitis. When this is due to partial obstruction of the common

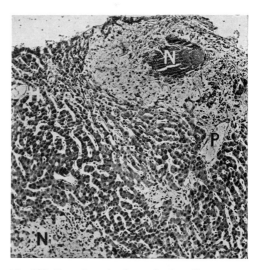

Fig. 208. Extra-hepatic obstructive jaundice. Necroses (N) of liver cells are seen in the periportal zones. The larger shows central bile staining. P=branch of portal vein; H=central hepatic vein. H & E, × 70.

duct by ball-valve calculus or traumatic stricture there may be intermittent high fever with rigors (*Charcot's intermittent biliary fever*).

The liver is enlarged. Nodularity may indicate malignancy; the gall bladder may be palpable or tender.

Other abdominal masses may indicate a primary lesion such as carcinoma of stomach or colon. Rectal examination and sigmoidoscopy may indicate carcinoma.

Haematological changes. Anaemia implies infection, blood loss or malignant disease. A polymorphonuclear leucocytosis suggests some complication such as cholangitis or underlying neoplastic disease.

In the febrile, blood cultures should be performed repeatedly. Septicaemias, especially due to Gram-negative organisms, are common.

Patients with partial biliary obstruction and cholangitis have a very high bacterial population in the bile, rivalling that of the colon [79]. Bacterial contamination of the small bowel leads to some of the features of the blind loop syndrome [80].

The *mitochondrial antibody test* for primary biliary cirrhosis is consistently negative.

Ultrasound (fig. 49) confirms dilated bile ducts in the liver and may indicate gall-stones or cancer of the pancreas.

Cholangiography

Intravenous techniques, even with infusion of contrast and tomography, are rarely satisfactory in the presence of extra-hepatic cholestasis.

Percutaneous techniques are very satisfactory in defining large bile ducts.

Endoscopic techniques are required if bile ducts are not dilated but choledocholithiasis, sclerosing cholangitis or a pancreatic cause is suspected. This specialist method is 70% successful in defining main bile and pancreatic ducts.

Aspiration liver biopsy

Needle liver biopsy can be performed safely in patients with cholestatic jaundice, however deep [68]. However, after intramuscular vitamin K therapy, the prothrombin time must not be prolonged more than three seconds over control values. The platelet count should exceed 80 000.

Histology is usually characteristic and readily distinguishes extra-hepatic cholestasis from hepatitis. The portal zones are the most diagnostic areas (fig. 207). They show oedema, bile duct reduplication, cubical epithelium and wide lumen, polymorph and mononuclear cells, some fibrosis and a well-defined limiting plate.

Interpretation of the histological appearances demands a skilled histopathologist. It is usually possible to distinguish appearances associated with obstruction to main bile ducts (fig. 207), viral hepatitis, alcoholism, drug-associated cholestasis, or primary biliary cirrhosis.

INTRA-HEPATIC CHOLESTASIS

The cause of the cholestasis lies within the liver, somewhere distal to the hepato-cellular microsomes and down to the major bile ducts. The general pathological, clinical and biochemical picture and general treatment are the same as cholestasis. Febrile cholangitis is absent and there is no pain apart from that which may be associated with the cause. The liver is not necessarily enlarged and is not tender. Bile ducts are not dilated within the liver and, histologically, biliary necrosis and bile duct multiplication are not seen (table 29).

Cholestasis with undilated intra-hepatic bile ducts (fig. 210) (table 30)

HEPATO-CELLULAR

The cholestasis is complex. There is primary injury to intracellular membranes. Leakage of bile salts through defective canaliculi leads to a reduction of bile salt-dependent bile flow. Inhibition of canalicular ATPase interferes with bile salt-independent secretion. Impaired uptake of bile salts by the injured hepatocyte results in loss in the urine. Finally impaired hydroxylation of cholesterol to bile acids in the endoplasmic reticulum reduces bile salt-dependent flow.

Cholestatic viral hepatitis (Chapter 15). The history of exposure and the nature of the prodromal symptoms may be helpful. The liver biopsy appearances are those of acute viral hepatitis. A 'whitewash', i.e. a profound fall in serum bilirubin value, follows five days of 30 mg prednisolone daily.

Acute alcoholic hepatitis (Chapter 19) can be cholestatic [67]. The history of alcohol abuse, the large tender liver and, often, vascular spiders on the skin are helpful points. Liver biopsy appearances are diagnostic.

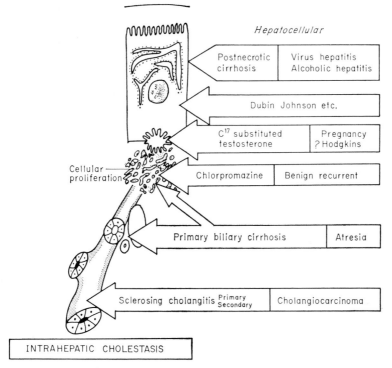

Fig. 209. Classification of intra-hepatic cholestasis according to possible major sites of involvement of the biliary tree (Sherlock 1966).

Drugs include the promazine group, long-acting sulphonamides and anti-thyroid drugs (Chapter 17). The history is important and liver biopsy appearances are usually diagnostic.

In some patients with *cryptogenic macronodular cirrhosis* cholestasis may be prominent.

SEX HORMONE CANALICULAR MEMBRANE CHANGES

Cholestatic reactions to oral contraceptives (Chapter 17) and in the last trimester of pregnancy (Chapter 24) fall into this group.

Table 30. Cholestasis with undilated intra-hepatic bile ducts.

Type	Diagnostic points
Hepato-cellular	
viral hepatitis	Onset typical. Liver biopsy. Steroid 'whitewash'.
alcoholic hepatitis	History. Large tender liver. Spiders. Liver biopsy.
drugs	History. Onset six weeks of starting. Liver biopsy.
Sex hormones (canalicular)	Hormone therapy. Remit on stopping. Liver biopsy.
Bile acids	All rare. Often familial.
Biliary	
intra-hepatic atresia	History. Age. Liver biopsy.
benign recurrent	Repeated. Cholangiography normal. Normal liver between attacks.
primary biliary cirrhosis	Female. Onset pruritus. Positive mitochondrial antibody. Raised serum IgM. Liver biopsy.
choledocholithiasis	History. Cholangiography. ERCP.
sclerosing cholangitis	Association ulcerative colitis. ERCP. Liver biopsy.

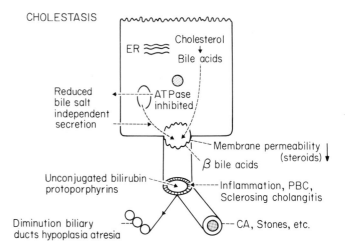

CHOLESTASIS

Fig. 210. Possible
mechanisms of cholestasis.
ER = endoscopic reticulum.

BILE ACIDS

Toxic bile acids have detergent effects on canalicular membranes and are inadequate as micelle formers.

Lithocholic acid [102] is a naturally occurring bile acid formed in the colon. The human liver probably metabolizes it when it is re-absorbed so preventing its injurious (cholestatic) action.

Monohydroxy bile acids, such as 3-beta-hydroxy-5-cholenate, accumulate in canalicular membranes and are cholestatic. They have been found in the bile of infants with established cholestasis, but their role as cause or effect is uncertain.

Coprostanic acid [49]. Two children from two families with cholestasis from birth were found to have this C27 alligator bile acid in bile. They soon died of cirrhosis. An enzyme catalysing C24 hydroxylation may be defective.

Byler's disease. This fatal intra-hepatic cholestasis has been reported in Amisch kindreds named Byler [21]. Death is usual before the age of eight. Inheritance is probably autosomal recessive. A defect in the biliary canalicular membrane is postulated. Conjugated bile acids cannot be excreted and this may be related to the cholestasis.

MISCELLANEOUS

Cholestasis in *severe bacterial infections*, particularly in childhood or post-operatively, is presumably hepato-cellular. A *nutritional* cholestasis develops in infants with hyperalimentation and pyloric obstruction. *Hodgkin's disease*, usually terminally, may be complicated by deep chole-

stasis. This is not necessarily due to excess haemolysis, hepatic infiltration or invasion of major bile ducts. The cause is unknown. A similar picture is sometimes seen with metastatic cancer of the liver or after successful marrow allograft [59].

Biliary precipitation of insoluble solutes. Unconjugated bilirubin may precipitate as intra-hepatic pigment stones or as inspissated bile in *cystic fibrosis.*

Protoporphyrins in *erythrocytic protoporphyria* may lead to precipitation in the canalicular ducts.

The cholestasis of *intra-hepatic atresia* (infantile cholangiopathy) (Chapter 23) is probably related to viral injury to intra-hepatic bile ducts.

Benign recurrent intra-hepatic cholestasis (see page 226).

Primary biliary cirrhosis (see page 227).

LARGE BILE DUCT DISEASE WITH UNDILATED INTRA-HEPATIC DUCTS

Finally some diseases which involve main bile ducts do not result in intra-hepatic biliary dilatation. Choledocholithiasis may be found without dilated intra-hepatic ducts if the stone has only recently migrated from the gall bladder, or if it has been present for months so that a secondary bacterial cholangitis has led to sclerosing cholangitis. Primary sclerosing cholangitis involves bile ducts inside and outside the liver.

Benign recurrent intra-hepatic cholestasis

This rare condition presents as multiple episodes of cholestatic jaundice [101]. Main bile duct obstruction must be excluded. The first patient described has now survived 22 episodes and three laparotomies [101]. Another patient has had 27 attacks over 38 years. The onset is with itching, occasionally an influenza-like illness and vomiting. Jaundice appears and persists for three to four months. Hepatic histology shows cholestasis, portal zone expansion, mononuclears and some liver cell degeneration, mainly centrizonal. Hepatic histology and liver function are normal in remission [101].

Aetiology. In favour of a genetic origin is the early onset, usually starting before the age of 10, and the familial incidence [15, 58, 96].

Study of a patient in the anicteric stage suggested enhanced bile acid synthesis and abnormal faecal bacteria [27]. Unusual bile acids were found in bile and faeces.

Environmental origins must be considered, for some of the patients have an allergic diathesis, rashes may be associated and the condition may recur at definite times in the year.

Treatment. The attacks are self-limiting and vary in duration. Corticosteroid treatment is probably of little benefit.

PRIMARY BILIARY CIRRHOSIS

This condition of progressive destruction of intra-hepatic bile ducts was first described in 1851 by Addison and Gull [1] and later by Hanot [48]. The association with high serum cholesterol levels and

Primary biliary cirrhosis

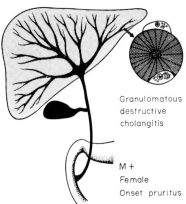

Granulomatous
destructive
cholangitis

M +
Female
Onset pruritus

Fig. 211. The features of primary biliary cirrhosis (Sherlock 1972).

skin xanthomas led to the term 'xanthomatous biliary cirrhosis' [65]. Ahrens and co-workers [3] termed the condition 'primary biliary cirrhosis'. However, in the early stages nodular regeneration is inconspicuous and cirrhosis is not present. The term 'chronic non-suppurative destructive cholangitis' [77] is a better one although too cumbersome to replace the popular 'primary biliary cirrhosis' (PBC).

Aetiology

The aetiology remains unknown, but immunological mechanisms have been invoked in the initiation of the bile duct injury. Histometric examinations show that bile ducts less than 70–80 μm in diameter are destroyed and particularly in the early stages [70].

There is an association with diseases believed to have an immunological basis, particularly the collagen diseases.

The histological reaction around injured bile ducts is predominantly monocytic with prominent lymphocytic accumulations. Granulomas, the hallmark of disturbed cell-based immunity, are present near damaged bile ducts. They can also be found in lymph nodes outside the liver, in the omentum and lungs [35]. Enlarged fleshy lymph nodes in the porta hepatis may even cause diagnostic difficulties at surgery.

Skin tests using tuberculin or dinitrochlorobenzene (DNCB) show that many patients with primary biliary cirrhosis are anergic [35]. Phyto-haemagglutinin-stimulated lymphocytes show impaired transformation, a good indication of depressed T lymphocyte function. Injury to bile ducts by sensitized T lymphocytes has been invoked as aetiological. However, using Chang cells as the target there was no evidence of specific T lymphocyte-mediated cytotoxicity in patients with primary biliary cirrhosis [98].

There is no relationship between results for the various serological auto-antibody markers, and particularly the mitochondrial antibody, and the aetiology of the disease. The disturbances in cell-mediated immunity seem to bear little relationship to severity. Four pre-symptomatic patients had normal mechanisms of delayed hypersensitivity [36]. This raises the possibility that the anergy is the result rather than the cause of the disease. The demonstrated disturbances in cell-mediated immunity in primary biliary cirrhosis may be an effect of the disease rather than aetiological.

Genetic factors

There seems to be familial clustering, and primary biliary cirrhosis has been reported in sisters, twins [13] and in mothers and daughters [95].

There is a significant increase in the incidence of serological antibodies, including the mito-chondrial antibody, in healthy relatives of patients with primary biliary cirrhosis [32, 39]. This raises the question of genetic and environmental factors or indeed interaction between the two.

The disease is not associated with any particular pattern of histocompatibility antigens [47]. This is in contrast to chronic active hepatitis and empha-sizes the differences between the two conditions.

Primary biliary cirrhosis as a graft-versus-host disease (fig. 212)

The bile duct destruction may be mediated via im-mune complex formation [93]. The sera of most patients with primary biliary cirrhosis show im-mune complexes by the C1q binding method [100]. The large complexes may fix complement and be responsible for tissue damage. Large com-plexes of this type, when injected into the tissues of animals, result in granuloma formation. It has been more difficult demonstrating immune com-plexes in the liver parenchyma.

In primary biliary cirrhosis C_3 is probably activated by the classical pathway, since the cata-bolism of C1q, a component exclusive to the classi-cal pathway, is five times greater than normal, but either normal or slightly increased in other forms of chronic liver disease [53]. The reason for the localization of the complexes in granulomas in the portal zones of the liver is unknown. The route is probably non-systemic. Neither are immune com-plexes likely to be found in the bile. It seems more probable that they are produced in the walls of bile ductules or surrounding tissue—a reaction in many ways analogous to an Arthus reaction. An antigen absorbed through the bile may combine with antibody derived from the portal circulation and result in formation of complexes in the bile ductule wall and interstitial space of the portal tracts. A spillover of complexes into the systemic circulation is incidental to the primary patho-genetic process but may explain the association of primary biliary cirrhosis with extra-hepatic condi-tions such as arthritis, vasculitis and glomerulo-nephritis. Such immune complexes might also con-tribute to the state of anergy.

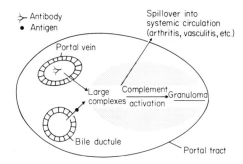

Fig. 212. Possible mechanisms of bile ductular injury in primary biliary cirrhosis (Thomas *et al* 1977).

Although this hypothesis describes a possible mechanism of bile duct damage and granuloma formation in primary biliary cirrhosis, the antigen involved and the way in which it enters the tissues of the portal zones of the liver are unknown.

Primary biliary cirrhosis may be visualized as a 'dry gland' syndrome with damage to the ductular epithelium of lacrimal and salivary glands, liver and pancreas. Additional extra-glandular features include scleroderma-like skin lesions, pigmen-tation, Raynaud's phenomenon and severe abnormalities of both humoral and cellular im-munity. Identical ductular and extraductular fea-tures, including abnormalities of the immune system with immune complex formation and macro-globulinaemia, are seen in chronic graft-versus-host disease following bone-marrow transplantation. In graft-versus-host reaction the immune response is to the histocompatibility-complex antigens which are present in high density on ductular epithelial cells of the biliary tree. A similar mechanism may be operative in primary biliary cirrhosis, either because of altered antigenicity of epithelial cell histocompatibility antigens or because of failure of the HLA-dependent T cell self-recognition system [30].

Clinical features

PRESENTATION [85]

Ninety per cent are female usually between the ages of 40 and 59 (range 32–72 years). The reason for the female predominance is unknown. The disease starts insidiously most frequently as pruritus without jaundice. Patients may be referred initially to dermatologists. Jaundice may never develop but in the majority appears within

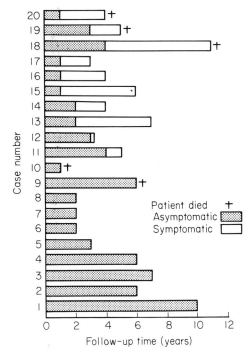

Fig. 213. The course of 20 patients with primary biliary cirrhosis diagnosed when asymptomatic. Note that one patient continued asymptomatic for 10 years (Long *et al* 1977).

six months to two years of the onset of pruritus. In about a quarter jaundice and pruritus start simultaneously. Jaundice preceding pruritus is extremely unusual and jaundice without pruritus at any time is very rare. The pruritus can start during pregnancy and be confused with idiopathic cholestatic jaundice of the last trimester.

Examination shows a well-nourished pigmented woman. Jaundice is slight or absent. The liver is usually enlarged and firm and the spleen palpable.

The patient may also be diagnosed when *asymptomatic* [64]. This may follow detection of hepatomegaly, a raised serum alkaline phosphatase level or a positive auto-antibody test at the time of examination for another or related condition such as rheumatoid arthritis. Such patients tend to be diagnosed younger; the earliest was 23 years old. They may be slightly pigmented and the liver may be enlarged.

COURSE

Earlier diagnosis has made the duration seem much longer. Even in the asymptomatic the

disease has probably been present for many years before diagnosis.

The rate of progress is very variable (fig. 213). Patients can remain asymptomatic for as long as 10 years. The development of symptoms in the asymptomatic cannot be predicted by biochemical tests or hepatic histology.

The course of those diagnosed with symptoms is 6–7 years (range 4–14 years) [82]. Prognosis is improving with better supportive care [81].

Serum bilirubin levels remain stable for a variable period (about four years) and then rise rapidly until death some two years later. The accelerated phase is marked by an increase in serum bilirubin of more than 2 mg per 100 dl on successive six-monthly samples [81].

Diarrhoea may be due to steatorrhoea. Weight loss is slow. In spite of the jaundice, patients feel surprisingly well and have a good appetite. The course is afebrile and abdominal pain is unusual.

Skin xanthomas (figs. 193–5) develop frequently and sometimes acutely, but many patients remain in the pre-xanthomatous state throughout their course; terminally xanthomas may disappear.

The skin may be thickened and tough over the fingers, ankles and legs. Pain in the fingers, especially on opening doors, and in the toes may be due to xanthomatous peripheral neuropathy [94]. There may be a butterfly area over the back which is inaccessible and escapes scratching [74].

The bone changes complicating chronic cholestasis are particularly profound in the deeply jaundiced (figs. 198, 200, 201). In the late stages the patient complains of backache and pain over the ribs sometimes with pathological fractures. These bone changes are enhanced by prolonged corticosteroid therapy.

Duodenal ulceration and haemorrhage are common.

Bleeding oesophageal varices may be a presenting feature (55, 103), even before nodules have developed in the liver. The portal hypertension is probably pre-sinusoidal. Haemorrhage from varices also accompanies the late cirrhotic stage [82].

Hepato-cellular carcinoma is a very rare termination, perhaps because a true nodular cirrhosis develops so late [56].

ASSOCIATED DISEASES

Non-hepatic disorders are found in 69% [43]. Associated collagen diseases include rheumatoid arthritis [12] and dermatomyositis. The CRST syndrome of calcinosis, Raynaud's phenomenon, sclerodactyly and telangiectasia may be present in whole or in part [75].

The 'sicca complex' of dry eyes and mouth with or without the arthritis complicating Sjögren's syndrome occurs in about 70% of fatal cases [42]. Auto-immune thyroiditis is another association.

Finger clubbing is common and occasionally hypertrophic osteoarthropathy (fig. 201) [28].

Renal complications include IgM-associated membranous glomerulonephritis [73] and renal tubular acidosis.

Weight loss may sometimes be explained by the steatorrhoea of coeliac disease [61].

Gall-stones, usually of pigment type, have been seen by endoscopy in 39% [91].

Biochemical findings

The serum reflects prolonged cholestasis with a serum bilirubin level usually between 1 and 5 mg/100 ml (fig. 214). The alkaline phosphatase is always raised, being three times the upper limit of normal in about 75% (fig. 215). The serum bilirubin level may fluctuate and may be within normal limits for some months. The serum alkaline phosphatase, however, continues elevated.

The serum IgM may be very high [8] but in a quarter is within normal limits on presentation [85] (fig. 216). Serum angiotensin converting enzyme (SACE) may rarely be increased [90].

Serum mitochondrial (M) test

Mitochondrial antibodies are non-organ specific and are demonstrated by immunofluorescence on renal tubules or by a sensitive complement fixation test. The antigen is a lipoprotein composed of mitochondrial inner membranes. They are present in the serum of over 96% of patients with primary biliary cirrhosis compared with 2–3% of those with mechanical bile duct obstruction (fig. 217) [22, 99]. The antibody is absent in the serum of patients with cholestasis associated with inflammatory bowel disease or with viral hepatitis or in a normal population. It is present in 30% of patients with chronic active hepatitis (HBsAg negative) and in 3% of those with connective tissue diseases.

The antibody may also be found in some patients with cryptogenic cirrhosis. These are usually middle-aged women who have some points in common with primary biliary cirrhosis in terms of hepatic and cholestatic biochemistry.

In a patient with cholestasis, a negative result means that primary biliary cirrhosis is not the correct diagnosis. A positive result in an icteric patient throws considerable doubt on whether the jaundice is due to a mechanical block to main bile passages.

Liver biopsy [77, 78, 85]

Stage 1: The florid duct lesion (fig. 219; see also fig. 218 in colour section). This is pathognomonic. Septal and larger interlobular bile ducts are damaged and surrounded by a dense infiltrate of lymphocytes, or epithelioid cells, plasma cells and a few eosinophils. Lymphoid aggregates with or without germinal centres may be found. Granulomas are often seen as poorly defined collections of histiocytes or as well-organized tuberculoid lesions without central necrosis. They are usually near a damaged duct in the portal tract. This damage is seen as swelling, proliferation and crowding of epithelial cells and as rupture. The portal tract is otherwise normal and the limiting liver cell plates are intact. Within the lobules there may be slight mononuclear cell infiltration and regenerative hyperplasia seen as double liver cell plates. Centrizonal cholestasis is often absent and rarely severe.

Stage 2: Ductular proliferation (fig. 220). Lesions are now more widespread but are less specific. There is fibrosis, acute and chronic inflammatory infiltration and ductular proliferation. Ducts are reduced and their place taken by ill-defined lymphoid aggregates which, together with the fibrosis and inflammation, give a rather characteristic appearance. Granulomas are less common. Periportal areas show a slight to moderate degree of liver cell necrosis, swelling and cholestasis, and liver cells may contain Mallory's hyalin [40]. Lipid laden histiocytes are sometimes seen.

Stage 3: Scarring (fig. 221). The inflammation subsides and relatively acellular septa extend from the portal tracts into and around the lobules. Lymphoid aggregates are still seen and periportal cholestasis may be severe. The appearances are not pathognomonic but can be interpreted as compatible.

Stage 4: Cirrhosis. Regeneration nodules are seen and the picture is of end-stage liver disease. The diagnosis may still be suggested by paucity of bile ducts or by accumulation of lymphocytes.

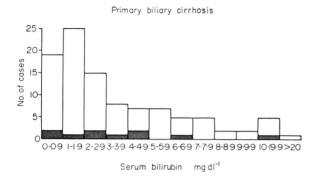

Primary biliary cirrhosis

Fig. 214. Serum bilirubin levels at presentation in 100 patients with primary biliary cirrhosis. Note that the serum bilirubin was less than 2 mg in 41%. Males are in hatched columns (Sherlock & Scheuer 1973).

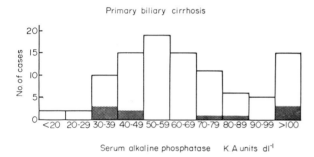

Primary biliary cirrhosis

Fig. 215. Serum alkaline phosphatase levels (normal 3–14 K.A. units) at presentation in 100 patients with primary biliary cirrhosis. The level exceeded 50 units in 71%. Males are in hatched columns (Sherlock & Scheuer 1973).

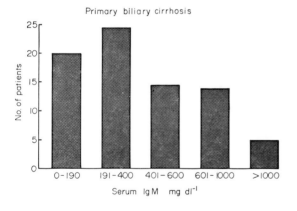

Primary biliary cirrhosis

Fig. 216. Serum immunoglobin M levels in 76 patients with primary biliary cirrhosis. Levels are usually raised but in 20 patients (26%) did not exceed the upper limit of normal of 190 mg/dl (Sherlock & Scheuer 1973).

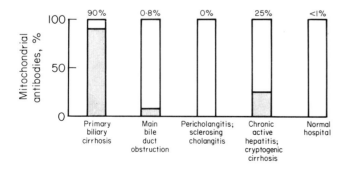

Fig. 217. The percentage incidence of positive serum mitochondrial antibodies in various hepato-biliary diseases and in a normal hospital population.

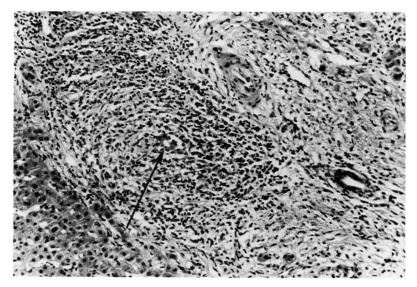

Fig. 219. Primary biliary cirrhosis. Diagnostic stage 1 lesion with damaged bile duct (arrow) surrounded by a mononuclear-cell infiltrate. H & E, × 120 (Sherlock & Scheuer 1973).

There is much overlap between the stages to the extent that stage 1 lesions are occasionally seen in stage 4 livers with well-established cirrhosis [44].

Although diagnosis is more confident with large, laparotomy liver biopsies than with needle ones, diagnosis nowadays is usually made on the small samples. Much depends on the skill and experience of the interpreter. The appearances of focal portal zone lymphocyte accumulations, 'biliary' type fibrosis, and peripheral cholestasis

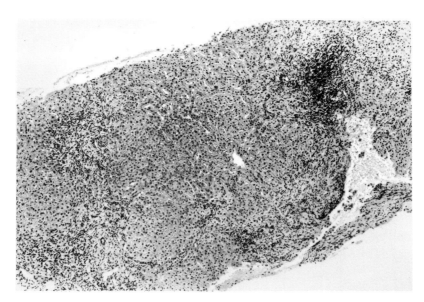

Fig. 220. Primary biliary cirrhosis, stage 2. Characteristic changes in this needle biopsy are fibrosis, ductular proliferation and presence of lymphoid aggregates. These appearances are regarded as compatible with the diagnosis rather than diagnostic. H & E, × 48 (Sherlock & Scheuer 1973).

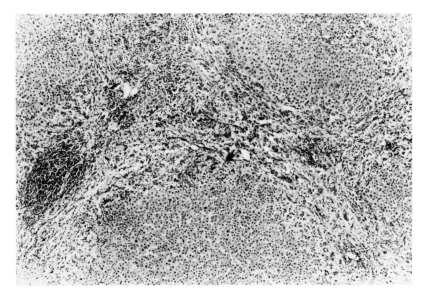

Fig. 221. Primary biliary cirrhosis, stage 3. There is scarring and septa contain lymphoid aggregates. Hyperplastic 'regeneration' nodules are beginning to develop. H & E, × 48 (Sherlock & Scheuer 1973).

are very suggestive of primary biliary cirrhosis. The distinction between diagnostic changes, i.e. destructive lesions of larger bile ducts, and compatible ones is very helpful. The report of 'compatible histology' can be slotted into place with clinical, biochemical and immunological findings to provide a diagnostic whole.

Diagnosis

This is suspected when a middle-aged woman presents with pruritus with or without mild jaundice. It is confirmed by a raised serum alkaline phosphatase level, sometimes a high serum IgM, a positive serum mitochondrial antibody test and diagnostic or compatible hepatic histology on needle biopsy. In the asymptomatic it may be suspected simply by a raised serum alkaline phosphatase level.

Visualization of the bile ducts by endoscopy [91], percutaneous cholangiography or, in the anicteric, by infusion cholangiography may be necessary in atypical patients. These include males and those with a negative serum mitochondrial antibody test, with inconclusive liver biopsy findings or with abdominal pain. Surgical exploration of the bile ducts is not necessary for diagnosis.

Primary biliary cirrhosis must be differentiated

from chronic cholestatic drug jaundice, primary and secondary sclerosing cholangitis and carcinoma of the hepatic duct (table 31) (figs. 222, 223).

Widespread tissue and hepatic granulomas may suggest sarcoidosis (table 31). The negative Kveim

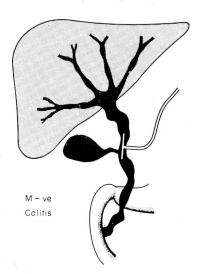

Sclerosing cholangitis

M – ve
Colitis

Fig. 222. The features of primary sclerosing cholangitis (Sherlock 1972).

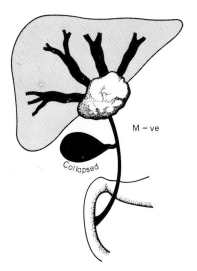

Carcinoma hepatic duct

M – ve

Collapsed

Fig. 223. The features of carcinoma of the hepatic ducts (Sherlock 1972).

test and positive serum mitochondrial antibody test are diagnostic.

Prognosis

The outlook when the patient is first seen may be unpredictable except that the disease is not curable at present. There seems to be no correlation between the extent and severity of the liver lesions and the duration of symptoms. The deeper the jaundice the worse the prognosis. Bleeding from oesophageal varices in the deeply jaundiced is particularly ominous [55].

The terminal stages last about one year and are marked by a rapid deepening of jaundice with disappearance of both xanthomas and pruritus. Serum albumin and total cholesterol levels fall. Oedema and ascites develop. The final events include episodes of hepatic encephalopathy with uncontrollable bleeding, usually from the oesophageal varices. An intercurrent infection, sometimes a Gram-negative septicaemia, may be terminal.

Treatment

The symptomatic management is that of chronic cholestasis (table 27), with intramuscular fat-soluble vitamins and calcium supplements particularly important. If bone thinning and pain are severe, intravenous calcium chloride must be given. Pruritus is controlled, usually with cholestyramine. Medium chain triglycerides may be helpful. The patient must be encouraged to lead as normal a life as possible, since the disease is compatible with a full domestic and professional

Table 31. Features distinguishing sarcoidosis from primary biliary cirrhosis (Stanley *et al* 1972).

Feature	Sarcoidosis	PBC
Sex (F:M)	Equal	8:1
Erythema nodosum	Yes	No
Uveitis	Yes	No
Pruritus	No	Yes
Xanthomas	No	Yes
Splenomegaly	Yes (in 12%)	Yes (in 50%)
Skin pigmentation	No	Yes
Steatorrhoea	No	Yes
Bilateral hilar lymphadenopathy	Yes	No
Kveim test	Positive (in 75%)	Always negative
Serum angiotensin converting enzyme	Yes	No
Depression of delayed-type hypersensitivity	Yes	Yes
Circulating mitochondrial antibodies	No	Yes
Calcium metabolism	Hypercalcaemia (vitamin D sensitivity)	Hypocalcaemia (steatorrhoea)
Alkaline phosphatase raised	Yes (minority)	Yes (majority)
Liver granulomas	Yes	Yes
Corticosteroids	Helpful	Contraindicated
Prognosis	Very good	Progressive disease

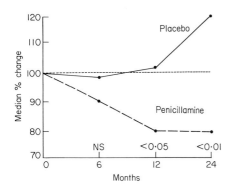

Fig. 224. Primary biliary cirrhosis. The median percentage change in immune complexes (^{125}IClq binding) in penicillamine- and placebo-treated patients with primary biliary cirrhosis (Epstein *et al* 1979) NS = not significant.

life for many years. Skilful make-up may be necessary to conceal facial icterus.

Corticosteroids increase bone thinning and are contraindicated.

Azathioprine in a controlled prospective trial did not improve liver function tests. Serial hepatic biopsies showed the development of cirrhosis equally in treated and untreated groups and survival was similar [50].

Liver copper levels in primary biliary cirrhosis can be as high as those found in Wilson's disease. Copper is toxic to liver cells and, as in Wilson's disease, removal by D-penicillamine would be expected to be beneficial. In addition D-penicillamine affects the immune system and this is the basis for its use in rheumatoid arthritis. D-penicillamine also prevents formation of some types

of cross-linkage between collagen molecules. Whether or not it might prevent collagen deposition in primary biliary cirrhosis cannot be predicted since the predominant type of cross-linking of this collagen has not been characterized. Prospective controlled trials have shown benefit for penicillamine-treated patients [19, 29, 51]. After one year liver copper levels fall, serum transaminase and immunoglobulin values are reduced over controls, and serum immune complexes fall significantly (figs. 224, 225, 226). Bilirubin concentration increases at a slower rate. Survival is prolonged.

The initial dose of D-penicillamine is 150 mg daily. This is built up to a maintenance dose of 600 mg daily over nine weeks. Unfortunately the side-effects of the drug are numerous. Nausea, vomiting and transient loss of taste are frequent. Skin rashes can usually be controlled by corticosteroids and the drug re-started; occasionally this may not be possible. Proteinuria and blood dyscrasias (neutropenia) and erythroid aplasia are more serious and necessitate stopping the drug.

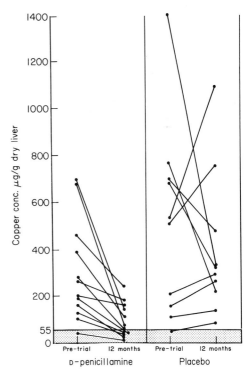

Fig. 226. Change in liver copper concentrations in control and D-penicillamine-treated patients over 12 months. The hatched area denotes the normal range (5–55 µg/g of dry liver) (Epstein *et al* 1979).

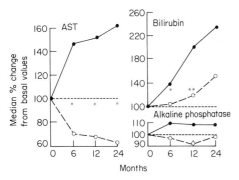

Fig. 225. Primary biliary cirrhosis. The median percentage change in serum aspartate transaminase (AST), total bilirubin and alkaline phosphatase in penicillamine-treated (open circle) and placebo-treated (closed circle) patients (Epstein *et al* 1979).

Urine tests and blood counts should be performed weekly for the first month and then monthly during therapy.

The decision to start D-penicillamine in an asymptomatic patient is difficult. It should certainly be used in the symptomatic, particularly if an increased hepatic copper concentration or urinary copper excretion after penicillamine have been found. Other forms of therapy under trial include cyclosporin A which is giving promising results but is nephrotoxic [76].

Portal–systemic shunts should be considered for bleeding oesophageal varices in those without hepato-cellular failure (deep jaundice and ascites). Such operations are tolerated well and the incidence of encephalopathy is low.

Gall-stones should be left *in situ* unless causing severe symptoms or present in the common bile duct. Cholecystectomy is rarely indicated and is badly tolerated.

KIDNEY FAILURE AND CHOLESTASIS

Following prolonged cholestasis or after its surgical relief, the patient may become oliguric, anuric and uraemic. The resulting coma is mixed hepatic and renal and it is often difficult to disentangle the precise sequence of events. However, in most instances, acute tubular necrosis (*intrinsic renal failure*) is the cause of the kidney failure, and has been precipitated by a prolonged, difficult operation, hypotension, haemorrhage with diminished renal blood flow, and sepsis such as peritonitis. The diminished renal and hepatic blood flow are contributory.

The kidneys of patients with cholestatic jaundice may be particularly prone to acute renal failure. Uraemia seems to complicate operations on deeply jaundiced patients more often than comparable operations on the non-jaundiced. Experiments on rats with obstructive jaundice support this hypothesis. Deep jaundice is particularly important [17]. Mannitol infusions should be given to maintain glomerular filtration immediately preoperatively and during the operation in every patient with deep cholestatic jaundice [18].

Examples of other conditions which cause simultaneous liver and kidney injury are carbon tetrachloride, paracetamol or tetracycline overdosage, Weil's disease and Gram-negative septicaemias; similarly any condition which causes

acute renal and hepatic necrosis such as shock or haemorrhage. The problem of renal failure in cirrhotic patients with ascites ('hepato-renal syndrome') is considered elsewhere.

REFERENCES

1. ADDISON T. & GULL W. (1851) On a certain affection of the skin—vitiligoidea—α plana β tuberosa. *Guy's Hosp. Rep.* **7**, 265.
2. AGORASTOS J., FOX C., HARRY D.S. *et al* (1978) Lecithin-cholesterol acyl transferase and the lipoprotein abnormalities of obstructive jaundice. *Clin. Sci. molec. Biol.* **54**, 369.
3. AHRENS E.H. Jr, PAYNE M.A., KUNKEL H.G. *et al* (1950) Primary biliary cirrhosis. *Medicine (Baltimore)* **29**, 299.
4. AJDUKIEWICZ A.B., AGNEW J.E., BYERS P.D. *et al* (1974) The relief of bone pain in primary biliary cirrhosis with calcium infusions. *Gut* **15**, 788.
5. ATKINSON M., NORDIN B.E.C. & SHERLOCK S. (1956) Malabsorption and bone disease in prolonged obstructive jaundice. *Q. J. Med.* **25**, 299.
6. BADLEY B.W.D., MURPHY G.M., BOUCHER I.A.D. *et al* (1970) Diminished micellar phase lipid in patients with chronic nonalcoholic liver disease and steatorrhea. *Gastroenterology* **58**, 781.
7. BERTHELOT P., ERLINGER S., DHUMEAUX D. *et al* (1970) Mechanism of phenobarbital-induced hypercholeresis in the rat. *Am. J. Physiol.* **219**, 809.
8. BEVAN G., BALDUS W.P. & GLEICH G.J. (1969) Serum immunoglobulin levels in cholestasis. *Gastroenterology* **56**, 1040.
9. BOYER J.L. (1971) Canalicular bile formation in the isolated perfused rat liver. *Am. J. Physiol.* **221**, 1156.
10. CALDWELL J.H., BUSH C.A. & GREENBERGER N.J. (1971) Interruption of the entero-hepatic circulation of digitoxin by cholestyramine. *J. clin. Invest.* **50**, 2638.
11. CAMERON R. & HOU P.C. (1962) *Biliary Cirrhosis.* Oliver & Boyd, London.
12. CHILD D.L., MATHEWS J.A. & THOMPSON R.P.H. (1977) Arthritis and primary biliary cirrhosis. *Br. med. J.* ii, 557.
13. CHOHAN M.R. (1973) Primary biliary cirrhosis in twin sisters. *Gut* **14**, 213.
14. COTTON P.B. (1977) E.R.C.P. *Gut* **18**, 316.
15. DA SILVA L.C. & DE BRITO T. (1966) Benign recurrent intrahepatic cholestasis in two brothers. *Ann. intern. Med.* **65**, 331.
16. DATTA D.V. & SHERLOCK S. (1966) Cholestyramine for long term relief of the pruritus complicating intrahepatic cholestasis. *Gastroenterology* **50**, 323.
17. DAWSON J.L. (1965) The incidence of postoperative renal failure in obstructive jaundice. *Br. J. Surg.* **52**, 663.
18. DAWSON J.L. & STIRLING G.A. (1964) Protective effect of mannitol on anoxic jaundiced kidneys. A histological study. *Arch. Path.* **78**, 254.
19. DEERING T.B., DICKSON E.R., FLEMING C.R. *et al*

(1977) Effect of D-penicillamine on copper retention in primary biliary cirrhosis. *Gastroenterology* **72,** 1208.

20. DESMET V.J. (1977) *Anatomy I: Hepatocyte-canaliculus in Liver and Bile.* Falk Symposium 23, p. 3. MTP, Lancaster.

21. DE VOS R., DE WOLF-PETERS C., DE SMET V. *et al* (1975) Progressive intrahepatic cholestasis (Byler's disease): case report. *Gut* **16,** 943.

22. DONIACH D. & WALKER J.G. (1974) Progress report. Mitochondrial antibodies (AMA). *Gut* **15,** 664.

23. DOOLEY J.S., DICK R., OLNEY J. *et al* (1979) Non-surgical treatment of biliary obstruction. *Lancet* ii, 1040.

24. DUBIN M., MAURICE M., FELDMAN G. *et al* (1978) Phalloidin-induced cholestasis in the rat: relation to changes in microfilaments. *Gastroenterology* **75,** 450.

25. ELIAS E. (1976) Progress report. Cholangiography in the jaundiced patient. *Gut* **17,** 80.

26. ELMSLIE R.G., THORPE M.E.C., COLMAN J.V.L. *et al* (1969) Clinical significance of white bile in the biliary tree. *Gut* **10,** 530.

27. ENDO T., UCHIDA K., AMURO Y. *et al* (1979) Bile acid metabolism in benign recurrent intrahepatic cholestasis. Comparative studies on the icteric and anicteric phases of a single case. *Gastroenterology* **76,** 1002.

28. EPSTEIN O., AJDUKIEWICZ A.B., DICK R. *et al* (1979) Hypertrophic hepatic osteoarthropathy. *Am. J. Med.* **67,** 88.

29. EPSTEIN O., DE VILLIERS D., JAIN S. *et al* (1979) Reduction of immune complexes and immunoglobulins induced by D-penicillamine in primary biliary cirrhosis. *New Engl. J. Med.* **300,** 274.

30. EPSTEIN O., THOMAS H.C. & SHERLOCK S. (1980) Primary biliary cirrhosis is a 'dry gland' syndrome with features of chronic graft versus host (GVH) disease. *Lancet* i, 1166.

31. ERLINGER S. (1978) Cholestasis: pump failure, microvilli defect, or both? *Lancet* i, 533.

32. FEIZI T., NACCARATO R., SHERLOCK S. *et al* (1972) Mitochondrial and other tissue antibodies in relatives of patients with primary biliary cirrhosis. *Clin. exp. Immunol.* **10,** 609.

33. FLEMING C.R., DICKSON E.R., HOLLENHORST R.W. *et al* (1975) Pigmented corneal rings in a patient with primary biliary cirrhosis. *Gastroenterology* **69,** 220.

34. FORKER E.L. & RUNYON B.A. (1978) Canalicular cholestasis. *Gastroenterology* **75,** 535.

35. FOX R.A., SCHEUER P.J., JAMES D.G. *et al* (1969) Impaired delayed hypersensitivity in primary biliary cirrhosis. *Lancet* i, 959.

36. FOX R.A., SCHEUER P.J. & SHERLOCK S. (1973) Asymptomatic primary biliary cirrhosis. *Gut* **14,** 444.

37. FRENCH S.W. (1976) Is cholestasis due to microfilament failure? *Hum. Pathol.* **7,** 243.

38. FROMMER D., MORRIS J., SHERLOCK S. *et al* (1977) Kayser–Fleischer-like rings in patients without Wilson's disease. *Gastroenterology* **72,** 1331.

39. GALBRAITH R.M., SMITH M., MACKENZIE R.M. *et al* (1973) High prevalence of seroimmunologic abnormalities in relatives of patients with active chronic hepatitis or primary biliary cirrhosis. *New Engl. J. Med.* **290,** 63.

40. GERBER M.A., ORR W., DENK H. *et al* (1973) Hepatocellular hyalin in cholestasis and cirrhosis: its diagnostic significance. *Gastroenterology* **64,** 89.

41. GIBSON W.R. & ROBERTSON H.E. (1939) So-called biliary cirrhosis. *Arch. Path.* **28,** 37.

42. GOLDING P.L., BOWN R., MASON A.M.S. *et al* (1970) 'Sicca complex' in liver disease. *Br. med. J.* iv, 340.

43. GOLDING P.L., SMITH M. & WILLIAMS R. (1973) Multisystem involvement in chronic liver disease: studies on the incidence and pathogenesis. *Am. J. Med.* **55,** 772.

44. GOUDIE R.B., MACSWEEN R.N.M. & GOLDBERG D.M. (1966) Serological and histological diagnosis of primary biliary cirrhosis. *J. clin. Pathol.* **19,** 527.

45. HADZIYANNIS S., SCHEUER P.J., FEIZI T. *et al* (1970) Immunological and histological studies in primary biliary cirrhosis. *J. clin. Path.* **23,** 95.

46. HAMILTON R.L., HAVEL R.J., KANE J.P. *et al* (1971) Cholestasis: lamellar structure of the abnormal human serum lipoprotein. *Science* **172,** 475.

47. HAMLYN A.N., MORRIS J.S. & SHERLOCK S. (1974) ABO blood groups, rhesus negativity and primary biliary cirrhosis. *Gut* **15,** 480.

48. HANOT V. (1876) *Étude sur une Forme de Cirrhose Hypertrophique de Foie (Cirrhose Hypertrophique avec Ictère Chronique).* J. B. Baillière, Paris.

49. HANSON R.F., ISENBERG J.N., WILLIAMS G.C. *et al* (1975) The metabolism of 3α, 7α, 12α-trihydroxy-5β-cholestan-26-oic acid in two siblings with cholestasis due to intrahepatic bile duct anomalies: an apparent inborn error of cholic acid synthesis. *J. clin. Invest.* **56,** 577.

50. HEATHCOTE J., ROSS A. & SHERLOCK S. (1976) A prospective controlled trial of azathioprine in primary biliary cirrhosis. *Gastroenterology* **70,** 656.

51. JAIN S., SAMOURIAN S., SCHEUER P.J. *et al* (1977) A controlled trial of D-penicillamine in primary biliary cirrhosis. *Lancet* i, 831.

52. JAIN S., SCHEUER P.J., ARCHER B. *et al* (1978) Histological demonstration of copper and copper-associated protein in chronic liver diseases. *J. clin. Path.* **31,** 784.

53. JONES E.A. (Moderator) (1979) Primary biliary cirrhosis and the complement system. *Ann. intern. Med.* **90,** 72.

54. KEHAYOGLOU A.K., HOLDSWORTH C.D., AGNEW J.E. *et al* (1968) Bone disease and calcium absorption in primary biliary cirrhosis with special reference to vitamin-D therapy. *Lancet* i, 715.

55. KEW M.C., VARMA R.R., DOS SANTOS H.A. *et al* (1971) Portal hypertension in primary biliary cirrhosis. *Gut* **12,** 830.

56. KRASNER N., JOHNSON P.J., PORTMAN B. *et al* (1979) Hepatocellular carcinoma in primary biliary cirrhosis: report of four cases. *Gut* **20,** 255.

57. KUNKEL H.G. & AHRENS E.H. Jr (1949) The relationship between serum lipids and the electrophoretic pattern, with particular reference to patients with primary biliary cirrhosis. *J. clin. Invest.* **28,** 1575.

58. LESSER P.B. (1973) Benign familial recurrent intrahepatic cholestasis. *Am. J. dig. Dis.* **18**, 259.

59. LIPSCHUTZ G.R., KATON R.M. & LEE T.G. (1977) Obstructive jaundice after bone marrow transplantation. *Gastroenterology* **73**, 565.

60. LLOYD-THOMAS H.G.L. & SHERLOCK S. (1952) Testosterone therapy for the pruritus of obstructive jaundice. *Br. med. J.* ii, 1289.

61. LOGAN R.F.A., FERGUSON A., FINLAYSON N.D.C. *et al* (1978) Primary biliary cirrhosis and coeliac disease. An association? *Lancet* i, 230.

62. LONG R.G. & SHERLOCK S. (1979) Vitamin D in chronic liver diseases. *Progress in Liver Disease*, vol. 6, p. 539, eds H. Popper and F. Schaffner. Grune and Stratton, New York.

63. LONG R.G., MEINHARD E., SKINNER R.K. *et al* (1978) Clinical, biochemical and histological studies of osteomalacia, osteoporosis and parathyroid function in chronic liver disease. *Gut* **19**, 85.

64. LONG R.G., SCHEUER P.J. & SHERLOCK S. (1977) Presentation and course of asymptomatic primary biliary cirrhosis. *Gastroenterology* **72**, 1204.

65. MACMAHON H.E. & THANNHAUSER S.J. (1949) Xanthomatous biliary cirrhosis (a clinical syndrome). *Ann. intern. Med.* **30**, 121.

66. MAGNANI H.N. & ALAUPOVIC P. (1976) Utilisation of the quantitative assay of lipoprotein X in the differential diagnosis of extrahepatic obstructive jaundice and intrahepatic diseases. *Gastroenterology* **71**, 87.

67. MORGAN M.Y., ROSS M.G.R., NG C.M. *et al* (1980) HLA-B8, immunoglobulins and antibody responses in alcohol-related liver disease. *J. clin. Pathol.* **33**, 488.

68. MORRIS J.S., GALLO G.A., SCHEUER P.J. *et al* (1975) Percutaneous liver biopsy in patients with large bile duct obstruction. *Gastroenterology* **68**, 750.

69. MURPHY G.M., ROSS A. & BILLING B.H. (1972) Serum bile acids in primary biliary cirrhosis. *Gut* **13**, 201.

70. NAKANUMA Y. & OHTA G. (1979) Histometric and serial section observations of the intrahepatic bile ducts in primary biliary cirrhosis. *Gastroenterology* **76**, 1326.

71. PAUMGARTNER G. (1977) *Physiology I: Bile Acid-dependent Bile Flow in Liver and Bile*, eds L. Bianchi, W. Gerok & K. Sickinger, Falk Symposium 23. MTP, Lancaster.

72. PHILLIPS M.J., ODA M., MAK E. *et al* (1975) Microfilament dysfunction as a possible cause of intrahepatic cholestasis. *Gastroenterology* **69**, 48.

73. RAI G.S., HAMLYN A.N., DAHL M.G.C. *et al* (1977) Primary biliary cirrhosis, cutaneous capillaritis and IgM-associated membranous glomerulonephritis. *Br. med. J.* i, 817.

74. REYNOLDS T.B. (1973) The 'Butterfly' sign in patients with chronic jaundice and pruritus. *Ann. intern. Med.* **78**, 545.

75. REYNOLDS T.B., DENISON E.K., FRANKL H.D. *et al* (1971) Primary biliary cirrhosis with scleroderma, Raynaud's phenomenon and telangiectasia: new syndrome. *Am. J. Med.* **50**, 302.

76. ROUTHIER G., EPSTEIN O., JANOSSY G. *et al* (1980) Effects of cyclosporin A on suppressor and inducer T lymphocytes in primary biliary cirrhosis. *Lancet* ii, 1223.

77. RUBIN E., SCHAFFNER F. & POPPER H. (1965) Primary biliary cirrhosis. Chronic non-suppurative destructive cholangitis. *Am. J. Pathol.* **46**, 387.

78. SCHEUER P.J. (1967) Primary biliary cirrhosis. *Proc. R. Soc. Med.* **60**, 1257.

79. SCOTT A.J. & KHAN G.A. (1967) Origin of bacteria in bile duct bile. *Lancet* ii, 790.

80. SCOTT A.J. & KHAN G.A. (1968) Partial biliary obstruction with cholangitis producing a blind loop syndrome. *Gut* **9**, 187.

81. SHAPIRO J.M., SMITH H. & SCHAFFNER F. (1979) Serum bilirubin: a prognostic factor in primary biliary cirrhosis. *Gut* **20**, 137.

82. SHERLOCK S. (1959) Primary biliary cirrhosis (chronic intrahepatic obstructive jaundice). *Gastroenterology* **31**, 574.

83. SHERLOCK S. (1966) Biliary secretory failure in man. The problem of cholestasis. *Ann. intern. Med.* **65**, 397.

84. SHERLOCK S. (1972) The problem of chronic cholestasis. *J. R. Coll. Surg. Ed.* **17**, 1.

85. SHERLOCK S. & SCHEUER P.J. (1973) The presentation and diagnosis of 100 patients with primary biliary cirrhosis. *New Engl. J. Med.* **289**, 674.

86. SIMON J.B. & POON R.W.M. (1978) Lipoprotein-X levels in extrahepatic versus intrahepatic cholestasis. *Gastroenterology* **75**, 177.

87. SKINNER R.K., LONG R.G., SHERLOCK S. *et al* (1977) 25-hydroxylation of vitamin D in primary biliary cirrhosis. *Lancet* i, 720.

88. SMALLWOOD R.A., WILLIAMS H.A., ROSENOER V.M. *et al* (1968) Liver copper levels in liver disease: studies using neutron activation analysis. *Lancet* ii, 1310.

89. STANLEY N.N., FOX R.A., WHIMSTER W.F. *et al* (1972) Primary biliary cirrhosis or sarcoidosis—or both. *New Engl. J. Med.* **287**, 1282.

90. STUDDY P., BIRD R., JAMES D.G. *et al* (1978) Serum angiotensin-converting enzyme (SACE) in sarcoidosis and other granulomatous disorders. *Lancet* ii, 1331.

91. SUMMERFIELD J.A., ELIAS E., HUNGERFORD G.D. *et al* (1976) The biliary system in primary biliary cirrhosis: a study by endoscopic retrograde cholangiopancreatography. *Gastroenterology* **70**, 240.

92. SUMMERFIELD J.A., ELIAS E. & SHERLOCK S. (1975) Effects of clofibrate in primary biliary cirrhosis, hypercholesterolaemia and gallstones. *Gastroenterology* **69**, 998.

93. THOMAS H.C., POTTER B.J. & SHERLOCK S. (1977) Is primary biliary cirrhosis an immune complex disease? *Lancet* ii, 1261.

94. THOMAS P.K. & WALKER J.G. (1965) Xanthomatous neuropathy in primary biliary cirrhosis. *Brain* **88**, 1079.

95. TONG M.J., NIES K.M., REYNOLDS T.B. *et al* (1976) Immunological studies in familial primary biliary cirrhosis. *Gastroenterology* **71**, 305.

96. TYGSTRUP N. & JENSEN B. (1969) Intermittent intrahepatic cholestasis of unknown etiology in five young males from the Faroe Islands. *Acta med. Scand.* **186**, 523.

97. VARCO R.L. (1947) Intermittent external biliary drainage for relief of pruritus in certain chronic disorders of liver. *Surgery* **21,** 43.

98. VIERLING J.M., NELSON D.L., STROBER W. *et al* (1977) In vitro cell-mediated cytotoxicity in primary biliary cirrhosis and chronic hepatitis. *J. clin. Invest.* **60,** 1116.

99. WALKER J.G., DONIACH D., ROITT I.M. *et al* (1965) Serological tests in diagnosis of primary biliary cirrhosis. *Lancet* i, 827.

100. WANDS J.R., DIENSTAG J.L., BHAN A.K. *et al* (1978) Circulating immune complexes and complement activation in primary biliary cirrhosis. *New Engl. J. Med.* **298,** 233.

101. WILLIAMS R., CARTTER M., SHERLOCK S. *et al* (1964) Idiopathic recurrent cholestasis: a study of the functional and pathological lesions in four cases. *Q. J. Med.* **33,** 387.

102. YOUSEF I.M., KAKIS G. & FISHER M.M. (1976) Lithocholate-induced intrahepatic cholestasis. *Gastroenterology* **70,** 996.

103. ZEEGEN R., STANSFELD A.G., DAWSON A.M. *et al* (1969) Bleeding oesophageal varices as the presenting feature in primary biliary cirrhosis. *Lancet* ii, 9.

PRIMARY SCLEROSING CHOLANGITIS

All parts of the biliary tract, including the gall bladder, are involved in a chronic fibrosing inflammatory process. Histologically the wall of the gall bladder or bile ducts shows a cellular infiltrate of lymphocytes, plasma cells and sometimes eosinophils, with varying degrees of fibrosis. A similar reaction can be seen in the portal zones with periductular inflammation and fibrosis and occasional desquamation of epithelium (figs. 227, 228). Rarely bile duct carcinoma may develop.

The degree of involvement of the different parts of the biliary tract varies from patient to patient. Changes in the portal zones led to the term 'pericholangitis'. However, pericholangitis probably does not exist as a clinical entity divorced from primary sclerosing cholangitis. It merely represents the involvement of small intra-hepatic ducts in the sclerosing process.

AETIOLOGY

Over three-quarters of patients also suffer from ulcerative colitis. The biliary disease follows the colitis, which is usually diffuse, mild and chronic. The colonic disease tends to decrease in intensity when the biliary tract condition becomes apparent. The disease has been related to portal toxaemia and to bacteraemia from the diseased colon [8]. Bacteria have been found in veins draining the colon of patients with ulcerative colitis [7]. Material reaching the liver in the portal vein may be drained from the interstitial spaces by portal lymphatics and a pericholangitis could thus arise. This explanation seems unlikely for the extent of the histological change is unrelated to whether or not the portal blood gives a positive bacteriological culture [7]. Culture of liver biopsies has given negative results. Moreover, the hepato-biliary features do not improve with broad-spectrum antibiotic therapy or after colectomy.

Other associations include Riedel's struma,

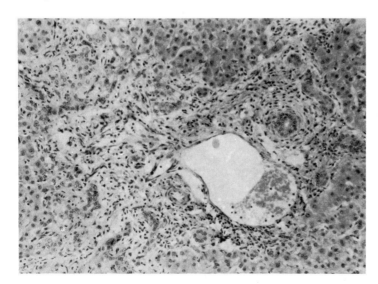

Fig. 227. Sclerosing cholangitis and pericholangitis. The portal zone is oedematous and expanded with proliferated bile ducts and an inflammatory cell infiltrate. H & E, × 160 (Thorpe *et al* 1967).

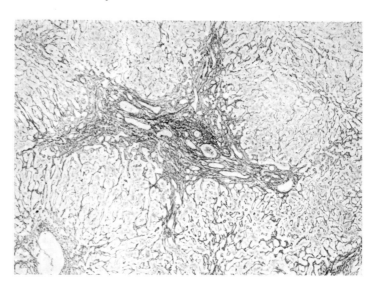

Fig. 228. Reticulin preparation of liver biopsy shows stellate expansion of portal zones (Thorpe *et al* 1967).

mediastinal and retro-peritoneal fibrosis, pancreatitis, orbital fibrosis, immuno-deficiency syndromes and Peyroni's disease [11, 14, 15, 17].

It is conceivable that toxic (deconjugated) bile acids, such as lithocholic acid, might be formed by bacterial action in the diseased colon. These could be absorbed into the portal blood and so excite pericholangitis. However, the liver metabolizes lithocholic acid with ease and this bile acid cannot be found in the bile and portal blood of patients with inflammatory bile disease [13].

CLINICAL FEATURES [5] (table 32)

Males are twice as commonly affected as females. They usually present between the ages of 25 and 45, but the disease has been seen in a girl of 10. The usual presentation is as cholangitis with inter-

Table 32. Symptoms at presentation in 29 patients with primary sclerosing cholangitis (Chapman *et al* 1980). *n*=number of patients.

Symptoms	*n*	%
Jaundice	21	72
Pruritus	20	69
Weight loss	23	79
Right upper quadrant pain	21	72
Acute cholangitis	13	45
Bleeding oesophageal varices	4	14
Malaise	1	3
Asymptomatic	2	7
Total	29	

mittent fever, rigors and jaundice. Icterus lasts weeks or months but occasionally as long as two years. Weight loss, pruritus and right upper quadrant pain are other features.

The patient may present as established cirrhosis with portal hypertension. This can develop [10] in those with asymptomatic pericholangitis and without cirrhosis. It is of pre-sinusoidal type and presumably related to the portal zone inflammation.

Finally the patient may be asymptomatic and without jaundice [4]. The diagnosis may be made incidentally when a raised serum alkaline phosphatase level is discovered.

Evidences of ulcerative colitis (but not regional ileitis, Crohn's disease) should be sought by barium enema, sigmoidoscopy and by rectal biopsy. The liver disease may appear long after the colitis, which in any case is mild to moderate. The liver disease does not correlate with the activity of the colitis, which tends to decrease when the cholangitis appears.

LABORATORY INVESTIGATIONS

Serum biochemical tests usually show cholestasis with alkaline phosphatase three times above normal and the serum immunoglobulin M (IgM) increased. Serum bilirubin values are variable. They can exceed 10 mg/dl, but this is unusual.

The serum mitochondrial antibody is always absent.

Eosinophilia is a rare finding.

LIVER BIOPSY [5] (table 33)

The portal zones are infiltrated with small and large lymphocytes, polymorphs and occasional macrophages and eosinophils (fig. 227). The interlobular ductules show a periductular inflammation with occasional epithelial desquamation. Intra-lobular inflammatory cell accumulations may be noted and the Kupffer cells are swollen and prominent. Cholestasis is inconspicuous unless jaundice is deep.

As the disease continues fibrosis develops in the portal tracts until the small ducts are surrounded by a cuff of fibrous tissue. The portal zones adopt a stellate appearance (fig. 228).

The appearances are not diagnostic, but the association of reduced numbers of bile ducts, ductular proliferation and substantial copper deposition [12] with piecemeal necrosis is very suggestive of primary sclerosing cholangitis and indicates the need for cholangiography [5].

Table 33. Histological findings in 29 patients with primary sclerosing cholangitis (Chapman *et al* 1980).

	−	+	+ +
Portal changes			
Inflammation	0	17	12
Bile duct diminution	12	10	7
Periductal fibrosis	18	9	2
Bile ductular proliferation	4	7	18
Lobular changes			
Piecemeal necrosis	10	8	11
Focal necrosis	11	18	0
Focal inflammation	12	17	0
Kupffer cell hyperplasia	5	11	13

CHOLANGIOGRAPHY [2, 3, 5]

Endoscopic retrograde cholangiography (ERCP) is the most successful technique although the bile ducts can often be visualized by percutaneous trans-hepatic cholangiography. The appearances are diagnostic with areas of irregular stricturing and dilatation (beading) of the intra-hepatic and extra-hepatic biliary tree (fig. 229). Cholangiograms may show involvement of the intra-hepatic ducts alone [1] or the extra-hepatic ducts alone.

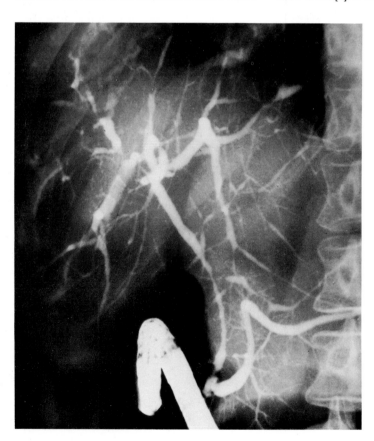

Fig. 229. ERCP in primary sclerosing cholangitis shows an irregular common bile duct and beading irregularities in the intra-hepatic bile ducts.

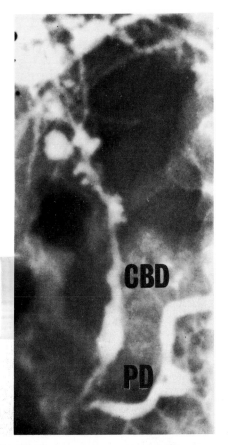

Fig. 230. Endoscopic retrograde cholangio-
pancreatography (ERCP) in sclerosing cholangitis.
The lower portion of the common bile duct (CBD)
is narrowed and intra-hepatic duct narrowing and
irregularity are also obvious. The pancreatic duct
(PD) is also visualized (Elias *et al* 1974).

DIAGNOSIS

Criteria for the diagnosis [16] of sclerosing cholangitis are: (1) diffuse generalized involvement of the
extra-hepatic ducts, (2) absence of previous biliary
surgery, (3) absence of gall-stones and (4)
exclusion of carcinoma of the bile ducts by a
reasonably long follow-up.

The cholangiographic appearances and the
negative mitochondrial antibody test distinguish
primary sclerosing cholangitis from primary
biliary cirrhosis.

Primary sclerosing cholangitis can present as
cryptogenic cirrhosis, the biliary lesions being unrecognized. The increased serum alkaline phosphatase provides the clue to the diagnosis and indicates cholangiography. The exclusion of a bile

duct carcinoma is difficult although the cholangiographic appearances of bile duct cancer with total
biliary obstruction of a nipple-like nature are
suggestive (fig. 231).

The differentiation from secondary sclerosing
cholangitis, due to such conditions as benign
post-operative biliary stricture or choledocholithiasis, depends on the history of previous surgery
or the demonstration of gall-stones.

PROGNOSIS

The main complications are recurrent acute cholangitis and bleeding from oesophageal varices.
The duration is very variable. Some patients can
be asymptomatic for as long as six years [4], while
others develop deep jaundice and liver failure and
are dead in a few months. In one series the mean
duration in 11 patients from onset of symptoms
to death was seven years [5].

An increased frequency of bile duct carcinoma
is recognized in patients with primary sclerosing
cholangitis.

TREATMENT

This is in general unsatisfactory. Corticosteroids
are not beneficial, but assessment of treatment in

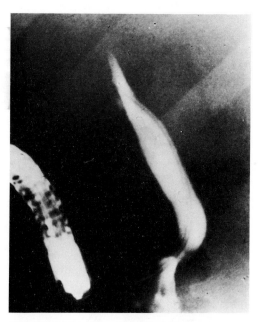

Fig. 231. ERCP in bile duct carcinoma shows the
common bile duct terminating in a nipple-like
deformity.

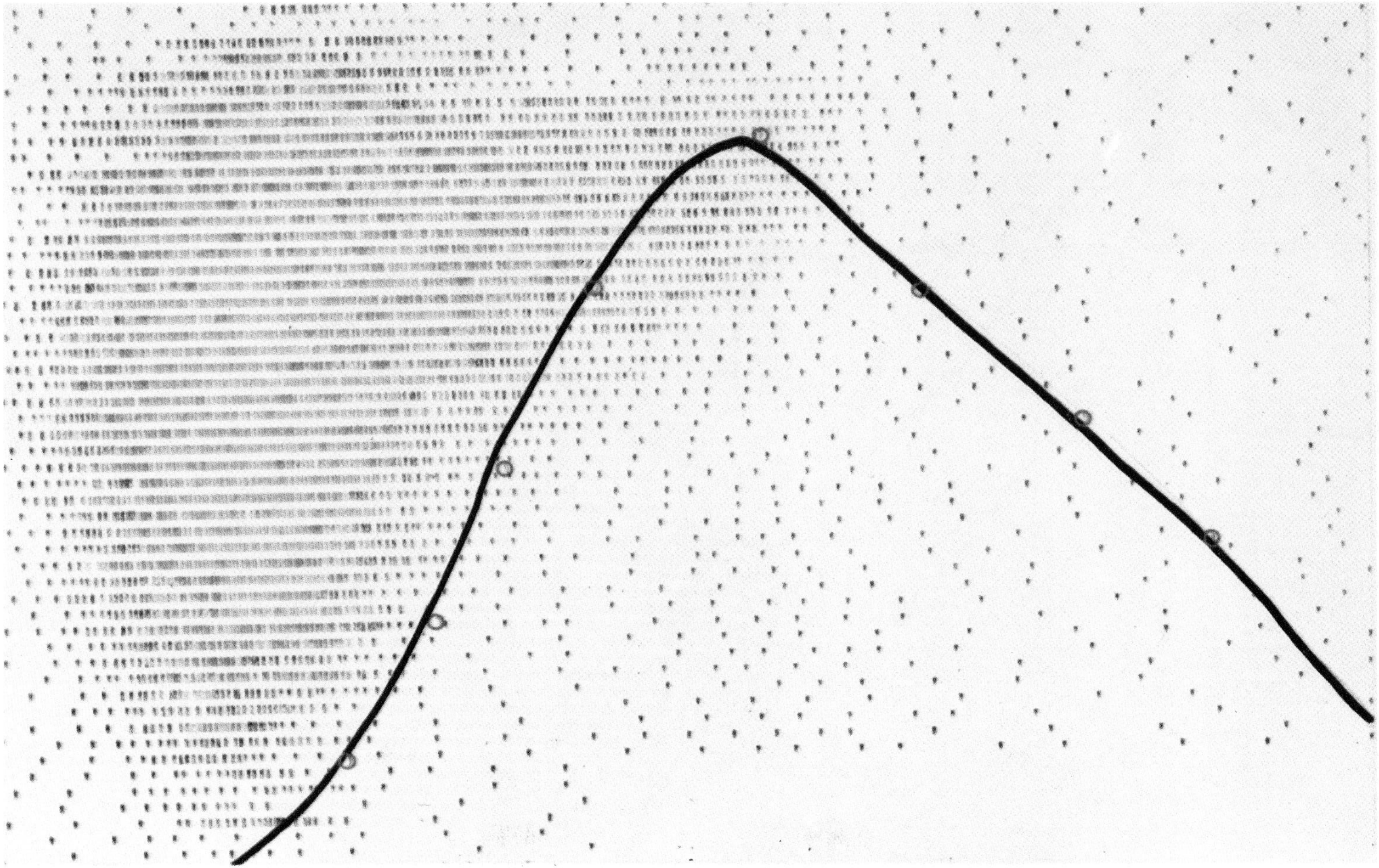

Fig. 40. Scintiscan of normal human liver using ^{198}Au. The costal margin is outlined.

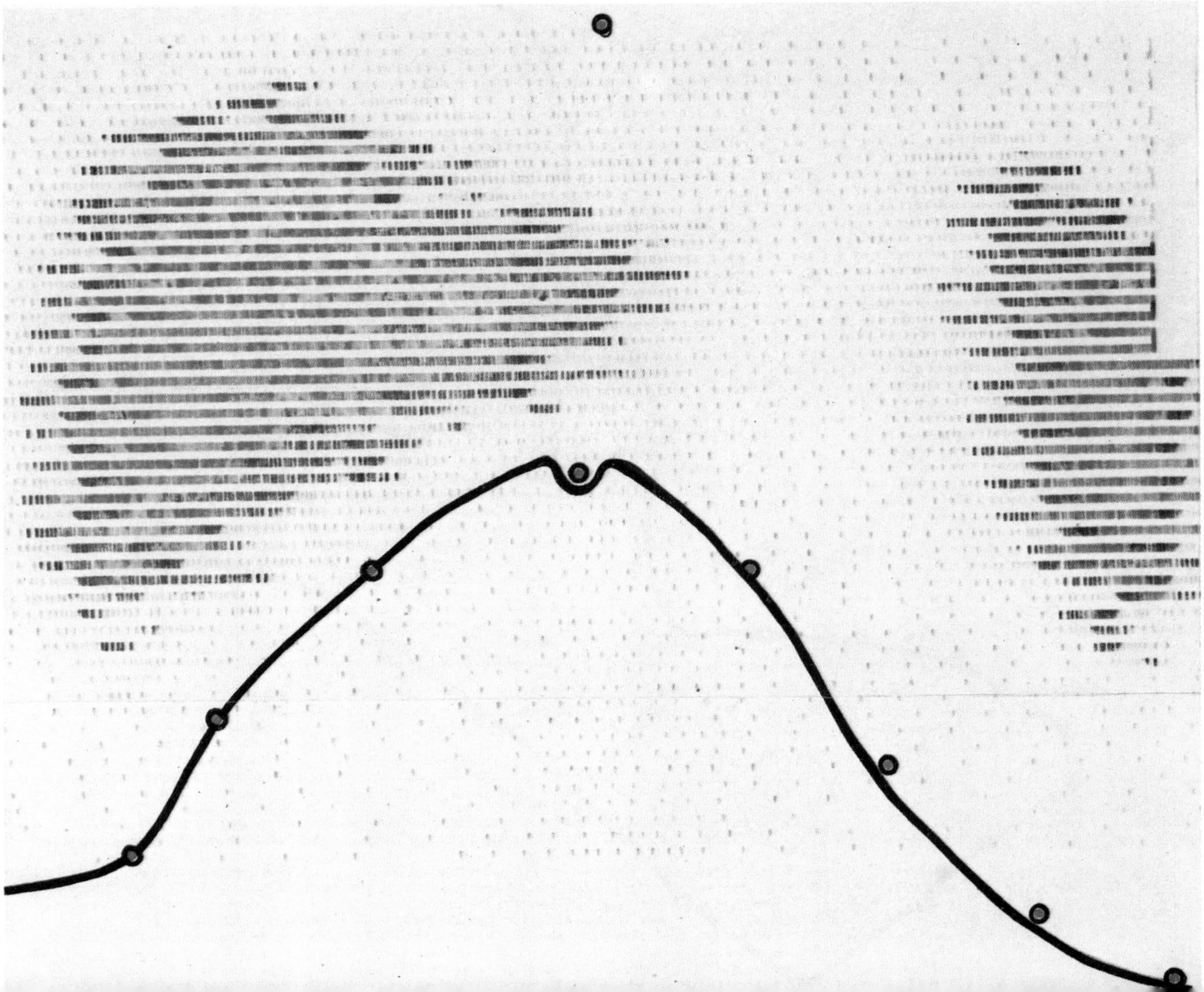

Fig. 41. Scintiscan using ^{198}Au in a patient with cirrhosis of the liver. Much of the isotope has been taken up by the spleen.

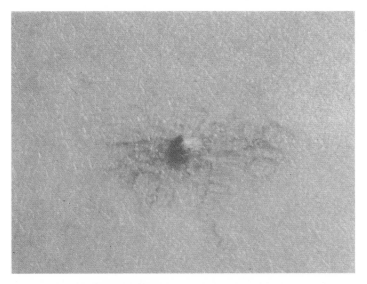

Fig. 74. A vascular spider. Note the elevated centre and radiating branches.

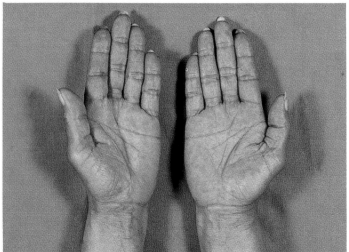

Fig. 76. Palmar erythema ('liver palms') in a patient with hepatic cirrhosis.

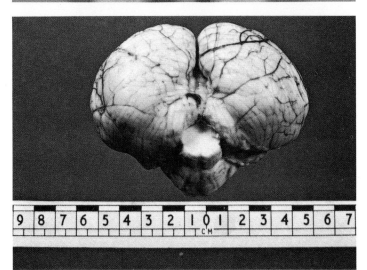

Fig. 84. Cerebral oedema in a patient who died in hepatic coma. Note the indented cerebellum.

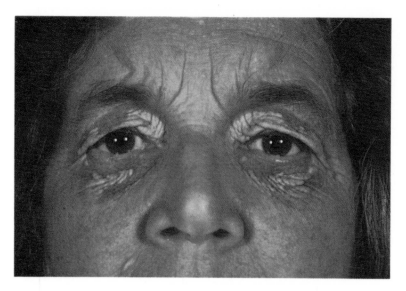

Fig. 193. Primary biliary cirrhosis. The patient shows xanthelasma and pigmentation.

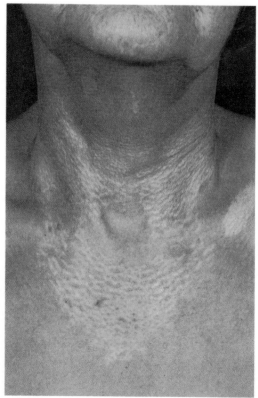

Fig. 194. Primary biliary cirrhosis. Xanthomatous skin lesions in the necklace area.

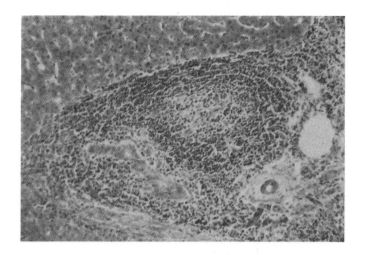

Fig. 218. Primary biliary cirrhosis. The portal zone contains a well-formed granuloma. An adjacent bile duct shows damage.

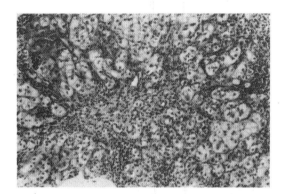

Fig. 255. Chronic active liver disease. The lobular architecture is completely disturbed. Isolated groups of liver cells, which often assume a rosette-like appearance, are separated by the septa of connective tissue. Remaining cells are large with clear cytoplasm. Lymphocytic and plasma cell infiltration is conspicuous. H & E, × 40 (Sherlock 1962).

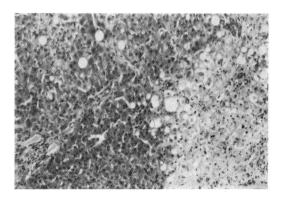

Fig. 285. Accidental carbon tetrachloride poisoning. To the right of the section liver cells are necrotic and show hydropic degeneration and fatty change. Surviving liver cells to the left of the section show occasional fatty change. The portal zones are unaffected (Sherlock 1962).

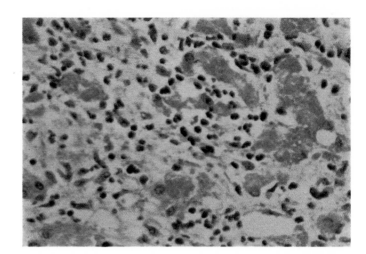

Fig. 316. Mallory's hyaline is shown as a pinkish deposit in the liver cell. H & E.

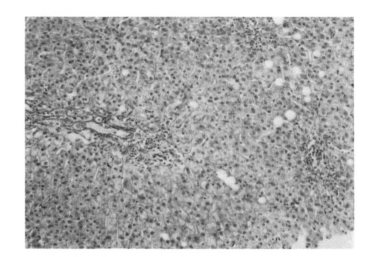

Fig. 317. Centrizonal areas show creeping alcoholic sclerosing hyaline necrosis. There is some periportal fatty change and the portal zones show cellularity. Trichrome, × 40.

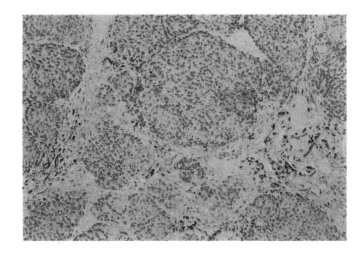

Fig. 324. The liver in idiopathic haemochromatosis. Cirrhosis is seen, the liver cells being filled with blue-staining iron pigment. Fibrous tissue is also infiltrated with iron. Perls, × 13.

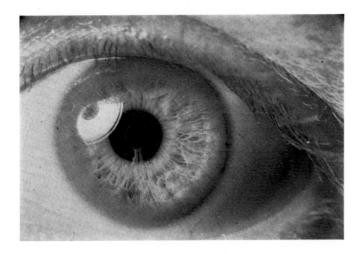

Fig. 334. Kayser–Fleischer ring. A brownish deposit is seen at the periphery of the cornea.

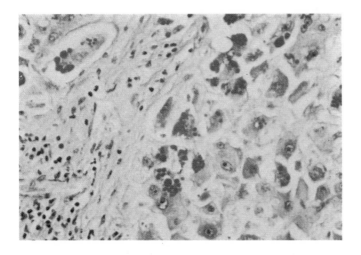

Fig. 344. α$_1$ anti-trypsin deficiency. Liver biopsy shows bright red deposits in periportal liver cells when stained by periodic acid Schiff after diastrase digestion. PAS, × 100.

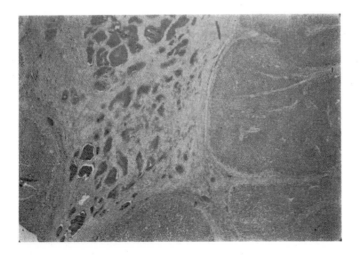

Fig. 346. The cirrhosis accompanying hereditary haemorrhagic telangiectasia. Note spaces filled with blood at the periphery of the lobules.

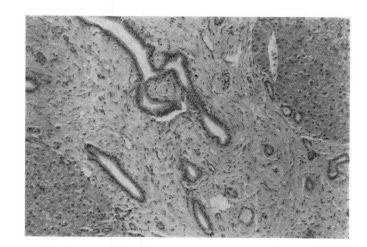

Fig. 358. Congenital hepatic fibrosis. Portal area shows dense mature fibrous tissue with a number of abnormal bile ducts. H & E, × 40.

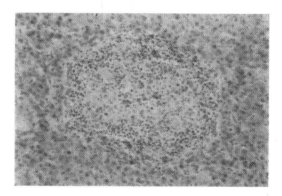

Fig. 361. Sarcoidosis. A well-demarcated granuloma is seen with surrounding lymphocytes and central, pale-staining epitheloid cells. H & E, × 84.

this rare disease is difficult because survival is variable and some patients remain asymptomatic for long periods. In view of the hazards of corticosteroids, accentuating osteoporosis in patients with cholestasis, these drugs should be avoided in primary sclerosing cholangitis.

In patients with ulcerative colitis removal of the colon does not influence the course of primary sclerosing cholangitis which can even become overt after colectomy.

Laparotomy is not required for diagnosis. Surgery is indicated in the minority of patients with complete main bile duct obstruction and to exclude bile duct carcinoma. Surgery may also be required to remove sludge and stones above strictures.

Intra-ductal prostheses (fig. 416) inserted transhepatically may be useful if strictures are tight and not susceptible to surgical relief [6, 9].

In view of the heavy copper deposition in the liver, D-*penicillamine* has been given. Analysis of a controlled trial now in progress will show whether or not it is beneficial.

Episodes of acute cholangitis are treated by antibiotics.

REFERENCES

1. BHATHAL P.S. & POWELL L.W. (1969) Primary intrahepatic obliterating cholangitis: a possible variant of 'sclerosing cholangitis'. *Gut* **10**, 886.
2. BLACKSTONE M.O. & NEMCHAUSKY B.A. (1978) Cholangiographic abnormalities in ulcerative colitis and associated pericholangitis which resembled sclerosing cholangitis. *Am. J. dig. Dis.* **23**, 579.
3. CELLO J.P. *et al* (1977) Cholestasis in ulcerative colitis. *Gastroenterology* **73**, 357.
4. CHAPMAN R.W.G. & SHERLOCK S. (1980) Asymptomatic primary sclerosing cholangitis. *Digestion.* In press.
5. CHAPMAN R.W.G., ARBORGH B.A.M., RHODES J.M. *et al* (1980) Primary sclerosing cholangitis— a review of its clinical features, cholangiography and hepatic histology. *Gut* **21**, 870.
6. DOOLEY J.S., DICK R., OLNEY J. *et al* (1979) Non-surgical treatment of biliary obstruction. *Lancet* ii, 1040.
7. EADE M.N. & BROOKE B.N. (1969) Portal bacteraemia in cases of ulcerative colitis submitted to colectomy. *Lancet* i, 1008.
8. KLECKNER M.S., STAUFFER M.H., BARGEN J.A. *et al* (1952) Hepatic lesions in the living patient with chronic ulcerative colitis as demonstrated by needle biopsy. *Gastroenterology* **22**, 13.
9. LUPINETTI M., MEHIGAN D. & CAMERON J.L. (1980) Hepato-biliary complications of ulcerative colitis. *Am. J. Surg.* **139**, 113.
10. MCCARTHY C.F. & READ A.E. (1962) Bleeding esophageal varices in ulcerative colitis. *Gastroenterology* **42**, 325.
11. RECORD C.O., EDDLESTON A.L.W.F., SHILKIN K.B. *et al* (1973) Intrahepatic sclerosing cholangitis associated with a familial immunodeficiency syndrome. *Lancet* ii, 18.
12. RITLAND S., ELGIO K., JOHANSEN O. *et al* (1979) Liver copper content in patients with inflammatory bowel disease and associated liver disorders. *Scand. J. Gastroenterol.* **14**, 711.
13. SIEGEL J.H., BARNES S. & MORRIS J.S. (1977) Bile acids in liver disease associated with inflammatory bowel disease. *Digestion* **15**, 469.
14. SMITH M.P. & LOE R.H. (1965) Sclerosing cholangitis. Review of recent case reports and associated diseases and four new cases. *Am. J. Surg.* **110**, 239.
15. VITERI A.L., HARDIN W.J. & DYCK W.P. (1979) Peyroni's disease and sclerosing cholangitis in a patient with ulcerative colitis. *Am. J. dig. Dis.* **24**, 490.
16. WARREN K.W., ATHANASSIADES S. & MONGE J.I. (1966) Primary sclerosing cholangitis. A study of forty-two cases. *Am. J. Surg.* **111**, 23.
17. WENGER J., GINGRICH G.W. & MEDELOFF J. (1965) Sclerosing cholangitis—a manifestation of systemic disease. *Arch intern. Med.* **116**, 509.

Chapter 15
Virus Hepatitis

The first reference to epidemic jaundice has been ascribed to Hippocrates. The earliest record in Western Europe is in a letter written in AD 751 by Pope Zacharias to St Boniface, Archbishop of Mainz. Since then there have been numerous accounts of epidemics, particularly during wars. Hepatitis was a problem in the Franco–Prussian War, the American Civil War and World War I. In World War II huge epidemics occurred, particularly in the Middle East and Italy [96].

Knowledge of virus hepatitis has expanded greatly in the last 10 years, and several excellent monographs on the subject have been published [9, 51, 80, 90, 95].

HEPATIC PATHOLOGY

The basic pathology of virus A, B and non-A, non-B hepatitis is virtually identical [23, 45].

The essential lesion is an acute inflammation of the entire liver [23, 75]. Hepatic cell necrosis is associated with leucocytic and histiocytic reaction and infiltration. The centres of the lobule show the necrosis most markedly and the portal tracts the greatest cellularity (figs. 232, 233). The sinusoids show hyperplasia of Kupffer cells, polymorphs and eosinophils. Surviving liver cells retain their glycogen. Fatty change is absent. Centrizonal liver cells may show eosinophilic change (*acidophil bodies*), ballooning pleomorphism and hyalinization, and giant multinucleated cells may be present. Mitoses are sometimes prominent. Centrizonal cholestasis may be found. Focal 'spotty' necrosis may be seen. Bile duct proliferation is usual and damage is an occasional feature [70]. Histological changes are found even before the development of jaundice.

The reticulin framework is usually well preserved even in the midst of extreme disorganization. This framework provides a scaffolding when the liver cells regenerate from without inwards, the cells adjoining the hepatic vein being the last to recover. Inflammatory cells disappear gradually from the portal tracts, and some new portal con-

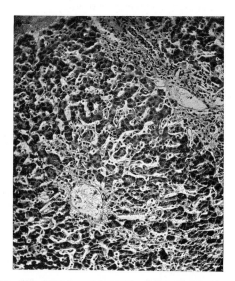

Fig. 232. Mild type A hepatitis. Cellular infiltration of portal zones and sinusoids and slight centrizonal disappearance and pleomorphism of liver cells. Best's carmine, × 90 (Sherlock 1946).

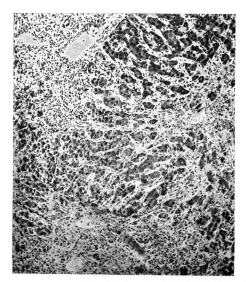

Fig. 233. Severe type B hepatitis. To the right of the section the centrizonal cells have disappeared and are replaced by cellular debris. The portal zones are heavily infiltrated, mainly by mononuclears. Best's carmine, × 65 (Sherlock 1946).

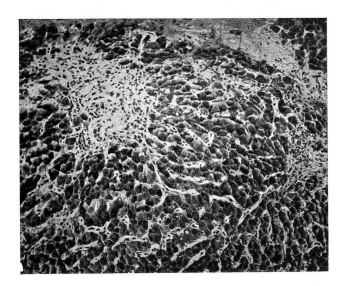

Fig. 234. Residual portal zone scarring seen 33 days after the onset of jaundice. Best's carmine, × 100 (Sherlock 1946).

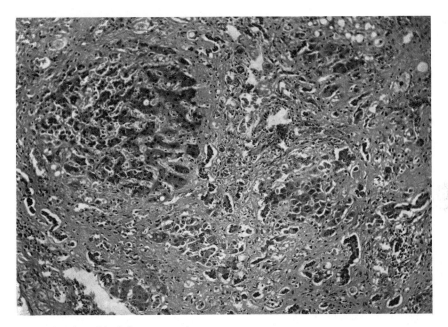

Fig. 235. Acute virus hepatitis. Sub-acute massive necrosis with nodular regeneration. H & E, × 120.

nective tissue can often be found for many months (fig. 234). During recovery reticulo-endothelial activity increases throughout, apparently a 'scavenger' phenomenon. A slight increase in stainable fat is seen. The Kupffer cells contain lipofuscin pigment and iron.

Occasionally the necrosis may be *confluent* (submassive), affecting substantial groups of adjacent liver cells, usually centrizonal.

In massive fulminant necrosis the whole lobule is involved. Macroscopically the liver is reduced in size, being smallest in those who died the soonest. It is flaccid and shrunken and the left lobe may be disproportionately atrophied. Nodular regeneration is seen in those surviving for more than two weeks (fig. 235). The cut surface shows a 'nutmeg' appearance, red areas of haemorrhage alternating with yellow patches of necrosis.

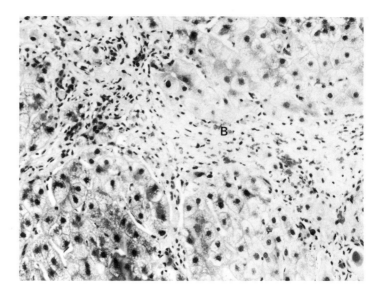

Fig. 236. Acute virus hepatitis. A passive septum (bridge) (B) has formed between portal and central areas. H & E, × 225.

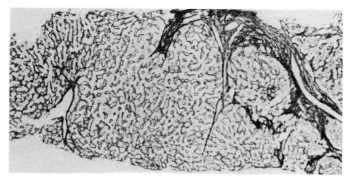

Fig. 237. Post-necrotic scarring. The liver biopsy specimen shows scarring, involving and extending from portal tracts. Reticulin, × 34.

Necrosis in life is always less than that seen in autopsy material as autolysis proceeds particularly rapidly in the presence of acute hepatitis.

If the confluent necrosis extends from centri-zonal areas to portal zones the reticulum collapses leaving connective tissue septa. This is termed *bridging* (fig. 236) [11]. Such bridging may be fol-lowed by the development of active fibrous septa, nodules and cirrhosis. More usually it is followed by scar formation (*post necrotic scarring*) (fig. 237).

Continuation of inflammatory activity and fibrosis in the portal zones with an undisturbed limiting plate gives the picture of *chronic persistent hepatitis.*

The portal zones may enlarge and become irregular. Liver cell necrosis is seen at the junction of the portal zone, and *active* septa extend into the lobule (see Chapter 16). This is *chronic active hepa-titis.* Evidence of recent acute hepatitis such as pleomorphism and cell dropout centrally may be seen.

Electron microscopy

This shows non-specific changes. The rough endo-plasmic reticulum is disrupted into vesicles and adherent ribosomes becomes detached. Large and irregular lysosomes develop which form auto-phagic vacuoles. The light cells represent ballooned cells and dark cells the eosinophilic bodies and de-hydrated remnants of hepatocytes. Mitochondria are clumped, forming hyaloplasmic blebs. Macro-phages have approached the sinusoidal cell sur-face.

During healing, the many polyribosomes form new profiles of endoplasmic reticulum and the smooth endoplasmic reticulum hypertrophies.

Changes in other organs

Regional lymph nodes are large. Splenomegaly is related to cellular proliferation and venous con-gestion. The bone marrow is moderately hypoplastic, but maturation is usually normal. Fatal marrow aplasia has, however, been reported [39]. The pathogenesis is obscure. In about 15% of fatal cases there is ulceration of the gastro-intestinal tract—particularly caecal.

The brain shows an acute non-specific degeneration of ganglion cells. Because of the short duration, the cerebral lesions of hepatic coma (Chapter 7) are rarely evident. Occasionally acute pancreatitis and myocarditis have been noted. Haemorrhages are found in most organs.

Virus hepatitis is a multi-system infection involving many organs.

CLINICAL TYPES

Note is taken of jaundiced contacts, recent travel, injections, tattooing, dental treatment, transfusions or ingestion of shell fish. All drugs taken in the previous two months are listed.

Hepatic involvement, to the extent of jaundice, is an *infrequent* complication of a rather common virus infection. The picture varies widely, ranging from slight malaise to a severe and fatal disease culminating in hepatic coma.

In general, type A, type B and non-A, non-B hepatitis run the same clinical course. Type B tends to be more severe and may be associated with a serum sickness-like syndrome (page 256).

The mildest attack is without symptoms and marked only by a rise in serum transaminase levels. Alternatively, the patient may still be anicteric but suffer gastro-intestinal and influenza-like symptoms. Such patients are likely to remain undiagnosed unless there is a clear history of exposure or the patient is being followed up after a blood transfusion. Increasing grades of severity are then encountered ranging from the icteric, from which recovery is usual, through to fulminant, fatal viral hepatitis.

The usual icteric attack in the adult is marked by a prodromal period, usually about three or four days even up to two or three weeks, during which the patient feels generally unwell, suffers digestive symptoms, particularly anorexia and nausea, and may, in the later stages, have a mild pyrexia. Rigors are unusual. An ache develops in the right upper abdomen. There is loss of desire to smoke or to drink alcohol. Malaise is profound and increases towards evening; the patient feels wretched.

Occasionally headache may be severe and, in children, its association with neck rigidity may suggest meningitis. Protein and lymphocytes in the CSF may be raised.

The prodromal period is followed by darkening of the urine and lightening of the faeces. This heralds the development of jaundice and symptoms decrease. The temperature returns to normal and there may be bradycardia. Appetite returns and abdominal discomfort and vomiting cease. Pruritus may appear transiently for a few days.

The liver is palpable with a smooth, tender edge in 70%. Heavy percussion over the right lower ribs posteriorly causes sickening discomfort. The spleen is palpable in about 20% of patients. This reflects portal hypertension and cellular infiltration.

The adult loses about 4 kg weight. A few vascular spiders may appear transiently.

After an icteric period of about one to four weeks the adult patient makes an uninterrupted recovery. In children, improvement is particularly rapid and jaundice mild or absent. The stools regain their colour. The appetite returns. After apparent recovery lassitude and fatigue persist for some weeks. Clinical and biochemical recovery is usual within six months of onset.

PROLONGED CHOLESTASIS

Occasionally, prolonged jaundice is of cholestatic type. Onset is acute, jaundice appears and deepens but, within three weeks, the patient starts to itch. After the first few weeks the patient feels well, gains weight and there are no physical signs apart from icterus and slight hepatomegaly. Jaundice persists for 8–29 weeks and recovery is then complete [30, 79].

Liver biopsy shows conspicuous cholestasis which tends to mask the definite, usually mild, hepatitis that is also present.

This type must be differentiated from surgical obstructive jaundice. The acute onset and only moderately enlarged liver are the most helpful points. Cholestatic drug jaundice is excluded by the history.

Prednisolone (30 mg daily for five days) may be diagnostically useful [fig. 238]. A fall in serum bilirubin level of more than 40% suggests a hepatitis. If doubt remains needle biopsy is helpful. Surgical exploration is to be avoided as it may precipitate hepato-cellular failure.

The prognosis is usually excellent with complete clinical recovery and restitution of a normal liver [79].

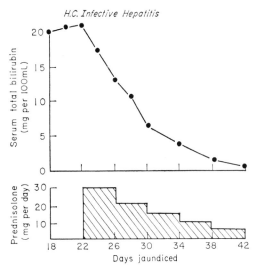

Fig. 238. Cholestatic virus hepatitis. Prednisolone therapy was associated with a fall in serum bilirubin values.

RELAPSES

These occur in 1.8–15%. In some the original attack is duplicated, usually in milder form, with prodromata, faecal pallor, bilinuria and jaundice. More often, the relapse is simply shown by an increase in serum transaminases and sometimes bilirubin. Hepatic histology is similar to that seen in the original attack. The relapse may be precipitated by premature activity or by taking large amounts of alcohol. Multiple episodes may occur. Recovery after relapses is usually complete. In some patients relapses may indicate progression to a chronic hepatitis.

FULMINANT HEPATITIS (Chapter 9)

This rare form of the disease usually overwhelms the patient within 10 days. It may develop so rapidly that jaundice is inconspicuous and the disease is confused with an acute psychosis or meningo-encephalitis. Alternatively, the patient, after a typical acute onset, becomes deeply jaundiced. Ominous signs are repeated vomiting, fetor hepaticus, confusion and drowsiness. The 'flapping' tremor may be only transient, but rigidity is usual. Coma supervenes rapidly and the picture becomes that of acute liver failure. Temperature rises, jaundice deepens and the liver shrinks. Widespread haemorrhages may be shown.

Leucocytosis may be found in contrast to the usual leucopenia of virus hepatitis. The biochemical changes are those of acute liver failure (Chapter 9). The height of the serum bilirubin and transaminase are poor indicators of prognosis. Transaminase levels may actually fall as the patient's clinical condition worsens. Blood coagulation is grossly deranged and a test of prothrombin is the best indicator of prognosis (figs. 29 and 96).

POST-HEPATITIS SYNDROME

Adult patients feel below par for variable periods after acute hepatitis. Usually this is a matter of weeks but it may extend to months. This is termed the post-hepatitis syndrome [81]. It is particularly common in the intelligent, perhaps because of their knowledge of the possible sequelae of hepatitis. Features are anxiety, fatigue, failure to regain weight, anorexia and alcohol intolerance, and right upper abdominal discomfort. The liver edge may be palpable and tender.

Serum transaminases may be raised up to three times normal. Too much attention should not be focused on them and they should not be repeated frequently. This exacerbates the anxiety and a 'transaminitis' is engendered. Serum globulin levels are normal.

Hepatic histology shows only mild, residual, portal zone cellularity and fibrosis with perhaps some fatty change in the liver cells. These features do not differ from those found in patients recovering normally who are now symptom-free. They rarely persist for longer than one year after the acute attack. In general, liver biopsy should not be performed too soon after acute hepatitis, certainly not less than six months, because of the difficulty in distinguishing the usual residual changes from an organic chronic hepatitis.

Treatment consists of reassurance after full investigation. If the acute attack has been type A, chronicity can be excluded.

Investigations

URINE AND FAECES

Bilirubin appears in the urine before jaundice. The urinary threshold for bilirubin varies in hepatitis. It is found before the serum level is raised; later it disappears although serum levels remain elevated.

Urobilinogenuria is found in the late pre-icteric phase. At the height of the jaundice, very little bilirubin reaches the intestine, so urobilinogen disappears. Its reappearance indicates commencing recovery. It persists in excess in gradually diminishing amounts until final recovery.

The onset of jaundice is marked by lightening of the faeces. There is moderate steatorrhoea. Reappearance of stool colour denotes impending recovery.

BLOOD CHANGES

Total serum bilirubin levels range widely. Deep jaundice generally implies a prolonged clinical course. An increase in conjugated pigment is early, even when the total bilirubin level is still normal.

Serum alkaline phosphatase level is usually less than three times the upper limit of normal. Serum albumin and globulin are quantitatively unchanged. The serum iron level is raised.

Serum immunoglobulins G and M are raised in about one-third of patients during the acute phase [2, 31].

Serum transaminase estimations are useful in early diagnosis, in detecting the anicteric case, and for detection of inapparent cases in epidemics. The peak level is found one or two days before or after onset of jaundice. Later in the course the level falls, even if the clinical condition is worsening. The estimation cannot be used prognostically. Values may remain elevated for six months in those who are recovering uneventfully.

In both type A and type B hepatitis antibody against smooth muscle is present, usually in low titre [32]. Mitochondrial antibody is absent [32].

HAEMATOLOGICAL CHANGES

The pre-icteric stage is marked by leucopenia, lymphopenia and neutropenia. These revert towards normal as jaundice appears. Some 5–28% show atypical lymphocytes (virucytes), resembling those seen in infectious mononucleosis. Acute Coombs' test positive haemolytic anaemia is a rare complication. Haemolysis is commonly precipitated in patients with glucose 6PD deficiency [15]. Aplastic anaemia is very rare and often fatal [39].

The *prothrombin time* is lengthened in the more severe cases and does not return completely to normal with vitamin K therapy.

The *sedimentation rate* of the red cells (ESR) is high in the pre-icteric phase, falls to normal with jaundice, and rises again when the jaundice subsides. It returns to normal with complete recovery.

NEEDLE LIVER BIOPSY

This is rarely indicated in the acute stage. It may occasionally be needed in older patients to differentiate from extra-hepatic cholestasis and from drug jaundice. It may be used to diagnose the presence and type of chronic complications but should not be performed less than six months after the acute episode else the distinction between the picture of normal recovery and chronic hepatitis may be impossible.

Differential diagnosis

In the *pre-icteric stage*, hepatitis can be confused with other acute infectious diseases, with acute surgical abdomen, especially acute appendicitis, and with acute gastro-enteritis. Bile in the urine, tender enlargement of the liver and a rise in serum transaminase values are the most helpful points. In type B the antigen appears transiently. The distinction from infectious mononucleosis is outlined in table 38.

In the *icteric stage*, the diagnosis must be made from surgical cholestasis. This is outlined in table 26.

The diagnosis of acute virus hepatitis from the drug-related disease depends largely on the history of taking the offending drugs.

Needle liver biopsy is valuable in the problem case. Attempts at surgical diagnosis are disastrous.

The distinction from Weil's disease is shown in table 66.

In the *post-icteric stage*, the diagnosis of organic from non-organic complications necessitates routine investigations for the diagnosis of chronic hepatitis, and these may include needle biopsy.

Prognosis

Type B infection carries the highest mortality. In a survey of 1675 cases in a group of Boston hospitals, 1 in 8 sufferers from transfusion hepatitis succumbed whereas only 1 in 200 died with the type A disease. As many non-icteric cases are not included in the statistics the overall mortality rate is undoubtedly very much lower.

Those who are elderly or in poor general health clearly have a poor prognosis. The commonest cause of fulminant viral hepatitis is type B, then type non-A, non-B, and rarely type A [1]. More males than females have type B. Fulminant hepatitis is rare in those less than 15 years old. The non-A, non-B patients tend to be more than 45. Survival rate is the same for males as for females. Survival for fulminant type B is 33% and for non-A, non-B 13%.

VIRUS A (HAV) HEPATITIS

The disease is due to a small 27 nm, cubically symmetrical, RNA enterovirus [34] (figs. 239, 240). The virus can be identified in the stool of sufferers from about two weeks before until one week after the onset of jaundice [24]. It has been transmitted to marmosets and chimpanzees and has been grown in foetal rhesus-cell culture and primary explants of marmoset's liver [72].

A serum antibody (anti-HAV) appears as the stool becomes negative for virus, reaches a maximum in several months and is detectable for many years (fig. 240). Positive diagnosis can be made by showing a rise in anti-HAV titres, but these can be detected in only about 50% of patients. Anti-HAV probably gives immunity from further infection with hepatitis A. The appearance of serum IgM anti-HAV is more helpful diagnostically and implies a recent infection. This antibody persists for only two to six months (fig. 241) [12, 21].

Chronic carriers have not been identified. Hepatitis A virus may be shown in human liver biopsies

by immunofluorescence during the acute stage [61].

Epidemiology

The disease occurs sporadically or in epidemic form and has an incubation time of 15–50 days. It is usually spread by the faecal–oral route. Parenteral transmission is rare if it ever occurs.

Age 5–14 is the group most affected and adults are often infected by spread from children.

With improving hygiene the prevalence is decreasing world wide. Young people, not previously exposed and visiting endemic areas, are increasingly becoming affected. In urban areas 29% (Switzerland) to 96.9% (Yugoslavia) of adults show circulating anti-HAV.

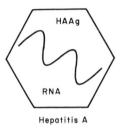

Fig. 240. Diagram of the hepatitis A virus shown as a hexagonal body containing single stranded RNA.

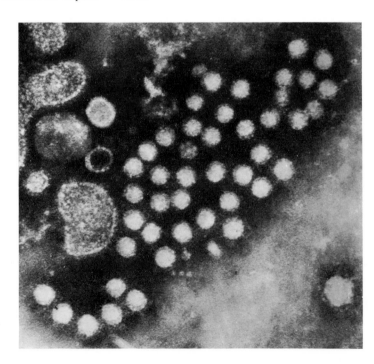

Fig. 239. Electron microscopy of hepatitis A antigen particles in faeces. These are shown as 22 nm spheres. × 250 000.

Table 34. Type A, type B, and non-A, non-B hepatitis contrasted.

	A	B	Non-A, non-B
Virus	RNA	DNA	DNA
Experimental animal	Marmoset	Chimpanzee	Chimpanzee
Tissue culture	Yes	No	No
Incubation (days)	15–20	50–60	7–50
Spread			
blood	No	Yes	Yes
faeces	Yes	No	No
saliva	Yes	Yes	No
vertical	No	Yes	No
Intra-family	Yes	Yes	Yes
Acute attack	Often mild	Severe	Mild
Onset	Acute	Insidious	Insidious
Serum sickness	No	Yes	No
Mortality	< 0.5%	1–5%	1–3%
Chronicity	No	10%	?20%
Liver cancer	No	Yes	?
Immunity			
homologous	Present	Present	?
heterologous	None	None	?
Antibody prevalence	60–70% (urban areas)	12–80% (geographic area)	?

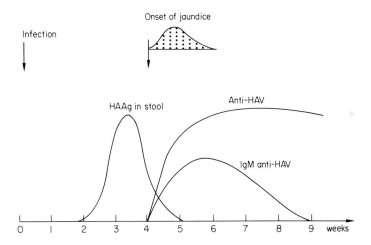

Fig. 241. Serology of hepatitis A infection.

Most sporadic cases follow person to person contact. Explosive water-borne and food-borne epidemics are described. In 1955, in Delhi, an epidemic followed floods and the diversion of sewage into a river, so contaminating the city water supply [63]. Chlorination of the water was increased but 335 000 cases of hepatitis were reported. Use of human sewage for soil fertilization can result in frozen-fruit-related epidemics.

Ingestion of raw clams and oysters from polluted waters is known to have caused three epidemics. Steaming the clams may not kill the virus for the temperature achieved inside the clams is not sufficiently high.

Contamination during preparation has resulted in transmission via other foods, including sandwiches, orange juice, potato salad and meat.

Clinical course

The hepatitis is usually mild, particularly in children where it is frequently anicteric, unrecognized and passed off as gastro-enteritis. The disease is more serious and prolonged in adults and may rarely be fulminant and fatal.

Prognosis

Prognosis is excellent, usually with full clinical recovery. Mortality rates in large epidemics are about one per 1000. The average young adult with icteric hepatitis can anticipate six weeks' illness and this will rarely exceed three months.

Chronicity does not develop. Follow-ups of large epidemics in World War I [19], the Korean conflict, and the Delhi outbreak [16] showed no long-term sequelae. Viral carriage is transient in faeces. The majority of adults have circulating antibodies and are immune.

TYPE B (HBV) HEPATITIS

In 1965, Blumberg and colleagues in Philadelphia found an antibody in two multiply-transfused haemophiliac patients which reacted with an antigen in a single serum in their panel and this came from an Australian Aborigine [10] (figs. 242, 243). Later the antigen was found in some 20% of patients with viral hepatitis. Because of its discovery in an aboriginal serum the antigen was called Australia antigen. In 1977, Blumberg was awarded the Nobel prize for his discovery. Australia antigen is now known to be the surface of the hepatitis B virion and is termed hepatitis B surface antigen (HBsAg).

Under the electron microscope three types of particle can be seen in hepatitis B serum: small 20 nm spheres, tubules 20 nm in diameter and 100 nm long, and the more complex 42 nm Dane

Table 35. Terminology of hepatitis A and B (WHO 1977).

HAV	Hepatitis A virus
Anti-HA	Antibody to hepatitis A virus
HBV	Hepatitis B virus
	The Dane particle
HBsAg	Hepatitis B surface antigen
HBcAg	Hepatitis B core antigen
HBeAg	The e antigen associated with hepatitis B infection and probably part of the core
Anti-HBs	Antibody to hepatitis B surface antigen
Anti-HBc	Antibody to hepatitis B core antigen
Anti-Hbe	Antibody to the e antigen

particles [20] (fig. 243). The Dane particle is the complete hepatitis B virus (HBV), whereas the small spheres and tubules are excess viral protein. The inner core remaining after detergent treatment of Dane particles is formed by the liver cell nucleus whereas the smaller particles are produced by multiplication in the cytoplasm [3].

The core of the Dane particle contains double stranded DNA, a DNA polymerase and core antigen (HBcAg). Another antigen, HBeAg, is probably part of the core (fig. 244). HBeAg has three specificities, HBeAg 1, 2, 3, of which HBeAg 3 is particularly associated with complete HBV viral replication [86].

HBsAg appears in the blood about six weeks after infection and has disappeared by three months [35] (fig. 245). Persistence for more than six months implies a carrier state [66]. It is usually

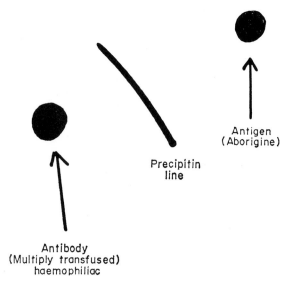

Fig. 242. Blumberg's discovery of Australia (hepatitis-associated) antigen. Antigen from a multiply-transfused haemophiliac reacted on an Ouchterlony plate with antigen from an Aborigine (Australian). Later, this antigen was demonstrated in the serum of patients with long incubation period hepatitis and termed hepatitis B antigen.

Antigen (Aborigine)

Precipitin line

Antibody (Multiply transfused) haemophiliac

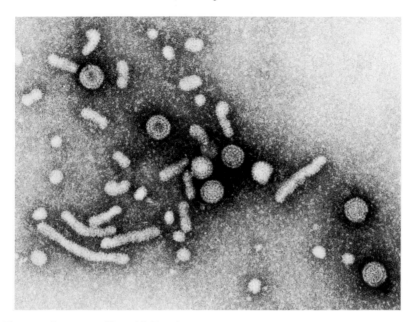

Fig. 243. Electron microscopy of hepatitis B antigen particles in blood. These are shown as spherical and tubular forms and the large Dane particles. × 250 000. (By courtesy of J.D. Almeida.)

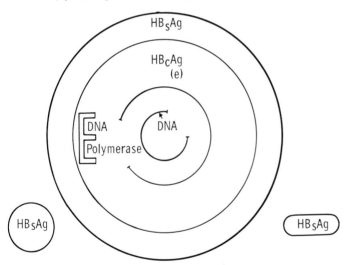

Fig. 244. Diagram of the virion of hepatitis B (HBV: Dane particle). The core contains DNA polymerase, double-stranded DNA, core antigen and e antigen. The surface consists of HBsAg. Spheres and tubules of HBsAg are free in the serum.

measured by RIA. Anti-HBs appears late, some three months after the onset of illness, and persists. Anti-HBs levels are rarely high and 10–15% of patients with acute type B hepatitis never develop antibody. Anti-HBs appears to confer immunity.

HBeAg appears after about one week of illness and has usually disappeared by two weeks. Persistence implies the carrier state and ongoing disease. Disappearance of HBeAg is followed by the appearance of anti-HBe which is present for many

months. HBeAg and anti-HBe are measured by RIA.

IgG antibody to the core antigen (anti-HBc) appears as the illness starts and persists for many months. It may be useful in diagnosing acute hepatitis B where tests for HBsAg are negative.

Specific DNA polymerase can be detected with difficulty by electron microscopy [52].

These markers are of some importance in diagnosing chronicity and identifying infectivity. Body

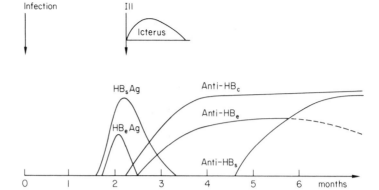

Fig. 245. Serology of hepatitis B infection (Frosner *et al* 1978).

fluids containing only HBsAg are not necessarily infectious and the presence of core markers is more significant. HBeAg and DNA polymerase imply ongoing infectivity. Continuing IgG HBcAb usually has the same meaning [44] but persistence of a IgM anti-HBc is more indicative of chronicity.

HBsAg may be shown stained orange with orcein in the hepatocytes of carriers and chronic hepatitis patients but not in the acute stage [22]. Electron microscopy and immune histology demonstrate HBcAg in nuclei and HBsAg in the membranes of liver cells [38]. Core markers are not found in the liver in the acute stage.

The disease has been transmitted to chimpanzees. The agent has not been grown in tissue culture.

Subdeterminants

HBsAg particles have surfaces that are antigenically complex [55]. This has led to the recognition of antigenic determinants [43].

a is a common determinant. Various combinations of other subdeterminants are designated d, y, w and r. The four major determinants are therefore adw, adr, ayw and ayr. Other variants are also described related to a, w and r [56]. Sub-types are useful epidemiologically. The sub-types are helpful in the sense that all cases in a single outbreak have been due to the same sub-type. Geographic differences exist in the predominant sub-type [55]. In Greece the main subdeterminant encountered is y; in France it is b. This is irrespective of clinical associations. The subdeterminant cannot be linked with any particular clinical entity.

Epidemiology (tables 36, 37)

Type B hepatitis is spread largely by whole blood and its products. Semen and saliva are also poss-

Table 36. Approximate percentage carrier rate for HBsAg (by RIA) in 'healthy' blood donors.

Scandinavia	0.1
United Kingdom	0.1
United States	0.1
Holland	0.2
Switzerland	0.2
Belgium	0.5
France	0.5
Spain	2.0
Southern Italy	3.0
Japan	3.0
Greece	5.0
South Africa	11.3
Taiwan	15.0
Singapore	15.0
Hong Kong	15.0

Table 37. Groups in which acute and chronic type-B hepatitis should be suspected.

Immigrants from Mediterranean countries, Africa or the Far East
Drug abusers
Homosexuals
Neonates of HBsAg, HBeAg-positive mothers
Hospital staff
Patients with
    renal failure
    reticuloses
    cancer
    organ transplants
Staff and patients of hospitals for mentally retarded
Post transfusion (paid donors)

ibly infectious. Other body fluids may contain HBsAg but not Dane particles and infectivity has not been established. The disease is transmitted parenterally or by intimate, often sexual, contact.

The carrier rate of HBsAg varies world wide from as low as 0.1–0.2% in Britain or the United States to more than 3% in Greece, Southern Italy and even up to 10–15% in Africa and the Far East (table 36). It is higher in urban than in rural areas. Immigrants with a high carrier rate, for instance Algerians in France and Vietnamese in Canada, increase the prevalence. Prevalence varies from area to area in the same country. In Northern Greece, for instance, the carrier rate is 7% compared with less than 3% in Athens [87]. If anti-HBs is measured, the rate of exposure to hepatitis B in any community is much higher [54]. There are thus millions of carriers of HBsAg all over the world. The majority are 'healthy', some suffer various forms of chronic hepatitis and some will develop cirrhosis and primary liver cancer.

How was the infection acquired? Vertical transmission, that is infection passing from a mother to the foetus or neonate, may be particularly important. The infection is usually not via the umbilical vein but from the mother at the time of birth and during close contact afterwards. The chance of transmission increases as term approaches and is greater with acute than chronic carriers. The mother is usually HBeAg positive. Antigenaemia develops in the baby within two months of birth and tends to persist [6].

In other areas the peak incidence is in childhood rather than in neonates and positive mothers are rare. In such countries, including Greece and Hong Kong, inter-family spread seems more likely. This may be by close contact such as kissing. Shared utensils, toothbrushes and razors may also be important. In the family group the sexual contacts of carriers are at risk. A carrier is more infectious if he has underlying acute or chronic liver disease than if the liver biopsy is normal [41]. Infectivity is greater from carriers who are HBeAg, DNA and HBc- and IgMAb-positive, indicating continuing viral replication [68].

Homosexuals are at risk of contracting hepatitis B (fig. 246). The number of their sexual contacts makes them an important means of spreading infection particularly in large urban areas such as Berlin, New York, London or San Francisco [42]. The mode of spread is uncertain and the type of sexual activity seems immaterial [59].

Blood-sucking arthropods such as mosquitoes or bed bugs may be important vectors, particularly in the tropics [13, 94]. However, there is no evidence that the virus replicates in the arthropod.

Infection in Swedish track-finders results from scratches acquired during the cross-country races and the communal washing afterwards [7].

Opportunities for parenteral infection include the use of unsterile instruments for dental treatment, ear piercing and manicures, neurological examination, prophylactic inoculations, subcutaneous injections, acupuncture, and tattooing (fig. 247) [60].

Parenteral drug abusers develop hepatitis from using shared, unsterile equipment. The mortality may be very high in this group. Multiple attacks are seen and chronicity is frequent. Liver biopsy may show, in addition to acute or chronic hepatitis, foreign material, such as chalk, injected with the illicit drug.

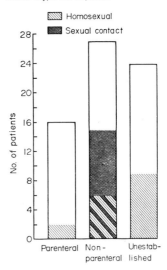

Fig. 246. The source of hepatitis B antigen infection in London. Note the high proportion where non-parenteral or unestablished sources of infection were found. Homo- or bisexual contact is an important source of spread (Heathcote & Sherlock 1973).

Blood transfusion in areas where routine screening of blood donors by radioimmunoassay is performed has caused hepatitis B, but this has largely been eliminated. It remains a problem in underdeveloped countries. Transmission is more likely if commercial blood from paid donors is used than when volunteer blood is transfused.

Hospital staff in contact with patients and especially patient's blood usually have a higher carrier rate than the general community. This applies particularly to staff on renal dialysis or oncology units. Patients are immuno-suppressed and, on contracting the disease, become chronic carriers [48]. Danger to the patient's attendant

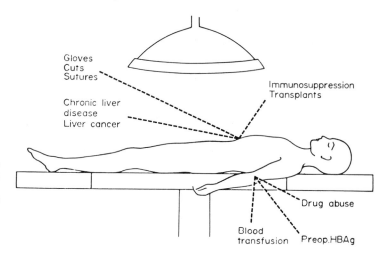

Fig. 247. The hepatitis hazard for hospital workers and particularly surgeons. This comes from skin lacerations and pricks when handling blood from a patient with a positive hepatitis B antigen test, especially those with chronic liver disease or cancer, those on immuno-suppression or having organ transplantation or abusing drugs. Care in handling all blood specimens is emphasized.

comes from contact with blood parenterally, such as from pricking or through skin abrasions. Surgeons and dentists may be particularly at risk in operating on patients with a positive HBsAg (fig. 247). Holes in gloves and cuts on hands are common. Wire sutures may be a particular hazard in penetrating the skin. Four surgeons developed hepatitis 80–105 days after performing procto-colectomy (with wire sutures) on a patient who developed a positive HBsAg [76]. Checks of 75 additional medical personnel who cared for the patient revealed no other cases of hepatitis. Other methods of casual contact in hospital are much less likely causes of infection.

Special care must be taken in transporting and handling *all* blood samples, but especially those coming from patients with hepatitis. These should be identified on the sample and the laboratory form.

Institutionalized mentally retarded children (especially with Down's syndrome) and their attendants have a high carrier rate [53].

Clinical course

The high carriage rate of serum HBsAg and anti-HBs in those who give no history of an acute attack of hepatitis suggests that subclinical episodes must be extremely frequent.

The usual clinical attack diagnosed in the adult tends to be more severe than for virus A or non-A, non-B infections. The overall picture is, however, similar.

In addition there may be features suggesting immune complex disease. This is shown in the pro-dromal period by a *serum sickness-like* syndrome.

This develops about a week before the onset of jaundice. It can be associated with an icteric or an anicteric attack. The syndrome has also been described with chronic hepatitis B [91].

Fever is usual. The skin lesion is urticarial, and rarely, in children, a papular acrodermatitis may be seen [37].

The arthropathy is symmetrical, non-migratory and affects small joints. Serum rheumatoid factor is negative.

These events can be related to circulating immune complexes containing HBsAg, anti-HBs and complement [85, 92]. Serum complement levels are reduced. Immunoglobulins, complement and HBsAg can be shown in vessel walls [26].

Extra-hepatic immune complex-related associations

These conditions are all associated with circulating immune complexes containing HBsAg. The accompanying liver disease is usually mild, at the most a chronic persistent hepatitis. The liver disease itself is not due to immune complex injury. The quantity of circulating immune complexes does not correlate with the severity of liver disease [71]. Turnover of the C_3 component of complement is not increased in acute type B hepatitis, and is less in chronic active than chronic persistent hepatitis [85]. Acute and chronic type B hepatitis can develop in patients with agammaglobulinaemia.

Polyarteritis (systemic necrotising vasculitis). This multi-system disease affects the gastrointestinal tract, peripheral and central nervous system. The course is similar to other types of polyarteritis.

Immune complexes containing HBsAg, IgG and complement have been found in the vascular lesions [64]. The presence of circulating complexes correlates with disease activity. As the lesions become less active, evidences of viral infection disappear [64].

The importance of hepatitis B virus in the whole picture of polyarteritis is probably low, perhaps representing some 10% of cases.

Glomerulonephritis. Membranous or membrano-proliferative glomerulonephritis has been found with chronic hepatitis B virus infection, either isolated or part of a generalized vasculitis [14]. The association is a rare one. Circulating HBsAg antigen–antibody complexes are found. Complexes containing HBsAg, IgG and C_3 are found in the glomeruli.

Polymyalgia rheumatica has been connected with hepatitis B infection [5], but the relationship is not clear cut [58].

Essential mixed cryoglobulinaemia. A patient with peripheral neuropathy and cryoglobulinaemia showed a cryoprecipitate with a high concentration of HBsAg. However, anti-HBsAg and complement were not found [57]. The relationship of hepatitis B to this condition has not been proved [27].

Hepatitis B carriers

Approximately 10% of patients contracting hepatitis B will not clear HBsAg from the serum within six months. Such patients become carriers and this state is likely to persist. Reversion to a negative HBsAg is rare but may develop in old age. Males are six times more likely to become carriers than females.

Persistence of antigen might be genetically determined. The dilemma of a person, such as a hospital worker, carrying the antigen and coming from an area where it is prevalent in apparently healthy persons is a very difficult one. The extent of his infectivity and the medico-legal implications of his employment are not yet clear. The HBsAg carrier of today must not replace the leper of yesterday. Hospital staff who develop HBsAg-positive hepatitis clear the antigen from the blood and are immune to type B hepatitis. They become particularly valuable members of staff. If they become carriers, the position is a difficult one. The extent of the infectivity of surgeons, dentists or indeed any hospital worker to patients and casual contacts has not been established but cannot be very great.

Although apparently healthy, carriers usually show histological changes on liver biopsy [47]. These run from simple non-specific minimal abnormalities through to chronic active hepatitis and cirrhosis [74]. The extent of the changes is not reflected by serum biochemical tests and may only be revealed by liver biopsy. A positive antigen test, however, can persist for many years without apparent clinical detriment.

The healthy carrier is said to show excess of the tubular and spherical antigen particles whereas the person incubating the disease or with an established chronic hepatitis shows more of the Dane particles, i.e. the complete virion [67, 69]. Serum HBcIgMAb and HBeAg positively indicate infectivity and ongoing disease. Mechanisms of chronicity are discussed in Chapter 16.

NON-A, NON-B HEPATITIS

The elimination of hepatitis A and hepatitis B from transfused blood did not eliminate post-transfusion hepatitis. Some of the cases were due to cytomegala infection, but the majority were due to another virus or viruses termed non-A, non-B. This infection now accounts for about 75% of post-transfusion hepatitis and possibly 15–20% of sporadic hepatitis, depending on the geographic location. Haemophiliacs receiving factor concentrates obtained from commercial sources are particularly at risk [18]. Non-A, non-B hepatitis is largely blood spread [25, 93]. It has also been reported with drug abuse, renal transplant recipients [93], in dialysis centres [36] and in donors used for plasmapheresis. It may affect recipients of commercial blood transfused at the time of coronary bypass surgery [4] (table 38). Waterborne epidemics in India resemble hepatitis A.

Table 38. Hepatitis after open heart surgery (Alter *et al* 1979).

	Transfused	Controls
Number	533	108
Hepatitis B	3	1
Non-A, non-B	43	0

Intra-familial spread has been described from Costa Rica [88]. Vertical transmission is also likely. The epidemiological pattern resembles type B hepatitis.

The agent has not been conclusively identified. It has been transmitted to chimpanzees [83]. These animals show double-walled 27 nm intranuclear particles, the nature of which is uncertain. An antigen appears within 7–10 days of infection. Antibody response is weak, and this may account for the difficulty in diagnosis. The identity of this agent remains uncertain [89] and some episodes may be modifications of type B.

Clinical course (fig. 248)

The incubation period is about seven weeks, although a short incubation type (one to four weeks) is also seen. The acute episode is usually mild and often anicteric. Extra-hepatic manifestations do not occur. Fulminant hepatitis is rare. The serum bilirubin and transaminase levels tend to be lower than with acute virus A or virus B infection. The serum immunoglobulin M is normal. The course may be prolonged, with serum transaminase levels waxing and waning for many months. A mild, chronic hepatitis develops in about a quarter, but this usually improves with time [8]. Circulating immune complexes may contribute [28]. Cirrhosis can develop.

In liver biopsies, in addition to the general

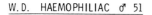

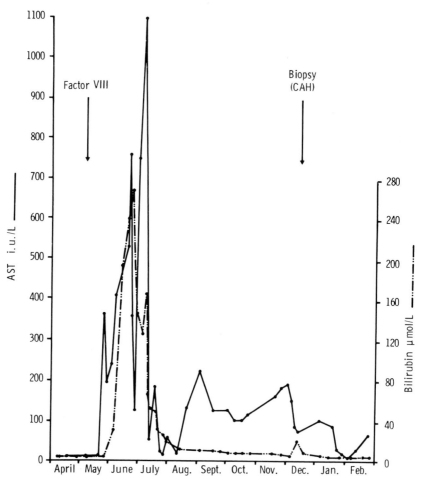

Fig. 248. W.D. haemophiliac patient developed acute hepatitis three weeks after a factor VIII concentrate known to cause non-A, non-B hepatitis. Serum HBsAg and hepatitis A IgM antibody were absent. Note very high serum bilirubin and aspartate (AST) levels. Serum bilirubin returned to normal, but aspartate transaminase fluctuated over the next seven months. Liver biopsy showed that a mild chronic active hepatitis (CAH) had developed. Normal AST = 5–15 i.u./1; normal bilirubin = 5–17 μmol/1.

features of acute virus hepatitis, the picture is one of marked sinusoidal and portal zone cellular infiltration, somewhat resembling infectious mononucleosis. Fatty change and evidence of bile duct damage may sometimes be seen [84].

Non-A, non-B hepatitis often progresses to a mild chronic hepatitis. The prognosis of this is, at the moment, uncertain but probably benign.

TREATMENT

Prevention

Compulsory notification leads to earlier detection and hence identification of methods of infection, for instance, food or water contamination.

VIRUS A

Control lies in perfect sanitation. The virus is particularly resistant to ordinary methods of water sterilization, including chlorination; boiling for 10 minutes is a safeguard. Ultimate control lies in general hygiene, safe disposal of faeces and control of insect vectors. The virus is excreted in the faeces for as long as two weeks before the appearance of jaundice. It is also probable that the anicteric patient may excrete the virus for a similar period. Virus may therefore be widely disseminated in a community before the diagnosis is made. For this reason isolation and quarantine of patients and contacts cannot be expected to influence significantly the spread of hepatitis.

Linen and other items of clothing soiled by patients should be autoclaved or boiled if this will not damage the fabric. Contamination of food, water and milk directly or indirectly by contacts or patients or by sewage should be prevented. Contacts need not be quarantined, but those who are food handlers should be given specific advice on personal hygiene.

VIRUS B

Virus B hepatitis is controlled by avoiding the use of blood products unless really indicated (one unit blood transfusions are never necessary). Where possible, sterile disposable equipment should be used for medical, dental and public health procedures and non-disposable equipment should be thoroughly washed and sterilized before use. This implies boiling for at least 10 minutes or subjecting to steam under pressure or to dry heat. Whole blood cannot be sterilized of the hepatitis virus. Routine thorough washing of endoscopes is sufficient to prevent infections [49].

All prospective blood donors should be screened for HBsAg by radioimmunoassay. This will not, of course, eliminate transfusion hepatitis, due to other hepatitis viruses, such as non-A, non-B.

Blood donors should be rejected if they have been in contact with hepatitis in the previous six months or if their blood is suspected of having been responsible for a case of post-transfusion hepatitis. The safest donor is one who has previously given blood many times without being responsible for a case of post-transfusion hepatitis.

Exclusion of commercial and HBsAg-positive donors reduces the frequency of post-transfusion hepatitis from 33% to 5%. Four of ten of the patients developing hepatitis were of non-A, non-B type, but six were HBsAg positive. Current tests, including radioimmunoassay, cannot detect all donors capable of transmitting hepatitis. The positive HBsAg donor with acute or chronic hepatitis may be more infectious than the so-called healthy carrier [41].

Immune-globulin prophylaxis (table 39) [77]

VIRUS A

Immune serum globulin (ISG) is effective in preventing or modifying type A virus hepatitis. When administered before or within one to two weeks of exposure in a dose of 0.02 ml/kg intramuscu-

Table 39. Immunoprophylaxis of virus hepatitis in adults.

Type	Globulin	Indication	Regime
A	Conventional	Close exposure to virus Travel to 'dirty' areas	3 ml within ten days 6 ml every six months
B	Immune	Exposure to HBsAg +ve blood Sexual consorts	5 ml within 48 hours and 28 days

larly it will prevent illness in 80–90% of those exposed. Because it may not suppress inapparent infection, long-lasting natural immunity may result.

It should be given to all close personal contacts who have not already had hepatitis A.

School contacts should not be given ISG routinely unless a school-centred outbreak exists. In institutions such as prisons or homes for the mentally subnormal epidemics frequently develop and patients and staff contacts of a patient with type A hepatitis should be given ISG. Routine prophylaxis of hospital personnel is not indicated, but sound hygiene should be insisted on. Office and work contacts do not need ISG.

When a common source of infection is identified, for instance food or water, ISG should be given to all exposed.

Short-term travellers (less than three months) on ordinary tourist routes do not require ISG. However, if they are travelling to the tropics or to developing countries and bypassing tourist routes, 0.02 ml/kg ISG should be given intramuscularly. If the journey is lasting longer than three months and in areas where hepatitis A is common, a single dose of 0.5 ml/kg is given and repeated every six months.

Preliminary testing of the person exposed for anti-HAV might be useful. If positive, ISG is not indicated.

VIRUS B

The position of hepatitis B immunoglobulin (HBIG) in prophylaxis is still confused [62]. Much depends on the anti-HBs titre of the preparation used. In a prospective double blind study on soldiers assigned to Korea, 5 ml immunoglobulin intramuscularly reduced the incidence of hepatitis, both HBsAg-positive and negative, for about six months [17]. The preparation used had a high anti-HBsAg titre. An HBIG globulin given to children receiving MS2 (analogous to type B) parenterally proved significantly protective [50]. Immunoglobulin also reduced hepatitis B infections in haemodialysis patients and staff [46].

Post-exposure prophylaxis reduces the incidence but prolongs the incubation period. Post-exposure prophylaxis with HBIG was effective for persons with accidental percutaneous exposure (needle stick) [78] and in post-exposure therapy of spouses and sexual partners of patients with acute hepatitis B [73].

Prior to giving HBIG the recipient must be tested for HBsAg and anti-HBs. If positive, immunoprophylaxis is not necessary. The dose of HBIG is 0.05–0.07 mg/kg, within two days of exposure and a similar dose 25–30 days later. This is used after single exposure to a large inoculum of HBsAg-positive material, such as by blood transfusion or for needle stick or mucosal contact with the infective material.

Infants born to mothers having hepatitis B in the last trimester of pregnancy or HBsAg positive at the time of delivery receive a high dose HBIG, 5 ml on the day of birth and every five weeks for six months [29].

Hepatitis B vaccines

The earliest vaccine was made in 1951 by boiling serum positive for HBsAg. It was shown to be effective, but not always safe [53]. Later vaccines have been prepared from HBsAg-positive donor plasma made uninfective by removing all Dane particles by treating with ammonium sulphate, pepsin and formaldehyde. The vaccine consists only of surface particles. Safety and potency are assessed in chimpanzees [82]. The vaccine is given at 0 and one month, and a third booster injection at six months (fig. 249). Over 90% seroconversion is achieved [82]. The vaccine will have a wide application to those at particular risk—especially patients and staff in dialysis and oncology units and in institutions for the mentally retarded. Dentists, homosexuals, parenteral drug abusers, babies born to hepatitis B-positive mothers and close contacts of carriers and sufferers may also benefit.

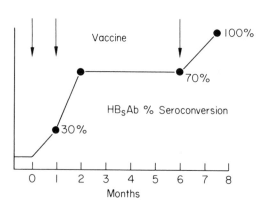

Fig. 249. The use of hepatitis B vaccine. Three injections result in about 93% seroconversion at eight months.

Genetic manipulation of the hepatitis B genome into *E. coli* may be another source of HBsAg for vaccine production.

The need for a vaccine is greatest in countries where the disease is most prevalent. These tend to be the countries with the least money to spend on health care, such as Greece, Spain, Africa and the Far East. The hepatitis B vaccine will have to be available to such countries. Its purchase will be justifiable, not only because it reduces human suffering, but also because it will reduce the cost of treating acute and chronic hepatitis and its long-term sequelae, particularly primary liver cancer.

Treatment of the acute attack

Treatment has little effect in altering the course. At the outset this is unpredictable and it is wise to treat all attacks as potentially fatal and to insist upon bed rest with bathroom privileges. Traditionally this is enforced until the patient is free of jaundice. A less strict regime may be possible if the patients are young, previously healthy, and are being treated in hospital. They can be allowed up when they feel well, regardless of the degree of jaundice. They rest after each meal. If symptoms return, the patient is immediately returned to bed rest. Selected patients treated along these liberal lines do not show an increased incidence of later complications [65].

Convalescence is not allowed until the patient is symptom-free, the liver no longer tender, and the serum bilirubin is less than 1.5 mg/100 ml. The period of convalescence should be twice the period spent in hospital or in bed at home.

The traditional low-fat, high-carbohydrate diet is popular because it has proved the most palatable to the anorexic patient. Apart from this, no benefit accrues from the rigid insistence upon a low-fat diet.

When the appetite returns, high protein intake may hasten recovery. Excess protein, however, is harmful to the severely ill patient in impending hepatic coma. The usual diet in hepatitis is composed of the food most appetizing to the patient. Supplementary vitamins, amino acids and lipotrophic agents are not necessary.

Corticosteroids do not alter the degree of liver necrosis, accelerate the rate of healing or assist in immunity in virus hepatitis. Hepatitis tends towards spontaneous recovery and any benefit is not sufficient to justify the routine use of this treatment. They do result in a rapid fall and a lower peak in the serum bilirubin concentration, and a more rapid reversion to normal of the transaminase tests. The drug must be continued into convalescence for premature withdrawal leads to relapse. A usual course is 30, 20, 15, 10 and 5 mg prednisolone, each dose being given for five days (duration of course 25 days). It should be reserved for the patient with prolonged cholestasis (fig. 238) or the patient who seems to be passing into a sub-acute stage with persistent jaundice, high serum globulin and transaminase values. The steroid 'whitewash' improves the morale of both patient and physician but probably has little effect on the healing of the liver [79].

Many patients with chronic hepatitis and a positive HBsAg have received corticosteroids during the acute attack [33]. This treatment may have helped to perpetuate the disease although this is not proven.

Corticosteroids in acute hepatitis may reduce the frequency of coma, but they favour relapses and chronicity.

Patients showing signs of acute hepato-cellular failure with pre-coma require more active measures and the regime described in Chapter 9 must be instituted.

FOLLOW-UP

The patient should be seen three to four weeks after discharge, and if necessary at monthly intervals for the next three months. Special attention should be paid to recurrence of jaundice and to the size of the liver and spleen. Tests should include serum bilirubin, globulin and transaminase levels, HBsAg if originally positive, and HBeAg.

The patient should not be questioned too closely about symptoms and feeling of weakness, for the 'post-hepatitis syndrome' can readily be induced by the physician. Exercise must be undertaken and within the limits of fatigue. Alcohol must be denied for six months and preferably one year afterwards. The patient often has little inclination for it and excessive consumption leads to relapses. Diet can be unrestricted.

Chronic organic sequelae

Hepatitis A infection never becomes chronic.

Exposure to HBV can have different results (fig. 250). Some are immune and have no clinical attack; they presumably have anti-HBV. In

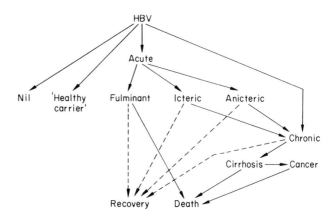

Fig. 250. The effect of
exposure to hepatitis B
virus (HBV).

others, an acute attack develops varying from
anicteric to fulminant. Previously normal persons
usually clear the antigen from the serum within
about four to six weeks from the onset of symptoms. Chronic liver disease is associated with
persistent antigenaemia [66]. In general, the
more florid and acute the original attack the less
likely are chronic sequelae.

If the patient survives a fulminant attack of viral
hepatitis, ultimate recovery is complete without
the development of chronic residuals. Chronicity
is more likely after the mildly icteric, anicteric or
relapsing episode and in those with immunological
incompetence such as neonates, sufferers from leukaemia and cancer, renal failure or those receiving
immunosuppressive treatment [33] (see Chapter
16).

REFERENCES

1. ACUTE HEPATIC FAILURE STUDY GROUP (1979)
   Etiology and prognosis in fulminant hepatitis.
   Gastroenterology **77**, A33.
2. AJDUKIEWICZ A.B., DUDLEY F.J., FOX R.A. *et al*
   (1972) Immunological studies in an epidemic of infective short-incubation hepatitis. *Lancet* i, 803.
3. ALMEIDA J.D., RUBENSTEIN D. & STOTT E.J. (1971)
   New antigen–antibody system in Australia-antigen-positive hepatitis. *Lancet* ii, 1225.
4. ALTER H.J. *et al* (1980) Non-A non-B hepatitis in
   cardiac surgery patients. In Vyas *et al* (see ref. 90).
5. BACON P.A., DOHERTY S.M. & ZUCKERMAN A.J.
   (1975) Hepatitis B antibody in polymyalgia rheumatica. *Lancet* ii, 476.
6. BEASLEY R.P., TREPO C., STEVENS C.E. *et al* (1977)
   The 'e' antigen and vertical transmission of hepatitis B surface antigen. *Am. J. Epidemiol.* **105**, 94.
7. BERG R., RINGERTZ O. & ESPMARK A. (1971) Australia antigen in hepatitis among Swedish track-
   finders. *Acta path. microbiol. Scand., Sect. B.* **79**,
   423.
8. BERMAN M., ALTER H.J., ISHAK K.G. *et al* (1979)

The chronic sequelae of non-A non-B hepatitis.
   Ann. intern. Med. **91**, 1.
9. BIANCHI L., GEROK W., SICKINGER K. *et al* (eds)
   (1980) *Virus and the Liver.* Falk Symposium 28.
   MTP, Lancaster. In press.
10. BLUMBERG B.S., ALTER H.J. & VISNICH S. (1965)
    A 'new' antigen in leukemia sera. *J. Am. med.
    Assoc.* **191**, 541.
11. BOYER J.L. & KLATSKIN G. (1970) Pattern of
    necrosis in acute viral hepatitis. *New Engl. J. Med.*
    283, 1063.
12. BRADLEY D.W., FIELDS H.A. & McCAUSTLAND
    K.A. (1979) Serodiagnosis of viral hepatitis A by
    a modified competitive binding radioimmunoassay
    for immunoglobulin M antihepatitis A virus. *J.
    clin. Microbiol.* **9**, 120.
13. BROTMAN B., PRINCE A.M. & GODFREY H.R.
    (1973) Role of arthropods in transmission of hepa-
    titis-B virus in the tropics. *Lancet* i, 1305.
14. BRZOSKO W.J., KRAWCZYŃSKI K., NAZAREWICZ T.
    et al (1974) Glomerulonephritis associated with
    hepatitis-B surface antigen immune complexes in
    children. *Lancet* ii, 477.
15. CHAN T.K. & TODD D. (1975) Haemolysis compli-
    cating viral hepatitis in patients with glucose-6-
    phosphate dehydrogenase deficiency. *Br. med. J.* i,
    131.
16. CHUTTANI H.K., SIDHU A.S., WIG K.L. *et al* (1966)
    Follow-up study of cases from the Delhi epidemic
    of infectious hepatitis 1955–6. *Br. med. J.* ii, 676.
17. CONRAD M.E. (1972) Endemic viral hepatitis in
    U.S. soldiers: causative factors and the effect of
    prophylactic gammaglobulin. *Canad. med. Assoc.
    J.* **106**, 456.
18. CRASKE J., DILLING N. & STERN D. (1975) An out-
    break of hepatitis associated with intravenous in-
    jection of factor VIII concentrate. *Lancet* ii, 221.
19. CULLINAN E.R., KING R.C. & RIVERS J.S. (1958)
    The prognosis of infective hepatitis. A preliminary
    account of a long-term follow-up. *Br. med. J.* i,
    1315.
20. DANE D.S., CAMERON C.H. & BRIGGS M. (1970)
    Virus-like particles in serum of patients with Aus-
    tralia-antigen-associated hepatitis. *Lancet* i, 695.
21. DECKER R.H., OVERBY L.R., LING C-M. *et al*
    (1979) Serologic studies of transmission of hepa-
    titis A in humans. *J. infect. Dis.* **139**, 74.

22. DEODHAR K.P., TAPP E. & SCHEUER P.J. (1975) Orcein staining of hepatitis B antigen in paraffin sections of liver biopsies. *J. clin. Pathol.*, **28**, 66.

23. DIBLE J.H., McMICHAEL J. & SHERLOCK S.P.V. (1943) Pathology of acute hepatitis. Aspiration biopsy studies of epidemic, arsenotherapy and serum jaundice. *Lancet* ii, 402.

24. DIENSTAG J.L., FEINSTONE S.M., KAPIKIAN A.Z. *et al* (1975) Faecal shedding of hepatitis-A antigen. *Lancet* i, 765.

25. DIENSTAG J.L., FEINSTONE S.M., PURCELL R.H. *et al* (1977) Non-A, non-B-post transfusion hepatitis. *Lancet* i, 560.

26. DIENSTAG J.L., RHODES A.R., BHAN A.K. *et al* (1978) Urticaria associated with acute viral hepatitis type B: studies of pathogenesis. *Ann. intern. Med.* **89**, 34.

27. DIENSTAG J.L., WANDS J.R. & ISSELBACHER K.J. (1977) Hepatitis B and essential mixed cryoglobulinemia. *New Engl. J. Med.* **297**, 946.

28. DIENSTAG J.L. *et al* (1979) Circulating immune complexes in non-A, non-B hepatitis. *Lancet* i, 1265.

29. DOSIK H. & JHAVERI R. (1978) Prevention of neonatal hepatitis B infection by high-dose hepatitis B immune globulin. *New Engl. J. Med.* **298**, 602.

30. DUBIN I.N., SULLIVAN B.H. Jr, LeGOLVAN P.C. *et al* (1960) The cholestatic form of viral hepatitis: experiences with viral hepatitis at Brooke Army Hospital during the years 1951 to 1953 *Am. J. Med.* **29**, 55.

31. DUDLEY F.J., O'SHEA M.J., AJDUKIEWICZ A. *et al* (1973) Serum autoantibodies and immunoglobulins in hepatitis-associated antigen (HAA)-positive and -negative liver disease. *Gut* **14**, 360.

32. DUDLEY F.J., O'SHEA M.J. & SHERLOCK S. (1973) Serum autoantibodies in hepatitis associated antigen (HAA) positive patients. *Clin. exp. Immunol.* **13**, 367.

33. DUDLEY F.J., SCHEUER P.J. & SHERLOCK S. (1972) Natural history of hepatitis-associated antigen-positive chronic liver disease. *Lancet* ii, 1388.

34. FEINSTONE S.M., KAPIKIAN A.Z. & PURCELL R.H. (1973) Hepatitis A: detection by immune electron microscopy of a virus-like antigen associated with acute illness. *Science* **182**, 1026.

35. FROSNER G.G., BRODERSEN M., PAPAEVANGELOU G. *et al* (1978) Detection of HBeAg and anti-HBe in acute hepatitis B by a sensitive radioimmunoassay. *J. med. Virol.* **3**, 67.

36. GALBRAITH R.M., DIENSTAG J.L., PURCELL J.L. *et al* (1979) Non-A non-B hepatitis associated with chronic liver disease in a haemodialysis unit. *Lancet* i, 957.

37. GIANOTTI F. (1973) Papular acrodermatitis of childhood: an Australian antigen disease. *Arch. Dis. Childh.* **48**, 794.

38. GUDAT F., BIANCHI L. & SONNABEND W. (1975) Pattern of core and surface expression in liver tissue reflects state of specific immune response in hepatitis B. *Lab. Invest.* **32**, 1.

39. HAGLAR L., PASTORE R.A., BERGIN J.J. *et al* (1975) Aplastic anemia following viral hepatitis. *Medicine (Baltimore)* **54**, 139.

40. HAUGAN R.K. (1979) Hepatitis after the transfusion of frozen red cells and washed red cells. *New Engl. J. Med.* **301**, 393.

41. HEATHCOTE J., GATEAU Ph. & SHERLOCK S. (1974) Role of hepatitis-B antigen carriers in nonparenteral transmission of the hepatitis-B virus. *Lancet* ii, 370.

42. HEATHCOTE J. & SHERLOCK S. (1973) Spread of acute type-B hepatitis in London. *Lancet* i, 1468.

43. HOLLAND P.V., PURCELL R.H., SMITH H. *et al* (1972) Subtyping of hepatitis-associated antigen (HBAg): simplified technique with counterelectrophoresis. *J. Immunol.* **109**, 420.

44. HOOFNAGLE J.H., GERETY R.J., NI L.Y. (1974) Antibody to hepatitis B core antigen: a positive indicator of hepatitis B virus replication. *New Engl. J. Med.* **290**, 1336.

45. INTERNATIONAL GROUP (1971) Morphological criteria in viral hepatitis. *Lancet* i, 333.

46. IWARSON S., AHLMÉN J., ERIKSSON E. *et al* (1977) Hepatitis B immune globulin in prevention of hepatitis B among hospital staff members. *J. infect. Dis.* **135**, 473.

47. KLINGE O., KABOTH U. & ARNOLD R. (1970) Liver histology in healthy carriers of Australia-SH antigen or antibodies. *Dtsch. med. Wschr.* **95**, 2583.

48. KNIGHT A.H., FOX R.A., BAILLOD R.A. *et al* (1970) Hepatitis associated antigen and antibody in haemodialysis patients and staff. *Br. med. J.* ii, 603.

49. KORETZ R.L. & CAMACHO R. (1979) Failure of endoscopic transmission of hepatitis B. *Dig. Dis. Sci.* **24**, 21.

50. KRUGMAN S. & GILES J.P. (1973) Viral hepatitis, type B (MS-2-strain). Further observations on natural history and prevention. *New Engl. J. Med.* **288**, 755.

51. KRUGMAN S. & GOCKE D.J. (1978) Viral hepatitis, Vol. XV. *Major Problems in Internal Medicine.* W.B. Saunders, Philadelphia.

52. KRUGMAN S., HOOFNAGLE J.H., GERETY R.J. *et al* (1974) Viral hepatitis B, DNA polymerase, and antibody to HB core antigen. *New Engl. J. Med.* **290**, 1331.

53. KRUGMAN S., OVERBY L.R., MUSHAHWAR I.K. *et al* (1979) Viral hepatitis type B: studies on natural history and prevention re-examined. *New Engl. J. Med.* **300**, 101.

54. LANDER J.J., HOLLAND P.V., ALTER H.J. *et al* (1972) Antibody to hepatitis-associated antigen. Frequency and pattern of response as detected by radioimmunoprecipitation. *J. Am. med. Assoc.* **220**, 1079.

55. LE BOUVIER G.L. (1973) Subtypes of hepatitis B antigen: clinical relevance? *Ann. intern. Med.* **99**, 894.

56. LE BOUVIER G.L. & WILLIAMS A. (1975) Serotypes of hepatitis B antigen (HBsAg); the problem of 'new' determinants as exemplified by 't'. *Am. J. med. Sci.* **270**, 165.

57. LEVO Y., GOREVIC P.D., KASSAB H.J. *et al* (1977) Association between hepatitis B virus and essential mixed cryoglobulinemia. *New Engl. J. Med.* **296**, 1501.

58. LIANG M., GREENBERG H., PINCUS T. *et al* (1976) Hepatitis-B antibody in polymyalgia rheumatica. *Lancet* i, 43.

59. LIM K.S., WONG V.T., FULFORD K.W.M. *et al* (1977) Role of sexual and non-sexual practices in the transmission of hepatitis B. *Br. J. ven. Dis.* **53**, 190.

60. LIMENTANI A.E., ELLIOT L.M., NOAH N.D. *et al* (1979) An outbreak of hepatitis B from tattooing. *Lancet* ii, 86.

61. MATHIESEN L.R. & THE COPENHAGEN HEPATITIS ACUTE PROGRAMME (1979) Immunofluorescence studies for hepatitis A virus and hepatitis B surface antigen and core antigen in liver biopsies from patients with acute viral hepatitis. *Gastroenterology* **77**, 623.

62. MAYNARD J.E. (1978) Passive immunisation against hepatitis B: a review of recent studies and comment on current aspects of control. *Am. J. Epidemiol.* **107**, 77.

63. MELNICK J.L. (1957) A water-borne urban epidemic of hepatitis. In *Hepatitis Frontiers*, p. 211. Little Brown, Boston.

64. MICHALAK T. (1978) Immune complexes of hepatitis B surface antigen in the pathogenesis of periarteritis nodosa: study of seven necropsy cases. *Am. J. Pathol.* **90**, 619.

65. NEFZGER M.D. & CHALMERS T.C. (1963) The treatment of acute infectious hepatitis. Ten-year follow-up of the effects of diet and rest. *Am. J. Med.* **35**, 299.

66. NIELSEN J.O., DIETRICHSON O., ELLING P. *et al* (1971) Incidence and meaning of persistence of Australia antigen in patients with acute viral hepatitis: Development of chronic hepatitis. *New Engl. J. Med.* **285**, 1157.

67. NEILSEN J.O., NEILSEN M.H. & ELLING P. (1973) Differential distribution of Australia-antigen associated particles in patients with liver diseases and normal carriers. *New Engl. J. Med.* **288**, 484.

68. PERRILLO R.P., GELB L., CAMPBELL C. *et al* (1979) Hepatitis BHe antigen, DNA polymerase activity and infection of household contacts with hepatitis B virus. *Gastroenterology* **76**, 1319.

69. POPPER H. & SCHAFFNER F. (1973) Hepatitis B antigen particles and prognosis in hepatitis. *New Engl. J. Med.* **288**, 518.

70. POULSEN H. & CHRISTOFFERSEN P. (1969) Abnormal bile duct epithelium in liver biopsies with histological signs of viral hepatitis. *Acta path. microbiol. Scand.* **76**, 383.

71. PRINCE A.M. & TREPO C. (1971) Role of immune complexes involving SH antigen in pathogenesis of chronic active hepatitis and polyarteritis nodosa. *Lancet* i, 1309.

72. PROVOST P.J. & HILLEMAN M.R. (1979) Propagation of human hepatitis A virus in cell culture *in vivo. Proc. Soc. exp. Biol. Med.* **160**, 213.

73. REDEKER A.G., MOSLEY J.W., GOCKE D.J. *et al* (1975) Hepatitis B immune globulin as a prophylactic measure for spouses exposed to acute type B hepatitis. *New Engl. J. Med.* **293**, 1059.

74. REINCKE V., DYBKJAER E., POULSEN H. *et al* (1972) A study of Australia-antigen-positive blood donors and their recipients, with special reference to liver histology. *New Engl. J. Med.* **286**, 867.

75. ROHOLM K. & IVERSEN P. (1939) Changes in the liver in acute epidemic hepatitis (catarrhal jaun-

dice) based on 38 aspiration biopsies. *Acta path. microbiol. Scand.* **16**, 427.

76. ROSENBERG J.L., JONES D.P., LIPITZ L.R. *et al* (1973) Viral hepatitis: an occupational hazard to surgeons. *J. Am. med. Assoc.* **223**, 395.

77. SEEFF L.B. & HOOFNAGLE J.H. (1979) Immunoprophylaxis of viral hepatitis. *Gastroenterology* **77**, 161.

78. SEEFF L.B., WRIGHT E.C., ZIMMERMAN H.J. *et al* (1978) Type B hepatitis after needle stick exposure: prevention with hepatitis B immune globulin. *Ann. intern. Med.* **88**, 285.

79. SHALDON S. & SHERLOCK S. (1957) Virus hepatitis with features of prolonged bile retention. *Br. med. J.* ii, 734.

80. SHERLOCK S. (ed.) (1980) Viral hepatitis. *Clinics in Gastroenterology.* W.B. Saunders, Philadelphia.

81. SHERLOCK S. & WALSHE V.M. (1946) The post-hepatitis syndrome. *Lancet* ii, 482.

82. SZMUNESS W., STEVENS C.E., HARLEY E.J., *et al* (1980) Hepatitis B vaccine: demonstration of efficacy in a controlled trial in a high-risk population in the United States. *New Engl. J. Med.* **303**, 833.

83. TABOR E., GERETY R.J., DRUCKER J.A. *et al* (1978) Transmission of non-A, non-B hepatitis from man to chimpanzee. *Lancet* i, 463.

84. THOMAS H.C., BAMBER M., ARBORGH B.A.M. *et al* (1981) The course of non-A, non-B hepatitis in haemophiliacs receiving factor VIII concentrates. *Gut.* In press.

85. THOMAS H.C., POTTER B.J., ELIAS E. *et al* (1979) Metabolism of the third component of complement in acute type B hepatitis. HB_s antigen positive glomerulonephritis, polyarteritis nodosum and HB_s antigen positive and negative chronic active liver disease. *Gastroenterology* **76**, 673.

86. TREPO C., VITVITSKI L., HANTZ O. *et al* (1980) Nature and significance of HBeAg specificities. In *Virus and the Liver.* MTP, Lancaster.

87. TRICHOPOULOS D., TABOR E., GERETY R.J. *et al* (1978) Hepatitis B and primary hepatocellular carcinoma in a European population. *Lancet* ii, 1217.

88. VILLAREJOS V.M., VISONA K.A., EDUARTE A. *et al* (1975) Evidence for viral hepatitis other than type A or type B among persons in Costa Rica. *New Engl. J. Med.* **293**, 1350.

89. VITVITSKI L., TREPO C., PRINCE A.M. *et al* (1979) Detection of virus associated antigen in serum and liver of patients with non-A non-B hepatitis. *Lancet* ii, 1263.

90. VYAS G.N., COHEN S.N. & SCHMID R. (eds) (1978) *Viral Hepatitis.* Franklin Institute Press, Philadelphia.

91. WANDS J.R., ALPERT E. & ISSELBACHER K.J. (1975) Arthritis associated with chronic active hepatitis. Complement activation and characterization of circulating immune complexes. *Gastroenterology* **69**, 1286.

92. WANDS J.R., MANN E., ALPERT E. *et al* (1975) The pathogenesis of arthritis associated with acute hepatitis-B surface antigen-positive hepatitis: complement activation and characterisation of circulating immune complexes. *J. clin. Invest.* **55**, 930.

93. WARE A.J., LUBY J.P., HOLLINGER B. *et al*

(1979) Etiology of liver disease in renal transplant patients. *Ann. intern. Med.* **91**, 364.

94. WILLS W., LONDON W.T., WERNER B.G. *et al* (1977) Hepatitis-B virus in bedbugs (*Climex hemipterus*) from Senegal. *Lancet* ii, 217.

95. WORLD HEALTH ORGANISATION (1977) Advances in viral hepatitis. *WHO tech. Report Series*, 602.

96. ZUCKERMAN A.J. (1997) The chronicle of viral hepatitis. *Bull. Hyg. Trop. Dis.* **54**, 113.

YELLOW FEVER

This acute infection is due to a group B arbovirus transmitted to man by the bite of infected mosquitoes. The virus cycle is a direct human one in urban yellow fever, or may involve wild monkeys in the jungle variety.

The two endemic regions are South America and equatorial Africa.

PATHOLOGY [5]

The characteristic lesions are principally in the liver, kidneys and heart. Liver cells show diffuse, non-inflammatory unicellular necrosis, mainly mid-zonal [1]. Scattered cells show distinctive acidophilic hyaline necrosis (Councilman bodies). Intranuclear acidophilic inclusions are occasionally found in man, but are frequent in infected monkeys.

Electron microscopy shows passage of granules of ribonucleoprotein from nucleus to cytoplasm where they aggregate to form rosettes which later give rise to spherical virus particles measuring 55–61 nm [2, 3].

With a recovery, regeneration is complete and chronicity does not result.

The *spleen* is enlarged with reticulo-endothelial proliferation; the *kidneys* show tubular necrosis; the *stomach* contains altered blood; and the *heart* is pale and flabby.

In endemic areas, the systematic study of the liver of patients dying with acute fever is important, because the lesions of yellow fever are diagnostic [6].

CLINICAL FEATURES

Following an incubation period of three to six days, the disease has a sudden onset with fever, chills, headache, backache, prostration and vomiting, often of altered blood. The blood pressure falls, haemorrhages become widespread, jaundice and albuminuria are conspicuous and there is a

relative bradycardia. Delirium proceeds to coma and death within nine days. If there is recovery the temperature becomes normal within this time and convalescence progresses rapidly and completely. There are no sequelae and life-long immunity follows. Apart from the classical course described, the majority of infections are probably milder, with no detectable jaundice and only a few constitutional symptoms.

Diagnosis [7]. Serum removed within the first three days of the illness is injected intracerebrally into mice and the development of encephalitis noted. Acute-phase and convalescent sera should be obtained for the demonstration of protective antibodies in mice. Prothrombin deficiency parallels the severity of the liver lesion [4]. The serum cholesterol level falls in the fatal case. Serum transaminases are increased relative to severity.

TREATMENT

There is no specific treatment. Death results principally from renal damage. The hepatic lesion is self-limited and of short duration and does not demand special treatment.

Prevention consists of vaccination and control of mosquitoes. It is necessary to be vaccinated at least 10 days before arrival in endemic areas. It should not be done concomitantly with primary smallpox vaccination, but either three days before or three weeks after a successful smallpox 'take'.

REFERENCES

1. BEARCROFT W.G.C. (1957) The histopathology of the liver of yellow-fever-infected rhesus monkeys. *J. Pathol. Bact.* **74**, 295.

2. BEARCROFT W.G.C. (1960) Electron-microscope studies on the liver cells of yellow-fever-infected rhesus monkeys. *J. Pathol. Bact.* **80**, 421.

3. BEARCROFT W.G.C. (1962) Studies on the livers of yellow-fever-infected African monkeys. *J. Pathol. Bact.* **83**, 49.

4. ELTON N.W., ROMERO A. & TREJOS A. (1955) Clinical pathology of yellow fever. *Am. J. clin. Pathol.* **25**, 135.

5. KLOTZ O. & BELT T.H. (1930) The pathology of the liver in yellow fever. *Am. J. Pathol.* **6**, 663.

6. SOPER F.L., RICKARD E.R. & CRAWFORD P.J. (1934) The routine post-mortem removal of liver tissue from rapidly fatal fever cases for the discovery of silent yellow fever foci. *Am. J. Hyg.* **19**, 549.

7. WORLD HEALTH ORGANISATION (1967) Arboviruses and human disease. *WHO tech. Report Series*, 369.

INFECTIOUS MONONUCLEOSIS

This virus infection is due to human herpes virus IV (Epstein–Barr) which excites a generalized reticulo-endothelial reaction. It largely affects adolescents and young adults and may mimic type A, type B, or non-A, non-B viral hepatitis.

HEPATIC HISTOLOGY [2, 5] (fig. 251)

The changes are seen within five days of the onset and reach their peak between the tenth and thirtieth days.

The sinusoids and portal tracts are infiltrated with large, mononuclear cells with deep-staining, basophil cytoplasm and fenestrated nuclei. Polymorphonuclear leucocytes and lymphocytes increase, and the Kupffer cells proliferate. The appearances may resemble those of leukaemia. The portal tract lesions resemble those of early A, B, or non-A, non-B viral hepatitis. The architecture of the liver is preserved.

Centrizonal necrosis is absent, although focal necroses may be randomly distributed. The liver cells are then replaced by acidophil remnants, with occasional, small dark nuclei. The necroses are not bile stained and there is no surrounding cellular reaction.

In later biopsies, binucleate liver cells and mitoses are conspicuous. The evidences of regeneration are out of proportion to cell necrosis. After clinical recovery, abnormal cells disappear although this may take as long as eight months. Portal zone fibrosis is not a sequel and cirrhosis is not a complication.

Overt jaundice is noted in 5–10% of sufferers. It is presumably due to damage to liver cells by the causative agent. Haemolysis may contribute [6]. Enlarged glands in the porta hepatis do not compress the common bile duct.

Fatal acute hepatic necrosis is a rare complication.

BIOCHEMICAL CHANGES

The total serum albumin level may be slightly decreased and the serum globulin value slightly elevated. Electrophoretic analysis shows a variable α_2-globulin and often abnormal proteins migrating between α_2 and β and between β and γ. The γ-globulin level is elevated.

Hyperbilirubinaemia is present in about one-half of patients. Serum transaminase values are raised to about 20 times the normal in 80% of patients. Values are usually less than those found in the early stages of an acute virus hepatitis. In about one-third the serum alkaline phosphatase value is increased, often more than the bilirubin [4].

Alkaline phosphatase and transaminase levels are found in those with severe, mononuclear round-cell infiltration in the hepatic sinusoids [3].

The heterophile antibody (Paul–Bunnell) reaction is positive. The disease is diagnosed conclusively by an increase in serum IgM antibodies against Epstein–Barr viral antigens.

DISTINCTION FROM VIRUS HEPATITIS
(table 40)

Although the diagnosis of virus hepatitis from infectious mononucleosis is usually easy, in an

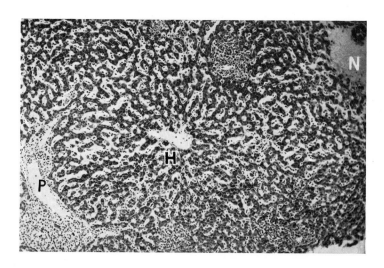

Fig. 251. Infectious mononucleosis. The sinusoids and portal tracts (P) are filled with mononuclear cells. H is a central hepatic vein. One small local necrosis (N) is seen in the upper right-hand corner. Best's carmine, × 70.

Table 40. Comparison of infectious mononucleosis and virus hepatitis.

	Infectious mononucleosis	Virus hepatitis
Epidemic history	Suggestive	Suggestive
Onset		
fever	+	+
anorexia	−	+
sore throat	+	−
rash	+	Rare
pruritus	−	+
Physical signs		
lymphadenopathy	+ +	±
jaundice	Mild, transient	Well-developed, persisting
liver	Enlarged; not usually tender	Enlarged and tender
spleen	Enlarged and tender	Enlarged but not tender
pale stools	−	+
dark urine	±	+ +
Peripheral blood		
leucocytes	Usually increased. Characteristic cells	Decreased, with relative lymphocytosis
Paul–Bunnell	+ ve	− ve
	(Heterophile antibodies not affected by guinea-pig kidney)	(If heterophile antibodies present, can be absorbed by guinea-pig kidney)
EB virus antibody	Present	Absent
HBsAg	− ve	+ ve, type B
Liver biopsy	Diffuse mononuclear infiltration. Focal necroses	Centrilobular 'spotty' necrosis Mononuclear infiltration

occasional instance of mild anicteric hepatitis or severe mononucleosis this may be impossible.

REFERENCES

1. GELB, D., WEST M. & ZIMMERMAN H.J. (1962) Serum enzymes in disease. IX. Analysis of factors responsible for elevated values in infectious mononucleosis. *Am. J. Med.* **33**, 239.
2. HOAGLAND R.J. & McCLUSKEY R.T. (1956) Hepatitis in mononucleosis. *Ann. intern. Med.* **43**, 1019.
3. KILPATRICK Z.M. (1966) Structural and functional abnormalities of liver in infectious mononucleosis. *Arch. intern. Med.* **117**, 47.
4. SHUSTER F. & OGNIBENE A.I. (1969) Dissociation of serum bilirubin and alkaline phosphatase in infectious mononucleosis. *J. Am. med. Assoc.* **209**, 267.
5. WADSWORTH R.C. & KEIL P.G. (1952) Biopsy of the liver in infectious mononucleosis. *Am. J. Pathol.* **28**, 1003.
6. WEBSTER S.G.P. (1968) Jaundice in infectious mononucleosis. *Br. med. J.* ii, 411.

OTHER VIRUSES

All viruses affect the liver in common with all other organs. The histological changes are usually non-specific, consisting of fatty change, or focal necrosis and lymphocytic infiltration of the portal zones. Biochemical tests are usually unchanged or show mild rises in transaminases. Occasionally the patient may be frankly icteric when the picture of type A, B, or non-A, non-B hepatitis is closely simulated.

Virus-related hepatitis is seen in those susceptible on account of a predisposing cause such as reticulosis, immuno-suppressive therapy, transplantation or blood transfusions. They are common in neonates (Chapter 23).

Cytomegalovirus

This type is due to human herpes virus type VI. In neonates it is usually inapparent. Confirmed disease in early infancy is rare. Sometimes, however, in association with the respiratory distress syndrome, cytomegalovirus may cause a devastating fatal pneumonitis [2].

In adults, the clinical picture may be of Paul–Bunnell-negative infectious mononucleosis [11]. Serum transaminase and alkaline phosphatase levels are increased and atypical lymphocytes are found in the peripheral blood. Occasionally, fatal, massive, hepatic necrosis develops [14].

The acute hepatitis may resemble type A, type B or non-A, non-B. The onset is similar, but pyrexia does not subside with the onset of jaundice. Icterus lasts two to three weeks and even up to three months.

Granulomatous hepatitis can develop in a previously normal adult evidenced by prolonged, unexplained fever without enlarged peripheral glands [5]. Liver biopsy shows non-caseating epithelioid granulomas.

It may present as a post-transfusion reaction.

The virus frequently affects the immuno-suppressed. After renal transplantation cytomegalovirus is a major cause of fever, leucopenia, pneumonitis, hepatitis, retinitis, encephalitis and even death. This probably represents a reactivation of endogenous virus.

Diagnosis is by isolation of virus from urine, saliva, or uterine cervix. The complement fixing antibodies rise, and CMV IgM antibodies can be found.

Herpes simplex

Human herpes virus types I and II affect all humans at some time during their lives.

In infants herpes hepatitis may be part of generalized herpetic disease.

In adults disseminated herpes simplex is very rare. It can, however, affect those with underlying diseases, on corticosteroid treatment or having renal transplants [1].

Fulminant herpes simplex hepatitis may also, very rarely, affect previously normal adults [6, 9]. Herpetic mucocutaneous lesions may be absent. The clinical picture is of fever, atypical lymphocytosis and finally fulminant hepatic failure with disseminated intravascular coagulation.

Liver biopsy shows confluent hepatic necrosis with intranuclear inclusions and the virus can be cultured from the liver.

Treatment is with anti-virals such as acyclovir.

Other viruses

Coxsackie virus B may cause hepatitis in the adult. Coxsackie virus, group A, type IV, has been isolated from the plasma of a child with hepatitis, and complement fixing antibodies appeared in the serum during convalescence.

Adenovirus has caused fulminant hepatitis in a young immuno-suppressed adult [4]. Intranuclear inclusions were confined to the liver.

Varicella hepatitis has been reported in a patient receiving corticosteroids.

Rubeola (measles) in adults may be associated with rises in serum transaminase levels [13].

HEPATITIS DUE TO EXOTIC VIRUSES

This term is applied to very dangerous, newly identified and unusual viruses where the liver appears to be the primary target [15]. They include Marburg, Lassa and Ebola viruses. They are becoming increasingly important as man encroaches into under-developed areas, as ecology changes and as a source of infection to medical or laboratory staff dealing with patients or their blood.

Lassa fever is due to an arena virus transmitted from rodents to man or from man to man. It is largely found in West Africa. The case fatality rate is 36–67%.

The liver shows eosinophilic necrosis of individual hepatocytes with little inflammation. Bridging necrosis is usual.

Marburg virus disease is due to an RNA virus transmitted by Vervet monkeys. In 1967, 27 cases of this disease occurred in persons in contact with Vervet monkeys in experimental institutes in Germany; five died [12]. Further patients have been reported from South Africa [10].

After an incubation of four to seven days the patients present with headache, pyrexia, vomiting, a characteristic rash, a haemorrhagic diathesis and central nervous system involvement. Serum transaminase levels are very high.

Liver pathology [3] shows single-cell acidophilic necrosis and Kupffer cell hyperactivity. This is followed by eccentric and radial extension of the necrosis, cytoplasmic inclusions and portal zone cellularity. A steatosis is noted in the severely affected. Virus can persist in the body for two to three months after initial infection [10].

Ebola virus infection resembles Marburg in clinical course, hepatic histology and electron microscopy [7]. It has been reported from Zaire and Sudan and has been transmitted to biologists working with it [8].

TREATMENT

There is no specific treatment for these exotic virus infections. Symptomatic measures are used and very strict precautions are necessary to avoid spread to contacts.

REFERENCES

1. ANURAS S. & SUMMERS R. (1976) Fulminary herpes simplex hepatitis in an adult: report of a case in renal transplant recipient. *Gastroenterology* **70**, 425.
2. BALLARD R.A., DREW L., HUFNAGLE K.G. *et al* (1979) Acquired cytomegalovirus infection in preterm infants. *Am. J. Dis. Childh.* **133**, 482.
3. BECHTELSHEIMER H., KORB G. & GEDIGK P. (1972) The morphology and pathogenesis of 'Marburgvirus' hepatitis. *Hum. Pathol.* **3**, 255.
4. CARMICHAEL G.P., ZAHRADNIK J.M., MOYER G.H. *et al* (1979) Adenovirus hepatitis in an immunosuppressed adult patient. *Am. J. clin. Pathol.* **71**, 352.
5. CLARKE J., CRAIG R.M., SAFFRO R. *et al* (1979) Cytomegalovirus granulomatous hepatitis. *Am. J. Med.* **66**, 264.
6. CONNOR R.W., LORTS G. & GILBERT D.N. (1979) Lethal herpes simplex virus type I hepatitis in a normal adult. *Gastroenterology* **76**, 590.
7. ELLIS D.S., SIMPSON D.I.H., FRANCIS D.P. *et al* (1978) Ultrastructure of Ebola virus particles in human liver. *J. clin. Pathol.* **31**, 201.
8. EMOND R.T.D., EVANS B., BOWEN E.T.W. *et al* (1977) A case of Ebola virus infection. *Br. med. J.* ii, 541.
9. ERON L., KOSINSKI K. & HIRSCH M.S. (1976) Hepatitis in an adult caused by herpes simplex virus type I. *Gastroenterology* **71**, 500.
10. GEAR J.S.S., CASSELL G.A., GEAR A.J. *et al* (1975) Outbreak of Marburg virus disease in Johannesburg. *Br. med. J.* iv, 489.
11. JORDON M.C., ROUSSEAU W.E., STEWART J.A. *et al* (1973) Spontaneous cytomegalovirus mononucleosis. *Ann. intern. Med.* **79**, 153.
12. MARTINI G.A., KNAUFF H.G., SCHMIDT H.A. *et al* (1968) Über eine bisher unbekännte, von Affen eingeschleppte Infektionskrankheit: Marburg-Virus-Krankheit. *Dtsch. med. Wschr.* **93**, 559.
13. NICKELL M.D., CANNADY P.B. Jr & SCHWITZER G.A. (1979) Subclinical hepatitis in rubeola infections in young adults. *Ann. intern. Med.* **90**, 354.
14. SCHUSTERMAN N.H., FRAUENHOFFER C. & KINSEY M.D. (1978) Fatal massive hepatic necrosis in cytomegalovirus mononucleosis. *Ann. intern. Med.* **88**, 810.
15. ZUCKERMAN A.J. & SIMPSON D.I.H. (1979) Exotic virus infections of the liver. In *Progress in Liver Diseases*, VI, eds H. Popper & F. Schaffner. Grune and Stratton, New York.

Chapter 16
Chronic Hepatitis

Slowly, over the last ten years, the concept has arisen of a spectrum of chronic inflammatory diseases of the liver, extending from acute hepatitis to chronic hepatitis and finally to cirrhosis. Recognition has depended on an explosion in the use of needle liver biopsy on which the diagnosis ultimately rests. Whatever the type of chronic hepatitis, the same basic underlying liver histology is seen. Superimposed are histological features relative to the aetiology. However, before needle liver biopsy can be recommended, the physician must be aware of the mode of presentation and of the associated laboratory findings which point to the diagnosis (table 41).

CLASSIFICATION

Chronic hepatitis is defined as a chronic inflammatory reaction in the liver continuing without improvement for at least six months.

Cirrhosis is defined as widespread fibrosis with nodule formation (Chapter 18). The normal zonal architecture of the liver cannot be recognized.

Chronic hepatitis was originally classified into two types—chronic persistent and chronic active (aggressive) [19]. This has proved to be an oversimplification of the problem; a further type, chronic lobular hepatitis, has been introduced and the chronic active form has been sub-divided into a mild and severe type (figs. 252, 253) [37, 57].

Chronic persistent hepatitis (fig. 254) is marked by expansion of the portal zone by mononuclear cells and some fibrosis. The limiting plate of liver cells between portal zones and liver cell columns is intact. Piecemeal necrosis of liver cells is not seen.

Chronic lobular hepatitis is sometimes termed prolonged or unresolved acute hepatitis. Many of the histological features resemble acute viral hepatitis, but the duration is greater than three months [53]. The picture is predominantly that of intra-lobular inflammation and necrosis. Piecemeal necrosis and bridging necrosis are not seen.

Chronic active hepatitis is marked by the presence of an inflammatory infiltrate, primarily of

Table 41. The investigation of suspected chronic hepatitis.

Presentation
Fatigue: generally unwell
Following blood donation—positive hepatitis B test
Following acute hepatitis—failure of recovery, whether clinical or biochemical or both
Abnormal liver function tests or positive hepatitis B antigen test at routine check-up
Abnormal physical findings— hepatomegaly ± splenomegaly
Jaundice

Careful *history* and *physical examination*

Routine laboratory tests
Liver function tests:
   bilirubin
   aspartate transaminase (SGOT)
   gammaglobulin
   albumin
   alkaline phosphatase
Haematology:
   haemoglobin
   white cell count
   platelet count
   prothrombin time
Hepatitis B surface antigen and hepatitis B antibody by radioimmunoassay

Special tests
Serum antibodies:
   nuclear
   smooth muscle
   mitochondrial
Serum ceruloplasmin and copper
Slit lamp cornea
'e' antigen
'e' antibody
Alpha fetoprotein

Needle liver biopsy
Haematoxylin and eosin and connective tissue stains
Skilled interpreter

lymphocytes and plasma cells, which greatly expands the portal areas. This inflammatory infiltrate extends into the liver lobule, causing erosion of the limiting plate and piecemeal necrosis.

The *severe form* is marked by fibrous septa extending into the liver cell columns with isolation of groups of liver cells in the form of rosettes (figs.

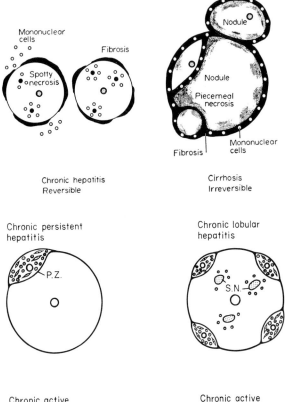

Chronic hepatitis
Reversible

Cirrhosis
Irreversible

Fig. 252. In chronic hepatitis the zonal architecture of the liver is preserved. In cirrhosis, nodular regeneration leads to loss of the essential hepatic architecture. Chronic hepatitis is essentially reversible, cirrhosis is not.

Chronic persistent hepatitis

Chronic lobular hepatitis

Chronic active hepatitis (mild)

Chronic active hepatitis (severe)

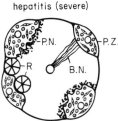

Fig. 253. Chronic hepatitis may be divided into three types. Chronic persistent and chronic lobular have a good prognosis. Chronic active is divided into a mild and a severe form. P.Z. = portal zone; S.N. = spotty necrosis; P.N. = piecemeal necrosis; B.N. = bridging necrosis.

256, 258; see colour section for fig. 255). Intra-hepatic 'bridging', either portal–central (fig. 236) or portal–portal, is seen.

The *milder form* (fig. 257) of chronic active hepatitis shows only slight erosion of the limiting plate with some piecemeal necrosis but without bridging or rosette formation.

This classification of chronic hepatitis is important in terms of prognosis. The chronic persist-ent and chronic lobular types do not progress to cirrhosis. Mild chronic active hepatitis may occa-sionally progress to cirrhosis but this is unusual. The severe chronic active hepatitis does so pro-gress and indeed cirrhosis may already be present, co-existing with the chronic active hepatitis.

Difficulties in liver biopsy interpretation [57]

Accurate categorization of the type of chronic hepatitis is clearly important because of the prog-nostic implications.

The liver lesion may vary in severity from place to place and this accounts for sampling errors which are particularly likely if the liver biopsy is small.

It can be difficult to distinguish periportal piece-meal necrosis from simple spill-over of inflamma-tory cells into the lobule, as in acute hepatitis.

If the patient is on corticosteroid therapy the in-flammatory reaction is reduced and a falsely optimistic interpretation may be made.

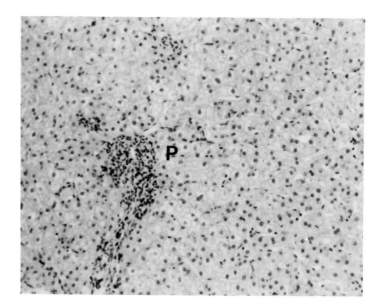

Fig. 254. Persistent hepatitis. Part of the liver biopsy, with inflamed expanded portal tract (P) but virtually no piecemeal necrosis. H & E, ×160 (Sherlock *et al* 1970).

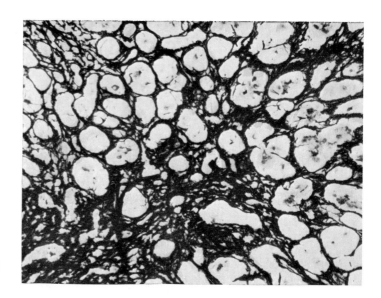

Fig. 256. Same case as fig. 255 (see colour section). Reticulin stains confirm the isolation of liver cells by bands of fibrous tissue, ×120 (Sherlock 1962).

In diseases with cholestasis, hepatocytes near the portal zones may swell and become necrotic. However, lymphocytes are relatively sparse, neutrophils prominent and hepato-cellular copper is often increased.

Difficulties in diagnosing cirrhosis on small samples are discussed in Chapter 18.

A skilled, experienced histopathologist is required to interpret these small samples.

CHRONIC PERSISTENT HEPATITIS

Aetiology and presentation

In many instances the aetiology is *unknown*. The patient presents with fatigue or when 'check-up' biochemical tests are found to be abnormal. Unexplained mild hepatomegaly is another mode of presentation. Patients are often males in the fourth or fifth decade.

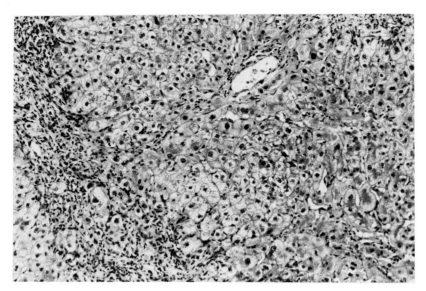

Fig. 257. Chronic active hepatitis. Part of a liver biopsy specimen, showing inflammation and piecemeal necrosis (*lower left*) and residual changes of acute hepatitis around a central vein (*upper right*). H & E, × 160 (Sherlock *et al* 1970).

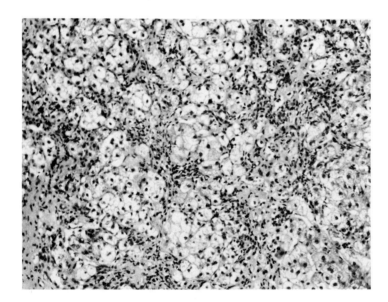

Fig. 258. Severe chronic active hepatitis with a positive hepatitis B antigen test. Shown are isolation of cell groups, fibrosis, and many plasma cells. The appearance is indistinguishable from active chronic hepatitis in patients not showing a positive hepatitis B antigen test. H & E, × 40.

Association with hepatitis B. These patients may come from geographic areas where carriage of hepatitis B is frequent or may be hospital workers in contact with blood. They may present as asymptomatic blood donors, found to be HBsAg positive.

Diagnosis may follow an acute attack of hepatitis with failure of HBsAg to be cleared from the blood. These patients are usually HBsAg and anti-HBc positive. Others may simply show anti-HBs alone. HBe is usually negative. HBsAg can be demonstrated histologically in the liver.

Hepatitis non-A, non-B [67]. This, at present ill-defined, condition can proceed to chronic persistent hepatitis. It is diagnosed by exclusion of hepatitis B and other known causes of chronic persistent hepatitis and by its relation to blood transfusion or exposure to blood products, such as factor 8, possibly contaminated with virus.

Alcohol. After recovery from an acute attack of

alcoholic hepatitis the portal zones may show inflammation persisting for some months.

Inflammatory bowel disease. Chronic persistent hepatitis may complicate longstanding chronic colonic disease, for instance ulcerative colitis, regional ileitis or infection with *E. histolytica* or *Salmonella.* Chronic persistent hepatitis may accompany infection with *Schistosoma mansoni* but here residua of ova are usually seen in the portal veins.

Clinical features

The patient may be asymptomatic. He may complain of fatigue, poor appetite, fat and alcohol intolerance and discomfort over the liver. These symptoms may only develop after the patient has been told he has chronic hepatitis.

Clinical examination may be normal or the liver edge may be tender. Physical signs of chronic liver disease, such as vascular spiders and splenomegaly, are absent.

Investigations

The serum bilirubin level is normal or slightly increased. Serum transaminase values may be elevated and values may continue to fluctuate up to about four times the normal limit for many years.

Serum alkaline phosphatase is usually normal.

Serum total globulin is usually within normal limits and the serum immunoglobulin G (IgG) is but slightly increased. This is a point of distinction from the active forms of chronic hepatitis.

Tests for serum hepatitis B antigen (HBsAg) should be performed.

In those with opportunities of contracting *Schistosoma mansoni* infection, evidences of this must be sought.

Needle liver biopsy

This is an invaluable method of confirming the diagnosis and particularly of distinguishing the persistent from the more serious forms of chronic hepatitis. The biopsy should not be performed until serum biochemical changes have lasted for at least six months. If the procedure is performed too soon the histological appearances may be difficult to distinguish from those of an acute attack of virus hepatitis which is recovering normally and which will not be persistent. If there is any diffi-culty in interpreting the first biopsy it may be prudent to wait six months and perform a second one.

Differential diagnosis

Chronic active hepatitis is distinguished by the physical signs of chronic liver disease and by the hyperglobulinaemia of polyclonal type. Needle biopsy appearances are helpful although mildly aggressive appearances in one portal zone with persistent hepatitis appearances in others can be extremely difficult to interpret. A longer period of follow-up with repeated needle biopsies of the liver may give a clear differentiation between the benign and the serious forms of chronic hepatitis.

Sclerosing cholangitis should be considered if the serum alkaline phosphatase is elevated. Endoscopic cholangiography is diagnostic.

Alcoholic liver disease is distinguished by the history of alcohol excess and by the physical stigmata of chronic alcoholism, including a large tender liver. Histologically, the biopsy may show the features of alcoholic liver disease. However, if the patient has abstained from alcohol for some time, such acute appearances may have vanished and the picture can be indistinguishable from other forms of chronic persistent hepatitis.

Gilbert's syndrome must be considered for both conditions can present after a hepatitis-like illness. Patients with Gilbert's syndrome show unconjugated hyperbilirubinaemia, normal serum transaminases and normal liver histology.

Treatment

This is by reassurance of the patient after the fullest possible investigations which may have to include needle biopsy of the liver.

Corticosteroid or immunosuppressant treatment, such as with azathioprine, should not be given. If these drugs have already been prescribed they must be withdrawn.

No specific dietary regime is indicated. In particular, there is no scientific justification for a low-fat diet, with avoidance of eggs and butter. Additional vitamins and 'liver tonics' are not necessary.

Alcohol can be permitted within reason provided it is believed that excess is unlikely in that individual and that the persistent hepatitis has not followed alcoholism.

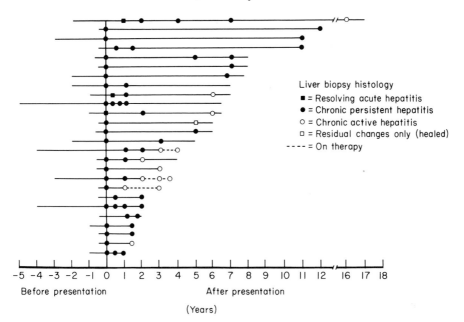

Liver biopsy histology
■ = Resolving acute hepatitis
● = Chronic persistent hepatitis
○ = Chronic active hepatitis
□ = Residual changes only (healed)
---- = On therapy

-5 -4 -3 -2 -1 0 1 2 3 4 5 6 7 8 9 10 11 12 16 17 18

Before presentation   After presentation

(Years)

Fig. 259. Chronic persistent hepatitis. Liver biopsies and length of observation in 26 patients. Mild chronic active hepatitis was seen histologically in nine. Cirrhosis did not develop (Chadwick *et al* 1979).

Prognosis

Twenty-six untreated patients were followed for 1–17 years (mean 5.6 years) (fig. 259) [10]. These patients did not develop any clinical features of chronic liver disease. Serial liver biopsies showed that nine patients progressed to a very mild chronic active hepatitis but none developed cirrhosis. In no case was there clinical or biochemical deterioration. Those who developed mild chronic active hepatitis were usually HBsAg positive and often 'e' antigen-positive.

CHRONIC LOBULAR HEPATITIS

This rare condition presents in much the same way as chronic persistent hepatitis. Patients, usually males, are diagnosed after an acute viral hepatitis-like illness [73]. Some may be due to non-A, non-B hepatitis. HBsAg is negative. The course is of remissions and relapses which are marked by elevations of serum transaminases. Serum auto-antibodies (smooth muscle and mitochondrial) may be positive.

There is an excellent clinical and biochemical response to prednisolone therapy and cirrhosis does not develop.

The differential diagnosis from other forms of chronic hepatitis can only be made by liver biopsy.

CHRONIC ACTIVE HEPATITIS

All types of chronic active hepatitis obey certain clinical, biochemical and histological criteria.

Clinically symptoms range from none to incapacitating exhaustion. Fluctuating hepatocellular jaundice is usual. Features of clinically diagnosable and symptomatic portal hypertension (ascites, bleeding oesophageal varices) are late features.

Biochemical tests show a variably elevated serum bilirubin level. Serum transaminase values are usually markedly increased and the gamma-globulin concentration is also elevated.

Hepatic histology shows the features of chronic active hepatitis.

Aetiology

A common clinical, biochemical and hepatic histological picture has been associated with more than one aetiological agent (fig. 260). Two main types have been identified (table 42). One is associated with persistence of hepatitis B infection while the

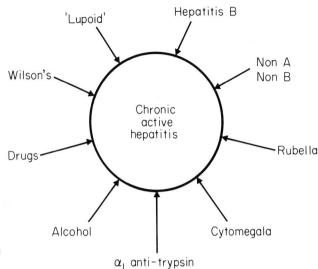

Fig. 260. The aetiology of chronic active hepatitis.

Table 42. Chronic active hepatitis: comparison of types negative and positive for hepatitis B surface antigen.

	'Lupoid' (HBsAg−ve)	Type B (HBsAg+ve)
Sex predominance	Female	Male
Age preference	15–25	Older males
	Menopause	Neonates
Serum HBsAg	Absent	Present
Autoimmune disease	Frequent	Rare
Serum gammaglobulin increase	Marked	Moderate
Smooth muscle antibody	High titre (70%)	Low or absent titre
LE cells	15%	Absent
Increased titre viral and bacterial antibodies	Yes	No
Liver membrane antibody	Present	Absent
Risk of primary liver cancer	Low	High
Response to corticosteroids	Good	Uncertain
Liver biopsy		
Shikata stain for HBsAg	−	+
'Ground glass' cells	−	+
Residual acute hepatitis	0	Frequent

other is associated with a negative result for hepatitis B, but has been termed 'lupoid' because of the association with a positive LE cell phenomenon in some 15% of patients (table 42). The two types will be described in detail. Non-A, non-B hepatitis can be followed by a chronic active hepatitis. In the neonate, and occasionally in the immuno-suppressed patient, other viral infections such as cytomegalovirus, may lead to chronic active hepatitis. Identical clinical, functional and morphological features may be found associated with some drug reactions, among them to oxyphenisatin found in

some laxatives, to methyl dopa and to isoniazid (Chapter 17). α_1 anti-trypsin deficiency may lead to a chronic hepatitis but more often presents as cholestasis in the neonate (Chapter 22). A liver biopsy in the alcoholic occasionally shows the picture of chronic active hepatitis (Chapter 19).

Immunological mechanisms of hepato-toxicity

Chronic active hepatitis is the liver disease *par excellence* where immunological factors are invoked in the perpetuation of the liver cell injury

[46]. Liver histology shows heavy infiltration by lymphocytes and plasma cells. This suggests a type four hypersensitivity reaction. Hyperglobulinaemia and circulating tissue antibodies are often present. In chronic active hepatitis it is postulated that the liver cells become injured by various agents. One such agent is hepatitis virus B. In the case of 'lupoid' chronic active hepatitis the injurious agent is unknown. Constituents of the injured liver cell so become antigenic. This leads to a self-perpetuating antigen–antibody reaction with resultant chronic liver disease [25]. Cell-mediated immunity to liver cell antigens has been demonstrated in chronic hepatitis and this process is mediated by sensitized lymphocytes and mononuclear cells. Peripheral blood lymphocytes from patients with chronic active hepatitis are cytotoxic towards other liver cells when tested in an *in vitro* microcytotoxicity assay [70].

Research has been directed in particular towards hepatitis B chronic active hepatitis for an antigen is available for study. Less information is available in chronic active hepatitis (non-B) where no such antigen has been identified. In hepatitis B the core antigen is produced in the nucleus of the hepatocyte. The surface is added in the cyto-

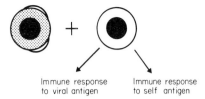

Fig. 262. The lymphocyte is sensitized both to viral and self antigen and mounts an immune response to both.

plasm and a portion of liver cell membrane is also introduced (fig. 261). The T lymphocyte is sensitized to both viral and membrane (self) antigen and an immune response is directed against both of them, so leading to lysis of the liver cell [25] (fig. 262)

Impairment of lymphocyte function may determine the outcome in type B viral hepatitis [25]. While this is defective, viral replication continues and a carrier state with or without chronic hepatitis results. Impaired T cell function is particularly important in such conditions as leukaemia, renal failure, in those receiving immuno-suppressive therapy and in neonates. With all these associations, acute type B hepatitis is likely to be followed by the carrier state. The type of lymphocyte involved and the interactions are difficult to unravel. Determination of lymphocyte populations in various types of chronic hepatitis has shown reduction in T cells in both HBsAg-positive and -negative chronic active hepatitis.

Null cells (i.e. not T, B or K) are increased. These results, however, may simply be secondary to liver damage. Suppressor lymphocytes moderate the activity of effector cells and so allow persistence of immune reactions to tissue antigens. Increased suppressor cell function is seen in patients with chronic active hepatitis [35] but cannot be related to the severity of the disease.

Failure of lysis of virally infected liver cells by T lymphocytes could have various mechanisms. It could be due to increased suppressor T cell function [29], to a defect in cytotoxic (K) lymphocytes, to blocking antibodies on the cell membrane [40], or to failure of recognition of genetic HLA markers displayed on the liver cell membrane (fig. 263).

In both HBsAg-positive and -negative chronic active hepatitis a candidate membrane-protein antigen has been termed liver specific protein (LSP) [49] (table 43). In the case of non-B chronic active hepatitis a liver membrane protein (LMP) is the postulated antigen. In this group a mem-

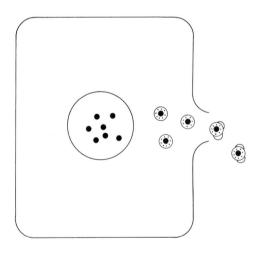

● Core antigen

⊙ Coat antigen (viral)

⌒ Membrane antigen (self)

Fig. 261. Hepatitis B. Core antigen is produced in the hepatocyte nucleus and coat antigen in the cytoplasm. The antigen leaving the liver cell also contains a membrane antigen.

Table 43. Chronic hepatitis: specific liver antibodies.

	Serum HBsAg +ve	HBsAg −ve
Liver specific protein (LSP)	+	+
Liver membrane protein (LMP)	0	+

brane-fixed IgG has been shown on hepatocytes [65] and continuing necrosis of liver cells is seen in patients with this antibody. It is not found in HBsAg-positive patients. These results support the existence of different pathogenetic mechanisms for chronic active hepatitis in the so-called 'lupoid' auto-immune type and in the hepatitis virus B induced type [49]. Cell-mediated immunity to both

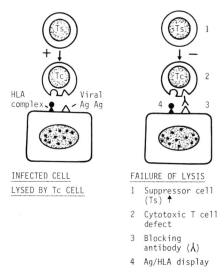

INFECTED CELL
LYSED BY Tc CELL

FAILURE OF LYSIS

1 Suppressor cell (Ts) ↑

2 Cytotoxic T cell defect

3 Blocking antibody (λ)

4 Ag/HLA display

Fig. 263. T lymphocyte lysis of infected hepatocytes and mechanisms of failure of lysis in chronic hepatitis. Ts = suppressor cell, Tc = cytotoxic cell (Thomas 1980).

membrane proteins has been shown in chronic active hepatitis. It is, of course, possible that chronic hepatitis may not be an immunologically perpetuated disease. The separation of primary events from immunological changes secondary to liver damage *per se* is almost impossible. The finding of mononuclear cells, toxic for liver-protein coated cells in five normal persons raises other problems [70]. At present, the mechanism of possible auto-immune chronic hepatitis, both HBsAg positive and negative, has not been solved.

CHRONIC ACTIVE 'LUPOID' (HBsAg-NEGATIVE) HEPATITIS

In 1950, Waldenström [71] drew attention to a chronic hepatitis occurring predominantly in young people, especially women. The syndrome has since been described under various titles [3, 7, 74]. None of the names is satisfactory and rather than dogmatize concerning aetiology, sex, age or pathology, all of which may vary, the term 'chronic active "lupoid" hepatitis' has been used.

Aetiology and pathogenesis

The aetiology is unknown. Immunological changes are conspicuous [46]. Serum gamma-globulin levels are grossly elevated. The finding of a positive LE cell test in about 15% led to the term 'lupoid hepatitis'. Antibodies against nuclei, smooth muscle and mitochondria are found in a high proportion of patients (table 44) [23]. An antibody to liver membrane protein has been shown [65]. This type of chronic active hepatitis is often referred to as 'auto-immune'.

Chronic active (lupoid) hepatitis is not the same as classical systemic lupus erythematosus, for the liver rarely shows any lesions in classical lupus. Moreover, the smooth muscle antibody and the mitochondrial antibody are not present in the blood of patients with systemic lupus erythematosus.

It is unlikely to be related to type B hepatitis, for markers of hepatitis B are consistently absent. Non-A, non-B seems unlikely for the chronic hepatitis found is not associated with circulating auto-antibodies in this condition.

There is an association with such conditions as pernicious anaemia and thyroiditis which are genetically related diseases. Family members of sufferers from 'lupoid' hepatitis show an increased incidence of serum auto-antibodies. The disease is associated with certain HLA antigens; 60% are HLA B8 positive (table 45) [30, 45]. The d locus antigen, DW3, may show an even stronger association [30, 47].

Table 44. Non-specific tissue antibodies in liver disease.

Disease	% positive serum antibodies against:		
	Smooth muscle	Mitochondria	Nuclei
Chronic active hepatitis			
HBsAg +ve	50*	0	0
HBsAg −ve	70	30	80
Primary biliary cirrhosis	50	98	24
'Cryptogenic' cirrhosis	40	25	38
Acute viral hepatitis			
type A	60†	0	2
type B	60†	0	0

* Low titre (1:10).
† Early. Titre usually low.

Increased antibody titres to measles and rubella are found in HBsAg-negative but not HBsAg-positive chronic active hepatitis [17]. The mechanism is unclear, but a defect in the antibody humoral and cellular lytic systems is possible.

Hepatic pathology

The lesion is a severe chronic active hepatitis. Activity is, however, variable from place to place and even in individual lobules. Near normal areas within the liver can sometimes be encountered.

Cellular infiltrates, largely lymphocytes and plasma cells, are seen in the portal zones and infiltrating between the liver cells. Aggressive septum formation isolates groups of liver cells as rosettes. Fatty change is inconspicuous. Areas of collapse may be seen. The connective tissue encroaches on the parenchyma. Cirrhosis develops rapidly and is usually of the macronodular type. The chronic hepatitis and the cirrhosis seem to develop almost simultaneously.

As time passes the activity subsides, the cellularity decreases, the piecemeal necrosis lessens and the fibrous tissue becomes denser. At necropsy in the longstanding case, the lesion appears that of an inactive cirrhosis. In most cases, however, careful search will reveal areas of piecemeal necrosis and rosette formation remaining at the periphery of a nodule.

Although inflammation and necrosis may subside completely during remissions, and the disease remain inactive for a variable interval, parenchymal regeneration appears inadequate as the perilobular architecture is not restored to normal and the pattern of injury remains detectable late in the disease.

Cirrhosis, although present in only one-third early in the disease, develops rapidly and is usually present two years after the onset [54]. Repeated episodes of necrosis with further stromal collapse and fibrosis lead to a more severe cirrhosis. Eventually the liver becomes small and grossly cirrhotic.

Clinical features

The condition is predominantly one of young people: half the patients present between 10 and

Table 45. The association of HLA–histocompatibility antigens with various liver diseases.

Disease	HLA association
Chronic active hepatitis	
HBsAg −ve	A1 B8 B12 DW3
HBsAg +ve	None
Primary biliary cirrhosis	None
Idiopathic haemochromatosis	A3 B7 B14
Alcoholic liver disease: males, severe	B8
Drug-related chronic active hepatitis	None

20 years old. A further peak of incidence is seen about the menopause. Three-quarters are female.

The onset is usually insidious, the patient feels generally off-colour and is then noticed to be jaundiced. In about a quarter, the disease seems to present as a typical attack of acute viral hepatitis [50]. It is only when the jaundice persists that the physician is alerted to the possibility of a more chronic liver disorder. Whether the disease does in fact commence as genuine viral hepatitis or present with intercurrent infection in a patient who

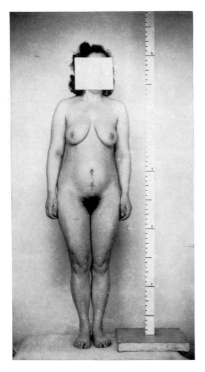

Fig. 264. Active juvenile cirrhosis. Well-developed girl with good nutrition.

is already suffering from chronic active hepatitis remains uncertain.

In most instances, the hepatic lesion on presentation does not agree with the stated duration of symptoms. Chronic active hepatitis must remain asymptomatic for some months or possibly years before jaundice becomes overt and the diagnosis is made. Patients may be recognized sooner if a routine medical examination reveals stigmata of liver disease or if, for some reason or another, biochemical tests of liver function are performed and found to be abnormal.

Although the serum bilirubin level is usually in-

creased, some are anicteric [50]. Frank jaundice is often episodic. Rarely, deep cholestatic jaundice is seen [16].

Amenorrhoea is usual and a return of the menses is a good sign. If a period does occur it may be associated with increase of symptoms and deepening of jaundice. Epistaxis, bleeding gums, and bruising with minimal trauma are other complaints.

Examination shows a tall girl, often above normal stature, well built and generally looking healthy (fig. 264). Spider naevi are virtually constant on face, necklace area or arms. They tend to be small and to come and go with changes in the activity of the disease. Livid cutaneous striae may be found on thighs, lateral aspect of the abdominal wall, and also, in severe cases, on upper arms, breasts and back (fig. 265). The face may be rounded even before administration of corticosteroids. Acne is prominent and hirsuties may be seen. The skin may show bruises.

Abdominal examination in the early stages shows a firm liver edge some 4 cm below the right costal margin. The left lobe may be disproportionately enlarged in the epigastrium; nodules are rarely palpable. In the later stages the liver shrinks and becomes impalpable and percussion confirms the decreased size. The spleen is almost universally enlarged. Ascites, oedema and hepatic encephalopathy are late features.

Recurrent episodes of active liver disease punctuate the course.

Associated conditions

Chronic active hepatitis of lupoid type is not a condition confined to the liver. The more careful the search the more likely is involvement of another organ to be detected. The association with conditions believed to have an auto-immune basis, such as Hashimoto's thyroiditis or Coombs'-positive haemolytic anaemia, has been partly responsible for the view that chronic active hepatitis represents an example of auto-aggression. It is uncertain how many of these associated conditions are related to the chronic active hepatitis and how many are coincidental.

In those particularly ill, usually with positive LE cells, there may be sustained pyrexia [54]. Such patients may also have an acute, recurrent, nondeforming migrating polyarthritis of large joints. In most cases pain and stiffness are present without marked swelling. The changes usually resolve completely.

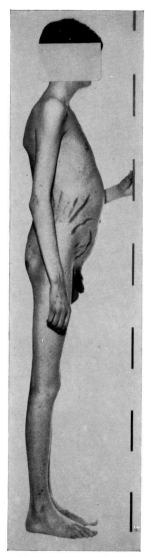

Fig. 265. Active chronic 'lupoid' hepatitis. Note tall boy with ascites and striae on abdominal wall and upper arms.

Subcutaneous striae have already been mentioned. A specific allergic capillaritis is characterized by active inflammatory papules with central crusting and lesions in the form of depressed scars [55]. More non-specific lesions include acne, erythematous lesions, lupus erythematosus type changes, papular eruptions and purpuric haemorrhages.

Splenomegaly may be present without portal hypertension, often with generalized lymphadenopathy, presumably part of the same process of lymphoid hyperplasia.

Renal biopsy often shows mild glomerulitis even in the absence of proteinuria and with a normal creatinine clearance [60]. Nodular deposits of immunoglobulins and complement have been found in the glomeruli [64]. Glomerular antibodies are present in about half the patients, but do not seem to relate to the extent of renal damage. Renal tubular acidosis is described and defect in urinary acidification, not related to serum immunological abnormality, may be found.

Pulmonary changes, including pleurisy and transitory pulmonary infiltrations and collapse, are found when the disease is active [54]. The mottled chest radiograph [11] may be related to dilated pre-capillary blood vessels. The high cardiac output of chronic liver disease would add to the pulmonary vascular plethora. Multiple pulmonary arteriovenous anastomoses are also found (Chapter 7). Fibrosing alveolitis is another possibility.

Primary pulmonary hypertension has been described in one patient with multi-system involvement [13].

Endocrine changes [59] include the Cushingoid appearance, acne, hirsuties and cutaneous striae seen in younger women even before corticosteroids are administered. Boys may develop gynaecomastia. Amenorrhoea is virtually constant. Hashimoto's thyroiditis may be seen [54] and other thyroid abnormalities include myxoedema and thyrotoxicosis [68]. Patients develop diabetes mellitus, before and after diagnosis of the chronic hepatitis [54].

Haematological findings of mild anaemia, leucopenia and thrombocytopenia are associated with an enlarged spleen ('hypersplenism'). A positive Coombs' test with haemolytic anaemia is another rare complication [54]. Auto-immune neutropenia with a serum immunoglobulin G antibody, specifically directed against neutrophils, has been demonstrated in one girl with chronic active hepatitis [5].

Ulcerative colitis tends to present with the chronic active hepatitis or to follow it.

The sicca complex of kerato-conjunctivitis sicca and a dry mouth is found in about one-half, less frequently than in primary biliary cirrhosis [32].

Biochemistry

The picture is of very active disease. Apart from the hyperbilirubinaemia of about 2–10 mg/dl, the serum gamma-globulin levels are very high (fig.

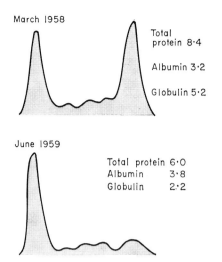

Fig. 266. Chronic active 'lupoid' hepatitis. Effect of corticosteroid treatment on the plasma proteins.

266). Electrophoresis shows a polyclonal gammopathy. Serum albumin is maintained until the later stages of clinical liver failure. Serum transaminases are very high. During the course, transaminases and gamma-globulin levels fall spontaneously.

Serum non-specific tissue antibodies (table 44)

Antinuclear factor. This is present in about 80% of patients with 'lupoid' chronic active hepatitis. The titres correlate with the serum gamma-globulin levels. It may be useful in evaluating prednisolone therapy. When ANF cannot be detected, treatment can be withdrawn with little fear of relapse [24].

Double-stranded DNA binding capacity. Elevated levels have been recorded in almost all types of liver disease, the highest in acute viral hepatitis and lowest in primary biliary cirrhosis [38]. The determination is of little practical value.

Smooth muscle antibody. This is detected in about 70% of patients with HBsAg-negative chronic active hepatitis. It is found in about 50% of patients with primary biliary cirrhosis. It is also present in low titre in patients with acute type A or B viral hepatitis or with infectious mononucleosis [23, 27]. Titres exceeding 1 in 40 are rare except in non-B chronic active hepatitis. The antibody is of IgM type. The antigen is related to the S actin or smooth and skeletal muscle. This is also present in cell membranes and in the contractile elements

(cytoskeleton) of the liver cell. Smooth muscle antibody can be regarded therefore as a result of liver cell injury.

Mitochondrial antibody. This antibody is present in 30% of patients with 'lupoid' type chronic active hepatitis, but its main role is in the diagnosis of primary biliary cirrhosis.

Liver membrane antibodies [65]. These may be found in the serum but the investigation is not performed routinely.

Haematology

Thrombocytopenia and leucopenia are frequent even before the late stage of portal hypertension and a very large spleen. A mild normochromic normocytic anaemia is also usual. The survival of erythrocytes is reduced, presumably related to splenic hyperfunction. Prothrombin time is often prolonged even in the early stages when hepatocellular function seems preserved.

Needle biopsy of the liver

This is very valuable but may prove impossible to perform because of the prothrombin time prolongation which is uncorrected by intramuscular vitamin K_1. If biopsy is possible the classical chronic active hepatitis is seen.

Differential diagnosis

The distinction from *chronic persistent hepatitis* usually depends on liver biopsy findings.

Needle liver biopsy and laparoscopy may be required to determine whether *cirrhosis* is also present.

The distinction from *hepatitis B-positive chronic active hepatitis* is made by testing for HBsAg.

The distinction from *Wilson's disease* is vital. A family history of liver disease is important. Presentation is often with haemolysis and ascites. The single mandatory investigation, however, is slit lamp examination of the cornea for Keyser–Fleischer rings. This should be performed in all patients under the age of 30 with HBsAg-negative chronic active hepatitis.

Confirmation of the diagnosis of Wilson's disease is made by finding a reduced serum copper and ceruloplasmin and increased urinary copper values. Liver copper is increased.

Ingestion of *drugs*, such as oxyphenisatin, methyl dopa or isoniazid, must be excluded.

Table 46. Significance between the difference in mortality in corticosteroid and control patients with chronic active hepatitis (Cook *et al* 1971)

Group	Total no. patients	Deaths from liver failure	Deaths from other causes	Total deaths
Corticosteroid	22	3	0	3
Control	27	13	2	15
Significance		5.09	–	7.45
(χ^1 with Yates' correction)		($p < 0.05$)		($p < 0.01$)

Chronic active hepatitis may co-exist with *ulcerative colitis*. Distinction must be made between the combination and *sclerosing cholangitis* where serum alkaline phosphatase values are markedly increased and serum smooth muscle antibodies absent. ERCP is diagnostic.

Alcoholic liver disease is usually seen in an older age group. The history, stigmata of chronic alcoholism and large tender liver are helpful diagnostic points. Liver histology shows fat, a rare association of chronic active hepatitis, alcoholic hyaline of Mallory, focal polymorph infiltration and maximally centrizonal liver damage.

Treatment

It is not surprising that drugs which alter immunological processes have been used therapeutically in this type of chronic active hepatitis. The most usual are the corticosteroids with or without azathioprine. In immunopathological conditions, corticosteroids probably act by reducing the damaging effects of antigen–antibody interaction at or near cell surfaces, as well as by a general nonspecific effect on the maintenance of cell integrity. The resulting decreased release of antigen could break a vicious cycle.

Three prospective controlled clinical trials have shown that corticosteroid treatment prolongs a life in severe chronic active hepatitis [14, 51, 61], although all the trials have imperfections [75] (table 46). Long-term follow-up of one trial confirmed that the benefit was particularly seen in the first two years (fig. 269) [42]. Well being is increased, appetite improves, fever and arthralgias are controlled. Biochemical changes are less constant, although serum bilirubin, transaminase and gamma-globulin levels usually fall. Serum albumin concentrations rise, so that after one year's treatment values are normal (fig. 268).

The effect on hepatic histology is variable and unconvincing, but there is unfortunately a large

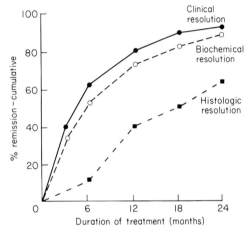

Fig. 267. The effect of prednisolone treatment in severe chronic active hepatitis (Summerskill *et al* 1975).

sampling error when needle biopsy specimens are used to assess this condition. Certainly progression from the stage of chronic hepatitis to cirrhosis does not seem to be prevented.

The indications for commencing prednisolone remain ill-defined.

If the patient is symptomatic, has very high serum transaminase and gamma-globulin levels and there is severe chronic active hepatitis on liver biopsy, the decision to start is easy. If symptoms are mild or absent and the biochemical tests are only modestly impaired, but the liver biopsy shows a definite chronic active hepatitis, the decision is less easy. Clinical judgement—a vague term—must be invoked. Liver biopsy must precede the commencement of therapy. If coagulation defects prohibit this procedure the biopsy must be done as soon as possible after a remission has been induced by corticosteroids.

The usual dose is 30 mg prednisolone for one week, reducing to a maintenance dose of 10–15 mg

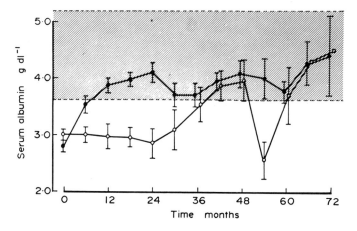

Fig. 268. Prospective controlled trial of prednisolone treatment in chronic active hepatitis. The treated patients (dark circles) show a significant increase in serum albumin concentration compared with a control over the first two years of treatment. At five years there was no statistical difference (Cook *et al* 1971).

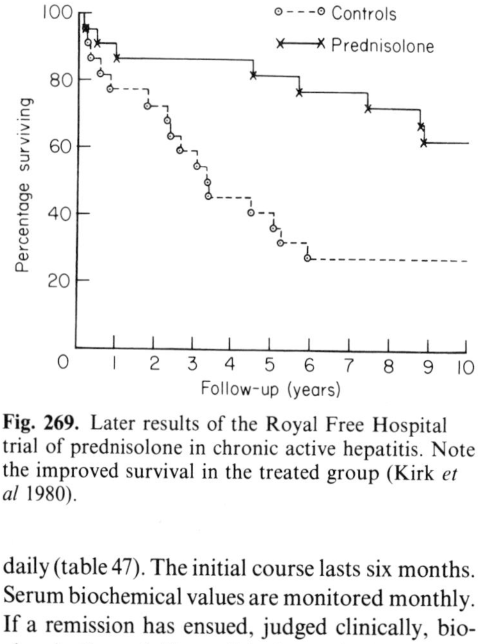

Fig. 269. Later results of the Royal Free Hospital trial of prednisolone in chronic active hepatitis. Note the improved survival in the treated group (Kirk *et al* 1980).

Table 47. Prednisolone in chronic active hepatitis.

First week
10 mg prednisolone three times a day (30 mg/day)

Second and third weeks
Reduce prednisolone to maintenance dose
  (10–15 mg/day)

Every month
Clinical check—liver tests

At six months
Full check—clinical and biochemical
Liver biopsy

Full remission
Withdraw prednisolone slowly
Re-start if relapse

No remission
If HBsAg +ve: stop therapy
If HBsAg −ve: continue maintenance dose for six
  more months, consider adding azathioprine
  (50 mg/day)

Maximum dose—20 mg prednisolone with 100 mg
  azathioprine
Maximum duration—usually three years

daily (table 47). The initial course lasts six months. Serum biochemical values are monitored monthly. If a remission has ensued, judged clinically, biochemically and if possible by a further needle biopsy of the liver, the drug should be tapered off slowly over a period of about two months. If activity has not abated, the prednisolone is continued. In general the usual course extends over two to three years. If the condition has not become inactive by that time, it is doubtful whether it is worth continuing the prednisolone. Disappearance of serum antinuclear factor may be a good indication of remission and for withdrawing the corticosteroid [24].

Prednisolone rather than prednisone should be given. Before it exerts its glucocorticoid effect prednisone has to be converted by 11-hydroxylation to prednisolone. This takes place largely in the liver. Blood levels are more predictable after prednisolone than prednisone and there may be a difficulty in the conversion in the presence of severely impaired liver function [47, 48]. Alternate day prednisolone treatment is not recommended as the incidence of serious complications is higher and histological remission less frequent [63].

Complications of treatment include facial mooning, acne, obesity, hirsuties and striae. These are particularly unwanted by female patients. More serious complications include growth retardation in those younger than 10 years, diabetes, bone thinning and serious infections. None is usually a problem if the dose of prednisolone is not more than 15 mg daily. If this is exceeded or serious complications have arisen, alternative measures must be considered.

If a remission has not ensued with 20 mg prednisolone daily, azathioprine (imuran) 50–100 mg daily may be added. It is not usually given routinely in the first instance. Continual use of such a drug over many months or even years has obvious disadvantages. However, it may be added if Cushingoid features are gross, if associated diseases such as diabetes prevent adequate doses of prednisolone or if other undesirable side-effects of prednisolone ensue at doses required to induce a remission. Azathioprine should never be given alone, as in controlled trials the results were no better than with placebo [63]. Azathioprine should not be given to young women wishing to become pregnant.

The later picture of cirrhosis is managed along the usual lines (Chapters 7, 8, 10, 11). Portal hypertension with bleeding oesophageal varices may raise the question of porta-caval anastomosis. This should never be done as a prophylactic procedure but only after significant bleeding from proven oesophageal varices. The incidence of hepatic encephalopathy after porta-caval anastomosis is greater in patients with cirrhosis following chronic hepatitis than in other forms of chronic liver disease. This may be related to the continuing activity of the disease; portal hypertension is relieved by the shunt, but the hepato-cellular necrosis continues unabated.

Course and prognosis

This is extremely variable. The course is a fluctuant one marked by episodes of deterioration when jaundice and malaise are enhanced. The ultimate effect of this continuing chronic active hepatitis is inevitably cirrhosis with very few exceptions.

In a long-term follow-up of patients in the Royal Free Hospital trial of prednisolone therapy the 10-year survival for the treated group was 63% compared with 27% in the control group ($P < 0.03$). The median survival was 12.2 years in the treated compared with 3.3 in the placebo group [42]. In the Mayo Clinic trial the five-year survival for the treated group was 93% [18]. Mortality is greatest during the first two years when the disease is most

active. Corticosteroid therapy prolongs life, but most patients reach the end stage of cirrhosis.

Oesophageal varices are an uncommon initial finding and do not develop quickly or bleed early after steroid treatment [18]. Nevertheless bleeding from oesophageal varices and hepato-cellular failure are the usual causes of death.

Pregnancy in patients with chronic active hepatitis is discussed later (Chapter 24).

CHRONIC ACTIVE HEPATITIS WITH POSITIVE HEPATITIS B ANTIGEN

The relationship between persistence of HBsAg and chronic liver disease is well recognized [26, 28, 52]. In many cases, perhaps the majority, the chronic liver disease is not preceded by a recognizable acute attack. In others the acute episode progresses directly to chronicity. In others, again, although the clinical picture at the apparent onset is of an acute illness, chronic hepatitis already exists.

About 10% of patients suffering acute type B hepatitis fail to clear HBsAg from the blood in 12 weeks and become chronic carriers [52].

Mechanisms of chronicity

These have already been discussed (page 276) (figs. 261, 262, 263). Progression depends on a combination of the background of the patient (particularly his immunological status) and on continuing replication of hepatitis B virus in the liver.

Those developing chronic hepatitis show a poor cell-mediated immune response to the virus [25, 26]. If the response is particularly poor, little or no liver damage ensues and the virus continues to proliferate in the presence of normal liver function. Such a patient would be an apparently healthy carrier. The livers of such patients have been shown to contain enormous amounts of HBsAg in the absence of hepato-cellular necrosis [34]. Serum levels of HBsAg are also high (fig. 270). Patients with a slightly better cell-mediated immune response show continuing hepato-cellular necrosis, but the response is insufficient to clear the virus and a chronic hepatitis results [25].

There is no evidence that any particular hepatitis B sub-type determines the clinical course.

There are no particular genetic (HLA) associations. Family clustering is probably environmental rather than genetic.

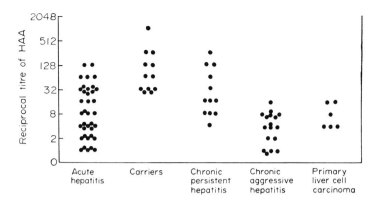

Fig. 270. The level of HBsAg (HAA) antigen in patients with a positive hepatitis B antigen test. 'Healthy' carriers show the highest levels and those with chronic aggressive hepatitis the lowest.

Predicting chronic type B hepatitis

Chronic hepatitis B has certain associations. Identification of them facilitates prediction of which patients, suffering from the acute disease, will progress to chronicity. Recognition of these associations also helps in the diagnosis of the patient with established chronic hepatitis.

The acute attack. Clinically the type of acute attack seems important. The patient having an explosive onset and deep jaundice usually recovers completely. Similarly, survivors of an attack of fulminant viral hepatitis seldom, if ever, develop progressive disease.

Patients receiving corticosteroids during the acute attack are also said to develop chronic hepatitis. In such circumstances the immunological response to the virus is reduced, hepato-cellular necrosis is mild but infection persists [28].

The relation of chronicity to premature and excessive exercise and over-indulgence in alcohol is largely anecdotal. These factors certainly seem to predispose to relapses but probably not to chronicity.

Age and sex. The very young and very old are at particular risk. The elderly have reduced absolute numbers of circulating T lymphocytes. Neonates are known to have impaired cellular immunity.

Chronic hepatitis B is found predominantly in males.

Serum biochemistry. Fluctuating serum transaminase levels are one of the least reliable measures of impending chronicity. A diagnosis based simply on an increase in serum transaminases is dangerous, engendering much concern in patients and physicians alike. Persistently increased serum immunoglobulin G is a more reliable indicator of continuing liver damage. Serum

bilirubin concentrations are unreliable; values may be normal despite progressive hepatitis. Alternatively, serum bilirubin may remain raised for months yet recovery is proceeding uneventfully.

Liver histology. Certain features suggest that chronic hepatitis will develop. Bridging necrosis whether portal–portal or portal–central (or both) is said to lead to cirrhosis [6]. If the portal inflammatory exudate spills over into the adjacent parenchyma, necrosis of hepatocytes ensues ('piecemeal necrosis'), connective tissue fibres accumulate and the limiting plate of the liver cell is eroded. This process continues on into chronic active hepatitis. However, during the acute stage no finding is absolute. Chronicity must not be diagnosed too soon after the acute attack of hepatitis. Because of sampling difficulties, more than one liver biopsy may be necessary.

HBsAg can be identified in liver cells by the 'ground glass' appearance of the cytoplasm. This is confirmed by Shikata's orcein staining [20]. This appearance suggests continuing infection although the correlation with severity of chronic hepatitis is not very close, the 'healthy' carrier showing the greatest number of antigen-containing cells. The demonstration of core antigen in the nuclei of hepatocytes suggests progression to a chronic state [4].

Hepatitis B markers. Continued presence of 'e' antigen in the blood suggests chronicity. On the other hand the demonstration of anti-e and anti-HBs are good signs. The presence of anti-HBc of IgM class suggests continuing viral replication, and association with chronic liver disease.

Clinical features

The patient presents the picture of a mild, slowly progressive, chronic active hepatitis. The features

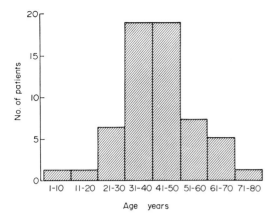

Fig. 271. The age at onset of symptoms or diagnosis in 59 patients with hepatitis B antigen-positive chronic liver disease (Dudley *et al* 1972).

suggesting an association with hepatitis B include origin from a country where the carriage rate of HBsAg is high, work in contact with human blood, patients having immuno-suppressive treatment, narcotic abuse, and homosexuality (table 37). Neonates born to an HBsAg-carrier mother can also develop chronic active hepatitis. There may be none of these associations.

The commonest sufferer is a male in the 30–50 age group (fig. 271).

The condition may be recognized as unresolved acute virus hepatitis, by fluctuating transaminase levels or by intermittent jaundice. The patient may be symptom-free with only biochemical evidence of continued activity.

In about one-half, presentation is as established chronic liver disease with jaundice, ascites or portal hypertension. Encephalopathy is unusual at presentation. The patient usually gives no history of a previous acute attack of hepatitis. Some present as primary liver carcinoma. Diagnosis may be made when a symptom-free person goes to donate blood.

Laboratory tests

Serum bilirubin, aspartate transaminase and gamma-globulin are only moderately increased (fig. 272). At time of presentation evidences of hepato-cellular disease are usually mild.

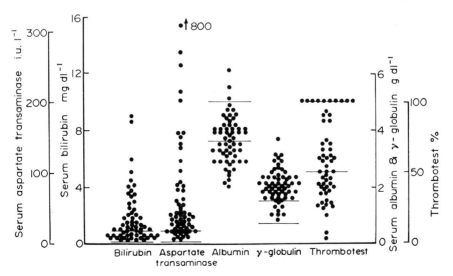

Fig. 272. Liver function tests of 59 hepatitis B antigen-positive patients when first seen at the Royal Free Hospital. Note that serum bilirubin, transaminase and gamma-globulin values are not particularly high and serum albumin is well maintained (Dudley *et al* 1972).

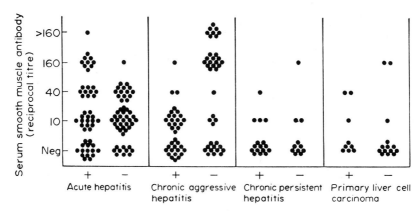

Fig. 273. Smooth muscle antibody titres in hepatitis B antigen-positive (+) and negative (−) patients with both acute and chronic liver disease. Note that the serum smooth muscle antibody titre tends to be higher in chronic active patients without the hepatitis B antigen (Dudley *et al* 1973).

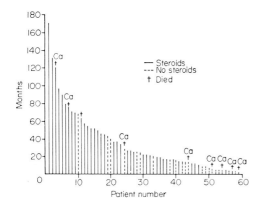

Fig. 274. Hepatitis B antigen chronic liver disease. Duration of disease in months after onset of symptoms. Ca=carcinoma. Note that most of the early deaths were related to hepato-cellular carcinoma. Thirty-three patients have been followed up for an average of two years without clinical or biochemical deterioration (Dudley *et al* 1972).

Smooth muscle antibody, if present, is in low titre (fig. 273) [27]. Serum mitochondrial antibody is negative.

Serum HBsAg is present, the titre being inversely proportional to the severity of the chronic hepatitis. In the later stages, HBsAg may be detected with difficulty in the blood yet the core antigen can be shown in the nuclei of the liver cells. 'e' antigen and anti-HBc are usually present.

Needle liver biopsy. This is essential to establish the diagnosis and, if possible, categorize the type of chronic hepatitis. Hepatic histology varies widely and includes chronic persistent and active cirrhosis and primary liver carcinoma. There are no constant diagnostic features for distinguishing this from other forms of chronic active or persistent hepatitis unless HBsAg is demonstrated as ground glass cells or by the orcein method [20, 34]. Cirrhosis is less frequent at presentation than in the 'lupoid' group.

Clinical and biochemical features correlate poorly with hepatic histology and biopsy is particularly important for assessing severity.

Treatment

PREDNISOLONE

Patients with HBsAg-positive chronic active hepatitis respond less well to prednisolone than do those who are HBsAg-negative. In the Mayo Clinic trial, clinical and biochemical remissions were less whereas treatment failures and deaths were greater in those patients with chronic active hepatitis where HBsAg was present [56] (fig. 275).

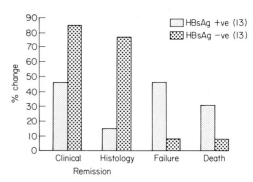

Fig. 275. The effect of prednisolone treatment in HBsAg-positive and -negative chronic active hepatitis. (Data from Schalm *et al* 1975.)

Table 48. Effect of prednisone on HBsAg-positive chronic active hepatitis (Scullard *et al* 1979).

	On prednisone	Off prednisone
DNA		
polymerase	1718± 359	489± 171
HBsAg	54± 8	24± 6
SGOT	50± 8	61± 8
HBeAg + ve	10	7

Viraemia may be increased as shown by a rise in serum DNA polymerase and HBsAg titres and with more patients remaining 'e' antigen-positive [58] (table 48). Another controlled trial showed that there were as many spontaneous, even complete, remissions with placebo as when prednisolone was given [44]. The use of prednisolone in HBsAg-positive chronic active liver disease is therefore controversial.

Prednisolone should be used only in those who are symptomatic and where the liver biopsy shows severe chronic active hepatitis. In such a patient, with severe abnormalities of both liver function and histology, there is no proven, available alternative. Some patients undoubtedly do improve with prednisolone therapy. The drug should be given for a trial period of three to six months and withdrawn if there is no improvement. Each patient has to be assessed individually. Patients having a mild histological picture on liver biopsy, and with only slight piecemeal necrosis, are usually managed conservatively in the first instance, with six-monthly checks and liver biopsies,

Table 49. Factors concerned in making the decision to treat chronic hepatitis (type B) with corticosteroids.

Factor	Yes	No
Age		
infant		/
old age		/
Concomitant disease (e.g. diabetes)		/
Long history of non-progressive liver		
disease		/
Severe symptoms	/	
High serum bilirubin, transaminase and		
gammaglobulin levels 'e' Ag − ve	/	
Liver biopsy		
chronic persistent hepatitis		/
marked piecemeal necrosis	/	
bridging	/	
rosettes	/	
'inactive' cirrhosis		/

as indicated, to assess progress. Other considerations contraindicating prednisolone therapy include advanced age or infancy, concomitant diseases, diseases such as diabetes, or a history of many years of non-progressive liver disease (table 49).

IMMUNOSTIMULANTS (fig. 276)

Corticosteroids suppress inflammation and reduce the activity of K lymphocytes. They do, however, favour viral replication. The defect in mounting a satisfactory immunological response to the virus must be corrected. Infected hepatocytes would then be destroyed as a result of a reaction in which non-infected cells would not take part.

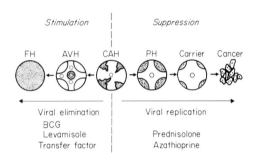

Fig. 276. Chronic HBsAg-positive hepatitis may be treated by immuno-suppression, but this favours viral replication and could predispose to hepatocellular carcinoma although this is unproven. Treatment by immuno-stimulation reduces virus but increases hepato-cellular necrosis. FH = fulminant hepatitis; AVH = acute virus hepatitis; CAH = chronic active hepatitis; PH = persistent hepatitis.

Levamisolone is an immunostimulant which increases the number of circulating T lymphocytes. Immunostimulation is shown by the development of cell-mediated immunity to hepatitis B antigen and by a rise in circulating HBsAg titres and transaminases as virus-infected hepatocytes are lysed [9]. However, clinical benefit does not ensue and this treatment has been abandoned.

Transfer factor converts null lymphocytes to functional T lymphocytes. Transfer factor, prepared from lymphocytes of patients who have recovered from acute hepatitis B, has been used to treat chronic active hepatitis, but the results have not been impressive [31, 39]. Rises in serum transaminases suggest necrosis of liver cells.

ANTI-VIRAL THERAPY

The aim is to eradicate the virus, improve liver function and reduce infectivity. Anti-viral therapy would clearly be the most satisfactory approach. Unfortunately, at the present time, no effective, inexpensive, anti-viral agent is available.

Interferons are small glycoproteins able to inhibit replication of a wide range of animal viruses. Two different interferons have been described, one produced in leucocytes, the other in fibroblasts. Administration both in man and in the chimpanzee has an inhibiting effect on replication

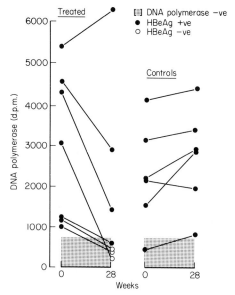

Fig. 277. The effect of arabinoside A on viral DNA polymerase in chronic HBsAg-positive hepatitis (Bassendine *et al* 1980).

of hepatitis B virus. When leucocyte interferon was given for less than two weeks, the changes were transient, but when two patients with chronic active hepatitis were given courses of three or more weeks a marked fall was noted in hepatitis B virus-associated DNA, in DNA polymerase and in core antigen. These improvements were maintained for some weeks after stopping treatment [33]. Human fibroblast interferon has also been used to reduce serum hepatitis B markers and transaminases in chronic active hepatitis [21, 41]. In one patient, fibroblast interferon also stimulated the immune response [22]. These results are promising, but interferons are difficult to prepare, in short supply and very costly. Until they are

more readily available, prepared perhaps by genetic manipulation, they will never solve the world-wide problem of the enormous numbers of patients with chronic hepatitis B infection.

Vidarabine (Arabinoside, ARA-A) is produced by fermentation of *Streptomyces antibioticus*. It acts as an analogue of the deoxyribonucleoside of adenine and has significant anti-viral activity *in vitro* against several DNA viruses. Preliminary results in the treatment of chronic HBsAg hepatitis have been promising [8]. In a controlled prospective trial, intravenous ARA-A reduced DNA polymerase in all patients with chronic hepatitis B liver disease (fig. 277) [2]. This indicates reduced viral replication and so less infectivity. In some, the effect was sustained and followed by a significant fall in circulating HBsAg, and in others hepatitis 'e' antigen was lost and anti-HBe developed. However, hepatitis B infection was not eradicated. A fall in serum transaminases was seen in those positive for HBe. ARA-A is easy to prepare and is not costly. An intramuscular preparation given twice daily over many weeks is under trial [72].

Prognosis

Progression is slow and insidious [28]. This is particularly so if the patient is asymptomatic and where the hepatic histology is that of a mild chronic active hepatitis. Such patients, with or without therapy, may go into remission, the histological picture becoming that of chronic persistent hepatitis. This is in contrast to the patients with the 'lupoid' type of chronic active hepatitis where, without therapy, there is a high mortality in the first two years. Once jaundice appears and decompensation (ascites, bleeding varices) is obvious, the outlook is as bad as in other forms of terminal cirrhosis (fig. 274).

Primary liver cancer is a dreaded complication. It should be suspected if the patient deteriorates suddenly with marked fatigue, right-upper quadrant pain, weight loss, oedema of the ankles and ascites (Chapter 28).

CHRONIC NON-A, NON-B HEPATITIS

Serial studies have shown that patients with acute non-A, non-B hepatitis progress to chronic liver disease. This applies to the blood transfusion-related [36], the blood factor-related [67] and the sporadic disease [1]. The incidence of chronicity seems to be about 30–40%.

Clinical features

Chronic hepatitis can follow both the long and short incubation types. Sexes are affected equally.

Chronicity may follow a clear-cut acute episode. It may develop insidiously and the acute episode would not have been recognized if the patient had not been under medical observation, for instance, after a blood transfusion.

A characteristic feature is the marked fluctuation in serum transaminase levels, extending over many months (fig. 248).

Serum auto-antibodies (ANF, smooth muscle and mitochondrial) are not detected. Serum immunoglobulin levels are normal. Serum markers for non-A, non-B infection are being evaluated, but none is currently available [69].

Liver histology [1] shows the general features of chronic hepatitis, usually of persistent or mild chronic active type. More specific histological features include fatty change and a disproportionate degree of sinusoidal cellular infiltration (fig. 278). Evidences of mild bile duct damage shown by irregular epithelium and infiltration by acute and chronic inflammatory cells may be seen.

Prognosis and course

This is marked by relapses and remissions associated with swings in serum transaminase values. Clinical progress is towards improvement, but cirrhosis has been reported.

Treatment

Reassurance and regular supervision at approximately three to six month intervals are required. More severe symptoms, biochemical abnormalities and hepatic histology may indicate prednisolone therapy (table 47). However, the role of prednisolone in this condition has not been fully evaluated.

DRUG-RELATED CHRONIC ACTIVE HEPATITIS

The whole picture of chronic active hepatitis can be related to drug reactions (Chapter 17). Such drugs include oxyphenisatin, methyl dopa, isoniazid and nitrofurantoin. Older females are affected

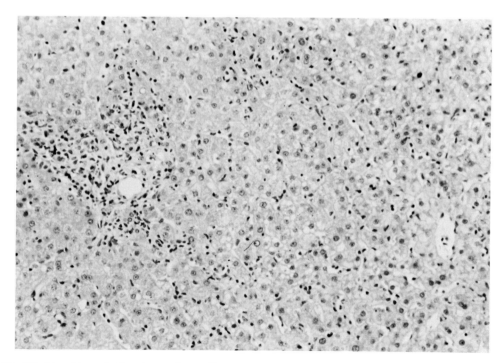

Fig. 278. Liver biopsy in chronic non-A, non-B hepatitis. Note marked sinusoidal cell infiltration ('lobular component') and fatty change in liver cells. H & E, ×208

most frequently. Clinical features include jaundice and hepatomegaly. Serum transaminase and globulin levels are raised and LE cells may be found in the blood. Liver biopsy shows chronic active hepatitis and even cirrhosis. Bridging hepatic necrosis is not so serious in this group [62].

Clinical and biochemical improvements follow drug withdrawal. Exacerbations of hepatitis follow re-exposure to the drug. Drug reactions must be considered in the aetiology of any patient with the clinical syndrome of chronic active hepatitis.

REFERENCES

1. BAMBER M., MURRAY A., THOMAS H.C. *et al* (1980) Clinical, serological and histological features of non-A, non-B hepatitis. *Gastroenterology* **79**, 1098A.
2. BASSENDINE M.F., CHADWICK R.G., SALMERON J. *et al* (1980) Treatment of HBsAg positive chronic liver disease with adenine arabinoside. In press.
3. BEARN A.G., KUNKEL H.G. & SLATER R.J. (1956) The problem of chronic liver disease in young women. *Am. J. Med.* **21**, 3.
4. BIANCHI L., ZIMMERLI-NING M. & GUDAT F. (1979) Viral hepatitis. In *Pathology of the Liver*, p. 164, eds R.N.M. Macsween, P.P. Anthony and P.J. Scheuer. Churchill Livingstone, Edinburgh.
5. BOXER L.A., YOKOYAMA M. & WIEBE R.A. (1972) Autoimmune neutropenia associated with chronic active hepatitis. *Am. J. Med.* **52**, 280.
6. BOYER K.L. (1976) Chronic hepatitis—a perspective on classification and determinants of prognosis. *Gastroenterology* **70**, 1161.
7. CATTAN R., VESIN P. & BODIN H. (1957) Cirrhoses dysprotéinémiques d'origine inconnue chez la femme. *Bull. Mém. Soc. méd. Hôp. Paris* **73**, 608.
8. CHADWICK R.G., BASSENDINE M.F., CRAWFORD E.M. *et al* (1978) HBsAg-positive chronic liver disease: inhibition of DNA polymerase activity by vidarabine. *Br. med. J.* **ii**, 531.
9. CHADWICK R.G., JAIN S., COHEN B.J. *et al* (1980) Levamisole therapy for HB$_s$Ag positive chronic liver disease. *Scand. J. Gastroenterol.* **15**, 973.
10. CHADWICK R.G., GALIZZI J., HEATHCOTE J. *et al* (1979) Chronic persistent hepatitis: hepatitis B virus markers and histological follow-up. *Gut* **20**, 372.
11. CHRISPIN A.R. & LESSOF L. (1965) The chest radiograph in 'juvenile' cirrhosis (active chronic hepatitis). *Br. J. Radiol.* **38**, 685.
12. COCHRANE A.M.G., MOUSSOUROS A., THOMSON A.D. *et al* (1976) Antibody-dependent cell-mediated (K-cell) cytotoxicity against isolated hepatocytes in chronic active hepatitis. *Lancet* i, 441.
13. COHEN N. & MENDELOW H. (1965) Concurrent 'active juvenile cirrhosis' and 'primary pulmonary hypertension'. *Am. J. Med.* **39**, 127.
14. COOK G.C., MULLIGAN R. & SHERLOCK S. (1971) Controlled prospective trial of corticosteroid therapy in active chronic hepatitis. *Q. J. Med.* **40**, 159.
15. COOK G.C., VELASCO M. & SHERLOCK S. (1968) Effect of corticosteroid therapy on bromsulphthalein excretion in active chronic hepatitis. *Gut* **9**, 270.
16. COOKSLEY W.G., POWELL L.W., KERR J.F. *et al* (1972) Cholestasis in active chronic hepatitis. *Am. J. dig. Dis.* **17**, 495.
17. CRIMMINS F.B., ADAMS D., ROSS M. *et al* (1980) Viral antibody titres in HBs antigen-positive and -negative chronic active hepatitis. *Scand. J. Gastroenterol.* **15**, 107.
18. CZAJA A.J., WOLF A.M. & SUMMERSKILL W.H.J. (1979) Development and early prognosis of esophageal varices in severe chronic active liver disease (CALD) treated with prednisone. *Gastroenterology* **77**, 629.
19. DE GROOTE J., DESMET V.J., GEDIGK P. *et al* (1968) A classification of chronic hepatitis. *Lancet* ii, 626.
20. DEODHAR K.P., TAPP E. & SCHEUER P.J. (1975) Orcein staining of hepatitis B antigen in paraffin sections of liver biopsies. *J. clin. Pathol.* **28**, 66.
21. DESMYTER J., RAY M.B., DE GROOTE J. *et al* (1976) Administration of human fibroblast interferon in chronic hepatitis-B infection. *Lancet* ii, 645.
22. DOLEN J.G., CARTER W.A., HOROSZEWICZ J.S. *et al* (1979) Fibroblast interferon treatment of a patient with chronic active hepatitis. *Am. J. Med.* **67**, 127.
23. DONIACH D., ROITT I.M., WALKER J.G. *et al* (1966) Tissue antibodies in primary biliary cirrhosis, active chronic (lupoid) hepatitis, cryptogenic cirrhosis and other liver diseases and their clinical implications. *Clin. exp. Immunol.* **1**, 237.
24. DOOLEY J.S., KIRK A.P., THOMAS H.C. *et al* (1979) Prediction of relapse following withdrawal of treatment in hepatitis B surface antigen-negative chronic active liver disease. *Gut* **20**, A954.
25. DUDLEY F.J., FOX R.A. & SHERLOCK S. (1972) Cellular immunity and hepatitis associated (Australia) antigen liver disease. *Lancet* i, 743.
26. DUDLEY F.J., GIUSTINO V. & SHERLOCK S. (1972) Cell-mediated immunity in patients positive for hepatitis-associated antigen. *Br. med. J.* iv, 574.
27. DUDLEY F.J., O'SHEA M.J., AJDUKIEWICZ A. *et al* (1973) Serum autoantibodies and immunoglobulins in hepatitis-associated antigen (HAA)-positive and -negative liver disease. *Gut*, **14**, 360.
28. DUDLEY F.J., SCHEUER P.J. & SHERLOCK S. (1972) Natural history of hepatitis-associated antigen-positive chronic liver disease. *Lancet* ii, 1388.
29. EDDLESTON A.L.W.F. & WILLIAMS R. (1974) Inadequate antibody response to HBsAg or suppressor T-cell defect in development of active chronic hepatitis. *Lancet* ii, 1543.
30. EDDLESTON A.L.W.F. & WILLIAMS R. (1979) HL-A system and liver disease. In *Progress in Liver Disease*, vol. VI, p. 285, eds H. Popper and F. Schaffner. Grune and Stratton, New York.
31. ELLIS-PEGLER R., SUTHERLAND D.C., DOUGLAS R. *et al* (1979) Transfer factor and hepatitis B: a double blind study. *Clin. exp. Immunol.* **36**, 221.
32. GOLDING P.L., BOWN R., MASON A.M.S. *et al* (1970) 'Sicca complex' in liver disease. *Br. med. J.* iv, 340.

33. GREENBERG H.B., POLLARD R.B., LUTWICK L.I. *et al* (1976) Effect of human leucocyte interferon on hepatitis B virus infection in patients with chronic active hepatitis. *New Engl. J. Med.* **295**, 517.

34. HADZIYANNIS S., VISSOULIS C., MOUSSOUROS A. *et al* (1972) Cytoplasmic localisation of Australia antigen in the liver. *Lancet* i, 976.

35. HODGSON H.J.F., WANDS J.R. & ISSELBACHER K.J. (1978) Alteration in suppressor cell activity in chronic active hepatitis. *Proc. natl. Acad. Sci. USA* **75**, 1549.

36. HOOFNAGEL J.H., GERETY R.J., TABOR E. *et al* (1977) Transmission of non-A, non-B hepatitis. *Ann. intern. Med.* **87**, 14.

37. INTERNATIONAL GROUP (1977) Acute and chronic hepatitis revisited. *Lancet* ii, 914.

38. JAIN S., MARKHAM R., THOMAS H.C. *et al* (1976) Double-stranded DNA binding capacity of serum in acute and chronic liver disease. *Clin. exp. Immunol.* **26**, 35.

39. JAIN S., THOMAS H.C. & SHERLOCK S. (1977) Transfer factor in the attempted treatment of patients with HB$_s$Ag-positive chronic liver disease. *Clin. exp. Immunol.* **30**, 10.

40. KAWANISHI H. & MACDERMOTT R.P. (1979) K-cell-mediated antibody-dependent cellular cytotoxicity in chronic active liver disease. *Gastroenterology* **76**, 151.

41. KINGHAM J.G.C., GANGULY N.K., SHAARI Z.D. *et al* (1978) Treatment of HBsAg-positive chronic active hepatitis with human fibroblast interferon. *Gut* **19**, 91.

42. KIRK A.P., JAIN S., POCOCK S. *et al* (1980) Late results of Royal Free Hospital controlled trial of prednisolone therapy in hepatitis B surface antigen-negative chronic active hepatitis. *Gut* **21**, 78.

43. KRUGMAN S. & GILES J.P. (1971) Viral hepatitis: new light on an old disease. *J. Am. med. Assoc.* **212**, 1019.

44. LAM K.C. & LAI C.L. (1979) Controlled prospective study on the effect of prednisolone in HBsAg-positive chronic active hepatitis (abstract). *EASL* 65.

45. MACKAY I.R. & MORRIS P.J. (1972) Association of autoimmune active chronic hepatitis, with HL-A1,8. *Lancet* ii, 793.

46. MACKAY I.R. & POPPER H. (1973) Immunopathogenesis of chronic hepatitis: a review. *Aust. N.Z. Med.* **1**, 79.

47. MACKAY I.R. & TAIT B.D. (1980) HLA associations with autoimmune-type chronic active hepatitis: identification of B8-DRW3 haplotype by family studies. *Gastroenterology* **79**, 95.

48. MADSBAD S., BJERREGAARD B., HENRIKSEN J.H. *et al* (1980) Impaired conversion of prednisone to prednisolone in patients with liver cirrhosis. *Gut* **21**, 52.

49. MEYER ZUM BUSCHENFELDE K-H., MANNS M., HÜTTEROTH T.H. *et al* (1979) LM Ag and LSP—two different target antigens involved in the immunopathogenesis of chronic active hepatitis? *Clin. exp. Immunol.* **37**, 205.

50. MISTILIS S.P. & BLACKBURN C.R.B. (1970) Active chronic hepatitis. *Am. J. Med.* **48**, 484.

51. MURRAY-LYON I.M., STERN R.B. & WILLIAMS R. (1973) Controlled trial of prednisone and azathioprine in active chronic hepatitis. *Lancet* i, 735.

52. NIELSEN J.P., DIETRICHSON O., ELLING P. *et al* (1971) Incidence and meaning of persistence of Australia antigen in patients with acute hepatitis: development of chronic hepatitis. *New Engl. J. Med.* **285**, 1157.

53. POPPER H. & SCHAFFNER F. (1971) The vocabulary of chronic hepatitis. *New Engl. J. Med.* **284**, 1154.

54. READ A.E., HARRISON C.V. & SHERLOCK S. (1963) 'Juvenile cirrhosis'; part of a system disease. The effect of corticosteroid therapy. *Gut* **4**, 378.

55. SARKANY I. (1966) Juvenile cirrhosis and allergic capillaritis of the skin. A hepatocutaneous syndrome. *Lancet* ii, 666.

56. SCHALM S.W., SUMMERSKILL W.H.J., GITNICK G.L. *et al* (1976) Contrasting features and responses to treatment of severe chronic active liver disease with and without hepatitis B$_s$ antigen. *Gut* **17**, 781.

57. SCHEUER P.J. (1980) *Liver Biopsy Interpretation*, 3rd edn. Baillière Tindall, London.

58. SCULLARD G.H., ROBINSON W.S., MERIGAN T.C. *et al* (1979) The effect of immunosuppressive therapy on hepatitis B viral infection in patients with chronic hepatitis. *Gastroenterology* **77**, 43A.

59. SHERLOCK S. (1958) Les 'troubles endocriniens' dans les affections hepatiques. *Rev. méd.-chir. Mal. Foie.* **33**, 63.

60. SILVA H., HALL E., HILL K.R. *et al* (1965) Renal involvement in active 'juvenile' cirrhosis. *J. clin. Pathol.* **18**, 157.

61. SOLOWAY R.D., SUMMERSKILL W.H., BAGGENSTOSS A.H. *et al* (1972) Clinical, biochemical, and histological remission of severe chronic active liver disease: a controlled study of treatments and early prognosis. *Gastroenterology* **63**, 820.

62. SPITZ R.D., KEREN D.F., BOITNOTT J.K. *et al* (1978) Bridging hepatic necrosis: etiology and prognosis. *Am. J. dig. Dis.* **23**, 1076.

63. SUMMERSKILL W.H.J., KORMAN M.G., AMMON H.V. *et al* (1975) Prednisone for chronic active liver disease: dose titration, standard dose, and combination with azathioprine compared. *Gut* **16**, 876.

64. SVEC K.H., BLAIR J.D. & KAPLAN M.H. (1967) Immunologic studies of systemic lupus erythematosus (SLE). Tissue bound immunoglobulins in relation to serum antinuclear immunoglobulins in systemic lupus and in chronic liver disease with LE cell factor. *J. clin. Invest.* **46**, 558.

65. TAGE-JENSEN U., ARNOLD W., DIETRICHSON O. *et al* (1977) Liver cell membrane autoantibody specific for inflammatory liver diseases. *Br. med. J.* i, 206.

66. TANNER A.R. & POWELL L.W. (1979) Corticosteroids in liver disease: possible mechanisms of action, pharmacology and rational use. *Gut* **20**, 1109.

67. THOMAS H.C., BAMBER M., MURRAY A. *et al* (1981) Short inoculation non-A, non-B hepatitis transmitted by factor VIII concentrates in patients with haemostatic disorders. *Gut*. In press.

68. THOMPSON W.G. & HART I.R. (1973) Chronic active hepatitis and Graves' disease. *Am. J. dig. Dis.* **18**, 111.

69. TREPO C., VITVITSKI A.M., PRINCE O. *et al* (1979) Demonstration in serum and liver of an antigen specific for long incubation non-A non-B hepatitis (HCAg). *Gastroenterology* **77**, 43A.

70. VOGTEN A.J.M., HADZICK N., SHORTER R.G., *et al* (1978) Cell-mediated cytotoxicity in chronic liver disease. *Gastroenterology* **74**, 883.

71. WALDENSTRÖM J. (1950) *Leber, Blutproteine und Nahrungseweiss Stoffwechs. Krh.*, Sonderband: XV, p. 8. Tagung, Bad Kissingen.

72. WELLER I.V.D., BASSENDINE M.F., MURRAY A.K. *et al* (1980) HBsAg-positive chronic liver disease: in-hibition of viral replication by highly soluble adenine arabinoside 5'-monophosphate, *Gastroenterology* **41**, 590.

73. WILKINSON S.P., PORTMANN B., COCHRANE A.M.G. *et al* (1978) Clinical course of chronic lobular hepatitis. *Q. J. Med.* **47**, 421.

74. WILLOCX R.G. & ISSELBACHER K.J. (1961) Chronic liver disease in young people. Clinical features and course in thirty-three patients. *Am. J. Med.* **30**, 185.

75. WRIGHT E.C., SEEFF L.B., BERK P.D. *et al* (1977) Treatment of chronic active hepatitis: an analysis of three controlled trials. *Gastroenterology* **73**, 1422.

Chapter 17
Drugs and the Liver

DRUG METABOLISM [31, 151]

The liver is particularly concerned with drug metabolism and especially drugs given orally (fig. 279). These must be lipid-soluble to have passed the membrane of the intestinal cell and must be converted to water-soluble (more polar) compounds for excretion via the urine or bile.

The main drug metabolizing system resides in the microsomal fraction of the liver cell (smooth endoplasmic reticulum). The enzymes concerned are cytochrome C reductase and cytochrome P-450. Reduced NADPH in the cell sap is a co-factor. The drug is rendered more polar by hydroxylation or oxidation. It is further made more polar by conjugation with such substances as glucuronic acid or sulphuric acid.

The drug metabolizing enzyme system may be induced, so increasing drug oxidation, by many lipid-soluble substances. These include barbiturates, alcohol, anaesthetics, hypoglycaemic and anticonvulsant agents, griseofulvin, rifampicin, glutethimide, phenylbutazone and meprobamate. At least 200 different substances may be enzyme inducers. Enlargement of the liver following the introduction of drug therapy can be related to enzyme induction. Inhibitors of the enzyme system include para-amino-salicylic acid. Two active drugs competing for the enzyme-binding site may lead to the drug with a lower affinity being metabolized more slowly and thus having a more prolonged action.

Factors determining whether the metabolized drug will be excreted ultimately in bile or urine are multiple and many are unclear. Highly polar substances are excreted unaltered in the bile and also those which become more polar after conjugation. Those with a molecular weight exceeding 200 are excreted in the bile. As the molecular weight gets smaller, the urinary route becomes more important.

Factors affecting hepatic drug metabolism

Removal of drugs by the liver depends on hepatic blood flow and on the ability of the hepatocyte to remove the drug as it perfuses through the sinusoids [82, 93]. In cirrhosis, impaired drug metabolism is related to extra- and intra-hepatic shunting and to failure of the liver cell [108]. A high degree of correlation exists between the half-life of a drug and the prothrombin time, serum albumin level, hepatic encephalopathy and ascites [32].

Chronic drug ingestion can induce drug metabolizing enzymes and so shorten the half-life of a drug in a patient with cirrhosis [64] (fig. 280).

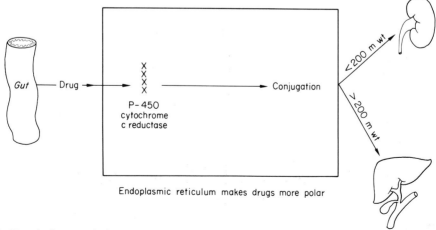

Fig. 279. Hepatic drug metabolism (Sherlock 1979).

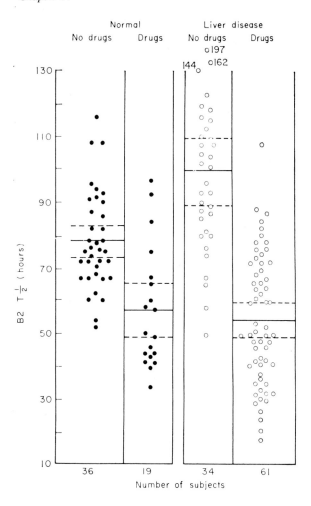

Fig. 280. The effect of preliminary treatment with drugs on the half-life of phenylbutazone. In those who were not pre-treated with drugs, the group of cirrhotics has a longer half-life than the controls. After pre-treatment there is no statistical difference in the half-life (Levi *et al* 1966).

Age. With increasing age there may be a decrease in drug clearance.

Sedatives. All commonly used sedatives are liable to precipitate hepatic encephalopathy in patients with liver disease. Oxazepam seems to be the safest [124].

The entero-hepatic circulation and the gut flora may also affect the quantity and nature of the drug or its metabolites presented to the liver.

Drugs causing interference with bilirubin metabolism

Drugs can affect bilirubin metabolism at any stage: in its production from haem, in its transport in the blood and through the liver cell, in its conjugation and in its canalicular excretion. These effects are relatively easy to investigate in man and the methods used in animals are usually applic-

able. Moreover, by and large, the response is predictable and reversible once the drug is stopped. These reactions are of little practical importance. They are rarely serious in the adult. In the neonate, however, a rise in unconjugated bilirubin in the brain is very important as this potentiates bilirubin encephalopathy (kernicterus). In the adult, those with an underlying tendency to, or actual, hyperbilirubinaemia will have their jaundice enhanced by any drug which interferes with bilirubin metabolism. This applies to such conditions as Gilbert's syndrome and chronic active hepatitis. Primary biliary cirrhosis, in its pre-icteric stage, may be made icteric by such drugs.

SERUM BINDING OF BILIRUBIN

Organic anions such as salicylates or sulphonamides compete with unconjugated bilirubin for

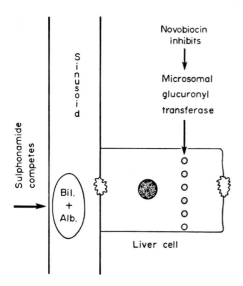

Fig. 281. Drugs given to neonates may compete with unconjugated bilirubin for serum albumin binding or may inhibit the microsomal conjugating enzymes (Sherlock 1972).

albumin binding and lead to its detachment (fig. 281). The unconjugated bilirubin can then reach the brain and, in neonates, can cause kernicterus. Infusions of albumin have been given therapeutically; these lower the cerebral but increase the serum unconjugated bilirubin level [22].

HAEMOLYTIC REACTIONS

These increase bilirubin production and so the load on the liver cell. This is rare as a single defect. In most instances the haemolysis is combined with a hypersensitivity reaction which decreases hepato-cellular function. Sulphonamides, for instance, can cause haemolysis but usually combined with generalized hypersensitivity. A haemolytic reaction may follow the use of para-aminosalicylate, phenacetin or quinine. Such drugs may also precipitate a haemolytic reaction in those having a genetically determined defect in the liver cell. In certain parts of the world, particularly in the Far East, glucose 6PD deficiency is a common cause of neonatal jaundice. The drug may be transmitted in the mother's milk. The toxic effects of synthetic vitamin K preparations given to neonates may partly be due to increased haemolysis.

INTERFERENCE WITH BILIRUBIN UPTAKE

Certain drugs interfere with the uptake of bilirubin into the liver cell and its transport to the microsomes for conjugation. This is true of the cholecystographic media. Rifampicin has a similar effect. The transport proteins may be decreased in the immature and this would make neonates particu-

larly susceptible to drugs that compete with bilirubin for transport. These drugs would potentiate kernicterus.

INTERFERENCE WITH BILIRUBIN CONJUGATION

The antibiotic novobiocin inhibits bilirubin glucuronyl transferase and the resultant unconjugated

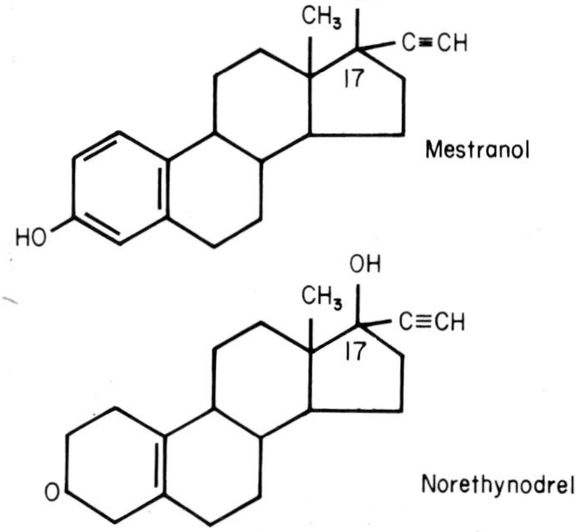

Fig. 282. The natural oestrogen, oestradiol, and the synthetic C_{17} substituted cholestatic derivatives, mestranol and norethynodrel.

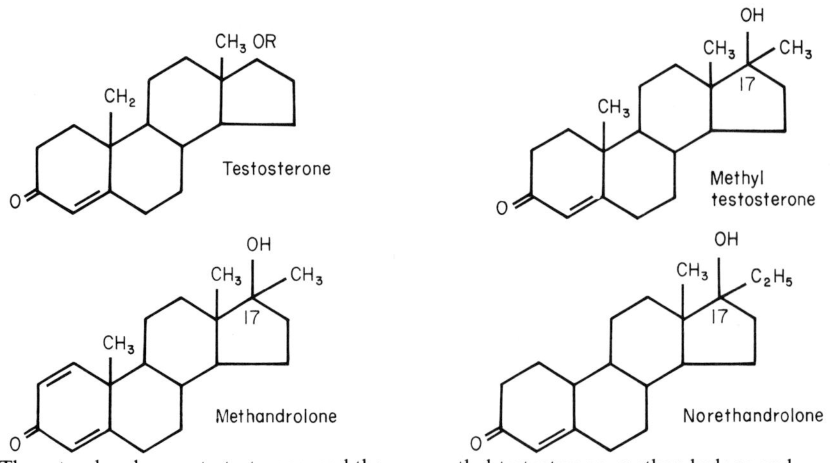

Fig. 283. The natural androgen, testosterone, and the synthetic C_{17} substituted cholestatic derivatives, methyl testosterone, methandrolone and norethandrolone.

hyperbilirubinaemia is particularly important in neonates [6] (fig. 281).

INTERFERENCE WITH CANALICULAR
EXCRETION

Cholestasis is known to follow ingestion of sex hormones, usually C_{17} substituted testosterones such as norethandrolone [97], methyltestosterone [142] or norethynodrel (figs. 282, 283). These are often contained in oral contraceptives (page 312). A similar cholestatic picture has followed organic arsenical therapy. The reaction is dose-dependent, benign and remits when the drug is stopped.

Light microscopy shows only mild cholestasis in liver cells, canaliculi and Kupffer cells. A portal zone reaction is absent. Electron microscopy shows variable changes in the canalicular microvilli which may be blunt and sparse. The Golgi apparatus is changed. Mitochondrial abnormalities have been noted [90]. The changes are not specific for this type of cholestasis.

The mechanism of cholestasis is extremely complicated. As both bilirubin and BSP (substances which are conjugated differently) appear in the blood in the conjugated form, the difficulty must be distal to the conjugating site in the microsomes. The drug might exert a direct toxic effect on the biliary secretory apparatus, namely the canaliculi, the canalicular membrane, the Golgi apparatus and mitochondria [97]. This could affect the flow of water into the bile and so cause cholestasis. An action on bile salts (taurocholate) excretion is also possible; this will interfere with micelle formation in the bile and so lead to cholestasis.

The prognosis is excellent. Phenobarbital may be tried to initiate a choleresis. Cholestyramine controls pruritus.

MECHANISMS OF DRUG HEPATOTOXICITY

Drugs seem rarely to cause damage by a direct action on the liver cell. Two other mechanisms are usually involved (fig. 284) [122]. The first is

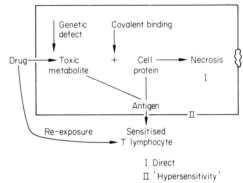

Fig. 284. The mechanisms of hepato-toxicity, direct, metabolic related and immunological hypersensitivity.

mediated by metabolite-related substances which combine covalently with cell proteins. The second is by the development of an immunological reaction to the drug which renders a constituent of the liver cell antigenic (fig. 284). In the case of some drugs, for instance paracetamol (acetaminophen), the metabolite-related injury seems particularly important. In others, for instance halothane, the immunological reaction may be predominant.

With many drugs the mechanism of the drug–liver reaction remains poorly understood.

Direct (metabolite-related) action

The hepatic drug metabolizing enzymes activate chemically stable drugs to produce potent alkylating, arylating or acylating agents. These bind covalently to liver macromolecules essential to the life of the liver cell and necrosis ensues [75]. The liver usually contains substances, such as glutathione, which are capable of preferentially conjugating with a toxic metabolite. It is only when the stores of these substances are exhausted that necrosis ensues.

The extent of the necrosis is increased by pretreatment with enzyme inducers, such as phenobarbital, and reduced by enzyme inhibitors.

The reaction is dose-dependent. Animal models exist. Other organs also suffer and renal damage is often the most important.

In mild cases, jaundice may be mild, slight and transient. Serum biochemical tests show marked rises in transaminases. Prothrombin time increases.

Light microscopy shows clear-cut centrizonal necrosis with scattered fatty change and little inflammatory reaction (see fig. 285 in colour section). Periportal fibrosis may sometimes be marked.

The problem, if this concept is correct, is to relate the extent of the liver injury to the small amounts of active metabolite released. The infrequency of the reaction compared with the many patients receiving the drug must also be explained.

Immunological reaction to the drug

Liver injury is unrelated to dose. Only a small proportion, usually about 1%, of those receiving the drug suffer liver injury. Children are usually unaffected. Associated phenomena may include fever, skin rashes and eosinophilia. Animal models do not exist. The diagnosis can only be confirmed by drug challenge. This is ethically unjustified if the original reaction has been a serious one. Familial reactions suggest hereditary factors which may influence the rate and form of metabolism of a drug. Microsomal enzyme activity is genetically determined. No relationship to HLA phenotypes has been shown.

The drug concerned is usually too small a molecule to become antigenic. The drug or its metabolite may act as a hapten combining with a normal membrane antigen. Alternatively, the drug or its metabolite may bind covalently to a liver macromolecule, so rendering it antigenic. Lymphocytes are sensitized and, on re-exposure, a delayed hypersensitivity reaction to the antigen is mounted and liver cell necrosis ensues. The reaction is unlikely to be self-perpetuating once the drug is removed.

TOXICITY OF INDIVIDUAL DRUGS

Carbon tetrachloride

This may be taken accidentally or suicidally. It may be inhaled, for instance in dry-cleaning or in filling fire extinguishers, or mixed in drinks.

The liver injury is induced by a toxic metabolite of microsomal origin which combines covalently with cell proteins and induces necrosis (fig. 286) [72]. The effect is enhanced by enzyme inducers such as alcohol and barbiturates and reduced by protein malnutrition which depresses drug metabolizing enzymes. This may explain the apparent resistance of those in under-developed countries to the hepato-toxic effects of carbon tetrachloride and similar compounds when used as vermifuges.

CLINICAL FEATURES

Jaundice develops within 48 hours. The liver may be enlarged and tender. Spontaneous haemorrhages reflect the profound hypoprothrombinaemia. Serum transaminase values are very high (fig. 287); the serum albumin level falls.

In severe cases acute renal failure overshadows hepatic destruction. Acute haemorrhagic gastritis is prominent. Since carbon tetrachloride is an anaesthetic the patient becomes increasingly drowsy.

PATHOLOGY

Centrizonal cells show hydropic degeneration marked by clear cytoplasm and pyknotic nuclei (fig. 285). Fatty change varies from a few droplets centrizonally to diffuse involvement of liver cells.

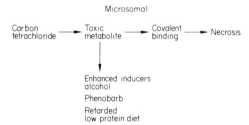

Fig. 286. Carbon tetrachloride liver injury mediated by a toxic metabolite (Sherlock 1979).

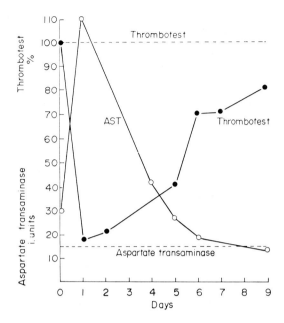

Fig. 287. Suicidal inhalation of carbon
tetrachloride in a young male. Note the
rapid fall in thrombotest with rise in
transaminase values. At six days they have
virtually resumed normal levels.

Polymorphonuclear infiltration of the portal zones
is slight, fibrosis is uncommon. With recovery the
liver pattern returns to normal.

PROGNOSIS

Death in the acute stage is due to kidney and not
liver failure. If the patient survives the acute episode there are no late hepatic sequelae. In rats one
oral dose of carbon tetrachloride causes acute
hepatic injury followed by complete recovery, but
repeated administration leads to cirrhosis. This
sequence is not seen in man. Liver cells may even
be more resistant with prolonged exposure.
Carbon tetrachloride is not an aetiological factor
in hepatic cirrhosis in man.

PROPHYLAXIS AND TREATMENT

Screening tests in workers should include routine
examination for liver enlargement and tenderness,
urine testing for urobilinogen and serum transaminase estimation.

Acute poisoning is treated by a high calorie,
high carbohydrate diet and the usual lines for
acute hepato-renal failure. Facilities for haemodialysis must be available.

RELATED COMPOUNDS

Other chlorinated hydrocarbons and benzol
derivatives may act similarly. Teenagers sniffing

cleaning fluid which contains trichlorethylene [2]
or glue containing toluene [86] suffer jaundice with
centrizonal liver necrosis and renal failure.

Chlorophenothane (DDT) in large doses causes
fatty change and hepato-cellular necrosis. It is a
potent enzyme inducer consumed as a food addi-
tive.

Benzene derivatives include trinitrotoluene
(TNT), dinitrophenol and toluene. The maximum
effect is on the bone-marrow with aplasia. The
liver may be involved acutely, but chronic sequelae
are rare.

Vinyl chloride

Workmen exposed to vinyl chloride monomer
over many years may develop hepato-toxicity [130]
(fig. 288). The earliest change is a sclerosis of portal

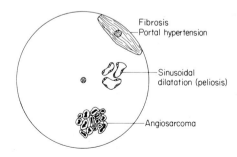

Fig. 288. Toxic effects of vinyl chloride, arsenic
and thorotrast on the liver.

venules in the portal zones of the liver with the clinical changes of splenomegaly and portal hypertension. Later associations include angiosarcoma of the liver and peliosis hepatis [5, 98].

Tetracyclines

Chlortetracycline and oxychlortetracycline interfere with protein synthesis. In 1963, six women in the last trimester of pregnancy were given large doses (3.5–6 g per day intravenously) of tetracycline for the treatment of pyelonephritis. Death followed in hepato-renal failure [117]. Autopsy showed a markedly fatty liver. Tetracyclines have been associated with fatty liver of pregnancy although the condition is also common without drug administration [94].

Tetracycline toxicity is especially likely when protein synthesis is under stress or impaired, as in pregnancy, or in protein undernutrition. Tetracycline may be inhibitory to protein synthesis particularly affecting the transport lipoproteins which remove triglyceride from the liver. It should be avoided during pregnancy although large doses intravenously are probably necessary for significant hepato-toxicity.

Oxacillin

This antibiotic frequently leads to an increase in serum transaminases which is usually reversible when the drug is withdrawn [14].

Muscarine

Acute liver failure follows ingestion of various *Amanita* mushrooms, including *A. phalloides* and *A. verna*. Three stages of illness can be recognized. The first, starting 8–12 hours after ingestion, consists of nausea, cramping abdominal pain and rice-water diarrhoea and lasts for three to four days. The second phase is characterized by apparent improvement. The third stage includes hepato-renal and central nervous system degeneration with massive cell destruction. The liver shows centrizonal necrosis without much inflammation. Fatty change is seen in fatal cases [141]. The condition is life-threatening although recovery can occur. The mushroom toxins, phalloidin and phalloin, are extremely lethal to liver cells.

Supportive measures are all that can be offered. Haemodialysis may be helpful.

Hycanthone

Hycanthone, used in the treatment of schistosomiasis, is hepato-toxic. Fatalities are seen particularly with overdose or in those with underlying liver diseases [16].

Paracetamol (acetaminophen)

Paracetamol is being used increasingly as a suicidal agent [8, 102]. About 10 g produces hepatic necrosis, but the dose actually ingested is difficult

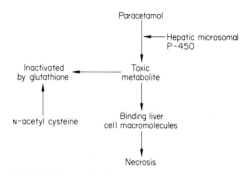

Fig. 289. The mechanism of paracetamol (acetaminophen) liver injury and of N-acetyl cysteine treatment (Sherlock 1979).

to assess because of early vomiting and unreliable histories.

The electrophilic metabolite of paracetamol preferentially conjugates with hepatic glutathione. When the glutathione is exhausted the paracetamol metabolite arylates essential nucleophilic macromolecules, so producing hepatic necrosis [76] (fig. 289).

CLINICAL FEATURES

Within a few hours of ingestion, the patient becomes nauseated and vomits. Consciousness is preserved. After about 48 hours recovery seems in progress; then the patient deteriorates and becomes jaundiced about the third or fourth day when the liver is tender. Serum transaminase and prothrombin levels are enormous. In the more seriously affected, deterioration is then rapid with the signs of acute hepatic necrosis (Chapter 7). Myocardial and renal damage and hypoglycaemia are prominent.

Hepatic histology shows centrizonal necrosis, some fatty change and very little inflammation [100]. Reticulin collapse may be confluent and massive, but cirrhosis is not a sequel.

PROGNOSIS

The overall mortality for 201 patients admitted to a general hospital was 3.5% [43]. A prothrombin ratio of 20% and hepatic coma are unfavourable prognostic signs. Severity can also be assessed by the paracetamol blood levels which should always be determined. The normal plasma half-life is two hours. If it exceeds four hours hepatic toxicity is likely, and if greater than 12 hours severe hepatic damage is probable. If the plasma level four hours after the overdose exceeds $300\,\mu g/ml$ there is 100% incidence of hepatic toxicity, and if less than $120\,\mu g/ml$ there is no danger. If the paracetamol level 12 hours after administration exceeds $50\,\mu g/ml$ hepatic toxicity is likely, and if less than $50\,\mu g/ml$ there is no danger [23, 99].

Chronic hepatitis. Long-term (about one year) exposure to paracetamol (within the therapeutic upper limit of 4 g daily) may lead to chronic hepatitis [12, 50]. Underlying liver disease may potentiate the effect [112].

TREATMENT

The stomach is washed out. The patient is admitted to hospital. Evidences of hepatic necrosis are delayed and early improvement should not give a sense of false security.

Forced diuresis and renal dialysis are not indicated as they do not increase the excretion of paracetamol or its metabolites already bound to tissues. The treatment of acute liver failure is outlined in Chapter 7.

Treatment is aimed at replenishing the glutathione reserves of the liver cell. Unfortunately the penetration of glutathione itself into liver cells is poor. Precursors of glutathione and glutathione-like substances have therefore been employed. They are necessary only when hepatic damage is likely. This is assessed by plasma levels. The patient's value is plotted against a line joining $200\,\mu g/ml$ at four hours, and $60\,\mu g/ml$ at 12 hours on a semi-log graph of concentration versus time [100]. If the patient's concentration is below this line, liver damage will be clinically insignificant and treatment can be stopped.

Cysteamine was the first drug used and methionine has also been given. They have been replaced by intravenous N-acetyl cysteine (Mucomist, Parvolex) [99]. This is rapidly hydrolysed to cysteine *in vivo*. It has fewer side-effects than cysteamine. It is very effective in preventing severe liver damage if administered up to eight hours after an overdose. Treatment after 15 hours is ineffective. The dose is 150 mg/kg in 200 ml 5% glucose over 15 minutes, followed by 50 mg/kg in 500 ml 5% dextrose over four hours and 100 mg/kg in one litre 5% dextrose over the next 16 hours (total dose 300 mg/kg in 20 hours).

Salicylates

Patients on salicylate therapy for acute rheumatic fever, juvenile and adult rheumatoid arthritis, and systemic lupus erythematosus, may develop acute hepatic injury and even chronic active hepatitis [39]. This may develop even with serum salicylate levels below 25 mg/100 ml [87].

Methotrexate

Methotrexate is first metabolized to 6-mercaptopurine. Hepato-toxicity results from a toxic metabolite of microsomal origin which induces fibrosis and ultimately cirrhosis (fig. 290) [1]. Primary liver cancer can develop [113]. Electron microscopy shows membrane whorls, lipid droplets and autophagic vacuoles [85].

This complication is likely to follow long-term therapy, usually for psoriasis [19] or leukaemia. A cumulative dose exceeding 2 g is especially dangerous [84]. Increased alcohol intake adds to the risk. Serum transaminases and, if possible, needle biopsy should be performed before starting and at regular (yearly) intervals during treatment; any abnormality is a contraindication to starting the drug and an indication to stop it. Repeated biopsies are helpful in following the course.

Other cytotoxic drugs

These drugs cause rises in serum transaminases and phosphatases if large amounts are given. Hepatic histology shows centrizonal necrosis. The pattern is of metabolite-related liver injury. This complication applies to such drugs as mithramycin, mitomycin and actinomycin.

More long-term use of cytotoxic agents, such as azathioprine, methotrexate, 6-mercaptopurine and cyclophosphamide, in recipients of renal transplants or in children with acute leukaemia leads to chronic hepatitis, fibrosis and portal hypertension [81].

Azathioprine may lead to cholestasis and, in recipients of liver transplants, this may cause con-

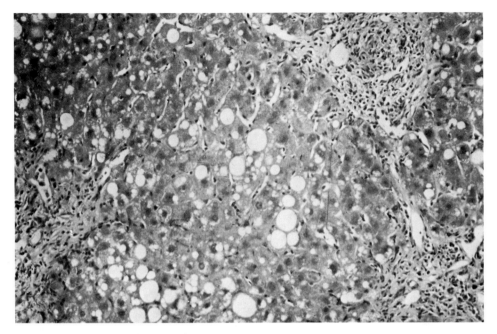

Fig. 290. Methotrexate liver injury. Zonal architecture is maintained. The portal zones are expanded with fibrous tissue and mononuclear cells. The hepatocytes show fatty change. H & E, × 65.

fusion with impending rejection and graft-versus-host reactions. Such cholestatic reactions should not be treated with azathioprine as this demands good hepato-cellular function for its metabolism to the active 6-mercaptopurine.

Arsenic

The organic, trivalent compounds are particularly poisonous. Arsenic trioxide 1% (Fowler's solution) given for long periods for the treatment of psoriasis has resulted in presinusoidal intra-hepatic portal hypertension [78, 137]. Arsenic in drinking water and drugs in India may be related to 'idiopathic' portal hypertension. The liver shows portal tract fibrosis and sclerosis of the thickened portal vein branches. Arsenic may damage intra-hepatic portal veins, producing the picture of hepato-portal sclerosis (fig. 288).

Manganese, gold, mercury and iron

These are also said to cause cirrhosis, but this must be exceedingly rare in man. Careful attention should be paid to other aetiological factors before these metals are incriminated.

Accidental ingestion of large quantities of ferrous sulphate is followed by haemorrhagic necrosis of the periportal zones of the liver.

Gold sodium thiomalate can cause cholestatic jaundice [34]. Eosinophilia may be noted. Liver biopsy shows cholestasis. Recovery is usual.

Phosphorus

The red form is relatively non-toxic but the yellow is extremely lethal, as little as 60 mg being fatal. It is usually taken accidentally or suicidally as rat poison or in fire crackers [71].

Acute poisoning causes nausea, vomiting and abdominal pain due to gastric irritation. Phosphorus may be found by gastric lavage. The patient's breath has a characteristic garlic odour and the faeces are frequently phosphorescent. Jaundice appears on the third or fourth day. The course may be fulminating with coma and death within 24 hours or, more usually, within the first four days. About half recover, but liver biopsy shows periportal fibrosis [41]. Ultimate recovery will probably be complete. There is no specific treatment.

Vitamin A

Chronic ingestion results in hepatomegaly, abnormal biochemical tests, portal hypertension and even cirrhosis [49]. The vitamin is stored in lipocytes (Ito cells). These may transform to fibroblasts.

Mineral oil

Chronic ingestion of mineral oils can lead to hepatic inflammation and scarring related to deposits in portal triads [11].

Physical agents

HYPERTHERMIA [54]

Heat-stroke is invariably accompanied by hepato-cellular damage. In 10% it is severe and may contribute to death. Pathologically it is marked by centrizonal degeneration or necrosis, congestion and cholestasis. Dilatation of portal venules is prominent in fatal cases. Biochemically there may be jaundice, increase in serum enzymes and a fall in prothrombin and albumin levels. The damage is due both to hypoxia and to direct thermal injury.

HYPOTHERMIA

Although the changes in experimental animals are impressive, in man they are inconspicuous. The effect of low temperatures on the liver is unlikely to be of serious consequence.

BURNS

Within 36–48 hours of burning, the liver shows changes very similar to those seen in carbon tetrachloride poisoning. These are reflected in minor changes in liver function tests.

IRRADIATION

Local irradiation of the liver causes a severe hepatitis. Two to six weeks following therapy the liver enlarges, ascites develops and jaundice may appear. The condition may be transient or death may ensue from liver failure. Histologically, centrizonal haemorrhage and congestion are seen with minimal hepato-cellular damage, but with loss of glucogen. The picture is that of damage to central hepatic veins which, in fact, show fibrosis and obliterate [105]. A form of veno-occlusive disease is so produced [105].

UNPREDICTABLE 'HYPERSENSITIVITY' TYPE DRUG REACTIONS

Only a very small proportion of patients taking the drug will have the reaction. There is no method of selecting who will be susceptible. The reaction is unrelated to dose but is commoner after multiple exposures to the drug. The onset is delayed about one week after exposure.

The pre-icteric period of gastro-intestinal symptoms resembles acute hepatitis and is followed by jaundice associated with pale stools and dark urine and an enlarged tender liver. Biochemical tests indicate hepato-cellular damage. Serum gamma-globulins are increased. Pathological changes in the liver resemble those of acute virus hepatitis [47]. The milder cases show spotty necrosis becoming more extensive and reaching a stage of diffuse massive liver injury and collapse; inflammatory infiltration is marked. There is a tendency towards transition to cirrhosis.

In those patients who recover, maximum serum bilirubin levels are reached after two to three weeks. The more seriously affected show a shrinking liver and die of hepatic failure. The mortality is high for those that are clinically recognized, higher than for sporadic virus hepatitis. If hepatic pre-coma or coma is reached the mortality is 70%.

Hepatic histology shows a picture virtually indistinguishable from that of acute virus hepatitis [47]. Milder cases show spotty necrosis becoming more extensive and reaching a stage of diffuse liver injury and collapse; inflammatory infiltration is marked. Chronic active hepatitis and macronodular cirrhosis may be sequels.

The drugs causing this type of reaction may do so by the production of toxic metabolites injurious to the liver *per se* or the metabolite may act as a hapten with cell protein, so inducing immunological liver injury (fig. 284). These mechanisms may apply to such drugs as isoniazid, methyl dopa, halothane and chlorpromazine. In others, such as erythromycin or nitrofurantoin, the reaction seems to be more a hypersensitivity one.

Isoniazid

This hydrazine, weak amine-oxidase inhibitor has been associated with severe hepato-toxicity. This followed its use alone in asymptomatic persons with positive tuberculin skin tests. In one serious outbreak, 19 of 2231 government employees in Washington developed clinical signs of liver disease within six months of starting isoniazid [38]. Thirteen subjects were jaundiced and two died.

The liver injury is metabolite-related (fig. 291). After acetylation the isoniazid is converted to a hydrazine which is changed by drug metabolizing enzymes to a potent acylating agent which produces liver necrosis [77]. Rapid acetylators are probably at particular risk of developing liver damage and this applies particularly to orientals, 90% of whom are fast acetylators [77]. Combination of the isoniazid with an enzyme inducer such

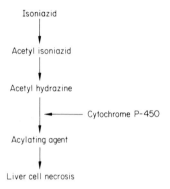

Fig. 291. The possible mechanism of isoniazid liver injury (Sherlock 1979).

as rifampicin increases the risk [73]. The combination of isoniazid and rifampicin can be particularly serious, leading to fulminant hepatitis [91]. Anaesthetic drugs may also enhance isoniazid toxicity. Para-amino salicylate, on the other hand, is an enzyme retarder, and this may account for the relative safety of the para-amino salicylate–isoniazid combination formerly used in the treatment of tuberculosis.

The possibility of immunological liver injury cannot be excluded. However, 'allergic' manifestations are not seen and the incidence of 12–20% developing subclinical liver injury is very high.

Elevated serum transaminase values are seen in 10% of all patients receiving isoniazid. There are usually no symptoms and the transaminases subside despite continued therapy.

CLINICAL FEATURES

Serious reactions commonly affect those more than 50 years old, usually female. After treatment

for about three months, non-specific symptoms develop, including anorexia and weight loss. These continue for one to four weeks before the onset of jaundice. The severity of hepatitis correlates with continuation of the drug during the prodromal period. There is a discrepancy between a well-looking patient and hepatic histological appearances.

The hepatitis usually resolves rapidly on stopping the drug, but if jaundice develops there is a 10% mortality.

Severity is greatly increased if the drug is continued after symptoms develop or serum transaminases rise. The mortality is 12% if overt liver damage develops [9]. The reactions are more serious if the patient presents after more than two months on the drug [9].

The *liver biopsy* may show spotty necrosis or extensive bridging necrosis and fibrosis. Continued administration leads to chronic active hepatitis and even cirrhosis [69]. This is probably non-progressive if the drug is withdrawn.

Rifampicin

In the majority of patients reporting with rifampicin hepato-toxicity, isoniazid has also been given [116]. Rifampicin on its own may cause a mild hepatitis, but this is unlikely to be serious or to have permanent effects on the liver. In some patients the drug has been continued and liver function and structure have returned to normal [116].

Methyl dopa

Asymptomatic increases in serum transaminases, which generally subside despite continued drug administration, are reported in 5% of those taking methyl dopa. This may be metabolite-related, for human microsomes can convert methyl dopa to a potent arylating agent [76]. An immunological mechanism is also possible, for methyl dopa is known to induce such reactions as direct Coombs' test positivity and a positive LE cell test.

The patient is often post-menopausal and has been on methyl dopa for one to four weeks. The reaction usually appears within the first three months. Prodromata include pyrexia and are short. The reaction is much more severe in those continuing the drug [109]. Liver biopsy shows bridging and multilobular necrosis. Death may occur in the acute state, but clinical improvement following drug withdrawal is usual [132]. Chronic active liver disease has been reported [69, 132]; this is probably not progressive. Cirrhosis has developed insidiously without a preceding acute hepatitic episode.

Halothane

There seems little doubt that, rarely, this anaesthetic causes hepatitis. Convincing evidence has come from challenge experiments such as that in an anaesthetist who developed clinical, biochemical and hepatic histological deterioration when rechallenged with halothane [57]. Two controlled prospective clinical trials have been reported. The first, from Oxford [133], reported liver function tests in women receiving multiple anaesthetics for the treatment of cancer of the uterine cervix. The second, from Southampton [148], in addition, studied men receiving multiple anaesthetics during the treatment of cancer of the bladder. In both there was an increased incidence of raised transaminase values in those receiving halothane. In the Oxford trial, four of 18 halothane-treated patients showed serum transaminase values exceeding 100 before the third radium treatment compared with none of the 21 in the control group who received a non-halothane anaesthetic. The delay between halothane anaesthesia and the diagnosis of the hepatic reaction, usually pyrexia, is at least seven days after a first exposure to halothane. Jaundice appears two to three days later. The patient may therefore have been discharged home from the hospital before the hepatic reaction appears. The anaesthetist has lost contact with the patient who is expecting to be unwell after a hospital admission. Many hepatic reactions to halothane are thus overlooked. Three liver biopsies were performed in the Oxford and Southampton trials on patients with increased serum transaminase values. These showed definite and sometimes severe acute hepatitis which would have been overlooked if the transaminases were not being monitored. The danger of such patients receiving further halothane anaesthetics is obvious.

MECHANISMS

The mechanisms of the hepato-toxicity remain obscure. Halothane is metabolized to trifluoroacetic acid, bromide and chloride. The first product of reductive metabolism is theoretically toxic and unstable. It could bind covalently with hepatic

metallo-enzymes of cellular protein and so lead to direct liver injury. In an animal model and in man, the three such reductive metabolites have been demonstrated [18]. In a rat with liver enzymes induced and receiving halothane plus 14% oxygen, the metabolites were increased at least fourfold while transaminases increased 10 times and the liver showed centrizonal necrosis. This would explain the potentiation of halothane hepato-toxicity by post-operative hypoxaemia. The metabolites are stored in adipose tissue and may be released later. Obesity is frequently associated with halothane hepatitis [79]. The hepatic histology in some patients is very suggestive of direct liver injury, the centrizonal necrotic area being particularly well demarcated and the liver cells sometimes containing fat (fig. 294).

The liver injury may be mediated immunologically. The association with multiple exposures, the pattern of fever and the occasional eosinophilia and skin rash would support this view. Smooth muscle antibodies may be present in low titre and a liver–kidney microsomal antibody is sometimes found [139]. Lymphocyte transformation with halothane has been described in subjects with halothane hepatitis [89], but this has not been confirmed [79]. Halothane macrophage migration inhibition factor tests have given positive results in patients with halothane hepatitis [101]. The sensitization to a halothane-altered rabbit liver cell component has been shown by the leucocyte migration tests in eight of 12 patients with halothane-associated hepatitis [136]. Halothane is a small molecule which binds poorly, if at all, with protein. Binding to a carrier protein is necessary before a small molecule can become immunogenic. In the case of halothane, covalent binding to protein has been considered obligatory before a hypersensitivity reaction can develop. It seems more likely that a metabolite of halothane binds to the carrier protein and so acts as an antigen. Idiosyncrasy might be expressed by the formation of excessive amounts of toxic metabolites or normal amounts of abnormally toxic ones.

CLINICAL FEATURES [59, 79, 95]

Halothane hepatitis is much more frequent after multiple anaesthetics. In 202 of 251 patients multiple halothane anaesthetics had been given and in 154 (75%) the exposure had been more than once in 28 days [46]. It is likely to affect patients having multiple surgical procedures. This is particularly so in gynaecological practice. It may complicate multiple orthopaedic or plastic operation and in ophthalmological practice as a complication of operations to correct strabismus. Obese, elderly females seem particularly at risk [79].

The first abnormal event is usually fever, usually with rigors, developing more than seven days (range 8–13) after the first operation and usually accompanied by malaise and non-specific gastro-intestinal symptoms, including right upper abdominal pain. After several exposures the temperature is noted 1–11 days post-operatively (fig. 292). Jaundice appears rapidly after the pyrexia, about 10–28 days after a single exposure and 3–17 days after multiple anaesthetics. This delay before jaundice, usually of about a week, is helpful

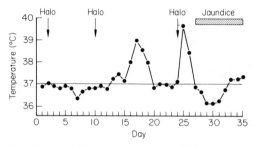

Fig. 292. Hepatitis associated with multiple exposures to halothane. Note the febrile response to the halothane anaesthetics. The patient became jaundiced after the third anaesthetic and rapidly became pre-comatose, developing deep coma on the fourth day and dying on the seventh day.

in excluding other causes of post-operative icterus. Early onset of jaundice is a bad sign [79]. Hepatomegaly and splenomegaly are rare. Clinicians must be alert to the possibility of halothane hepatitis in any patient with post-operative pyrexia.

The total white cell count is usually normal, but there may be an absolute eosinophilia. Serum bilirubin levels may be very high, particularly in fatal cases, but are under 10 mg in 40%. The condition may be anicteric. Serum transaminases are in the range found in viral hepatitis. An occasionally high serum alkaline phosphatase level may be seen. If the patient becomes icteric the mortality is very high. Altogether 139 of 310 patients in one series died (46%) [46]. If coma ensues and the one stage prothrombin time falls markedly in spite of intramuscular vitamin K therapy, the condition is virtually hopeless. The mortality is obviously less in the anicteric cases.

Those that recover probably show no late chronic effects despite marked 'bridging' necrosis in the acute stage [74].

HEPATIC CHANGES

At autopsy the liver is usually shrunken and weighs 1000 g or less.

Histological changes may be virtually indistinguishable from those of acute viral hepatitis (fig. 293). The leucocytic infiltration in the sinusoids, granulomas and fatty change in the liver cells, however, sometimes suggest a drug aetiology [59].

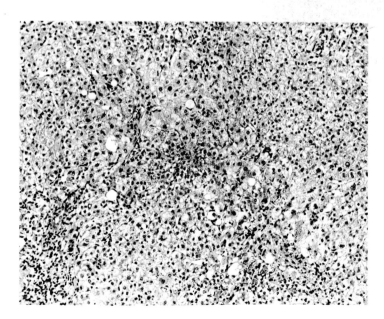

Fig. 293. Halothane-associated hepatitis. Hepatic histology shows cellular infiltration largely with mononuclear cells. Centrizonal areas show necrosis and cell swelling. Liver cell columns are disorganized. The appearances are virtually identical with those of acute virus hepatitis. H & E, × 96.

Alternatively the picture in the first week may be that of metabolite-related liver injury. A zonal type of massive necrosis involves the central two-thirds or more of each lobule (fig. 294).

In those who survive at least one week, the necrotic cells are almost completely absorbed, leaving behind many lipochrome-filled macrophages and either dilated sinusoids or a collapsed ischaemic centrizonal area in which are condensed stroma and collagen fibres.

In the regenerative stage, usually two or more weeks after the onset of jaundice, the necrotic debris in the centrizonal areas has disappeared and the connective tissue framework is rather compressed. Lipochrome-filled macrophages are still present together with a few lymphocytes. The characteristic feature is the presence of regeneration in the peripheral areas.

Interesting differences have therefore been shown both by light and electron microscopy [59] between halothane and viral hepatitis. The detection of such differences, however, depends largely on the experience of the pathologist. In the individual case there is no absolute diagnostic difference between the two conditions and usually only a tentative conclusion can be drawn concerning the aetiology of the hepatitis [95].

CONCLUSIONS

Halothane anaesthesia should not be repeated if there is the slightest suspicion of even a very mild reaction after the first anaesthetic. In view of its otherwise desirable properties it may be used on a single occasion for operations such as porta-caval shunt. There is no increased likelihood of a patient with underlying liver disease having an adverse reaction. There is no indication of the duration of hypersensitivity to halothane. Increased alertness to the significance of delayed post-operative pyrexia may allow diagnosis of the milder cases. The complication is certainly rare, although it is difficult to quote accurate figures. There is no doubt that halothane is a valuable anaesthetic for major operations. Its place in minor surgery, particularly if repeated, might be questioned.

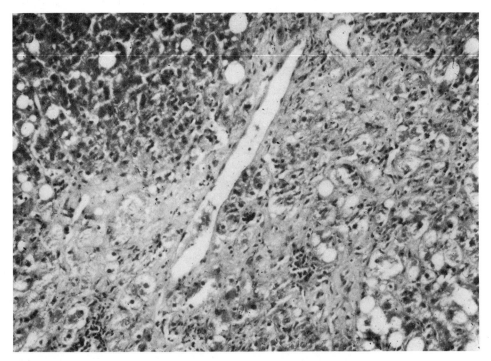

Fig. 294. Halothane liver injury. Centrizonal area shows well-defined necrosis without inflammatory reaction. Hepatocytes show fatty change. H & E, × 220.

Methoxyfluorane

Hepatic reactions have also been reported after another halogenated ether anaesthetic, methoxy-fluorane (penthrane), usually with repeated administration. It has been reported in an operating room nurse [52]. The picture is very similar to that of halothane hepatitis [58].

Chlorpromazine

Chlorpromazine jaundice has a strong immuno-logical association. Only 1–2% of those taking the drug develop cholestasis. The reaction is unrelated to dose and in 80–90% the onset is in the first four weeks. There may be associated hypersensitivity. Excess eosinophils may be found in the liver. The liver biopsy shows not only cholestasis but also a cellular reaction within the portal zones.

Evidence is accumulating that chlorpromazine is also directly hepato-toxic. Histologically, damage to liver cells may be noted in almost every patient. Chlorpromazine produces a dose-related enzyme release from Chang liver cells and liver slices [25]. It inhibits bile salt-independent biliary flow in the monkey [111] and in the isolated perfused rat liver [129]. The drug is an ampiphilic cationic detergent, and can insert itself into the lipid bilayer of cell membranes. The drug forms free radicals which can bind covalently to cellular components and so could induce liver injury. The liver cell has two inbuilt safeguards: first, the production of a more stable chlorpromazine sulphoxide, and second, the protective action of hepatic glutathione (fig. 295).

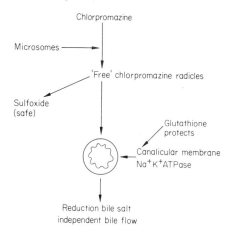

Chlorpromazine

Microsomes ⟶

'Free' chlorpromazine radicles

Sulfoxide (safe)

Glutathione protects

Canalicular membrane Na$^+$K$^+$ATPase

Reduction bile salt independent bile flow

Fig. 295. The possible mechanisms of chlorpromazine cholestasis (after Samuels and Carey 1978) (Sherlock 1979).

Using isolated liver membranes enriched with bile canaliculi, chlorpromazine-free radicles markedly inhibit Na$^+$-K$^+$-ATPase at much lower concentrations than chlorpromazine itself [114]. Such an inhibition would account for the reduction of bile salt-independent biliary flow which depends on Na$^+$-K$^+$-ATPase. This might, in part, account for cholestasis. It would not entirely explain it, for the histological and electron microscopical picture of the liver is not simply that of canalicular membrane injury.

Other effects of chlorpromazine, such as the delay in onset of jaundice, the extra-hepatic manifestations and the lack of a dose relationship, remain unexplained. There may be an individual idiosyncrasy in the production of free chlorpromazine radicles or in chlorpromazine sulphoxide formation or even in glutathione metabolism. It is also possible that chlorpromazine or one of its metabolites may induce alterations in the liver cell membrane so that it becomes antigenic.

CLINICAL PICTURE

The onset may simulate viral hepatitis, prodromata lasting some four to five days. Anorexia is rarely so absolute and prostration is never so great. Cholestatic jaundice appears concurrently or within a week of the systemic reaction and lasts some one to four weeks. Pruritus may precede jaundice. Recovery is usually complete [143].

Serum biochemistry shows the features of cholestatic jaundice. A sustained rise in alkaline phosphatase values may be the only change [13].

An eosinophilia may be seen in the peripheral blood in the very early stages.

HEPATIC CHANGES

Light microscopy shows cholestasis and, in the portal zones, a marked cellular reaction with mononuclear cells and eosinophils prominent (fig. 296). The reaction is not merely a cholestatic one. Even in the uncomplicated case a certain amount of damage to liver cells can be noted (fig. 297). 'Feathery' degeneration of liver cells, focal cell necrosis with cellular reaction, mild fatty change, anisocytosis and mitoses are all seen. Ballooned liver cells, peripheral vacuolation and hyaline deposits may also be noted [104]. Damage to the liver is greater than that observed with simple obstruction to main bile ducts.

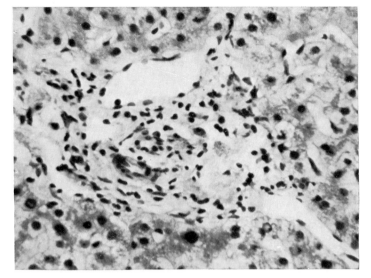

Fig. 296. Cholestatic jaundice following chlorpromazine. Same case as fig. 297. Portal zone shows a slight increase in cellularity, mainly mononuclear. A few eosinophils could also be demonstrated. H & E, ×275.

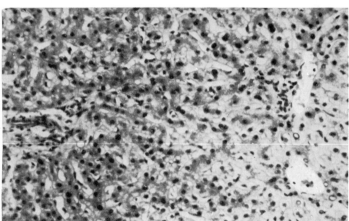

Fig. 297. Cholestatic jaundice following chlorpromazine. Same case as fig. 296. The zonal architecture is maintained intact. The centrizonal area shows heavy bile stasis. Liver cells, especially centrizonally, show patchy, often feathery necrosis with evidence of regeneration shown by variation in cell and nuclear size. The portal zones are virtually normal. H & E, ×72 (Sherlock 1972).

PROGNOSIS AND TREATMENT

Jaundice of the chlorpromazine type rarely proves fatal although an occasional death from hepato-cellular failure is reported [150].

Occasionally jaundice is more prolonged, lasting more than three months and even up to three years. The clinical picture is of prolonged chole-static jaundice with steatorrhoea and weight loss. The biochemical changes include the early appearance of very high serum alkaline phosphatase and cholesterol levels. The clinical picture simulates primary biliary cirrhosis. The onset is, however, much more explosive and in contrast to primary biliary cirrhosis, which is inevitably progressive, recovery almost always ensues. In two patients biliary cirrhosis is said to have developed six years and four years after the onset.

The diagnosis is not easy in these chronic cases for hepatic histology may be difficult to interpret. Retrograde or percutaneous cholangiography may be necessary to exclude mechanical biliary obstruction. The mitochondrial antibody test for primary biliary cirrhosis is negative or in low titre.

In the usual case of chlorpromazine jaundice no active treatment is required and recovery is complete. Corticosteroids do not affect the clinical course.

OTHER CAUSES

An essentially similar picture can complicate therapy with other phenothiazine derivatives such as promazine [53] or prochlorperazine, mepazine or trifluoperazine [62]. It can also complicate treatment with non-phenothiazine drugs including oral hypoglycaemic agents such as chlorpropamide [106], organic arsenicals [44] and gold [115].

OTHER DRUGS

A large number of drugs cause hepatic reactions of 'hypersensitivity' type and of variable severity, with or without jaundice [66]. The reaction usually appears within four weeks of starting therapy and is most frequent with multiple exposures. Liver histology shows focal, spotty necrosis of liver cells, with a mononuclear and sometimes eosinophilic reaction in the portal zones. Granulomas are sometimes found.

Oxyphenisatin

Oxyphenisatin, a constituent of many laxatives, has been associated with hepato-cellular damage [107]. The number of reported cases of liver damage is small so the reaction must be hypersensitivity and not only direct hepato-toxicity. Challenge with a small dose of 50 mg leads to rapid increases in serum bilirubin and transaminase values [17].

The reaction may present as an acute hepatitis or as chronic active hepatitis. Biochemical features include hypergammaglobulinaemia and raised serum transaminase values. The LE cell test may be positive. Hepatic histology shows a chronic active hepatitis. Recovery follows withdrawal of the drug.

Laxatives containing oxyphenisatin have now been withdrawn in most parts of the world [17], but are still on sale in some parts of Europe and in South America.

Sulphonamides

These drugs, particularly the long-acting ones, can cause hepatitis. Widespread granulomas may be found.

Sulfasalazine

The hepatic reaction is usually part of a systemic hypersensitivity one [51, 126]. It resembles that seen with sulphonamides.

Trimethoprim-sulfamethoxazole

This combination can cause intra-hepatic cholestasis [80].

Erythromycin

Hepatic reactions are usually associated with the estolate, but the proprionate and ethylsuccinate have also been incriminated [68, 138, 149].

The onset is one to four weeks after starting therapy with right upper quadrant pain, which may be severe, stimulating biliary disease, fever, itching and jaundice. The blood may show eosinophilia and atypical lymphocytes.

Liver biopsy shows cholestasis, hepato-cellular injury and acidophil bodies. Portal zones show the bile duct wall to be infiltrated with leucocytes and eosinophils and the bile duct cells may show mitoses. At autopsy the gall bladder has been shown to be inflamed.

Nitrofurantoin

This drug has been associated with cholestatic jaundice [29]. It has also rarely been related to chronic active hepatitis developing insidiously, usually in women, four weeks to 11 years after starting the drug [10, 119].

The serum albumin is reduced while gammaglobulin is increased. Serum nuclear antibodies and smooth muscle antibodies are positive.

Patients usually improve when the drug is stopped. Cirrhosis, however, can develop and patients may die with fatal progressive liver failure. The mechanism may be direct cytotoxicity to the parent compound or to a metabolite. Association with a lupus-like syndrome with positive lymphocyte transformation [10] suggests that an immunological mechanism may also be concerned. Chronic hepatitis has developed [45].

Anti-convulsants

Severe hepatitis-like reactions complicate therapy with many anti-convulsants. The reactions are probably of 'hypersensitivity' type.

Diphenylhydantoin (*Dilantin*) [63] usually affects adults. The onset is one to five weeks after starting treatment as a serum sickness-like syndrome. Massive hepatic necrosis can develop and there is a 50% mortality in those developing jaundice. Occasionally the picture is of an infectious mononucleosis-like disease.

Dantrolene is a phenytoin derivative used to treat spasticity. In one study 19 (1.8%) of 1044 patients taking the drug for more than 60 days developed abnormal biochemical tests. Six became jaundiced and three died [135]. Challenge caused recurrence of the liver damage [135]. Hepatic histology showed acute hepatitis, massive hepatic necrosis [24] and a cholangitic picture has also been seen [146]. Chronic active hepatitis and cirrhosis may follow its prolonged use. There is a disparity between clinical severity and the hepatic histological picture [146].

Sodium valproate has been associated with severe, often fatal, hepatocellular reactions [127]. Histologically the picture is of hepatitis with microvesicular lipid accumulations and cholestasis.

Anti-inflammatory drugs

Salicylates (page 302).

Phenylbutazone is associated with a high incidence of general hypersensitivity reactions. Hepatitis is rather uncommon and is usually found with evidence of a general reaction. Sometimes cholestasis may develop.

A granulomatous reaction simulating sarcoidosis has also been reported [48].

Allopurinol can be associated with a hepatic reaction which can include granulomas [128].

Methimazole and carbimazole

These have been implicated in producing hypersensitivity hepatic injury. [67].

Imipramine

In general, the tricyclic anti-depressants are very free from hepato-toxic effects. A promazine-type jaundice, however, has been reported following imipramine [123], which is perhaps not surprising in view of the structural resemblance of imipramine to the phenothiazines.

Quinidine [61]

The reaction is marked by fever 6–12 days after starting treatment. Liver biopsy shows hepatocellular necrosis and granulomas may be found.

Ticrynafen (Salacryn)

This uricosuric diuretic is associated with hepatotoxicity. It is diagnosed one to three months after starting by fever, malaise and abdominal pain. Transaminases are very high. The jaundice develops in 60% [35].

Perhexiline maleate

Prolonged use of this anti-anginal drug has been associated with a hepatic reaction resembling alcoholic hepatitis [7, 65]. Changes include fat and fibrosis. Mallory's bodies are seen in periportal hepatocytes. The liver cells show a brown lysosomal pigment having an electron microscopical laminar structure resembling that seen in hereditary phospholipidosis.

The changes usually remit when the drug is stopped. However, cirrhosis has been reported [92].

HEPATIC REACTIONS TO ORAL CONTRACEPTIVES

Cholestasis [121]

Sex hormones contained in oral contraceptives are potentially cholestatic. They are usually C_{17} substituted testosterones. They include norethandrolone, methylestranolone, norethindrone, methandrenone, norethisterone, mestranol and norethyndrol. The reaction has, however, been reported with methylandrostenolone which lacks a C_{17} substitution. Moreover, the sufferers tend also to exhibit cholestasis during pregnancy where the natural oestrogens and progestins are not C_{17} substituted. The cause is unlikely to be abnormal metabolism of the hormone but is probably an exaggeration of the mild cholestatic effect seen in normal late pregnancy or in normal women given sex hormones.

Cholestasis is probably related to the effect of oestrogen on the permeability of the canalicular membrane [36, 125]. A block in biliary micelle formation has also been suggested [97]. Sex hormones may also affect the cytoskeleton of the liver cell with failure of the pericanalicular microfilaments to contract [96].

Cholestasis is rare in relation to the millions of women taking sex hormones. The continual reduction of the dose of active hormone is further lessening this complication.

Genetic susceptibility may account for the geographic distribution of the reports of jaundice following 'the Pill'. Most come from Scandinavia, northern Europe and Chile. Cholestatic jaundice of pregnancy is particularly common in these countries [88, 121, 131]. There is a familial incidence. Those developing it are the same subjects as would develop cholestasis in the last trimester of pregnancy. Genetic predisposition remains unexplained; it might be due to an increased sensitivity of the bile secreting mechanism in the hepatocyte to steroid or to a decreased capacity of drug metabolizing enzymes in the liver cell.

Clinical features

The jaundice appears during the first or second cycle and rarely after the third. Malaise, nausea and anorexia precede icterus. Bilirubinaemia is variable but often exceeds 10 mg/dl. Serum alkaline phosphatase levels are raised. Serum transaminase values are variable but may exceed five times normal in about one-third of cases.

The cholestatic effects are enhanced in those with biliary excretory failure. Patients with Dubin-Johnson syndrome show an accentuation of bilirubinaemia without change in serum alkaline phosphatase levels. Patients with pre-symptomatic primary biliary cirrhosis may develop pruritus. The sex hormones are usually contraindicated in patients with chronic liver disease.

Theoretically, patients with acute hepatitis who continue to take oral contraceptives should develop deep jaundice and pruritus. This is not always so, for in a controlled trial, women taking oral contraceptives during the course of acute hepatitis had an illness of similar severity to matched controls [118]. A woman convalescent from viral hepatitis may resume use of 'the Pill' as soon as she wishes.

Liver biopsy shows normal architecture; there is centrizonal necrosis and occasional liver cell necrosis with surrounding reactions. Electron microscopy shows cholestasis and hepato-cellular damage [90].

Prognosis is excellent. The patient recovers when the drug is stopped. Recurrence is liable to follow resumption of oral contraceptives. The patient may develop cholestasis in a subsequent pregnancy.

Gall-stones (page 478).

Hepatic venous thrombosis (Budd–Chiari syndrome) (page 181).

Hepatic tumours

The association of hepatic adenoma, a hitherto very rare benign tumour, with oral contraceptives was first suggested in 1973 [3]. By 1977, 237 published cases were reviewed [56]. The association is a rare one, believed to be about 3–4 per 100 000 long-term users of oral contraceptives in the United States [110]. In the United Kingdom, with approximately 1.5 million 'Pill' users, this would mean 50 patients annually. Prolonged use seems important in determining the risk, which increases dramatically with duration of use, particularly after 48 months [26]. Complication seems associated with oral contraceptives containing mestranol but, as this is the most frequent constituent, the connection is not unexpected [56]. The use of pills with high hormone content and in women over the age of 30 may increase the risk of adenoma [110].

Familial adenomas have been described, the sufferers never having taken oral contraceptives [37].

MECHANISMS [120, 121]

The mechanism of tumour formation is complex (fig. 298). The oestrogens might be directly carcinogenic, which is unlikely. Oral contraceptives, as enzyme inducers, might potentiate the carcinogenesis of certain compounds by increasing their

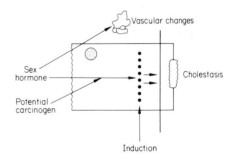

Fig. 298. Possible mechanisms of hepatic tumour production by sex hormones (Sherlock 1979).

rate of conversion to toxic (?carcinogenic) metabolites. Cholestatic properties of steroids might enhance the potentially carcinogenic action of substances normally excreted in the bile. Concomitant drugs might act as additional enzyme inducers; in a Swedish series of 28 patients with focal nodular hyperplasia, two patients were epileptics and three diabetic [40]. The vascular changes probably represent part of the general vasodilatation associated with sex hormones and are analogous both to the vascular spiders developing in the skin and to the endometrial arterial hypertrophy found in pregnancy.

TYPES OF TUMOUR [60]

Adenomas. These smooth, encapsulated tumours are usually single but may be multiple. They are about 8–10 cm in diameter, usually subcapsular and sometimes pedunculated. They are most frequent in the right lobe. Microscopically the

tumour consists of sheets of near-normal liver cells without portal tracts or central veins. Bile ducts are conspicuously absent (figs. 299, 300).

Focal nodular hyperplasia (fig. 301). This well-circumscribed, unencapsulated lesion presents as a nodular mass in an otherwise normal liver. The

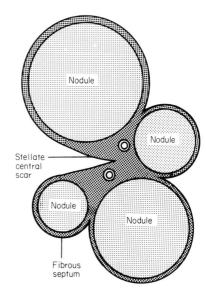

Fig. 301. The structure of focal nodular hyperplasia.

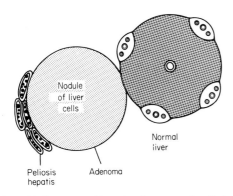

Fig. 299. Structure of hepatic adenoma and peliosis hepatis compared with normal liver.

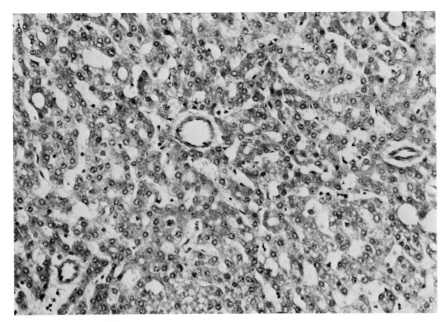

Fig. 300. Hepatic adenoma. The appearance is of sheets of near normal liver cells without portal tracts. H & E, × 185.

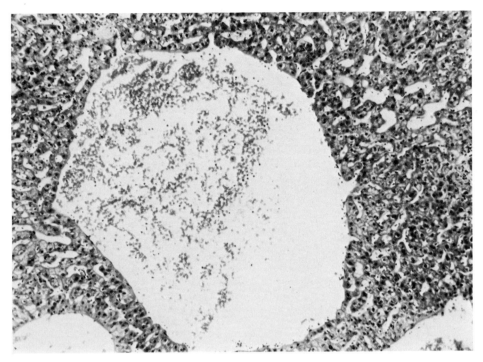

Fig. 302. Peliosis hepatis. A dilated blood space is seen with no clear-cut wall. H & E, × 107.

lesion is commonly subcapsular but can be pedunculated and can occur in either lobe. The lesions vary in size between 1 and 15 cm and may be multiple.

On cut section, a stellate, central scar is seen from which septa radiate, sub-dividing the mass into nodules which simulate cirrhosis.

Histologically, the central core consists of fibrous tissue and proliferating bile ducts. The hepatocytes are normal.

Hepato-cellular carcinoma. Association of hepato-cellular carcinoma with oral contraceptives is exceedingly rare but has been reported [20, 42, 83].

Cholangiocarcinoma has been reported [28].

Vascular lesions may accompany adenoma or focal nodular hyperplasia or may be seen alone. Large arteries and veins are present in excess. Sinusoids are focally dilated. Sometimes the blood spaces are particularly large and without endothelial linings. This is termed *peliosis hepatis* (fig. 302). Peliosis has been described in the absence of nodular lesions in patients taking oral contraceptives [147] and in men having androgenic and anabolic steroids. Peliosis has been reported in the recipients of renal transplants, perhaps

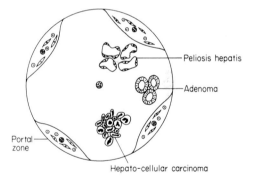

Fig. 303. The possible toxic effects of sex hormones on the liver.

due to azathioprine blocking blood flow from the sinusoids [21].

CLINICAL FEATURES [60, 121]

The tumour may be symptomless and discovered incidentally at autopsy or at the time of surgery for another condition. This presentation is particularly true for focal nodular hyperplasia.

The patient may present with a right upper quadrant mass.

Haemorrhage into the tumour, or infarction, leads to abdominal pain and the tumour is tender.

Rupture is associated with the symptoms and signs of acute intraperitoneal bleeding.

Serum biochemical tests may be normal. Necrosis and rupture are associated with increases in transaminases and alkaline phosphatase. Serum α fetoprotein is not increased.

Needle liver biopsy is contraindicated because of the vascular nature of the tumour.

LOCALIZATION

Ultrasound is useful. Technetium scans usually demonstrate the filling defect. However, both this method and the CT scan may fail to demonstrate the tumour when it closely resembles normal liver.

Arteriography (figs. 304, 305) shows stretching of the feeding arteries around the mass with branches penetrating the tumour from the periphery. Irregular vessels course through the lesion. Areas of haemorrhage may be demonstrated. There is a marked capillary blush.

Combined angiography and liver scan may be helpful in distinguishing between focal nodular hyperplasia, which is hypervascular and exhibits normal uptake on the scan, and liver cell adenoma, which is hypovascular and cold on a scan [60].

MANAGEMENT

Women who take oral contraceptives, particularly for many years, should be warned of the possibility of tumours developing and encouraged to examine their abdomens regularly.

Hepatic angiography may be useful for follow-up [4].

The temptation to operate on space-filling

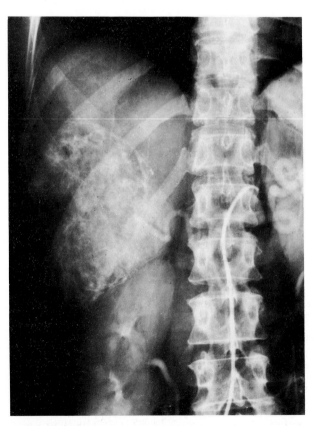
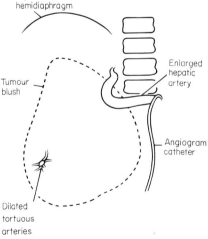

Fig. 304. Hepatic adenoma related to oral contraceptives. Late stage of coeliac angiogram shows abnormal vascularity in the tumour in the lower part of the right lobe of the liver.

lesions in the liver is almost overwhelming to some surgeons. However, in most uncomplicated cases it is advisable to be conservative. If, when operating for intraperitoneal haemorrhage, multiple tumours are found, all cannot be removed. If the tumour is diagnosed but there are no complications, it should be left in situ and sex hormones stopped. Tumours may regress [27, 103] although this is not always the case [70]. Women must be warned of the possibility of rupture and the significance of any unexplained right upper quadrant pain or swelling in the abdomen. Rupture becomes more likely in pregnancy. Liver ultrasound or scan should be repeated every six months.

Surgery may be needed for complications, particularly intraperitoneal or intratumour bleeding with severe abdominal pain and anaemia. Hepatic arteriography is particularly valuable in planning surgery. Local resection of the tumour is advised in amounts sufficient to control haemorrhage [140]. In some instances hepatic lobectomy may be needed.

Androgenic hormones

Adenoma, peliosis and particularly hepato-cellular carcinoma may complicate long-term use of C_{17} substituted testosterones. Angiosarcoma has also been associated [30]. These hormones may be given for the treatment of aplastic anaemia [33], hypopituitarism, eunuchoidism [55], impotency or in female trans-sexuals [144].

Hepato-cellular cancer of a rather benign type is much more frequent with male than with female hormone therapy, perhaps due to the much larger doses needed. The incidence of hepatic abnormality is particularly high; in one series, 19 of 60 patients given methyl testosterone showed abnormal liver function tests [144].

INDIVIDUAL VARIATION AND PREDICTION OF HEPATO-TOXICITY [134]

Drug testing must always be done on both an acute and chronic basis and on more than one species

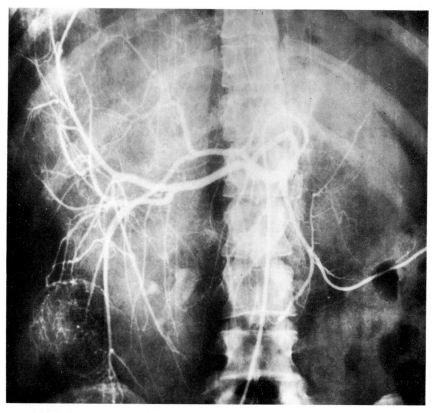

Fig. 305. Hepatic adenoma related to oral contraceptives. Coeliac angiogram shows stretching of branches of the hepatic artery around a relatively avascular lesion in the upper part of the right lobe of the liver.

or strain. Both the drug and its known metabolites must be used. Bilirubin Tm and light and electron microscopy of liver are essential. The albumin binding properties of the drug must be noted. The role of the drug as an hepatic enzyme-inducer should also be studied. Clinical trials must include regular pre- and post-treatment estimations of serum bilirubin and transaminase levels. Liver biopsies examined by light and electron microscopy, on a volunteer basis, are essential once the possibility of hepato-toxicity is raised.

The role of the drug which causes transient rises in transaminases and apparently no other hepatic effects remains obscure. Many valuable drugs in widespread use fall into this category. In many instances challenge is the only method of linking a drug with a hepatic reaction, but if its consequence is likely to be serious, this is ethically impossible.

AGE

The neonate is susceptible to drugs which interfere with bilirubin metabolism. The effects of unconjugated hyperbilirubinaemia are serious, for bilirubin encephalopathy may follow. Hepatitic reactions are rare in children.

NUTRITION

The elderly or undernourished patient with decreased or stressed protein synthesis reacts poorly to hepato-toxins which depress protein synthesis further. This also applies to the pregnant woman whose synthetic powers may already be stretched to capacity.

DISEASE

If hepatic detoxication is reduced, a drug, even if given in normal doses, may be hazardous. This may be illustrated by a patient with severe migraine who was taking large doses of ergot when she developed severe acute virus hepatitis [145]. The ergot was continued but was not detoxicated so that severe gangrene of all the extremities developed and she ultimately died.

The amino acid methionine can induce coma in those with cirrhosis but not in normal subjects.

Renal disease, for instance pyelonephritis, is probably important in potentiating the hepatotoxicity of tetracyclines.

PREVIOUS DRUG THERAPY

This is particularly important as regards enzyme induction which may facilitate hepatic handling of drugs. The importance of noting all drugs being taken by an individual who develops liver damage must be stressed.

REFERENCES

1. ALMEYDA J., BARNARDO D., BAKER H. *et al* (1972) Structural and functional abnormalities of the liver before and during methotrexate therapy. *Br. J. Dermatol.* **87**, 623.
2. BAERG R.G. & KIMBERG D.V. (1970) Centrilobular hepatic necrosis and acute renal failure in 'solvent sniffers'. *Ann. intern. Med.* **73**, 713.
3. BAUM J.K., BOOKSTEIN J.J., HOLTZ F. *et al* (1973) Possible association between benign hepatomas and oral contraceptives. *Lancet* ii, 926.
4. BENEDICT K.T. Jr, CHEN P.S., JANOWER M.L. *et al* (1979) Contraceptive-associated hepatic tumor. *Am. J. Roentgenol.* **132**, 452.
5. BERK P.D., MARTIN J.F., YOUNG R.S. *et al* (1976) Vinyl chloride-associated liver disease. *Ann. intern Med.* **84**, 717.
6. BERTHELOT P. (1973) Mechanisms and prediction of drug-induced liver disease. *Gut* **14**, 332.
7. BETRAND L., BALDET P., BLANC F. *et al* (1978) Hépatite cirrhogène au maleate de perhexiline. *Ann. Méd. Interne* **129**, 565.
8. BLACK M. (1980) Acetaminophen hepatotoxicity. *Gastroenterology* **78**, 382.
9. BLACK M., MITCHELL J.R., ZIMMERMAN H.J. *et al* (1975) Isoniazid-associated hepatitis in 114 patients. *Gastroenterology* **69**, 289.
10. BLACK M., RABIN L. & SCHATZ N. (1980) Nitrofurantoin-induced chronic active hepatitis. *Ann. intern. Med.* **92**, 62.
11. BLEWITT R.W., BRADBURY K., GREENALL M.J. *et al* (1977) Hepatic damage associated with mineral oil deposits. *Gut* **18**, 476.
12. BONKOWSKY H.L., MUDGE G.H. & MCMURTRY R.J. (1978) Chronic hepatic inflammation and fibrosis due to low doses of paracetamol. *Lancet* i, 1016.
13. BREUER R.I. (1966) Chlorpromazine hepatotoxicity manifested by a selective and sustained rise of serum alkaline phosphatase activity. *Am. J. dig. Dis.* n.s. **10**, 727.
14. BRUCKSTEIN A.H. & ATTIA A.A. (1978) Oxacillin hepatitis. Two patients with liver biopsy and review of the literature. *Am. J. Med.* **64**, 519.
15. CHAN C.K. & DETMER D.E. (1977) Proper management of hepatic adenoma associated with oral contraceptives. *Surg. Gynecol. Obstet.* **144**, 703.
16. COHEN C. (1978) Liver pathology in hycanthone hepatitis. *Gastroenterology* **75**, 103.
17. COOKSLEY W.G.E., COWEN A.E. & POWELL L.W. (1973) The incidence of oxyphenisatin ingestion in active chronic hepatitis: a prospective controlled study of 29 patients. *Aust. N.Z. J. Med.* **3**, 124.

18. Cousins M.J., Gourlay G.K., Sharp J.H. *et al* (1978) Halothane hepatitis. *Lancet* ii, 1197 (letter).

19. Dahl M.G.C., Gregory M.M. & Scheuer P.J. (1971) Liver damage due to methotrexate in patients with psoriasis. *Br. med. J.* i, 625.

20. Davis M., Portmann B., Searle M. *et al* (1974) Histological evidence of carcinoma in a hepatic tumour associated with oral contraceptives. *Br. med. J.* iv, 496.

21. Degott C., Rueff B., Kreis H. *et al* (1978) Peliosis hepatitis in recipients of renal transplants. *Gut* 19, 748.

22. Diamond I. (1966) Kernicterus: revised concepts of pathogenesis and management. *Pediatrics* 38, 539.

23. Dixon M.F., Nimmo J. & Prescott L.F. (1971) Experimental paracetamol-induced hepatic necrosis: a histopathological study. *J. Pathol.* 103, 225.

24. Donegan J.M., Donegan W.L. & Cohen E.B. (1978) Massive hepatic necrosis associated with dantrolene therapy. *Amer. J. dig. Dis.* 23, 48 S.

25. Dujovne C.A. & Zimmerman H.J. (1969) Cytotoxicity of phenothiazines on Chang liver cells as measured by enzyme leakage. *Proc. Soc. exp. Biol. Med.* 131, 583.

26. Edmondson H.A., Henderson B. & Benton B. (1976) Liver-cell adenomas associated with use of oral contraceptives. *New Engl. J. Med.* 294, 470.

27. Edmondson H.A., Reynolds T.B., Henderson B. *et al* (1977) Regression of liver cell adenomas associated with oral contraceptives. *Ann. intern. Med.* 86, 180.

28. Ellis E.F., Gordon P.R. & Gottlieb L.S. (1978) Oral contraceptives and cholangiocarcinoma. *Lancet* i, 207 (letter).

29. Ernaelstein D., & Williams R. (1981) Jaundice due to nitrofurantoin *Gastroenterology*. In press.

30. Falk H., Thomas L.B., Popper H. *et al* (1979) Hepatic angiosarcoma associated with androgenic–anabolic steroids. *Lancet* ii, 1120.

31. Farber E. & Fisher M.M. (eds) (1979) *Toxic Injury of the Liver*, Parts A and B. Marcel Dekker Inc., New York.

32. Farrell G.C., Cooksley W.G.E., Hart P. *et al* (1978) Drug metabolism in liver disease: identification of patients with impaired hepatic drug metabolism. *Gastroenterology* 75, 580.

33. Farrell G.C., Joshua D.E., Uren R.F. *et al* (1975) Androgen-induced hepatoma. *Lancet* i, 430.

34. Favreau M., Tannenbaum H. & Lough J. (1977) Hepatic toxicity associated with gold therapy. *Ann. intern. Med.* 87, 717.

35. FDA Drug Bulletin (1980) Ticrynafen recalled. *FDA Drug Bull.* xx, 3.

36. Forker E.L. (1969) The effect of estrogen on bile formation in the rat. *J. clin. Invest.* 48, 654.

37. Foster J.H., Donohue T.A. & Berman M.M. (1978) Familial liver-cell adenoma and diabetes mellitus. *New Engl. J. Med.* 299, 239.

38. Garibaldi R.A., Drusin R.E., Ferebee S.H. *et al* (1972) Isoniazid-associated hepatitis: report of an outbreak. *Am. Rev. resp. Dis.* 106, 357.

39. Goldenberg D.L. (1974) Aspirin hepatotoxicity. *Ann. intern. Med.* 80, 773.

40. Grabowski M., Stenram U. & Bergqvist A. (1975) Focal nodular hyperplasia of the liver, benign hepatomas, oral contraceptives and other drugs affecting the liver. *Acta pathol. microbiol. Scand.* Sect. A. 83, 615.

41. Greenburger N.J., Robinson W.L. & Isselbacher K.J. (1964) Toxic hepatitis after the ingestion of phosphorus with subsequent recovery. *Gastroenterology* 47, 179.

42. Ham J.M., Stevenson D. & Liddelow A.G. (1978) Hepatocellular carcinoma possibly induced by oral contraceptives. *Amer. J. dig. Dis.* 23, 38 S.

43. Hamlyn A.N., Douglas A.P. & James O. (1978) The spectrum of paracetamol (acetaminophen) overdose, clinical and epidemiological studies. *Postgrad. med. J.* 54, 400.

44. Hanger F.M. Jr & Gutman A.B. (1940) Postarsphenamine jaundice, apparently due to obstruction of intrahepatic biliary tract. *J. Am. med. Assoc.* 115, 263.

45. Hatoff D.E., Cohen M., Schweigert B.F. *et al* (1979) Nitrofurantoin: another cause of drug-induced chronic active hepatitis? *Am. J. Med.* 67, 117.

46. Inman W.H.W. & Mushin W.W. (1978) Jaundice after repeated exposure to halothane: a further analysis of reports to the committee on safety of medicines. *Br. med. J.* ii, 1455.

47. International Group (1974) Guidelines for diagnosis of therapeutic drug-induced liver injury in liver biopsies. *Lancet* i, 854.

48. Ishak K.G., Kirchner J.P. & Dhar J.K. (1977) Granulomas and cholestatic–hepatocellular injury associated with phenylbutazone. *Am. J. dig. Dis.* 22, 611.

49. Jacques E.A., Buschmann R.J. & Layden T.J. (1979) The histopathologic progression of vitamin A-induced hepatic injury. *Gastroenterology* 76, 599.

50. Johnson G.K. & Tolman K.G. (1977) Chronic liver disease and acetaminophen. *Ann. intern. Med.* 87, 302.

51. Kanner R.S., Tedesco F.J. & Kalser M.H. (1978) Azulfidine (sulfasalazine)-induced hepatic injury. *Am. J. dig. Dis.* 23, 956.

52. Katz S. (1970) Hepatic coma associated with methoxyflurane anesthesia. *Am. J. dig. Dis.* 15, 733.

53. Kemp J.A. (1957) Jaundice occurring during administration of promazine. *Gastroenterology* 32, 937.

54. Kew M., Bersohn I., Seftel H. *et al* (1970) Liver damage in heatstroke. *Am. J. Med.* 49, 192.

55. Kew M.C., Coller B.V., Prowse C.M. *et al* (1976) Occurrence of primary hepatocellular cancer and peliosis hepatis after treatment with androgenic steroids. *S. Afr. med. J.* 50, 1233.

56. Klatskin G. (1977) Hepatic tumors: possible relation to use of oral contraceptives. *Gastroenterology* 73, 386.

57. Klatskin G. & Kimberg D.V. (1969) Recurrent hepatitis attributable to halothane sensitisation in an anesthetist. *New Engl. J. Med.* 280, 515.

58. Klein N.C. & Jeffries G.H. (1966) Hepatotoxicity after methoxyflurane administration. *J. Am. med. Assoc.* 197, 1037.

59. KLION F.M., SCHAFFNER F. & POPPER H. (1969) Hepatitis after exposure to halothane. *Ann. intern. Med.* **71**, 467.

60. KNOWLES D.M., CASARELLA W.J., JOHNSON P.M. *et al* (1978) The clinical, radiologic and pathologic characterization of benign hepatic neoplasms. *Medicine (Baltimore)* **75**, 223.

61. KOCH M.J., SEEFF L.B., CRUMLEY C.E. *et al* (1976) Quinidine hepatotoxicity: a report of a case and review of the literature. *Gastroenterology* **70**, 1136.

62. KOHN N. & MYERSON R.M. (1961) Cholestatic hepatitis associated with trifluoperazine. *New Engl. J. Med.* **264**, 549.

63. LEE T.J., CARNEY C.N., LAPID J.L. *et al* (1976) Diphenylhydantoin-induced hepatic necrosis. *Gastroenterology* **70**, 422.

64. LEVI A.J., SHERLOCK S. & WALKER D. (1968) Phenylbutazone and isoniazid metabolism in patients with liver disease in relation to previous drug therapy. *Lancet* i, 1275.

65. LEWIS D., WAINWRIGHT H.C., KEW M.C. *et al* (1979) Liver damage associated with perhexiline maleate. *Gut* **20**, 186.

66. LUDWIG J. (1979) Drug effects on the liver: a tabular compilation of drugs and drug-related hepatic diseases. *Dig. Dis.* **24**, 785.

67. LUNZER M., HUANG S-N., GINSBURG J. *et al* (1975) Jaundice due to carbimazole. *Gut* **16**, 913.

68. LUNZER M.R., HUANG S.N., WARD K.M. *et al* (1975) Jaundice due to erythromycin estolate. *Gastroenterology* **68**, 1284.

69. MADDREY W.C. & BOITNOTT J.K. (1977) Drug-induced chronic liver disease. *Gastroenterology* **72**, 1348.

70. MARIANI A.F., LIVINGSTONE A.S., PEREIRAS R.V. Jr *et al* (1979) Progressive enlargement of an hepatic cell adenoma. *Gastroenterology* **77**, 1319.

71. MARIN G.A., MONTOYA C.A., SIERRA L. *et al* (1971) Evaluation of corticosteroid and exchange-transfusion treatment of acute yellow-phosphorus intoxication. *New Engl. J. Med.* **284**, 125.

72. MCLEAN A.E.M. & MCLEAN E.K. (1969) Diet and toxicity. *Br. med. Bull.* **25**, 278.

73 MIGUET J.P., MAVIER P., SOUSSY C.J. *et al* (1977) Induction of hepatic microsomal enzymes after brief administration of rifampicin in man. *Gastroenterology* **72**, 924.

74. MILLER D.J., DWYER J. & KLATSKIN G. (1978) Halothane hepatitis: benign resolution of a severe lesion. *Ann. intern. Med.* **89**, 212.

75. MITCHELL J.R. & JOLLOW D.J. (1975) Metabolite activation of drugs to toxic substances. *Gastroenterology* **68**, 392.

76. MITCHELL J.R., NELSON S.D., THORGEIRSSON S.S. *et al* (1976) Metabolic activation: biochemical basis for many drug-induced liver injuries. In *Progress in Liver Diseases*, vol. V, p. 259, eds H. Popper & F. Schaffner. Grune and Stratton, New York.

77. MITCHELL J.R. *et al* (1976) Isoniazid liver injury: clinical spectrum, pathology and probable pathogenesis. *Ann. intern. Med.* **84**, 181.

78. MORRIS J.S., SCHMID M., NEWMAN S. *et al* (1974) Arsenic and non-cirrhotic portal hypertension. *Gastroenterology* **66**, 86.

79. MOULT P.J.A. & SHERLOCK S. (1975) Halothane-related hepatitis. A clinical study of twenty-six cases. *Q. J. Med.*, **44**, 99.

80. NAIR S.S., KAPLAN J.M., LEVINE L.H. *et al* (1980) Trimethoprim-sulfamethoxazole-induced intrahepatic cholestasis. *Ann. intern. Med.* **92**, 511.

81. NATAF C., FELTMANN G., LEBREC D. *et al* (1979) Idiopathic portal hypertension (perisinusoidal fibrosis) after renal transplantation. *Gut* **20**, 531.

82. NEAL E.A., MEFFIN P.J., GREGORY P.B. (1979) Enhanced bioavailability and decreased clearance of analgesics in patients with cirrhosis. *Gastroenterology* **77**, 96.

83. NEUBERGER J., PORTMANN B., NUNNERLEY H.B. *et al* (1980) Oral-contraceptive-associated liver tumours: occurrence of malignancy and difficulties in diagnosis. *Lancet* i, 273.

84. NYFORS A. (1977) Liver biopsies from psoriatics related to methotrexate therapy. *Acta pathol. microbiol. Scand.*, Sect. A, **85**, 511.

85. NYFORS A. & HOPWOOD D. (1977) Liver ultra-structure in psoriatics related to methotrexate therapy. *Acta pathol. microbiol. Scand.*, Sect. A. **85**, 787.

86. O'BRIEN E.T., YEOMAN W.B. & HOBBY J.A.E. (1971) Hepatorenal damage from toluene in a 'glue sniffer'. *Br. med. J.* ii, 29.

87. O'GORMAN T. & KOFF R.S. (1977) Salicylate hepatitis. *Gastroenterology* **72**, 726.

88. ORELLANA-ALCALDE J.M. & DOMINGUEZ J.P. (1966) Jaundice and oral contraceptive drugs. *Lancet* ii, 1278.

89. PARONETTO F. & POPPER H. (1970) Lymphocyte stimulation induced by halothane in patients with hepatitis following exposure to halothane. *New Engl. J. Med.* **283**, 277.

90. PEREZ V., GORODISCH S., DE MARTIRE J. *et al* (1969) Oral contraceptives: Long-term use produces fine structural changes in liver mitochondria. *Science* **165**, 805.

91. PESSAYRE D., BENTATA M., DEGOTT C. *et al* (1977) Isoniazid-rifampicin fulminant hepatitis. *Gastroenterology* **72**, 284.

92. PESSAYRE D., BICHARA M., FELDMANN G. *et al* (1979) Perhexiline maleate-induced cirrhosis. *Gastroenterology* **76**, 170.

93. PESSAYRE D., LEBREC D., DESCATOIRE V. *et al* (1978) Mechanism for reduced drug clearance in patients with cirrhosis. *Gastroenterology* **74**, 566.

94. PETERS R.L., EDMONDSON H.A., MIKKELSEN W.P. *et al* (1967) Tetracycline-induced fatty liver in non-pregnant patients: a report of six cases. *Am. J. Surg.* **113**, 622.

95. PETERS R.L., EDMONDSON H.A., REYNOLDS T.B. *et al* (1969) Hepatic necrosis associated with halothane anesthesia. *Am. J. Med.* **47**, 748.

96. PHILLIPS M.J., ODA M., MAK E. *et al* (1975) Microfilament dysfunction as a possible cause of intrahepatic cholestasis. *Gastroenterology* **69**, 48.

97. POPPER H., SCHAFFNER F. & DENK H. (1976) Molecular pathology of cholestasis. In *The Hepatobiliary System*, p. 605, ed. W. Taylor. Plenum, New York.

98. POPPER H., THOMAS L.B., TELLES N.C. *et al* (1978) Development of hepatic angiosarcoma in man in-

duced by vinyl chloride, thorotrast and arsenic. *Am. J. Pathol.* **92,** 349.

99. PRESCOTT L.F., ILLINGWORTH R.N., CRITCHLEY J.A.J.H. *et al* (1979) Intravenous N-acetylcysteine: the treatment of choice for paracetamol poisoning. *Br. med. J.* ii, 1097.

100. PRESCOTT L.F., WRIGHT N., ROSCOE P. *et al* (1971) Plasma paracetamol half-life and hepatic necrosis in patients with paracetamol overdosage. *Lancet* i, 591.

101. PRICE G.D., GIBBS A.R. & JONES-WILLIAMS W.J. (1977) Halothane macrophage inhibition factor test in halothane-associated hepatitis. *J. clin. Pathol.* **30,** 312.

102. PROUDFOOT A.T. & WRIGHT N. (1970) Acute paracetamol poisoning. *Br. med. J.* iii, 557.

103. RAMSEUR W.L. & COOPER R. (1978) Asymptomatic liver cell adenomas. Another case of resolution after discontinuation of oral contraceptive use. *J. Am. med. Assoc.* **239,** 1647.

104. READ A.E., HARRISON C.V. & SHERLOCK S. (1961) Chronic chlorpromazine jaundice: with particular reference to its relationship to primary biliary cirrhosis. *Am. J. Med.* **31,** 249.

105. REED G.B. Jr. & COX A.J. Jr (1966) The human liver after radiation injury. A form of veno-occlusive disease. *Am. J. Pathol.* **48,** 597.

106. REICHEL J., GOLDBERG S.B., ELLENBERG M. *et al* (1960) Intrahepatic cholestasis following administration of chlorpropamide: report of a case with electron microscopic observations. *Am. J. Med.* **28,** 654.

107. REYNOLDS T.B., LAPIN A.C., PETERS R.L. *et al* (1970) Puzzling jaundice. Probable relationship to laxative ingestion. *J. Am. med. Assoc.* **211,** 86.

108. ROBERTS R.K., BRANCH R.A., DESMOND P.V. *et al* (1979) The influence of liver disease on drug disposition. *Clin. Gastroenterol.* **8,** 105.

109. RODMAN J.S., DEUTSCH D.J. & GUTMAN S.I. (1976) Methyl dopa hepatitis. A report of six cases and review of the literature. *Am. J. Med.* **60,** 941.

110. ROOKS J.B., ORY H.W., ISHAK K.G. *et al* (1979) Epidemiology of hepatocellular adenoma. The role of oral contraceptive use. *J. Am. med. Assoc.* **242,** 644.

111. ROS E., SMALL D.M. & CAREY M.C. (1972) Effects of chlorpromazine hydrochloride on bile flow, bile salt synthesis, and biliary lipid secretion in the primate. In *Bile Acid Metabolism in Health and Disease*, p. 219, eds G. Paumgartner & A. Stiehl. MTP, Lancaster.

112. ROSENBERG D.M. & NEELON F.A. (1978) Acetaminophen and liver disease. *Ann. intern. Med.* **88,** 129.

113. RUYMANN F.B., MOSIJCZUK A. & SAYERS R.J. (1977) Hepatoma in a child with methotrexate-induced hepatic fibrosis. *J. Am. med. Assoc.* **238,** 2631.

114. SAMUELS A.M. & CAREY M.C. (1978) Effects of chlorpromazine hydrochloride and its metabolites on Mg^{2+}- and $Na^+ K^+$-ATPase activities of canalicular-enriched rat liver plasma membranes. *Gastroenterology* **74,** 1183.

115. SCHENKER S., OLSON K.N., DUNN D. *et al* (1973)

116. SCHEUER P.J., SUMMERFIELD J.A., LAL S. *et al* (1974) Intrahepatic cholestasis due to therapy of rheumatoid arthritis. *Gastroenterology* **64,** 622.

116. SCHEUER P.J., SUMMERFIELD J.A., LAL S. *et al* (1974) Rifampicin hepatitis. A clinical and histological study. *Lancet* i, 421.

117. SCHULTZ J.C., ADAMSON J.S. Jr, WORKMAN W.W. *et al* (1963) Fatal liver disease after intravenous administration of tetracycline in high dosage. *New Engl. J. Med.* **269,** 999.

118. SCHWEITZER I.L., WEINER J.M., MCPEAK C.M. *et al* (1975) Oral contraceptives in acute viral hepatitis. *J. Am. med. Assoc.* **233,** 979.

119. SHARP J.R., ISHAK K.G. & ZIMMERMAN H.J. (1980) Chronic active hepatitis and severe hepatic necrosis associated with nitrofurantoin. *Ann. intern. Med.* **92,** 14.

120. SHERLOCK S. (1975) Progress report. Hepatic adenomas and oral contraceptives. *Gut* **16,** 753.

121. SHERLOCK S. (1979) Hepatic effects of steroid sex hormones. In *Toxic Injury of the Liver*, eds E. Farber & M.N. Fisher. Marcel Dekker Inc. New York.

122. SHERLOCK S. (1979) Hepatic reactions to drugs. *Gut* **20,** 634.

123. SHORT M.H., BURNS J.M. & HARRIS M.E. (1968) Cholestatic jaundice during imipramine therapy. *J. Am. med. Assoc.* **206,** 179.

124. SHULL H.J., WILKINSON G.R., JOHNSON R. *et al* (1976) Normal disposition of oxazepam in acute viral hepatitis and cirrhosis. *Ann. intern. Med.* **84,** 420.

125. SIMON F.R. (1978) Effects of estrogens on the liver. *Gastroenterology* **75,** 512.

126. SOTOLONGO R.P., NEEFE L.I., RUDZKI C. *et al* (1978) Hypersensitivity reactions to sulphasalazine with severe hepatoxicity. *Gastroenterology* **75,** 95.

127. SUCHY F.J., BALISTRERI W.F., BUCHINO J.J. *et al* (1979) Acute hepatic failure associated with the use of sodium valproate. *New Engl. J. Med.* **300,** 962.

128. SWANK L.A., CHEJFEC G. & NEMCHAUSKY B.A. (1978) Allopurinol-induced granulomatous hepatitis with cholangitis and a sarcoid-like reaction. *Arch. intern. Med.* **138,** 997.

129. TAVALONI N., REED J.S. & BOYER J.L. (1976) Chlorpromazine (CPZ) inhibits bile acid independent flow (BAIF) in the isolated perfused rat liver (IPRL). *Gastroenterology* **71,** 931 (abstr.).

130. THOMAS L.B., POPPER H., BERK P.D. *et al* (1975) Vinyl-chloride induced liver disease. From idiopathic portal hypertension (Banti's syndrome) to angiosarcomas. *New Engl. J. Med.* **292,** 17.

131. THULIN K.E. & NERMARK J. (1966) Seven cases of jaundice in women taking an oral contraceptive, Anovlar. *Br. med. J.* i, 584.

132. TOGHILL P.J., SMITH P.G., BENTON P. *et al* (1974) Methyl dopa liver damage. *Br. med. J.* iii, 545.

133. TROWELL J., PETO R. & CRAMPTON-SMITH A. (1975) Controlled trial of repeated halothane anaesthetics in patients with carcinoma of the uterine cervix treated with radium. *Lancet* i, 821.

134. US DEPARTMENT OF HEALTH, EDUCATION AND WELFARE (1980) *Guidelines for Detection of Hepatotoxicity Due to Drugs and Chemicals*, eds. C.S.

Davidson, C.M. Levy & E.C. Chamberlayne, NIH Publication No. 79–313.

135. UTILI R., BOITNOTT J.K. & ZIMMERMAN H.J. (1977) Dantrolene-associated hepatic injury. *Gastroenterology* **72**, 610.

136. VERGANI D., TSANTOULAS D., EDDLESTON A.L.W.F. *et al* (1978) Sensitisation to halothane-altered liver components in severe hepatic necrosis after halothane anaesthesia. *Lancet* ii, 801.

137. VIALLET A., GUILLAUME E., CÔTÉ J. *et al* (1972) Presinusoidal portal hypertension following chronic arsenic intoxication. *Gastroenterology* **62**, 177.

138. VITERI A.L., GREENE J.F. & DYCK W.P. (1979) Erythromycin ethylsuccinate-induced cholestasis. *Gastroenterology* **76**, 1007.

139. WALTON B., SIMPSON B.R., STRUNIN L. *et al* (1976) Unexplained hepatitis following halothane. *Br. med. J.* i, 1171.

140. WEIL R. III, KOEP L.J. & STARZL T.E. (1979) Liver resection of hepatic adenoma. *Arch. Surg.* **114**, 178.

141. WEPLER W. & OPITZ K. (1972) Histologic changes in the liver biopsy in amanita phalloides intoxication. *Hum. Pathol.* **3**, 249.

142. WERNER S.C., HANGER F.M. & KRITZLER R.A. (1950) Jaundice during methyl testosterone therapy. *Am. J. Med.* **8**, 325.

143. WERTHER J.L. & KORELITZ B.I. (1957) Chlorpromazine jaundice : analysis of twenty-two cases. *Am. J. Med.* **22**, 351.

144. WESTABY D., OGLE S.J., PARADINAS F.J. *et al* (1977) Liver damage from long term methyltestosterone. *Lancet* ii, 261.

145. WHELTON M.J., ALLAWAY A., STEWART A. *et al* (1968) Ergot poisoning in acute hepatic necrosis. *Gut* **9**, 297.

146. WILKINSON S.P., PORTMANN B. & WILLIAMS R. (1979) Hepatitis from dantrolene sodium. *Gut* **20**, 33.

147. WINKLER K. & POULSEN H. (1975) Liver disease with periportal sinusoidal dilatation. A possible complication to contraceptive steroids. *Scand. J. Gastroenterol.* **10**, 699.

148. WRIGHT R., EADE O.E., CHISHOLM M. *et al* (1975) Controlled prospective study of the effect on liver function of multiple exposure to halothane. *Lancet* i, 817.

149. ZAFRANI E.S., ISHAK K.G. & RUDZKI C. (1979) Cholestatic and hepatocellular injury associated with erythromycin esters. *Dig. Dis. Sci.* **24**, 385.

150. ZELMAN S. (1959) Liver cell necrosis in chlorpromazine jaundice (allergic cholangiolitis). A serial study of twenty-six needle biopsy specimens in nine patients. *Am. J. Med.* **27**, 708.

151. ZIMMERMAN H.J. (1979) *Hepatotoxicity. The Adverse Effects of Drugs and Other Chemicals on the Liver.* Appleton-Century-Crofts, New York.

Chapter 18
Hepatic Cirrhosis

Definition

Cirrhosis is defined anatomically as a diffuse process with fibrosis and nodule formation [1]. It has followed hepato-cellular necrosis. Although the causes are many, the end result is the same.

Fibrosis is not synonymous with cirrhosis. Fibrosis may be centrizonal in heart failure, or periportal in bile duct obstruction and congenital hepatic fibrosis (fig. 306) or interlobular in granulomatous liver disease, but without a true cirrhosis.

Nodule formation without fibrosis, as in Felty's syndrome, or partial nodular transformation (fig. 306), is not cirrhosis.

The relation of chronic active hepatitis to cirrhosis is discussed in Chapter 16.

Production of cirrhosis

The responses of the liver to necrosis are strictly limited; the most important are collapse of hepatic lobules, formation of diffuse fibrous septa, and nodular regrowth of liver cells. Thus, irrespective of the aetiology, the ultimate histological pattern of the liver is the same, or nearly the same [24]. Necrosis may no longer be apparent by the time the cirrhotic liver is examined.

When the liver cells become necrotic, the reticulin framework collapses with approximation of portal and central zones (bridging) (fig. 307). Some cells regrow to form nodules of various sizes. The nodules distort the hepatic vascular tree; portal blood flow is impeded and portal hypertension results (figs. 143, 151).

Sinusoids persist at the periphery of the regenerating nodules at the site of the portal–central bridges. Portal blood is diverted past functioning liver tissue leading to vascular insufficiency at the centre of the nodules (zone III) and even to persistence of the cirrhosis after the initial causative injury has been controlled. Basement membranes form in the Disse space, so impeding metabolic exchange with the liver cells.

Congenital hepatic fibrosis

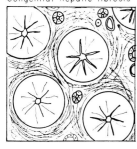

Partial nodular transformation

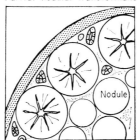

Cirrhosis

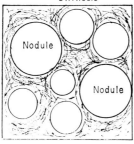

Fig. 306. Cirrhosis is defined as widespread fibrosis and nodule formation. Congenital hepatic fibrosis consists of fibrosis without nodules. Partial nodular transformation consists of nodules without fibrosis.

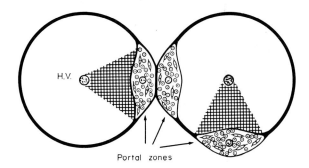

Fig. 307. Bridging necrosis and fibrosis is often pre-cirrhotic and the site of internal portal–systemic shunts.

Portal zones

New fibroblasts form round necrotic liver cells and proliferated ductules. The fibrosis (collagen) progresses from a reversible to an irreversible state where acellular permanent septa have developed in the portal zones and hepatic parenchyma. The distribution of the fibrous septa varies with the causative agent. In haemochromatosis the iron excites portal zone fibrosis. In alcoholism, the fibrosis is predominantly centrizonal.

The role of collagen [19, 25]

Collagen is a heterogeneous class of extracellular proteins characterized by a unique amino acid composition (about 30% glycine, 20% proline + hydroxyproline and a variable content of hydroxylysine). There are four distinct types (table 50). The cirrhotic liver shows an increase in all collagen types irrespective of aetiology. The ratio of type I to type III increases with the quantity of collagen formed. This may reflect duration of chronicity: type III is abundant in foetal tissue, whereas type I increases during ageing. The increased collagen is harmful by disrupting the hepatic architecture and by converting sinusoids to capillaries, so impeding metabolic exchange through basement membranes between liver cells and the blood.

In cirrhosis synthesis of collagen is increased, as shown by the hepatic prolyl hydroxylase level— the enzyme that controls production. This increase is due both to a greater collagen synthesis per fibroblast and to an increase in the number of collagen-producing cells.

Hepato-cellular necrosis is the stimulus to collagen formation. The factors concerned are not known. Necrotic cells could produce a stimulating factor or there might be a pre-formed inactive precursor in plasma. Lactic acidosis, as in alcoholic liver injury, may be a stimulating factor [25].

Macrophages may release a factor(s) which induces fibroblast proliferation and also increases hydroxyproline production by fibroblasts.

The perisinusoidal fat storage cell, the *Ito cell*, may change into a fibroblast and be responsible for intralobular collagen formation.

Fibronectin is a glycoprotein present in soluble form in the plasma and as an insoluble protein on the surface of liver cells. It binds the collagen and forms part of the extracellular matrix. Together with collagen, it is deposited in areas of liver cell damage as early as one hour after the injury. With collagen it may function in directing and organizing hepatocyte growth during the healing response.

Table 50. The types of collagen.

Type	Site	Stained by
I	Portal zones, central zones, broad scars	Van Giesen
II	Sinusoids (elastic tissue)	Elastin
III	Reticulin fibres (sinusoids, portal zones)	Silver
IV	Basement membranes	Periodic-acid Schiff (PAS)

CLASSIFICATION

Morphological

Three anatomical types are recognized: micronodular, macronodular and mixed, the liver showing both micro- and macronodular features [20].

Micronodular (regular, monolobular) is characterized by thick, regular septa, by regenerating small nodules varying little in size and by involvement of every lobule (figs. 308, 310). It is often associated with persistence of the injurious agent. The micronodular liver may represent impaired capacity for regrowth as in alcoholism, malnutrition, old age or anaemia.

Macronodular is characterized by septa and nodules of variable sizes and by normal lobules in the larger nodules (figs. 309, 311). Previous collapse is shown by juxtaposition in the fibrous scars of three or more portal tracts. Regeneration is reflected by large cells with large nuclei and by cell plates of varying thicknesses.

Vigorous regrowth in a micronodular cirrhosis results in a macronodular or mixed appearance.

Aetiology

The following are usually accepted:

1. Viral hepatitis
   types B, non-A non-B.
2. Alcohol
3. Metabolic
   e.g. haemochromatosis, Wilson's disease, α_1 anti-trypsin deficiency, type IV glycogenosis, galactosaemia, congenital tyrosinosis.
4. Prolonged cholestasis
   intra- and extra-hepatic.
5. Hepatic-venous outflow obstruction
   e.g. veno-occlusive disease, Budd–Chiari syndrome, constrictive pericarditis.
6. Disturbed immunity
   'lupoid' hepatitis.
7. Toxins and therapeutic agents
   e.g. methotrexate, isoniazid, methyl dopa.
8. Intestinal bypass.
9. Indian childhood cirrhosis.

Other possible factors to be considered include:

Malnutrition (Chapter 22).

Infections. Malarial parasites do not cause cirrhosis. The co-existence of malaria and cirrhosis probably reflects malnutrition, virus hepatitis and toxic factors in the community.

Syphilis causes cirrhosis in neonates but not in adults.

In schistosomiasis, the ova excite a fibrous tissue reaction in the portal zones. The association with cirrhosis in certain countries is probably related to other aetiological factors.

Granulomatous lesions Focal granuloma in such

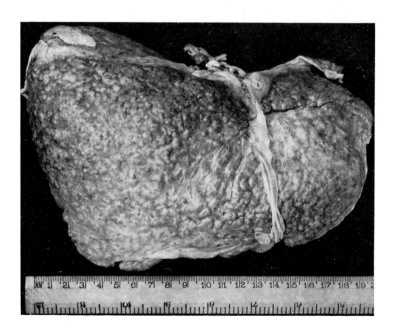

Fig. 308. The small, finely nodular liver of micronodular cirrhosis.

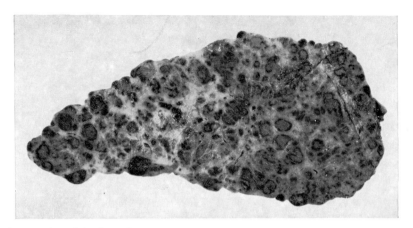

Fig. 309. The coarsely nodular liver of
macronodular cirrhosis.

conditions as brucellosis, tuberculosis and sarcoidosis heal with fibrosis, but the liver does not show
nodular regrowth.

Cryptogenic cirrhosis. The aetiology is unknown and this is clearly a heterogeneous group.
Its incidence varies in different parts of the world;
in the United Kingdom it is about 30% whereas
in other areas such as France or in urban parts of
the United States where alcoholism is prevalent
the level drops. As specific diagnostic criteria
appear, so the percentage falls. The advent of
HBsAg transferred many previously designated
cryptogenic cirrhotics to the post-hepatitic group.
Estimations of serum smooth muscle and mitochondrial antibodies and better interpretation of
liver histology separate others into the chronic

active hepatitis–primary biliary cirrhosis category.
Some of the remainder may be alcoholics who
deny alcoholism or have forgotten that they ever
consumed alcohol. There remains a hard core of
patients in whom the cirrhosis remains cryptogenic and aetiological diagnosis in these awaits the
advent of further specific criteria.

Mechanisms are discussed in individual chapters. The clinical and pathological picture may be
that of 'chronic active hepatitis' which has proceeded to cirrhosis (fig. 252) (Chapter 16).

Functional

An assessment of hepatic function should always
be attempted.

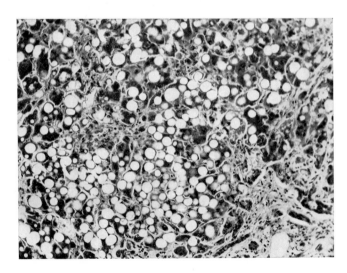

Fig. 310. Micronodular
cirrhosis. Gross fatty
change. The liver cells are
often necrotic. Fibrous septa
dissect the liver. H & E,
× 135.

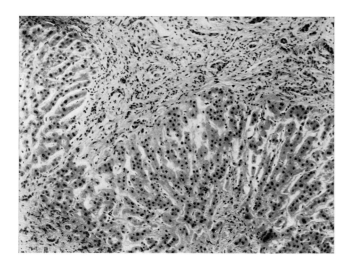

Fig. 311. Macronodular cirrhosis. Nodules of regenerating liver cells of different sizes are intersected by fibrous bands of various widths containing proliferating bile ducts. Fatty change is not seen. H & E, × 135.

Liver failure (Chapters 7, 8, 9, 10) is estimated by such features as jaundice, ascites, encephalopathy, low serum albumin, raised transaminase levels and a prothrombin deficiency not corrected by vitamin K.

Portal hypertension (Chapter 11) is shown by splenomegaly, oesophageal varices and by the newer methods of measuring portal pressure.

Activity is assessed by serial clinical, biochemical and histological observations, and classified whether progressing, regressing or stationary.

Examples of classification

In every patient, diagnosis must be in terms of aetiology, morphology and hepatic function. Examples of such complete diagnoses are:

1. Macronodular cirrhosis following type B hepatitis with liver cell failure and portal hypertension. Progressing.
2. Micronodular cirrhosis in an alcoholic with liver cell failure and minimal portal hypertension. Regressing.
3. Mixed micronodular and macronodular cirrhosis following bile duct stricture with minimal liver cell failure and portal hypertension. Progressing.

CLINICAL CIRRHOSIS

Cirrhosis, apart from other features peculiar to the cause, results in two major events, hepato-cellular failure (Chapters 7, 8, 9, 10) and portal hyper-

tension (Chapter 11). Prognosis and treatment depend on the magnitude of these two factors. In clinical terms, the types are either 'latent and well compensated' or 'active and decompensated'. In addition, cirrhosis, whatever its type, has certain clinico-pathological associations.

It is difficult to associate the clinical picture with the underlying pathology although there are certain similarities. In Europe and the United States, post-hepatitic cirrhosis, cirrhosis of the alcoholic, chronic active hepatitis, and cryptogenic cirrhosis account for the majority. The age and sex distribution of the various types differ [28].

The terminal stages of the various types may be identical and differences must not be stressed. The aetiological distinction, however, is important both for prognosis and for specific treatment such as alcohol withdrawal, venesection in haemochromatosis or prednisolone in chronic active hepatitis. Finally, comparison of cirrhosis in different parts of the world must allow for different aetiologies, although the basic pattern of liver cell failure and portal hypertension may be similar. Results of treatment of one type cannot be compared with those for another.

Clinical and pathological associations

1. Splenomegaly and abdominal wall venous collaterals usually indicate *portal hypertension*.

2. Chronic relapsing *pancreatitis* and pancreatic calcification are often associated with alcoholism.

3. *Gastro-intestinal*. Varices may collapse and be overlooked at autopsy. Peptic ulcer is frequent

with cirrhosis of alcoholics. Intestinal absorption of glucose and protein loss into the gastro-intestinal tract are normal [15]. Taste and smell acuity may be reduced [8].

4. *Steatorrhoea* is frequent even in the absence of pancreatitis or alcoholism. It can be related to reduced hepatic bile salt secretion and hence to a low micellar phase lipid concentration in the bile [2].

5. *Abdominal herniae* are common with ascites. They should not be repaired unless endangering life or unless the cirrhosis is very well compensated.

6. *Primary liver cancer* is frequent with all forms of cirrhosis except the biliary and cardiac types. Metastatic cancer is said to be rare, due to the reduced frequency of extra-hepatic carcinoma in cirrhosis [12, 26]. However, when groups of patients with cancer with and without cirrhosis were compared the incidence of hepatic metastases was the same in each group.

7. *Gall-stones.* In a survey of autopsy records, gall-stones were found in 29.4% of the cirrhotic patients (irrespective of the type) and 12.8% of the non-cirrhotic population [6, 22]. This increase does not seem to be related to lithogenic (low cholesterol-holding) bile [34]. Pigment stones due to abnormal bilirubin metabolism are frequent. When discovered, surgical intervention should be avoided unless life-saving, for the patient is potentially a poor operative risk.

8. *Digital clubbing* and *hypertrophic osteoarthropathy* may complicate cirrhosis, especially biliary [11].

9. *Parotid gland enlargement* and *Dupuytren's contracture* are seen in some alcoholic patients with cirrhosis.

10. *Renal.* Changes in intrarenal circulation, and particularly a redistribution of blood flow away from the cortex, are found in all forms of cirrhosis. This predisposes to the *hepato-renal syndrome.* Intrinsic renal failure follows periods of hypotension and shock.

Glomerular changes include a thickening of the mesangial stalk and to a lesser degree of the capillary walls [3, 5] (cirrhotic glomerular sclerosis). Deposits of IgA are most frequent. These are usually found with alcoholic liver disease. The pathogenesis is not certain. The changes are usually latent, but occasionally associated with proliferative changes and the clinical manifestations of glomerular involvement.

11. *Infections.* Tuberculosis has, in general,

decreased but tuberculous peritonitis is still encountered and is often unsuspected [7]. Respiratory infections have also lessened in severity.

Septicaemia should always be considered in patients developing pyrexia or deteriorating for no obvious reason. Spontaneous bacterial peritonitis should also be suspected. Missed diagnosis is frequent.

12. *Cardiovascular.* Cirrhotics are less liable to coronary and aortic atheroma than the rest of the population [23]. At autopsy, the incidence of myocardial infarction is about a quarter of that among total cases examined without cirrhosis [14].

Hypertension is unusual, perhaps due to the protection of a circulating vasodilator.

13. *Genetic factors.* A study of nineteen siblings of thirty-eight probands in Denmark failed to show a familial predisposition to cirrhosis [10].

14. *Eye signs.* Lid retraction and lid lag is significantly increased in patients with cirrhosis compared with a control population [29].

There is no evidence of thyroid disease. Serum-free thyroxin is not increased [13].

Histocompatibility antigens (HLA) [9] (table 45)

There is an association with HLA B8 and HBsAg-negative chronic active hepatitis, 60% of patients with this condition being HLA B8-positive. The patients who are positive tend to be female, less than 40 years old, have a remission with corticosteroid therapy and show positive non-specific serum antibody tests and high serum gamma-globulins. This association does not apply to HBsAg-positive chronic active hepatitis. The D locus antigen DW3 may show an even stronger association with non-B chronic active hepatitis than does lupus B8.

In males with alcoholic hepatitis and cirrhosis, but not with less severe liver disease, there is an increased incidence of HLA B8 [21].

In idiopathic haemochromatosis, there is an association with HLA B3, B7 and 14 (Chapter 20). This observation may be useful in detecting family members at risk of developing the disease.

In primary biliary cirrhosis, there is no association with HLA B8, nor indeed with any particular histocompatibility antigen. This is against the concept of an overlap between hepatitis B antigen-negative chronic active hepatitis and primary biliary cirrhosis based on co-existence in one patient or among related family members.

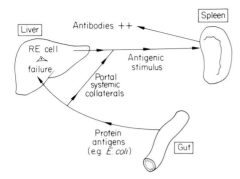

Fig. 312. A possible mechanism for the increased serum antibody (and globulin) levels in cirrhosis. Protein antigens from the gut bypass reticulo-endothelial (RE, Kupffer) cells in the liver and produce an antigenic stimulus to other organs, particularly the spleen, so increasing serum antibodies.

In general, detection of HLA types are not of practical importance in the investigation of patients with liver disease. They may be useful in family studies and in protection of relatives at risk of developing genetically related diseases.

Hyperglobulinaemia

Elevation of the total serum globulin, and particularly gamma, level is a well-known accompaniment of most forms of chronic liver disease. Electrophoresis of the serum proteins shows a polyclonal gamma response, but rarely a monoclonal picture may be seen. The increased gammaglobulin values may be related in part to increased tissue auto-antibodies, such as smooth muscle antibody. However, the major factor seems to be failure of the damaged liver to clear intestinal antigen (fig. 312). Patients with cirrhosis show increased serum antibodies to gastro-intestinal tract antigens, particularly *E. coli* [4, 32, 33]. Such antigens bypass the liver through portal–systemic channels or through the internal shunts developing round the cirrhotic nodule. The hepatic phagocyte [18] probably functions normally. Once in the systemic circulation these intestinal antigens provoke an increased antibody response from such organs as the spleen. Systemic endotoxaemia may arise similarly [16]. Suppressor T lymphocyte function is depressed in chronic liver disease and this would reduce the suppression of B lymphocytes and so favour antibody production [31].

CLINICALLY LATENT CIRRHOSIS

The disease may be discovered at a routine examination or biochemical screen or at operation

Table 51. General investigations in the patient with cirrhosis (see also table 20).

Occupation, age, sex, domicile

Clinical history
  Weakness and weight loss
  Anorexia and flatulent dyspepsia
  Abdominal pain
  Jaundice. Colour of urine and faeces
  Swelling of legs or abdomen
  Haemorrhage—nose, gums, skin, alimentary tract
  Loss of libido
Past health: Jaundice, hepatitis, drugs ingested
Social
  Hereditary. Alcohol consumption

Examination
  Nutrition, fever, fetor hepaticus, jaundice, pigmentation, purpura, finger clubbing, white nails, vascular spiders, palmar erythema, gynaecomastia, testicular atrophy, distribution of body hair. Parotid enlargement. Dupuytren's contracture. Blood pressure
  Abdomen: ascites, abdominal wall veins, liver, spleen
  Peripheral oedema
  Neurological changes: mental functions, stupor, tremor

Special investigations
Biochemical:
  Urine—urobilinogen qualitative test
  Serum—bilirubin concentration
            alkaline phosphatase concentration
            albumin and globulin concentration
            electrophoresis of proteins
            transaminase concentration
If ascites present: serum sodium, potassium, bicarbonate, chloride and urea levels
            Weigh daily
            24-hour urine volume and sodium excretion
Serum immunological:
  Smooth muscle, mitochondrial and nuclear antibodies
  Hepatitis-B antigen (HBsAg) (other markers of hepatitis, page 252)
  α_1 fetoprotein
Haematology:
  Haemoglobin, absolute values, leucocyte and platelet count, prothrombin time
Endoscopy
Radiology:
  Barium swallow and meal
Aspiration liver biopsy if blood coagulation permits
EEG. If neuropsychiatric changes
Hepatic scan or ultrasound

undertaken for some other condition. Cirrhosis may be suspected if the patient has mild pyrexia, vascular spiders, palmar erythema, or unexplained epistaxis or oedema of the ankles. Firm enlargement of the liver and splenomegaly are helpful diagnostic signs. Vague morning indigestion and flatulent dyspepsia may be early features in the alcoholic cirrhotic. Confirmation should be sought by biochemical tests and, if necessary, by aspiration liver biopsy.

Biochemical tests may be quite normal in this group. The most frequent changes are a slight increase in the serum transaminase or gamma GT level and a constant excess of urobilinogen in the urine. The two-hour post-prandial plasma 'total' bile acid level is usually increased [30].

Diagnosis is confirmed by *aspiration liver biopsy*.

These patients may remain compensated until they die from another cause. Some proceed, in a period from months to years, to the stage of hepato-cellular failure. In others the problem is of portal hypertension with oesophageal bleeding. Portal hypertension may present even with normal liver function tests. The course in the individual patient is very difficult to predict.

DECOMPENSATED CIRRHOSIS

The patient usually seeks medical advice because of ascites and/or jaundice. General health fails with weakness, muscle wasting and weight loss. Continuous mild fever (37.5–28 °C) is often due to Gram-negative bacteriaemia, to continuing hepatic cell necrosis or to a complicating liver cell carcinoma. Fetor hepaticus may be present. Cirrhosis is the commonest cause of hepatic encephalopathy.

Jaundice implies that liver cell destruction exceeds the capacity for regeneration and is always serious. The deeper the jaundice the greater the inadequacy of the liver cell function.

The skin may be pigmented, due to increased amounts of melanin. Clubbing of the fingers is occasionally seen. Purpura over the arms, shoulders and shins may be associated with a low platelet count. Spontaneous bruising and epistaxes reflect a prothrombin deficiency. The circulation is over-active. The blood pressure is low. Sparse hair, vascular spiders, palmar erythema, white nails and gonadal atrophy are common.

Ascites is usually preceded by abdominal distension. Oedema of the legs is frequently associated.

The liver may be enlarged, with a firm regular edge, or contracted and impalpable. The spleen may be palpable.

The differential diagnosis of ascites, hepatic encephalopathy, and jaundice are described in Chapters 8, 10, 13.

Laboratory findings

Urine. Urobilinogen is present in excess; bilirubin is also present if the patient is jaundiced. The urinary sodium excretion is diminished in the presence of ascites, and in a severe case less than 4 mEq are passed daily.

Serum biochemical changes. In addition to the raised serum bilirubin level, albumin is depressed and gamma-globulin raised. The percentage of esterified cholesterol is depressed. The serum alkaline phosphatase is usually raised to about twice normal; very high readings are occasionally found. Serum transaminase values may be increased.

Haematology. There is usually a mild normocytic, normochromic anaemia; it is occasionally macrocytic. Gastro-intestinal bleeding leads to hypochromic anaemia. The leucocyte and platelet counts are reduced ('hypersplenism'). The prothrombin time is prolonged and does not return to normal with vitamin K therapy. The bone-marrow is macro-normoblastic. Plasma cells are increased in proportion to the hyperglobulinaemia.

Needle biopsy diagnosis [1, 27] (table 52)

If there are no contraindications, such as ascites or a coagulation defect, this should always be done. It may give a clue to aetiology and to activity. Serial biopsies are useful in assessing progress.

Diagnosis may be difficult, especially when Menghini type needles are used. These tend to aspirate the soft parenchyma, leaving fibrous tissue behind. Large nodules provide a special difficulty in interpretation. Fragmentation of the specimen before and after processing, with fibrous tissue at the margins of the fragments, suggests cirrhosis. If fibrosis is scanty, reticulin and collagen stains are essential (table 50).

Helpful diagnostic points include absence of portal tracts, abnormal vascular arrangements in

Table 52. Histopathology and aetiology of cirrhosis.

Aetiology	Morpho-logical pattern	Fat	Cholestasis	Iron	Copper	Acido-philic bodies	PAS-positive globules	Mallory's hyalin	Ground-glass hepato-cytes
Viral hepatitis	macro- or micronodular	−	−	−	−	+	−	−	+
Alcoholism	micro- or macronodular	+	±	±	−	±	−	+	−
Haemochromatosis	micronodular	±	−	+	−	−	−	−	−
Wilson's disease	macronodular	±	±	−	+	+	−	+	−
α$_1$ anti-trypsin deficiency	micro- or macronodular	±	±	−	±	±	+	±	−
Primary biliary	biliary	−	+	−	+	−	−	±	−
Venous outflow obstruction	reversed	−	−	−	−	−	−	−	−
Intestinal bypass operation	micronodular	+	−	−	−	±	−	±	−
Indian childhood	micronodular	−	±	−	+	−	−	+	−

− usually absent; ± may be present; + usually present.

the specimen, the presence of nodules with fibrous septa, variability in liver cell size and appearance in different areas, and thickened liver cell plates.

PROGNOSIS

Cirrhosis is usually believed to be irreversible [24], but there is no doubt that fibrosis may regress as seen in treated haemochromatosis or Wilson's disease and the concept of irreversibility is not proven.

Cirrhosis need not be a progressive disease. With therapy the downhill progress may be checked. The following points are useful prognostically:

1. *Aetiology.* Alcoholic cirrhotics, if they abstain, respond better than those with 'cryptogenic' cirrhosis.
2. If decompensation has followed haemorrhage, infection or alcoholism, the prognosis is better than if it is spontaneous, because the *precipitating factor* is correctable.
3. The *response to therapy.* If the patient has failed to improve within one month of starting hospital treatment, the outlook is poor.
4. *Jaundice*, especially if persistent, is a serious sign.
5. *Neurological complications.* The significance

depends on their mode of production. Those developing in the course of progressive hepato-cellular failure carry a bad prognosis, whereas those developing chronically and associated with an extensive portal–systemic collateral circulation respond well to dietary protein restriction.

6. *Ascites* worsens the prognosis, particularly if large doses of diuretics are needed for control.
7. *Liver size.* A large liver carries a better prognosis than a small one because it is likely to contain more functioning cells.
8. *Haemorrhage from oesophageal varices.* Portal hypertension must be considered together with the state of the liver cells. If function is good, haemorrhage may be tolerated: if poor, hepatic coma and death are probable.
9. *Biochemical tests.* If the serum albumin is less than 2.5 g the outlook is poor. Hyponatraemia (serum sodium < 120 mEq/1) if unrelated to diuretic therapy is grave.

   Serum transaminase and globulin levels are no guide to prognosis.
10. Persistent *hypoprothrombinaemia* with spontaneous bruising is serious.
11. Persistent hypotension (systolic BP < 100 mmHg) is serious.
12. *Hepatic histological changes.* Sections are useful in evaluating the extent of necrosis and of inflammatory infiltration. A fatty liver responds well to treatment.

CONCLUSIONS

The prognosis is determined by the extent of hepato-cellular failure. Jaundice, spontaneous bruising and ascites, resistant to treatment, are grave signs. If specific treatment is available the outlook is better.

TREATMENT

The management of the *well-compensated* cirrhotic is that of the early detection of hepato-cellular failure. The principles of an adequate mixed diet and avoidance of alcohol should be explained.

A diet of 1 g protein/kg body weight is adequate unless the patient is obviously malnourished. Additional choline or methionine or various 'liver tonics' are unnecessary. The avoidance of butter and other fats, eggs, coffee or chocolate is not of any therapeutic value.

The onset of hepato-cellular failure with oedema and ascites demands sodium restriction and diuretics (Chapter 10); complicating encephalopathy is an indication for a lowered protein intake (Chapter 8).

Portal hypertension may demand surgical intervention (Chapter 11).

The therapy of cirrhosis may reside in switching off collagen synthesis. *Penicillamine* inhibits the formation of cross-links in collagen. Its use in hepatic cirrhosis remains uncertain, and toxic effects are numerous. *Colchicine* inhibits assembly of collagen and increases collagenase production. Randomized trial of its use is in progress and beneficial results are suggested [17]; again this is a toxic drug. *Corticosteroids* are anti-inflammatory and inhibit the activity of prolyl hydroxylase. They inhibit collagen synthesis but also inhibit procollagenase.

Corticosteroid therapy in chronic active hepatitis is discussed in Chapter 16.

REFERENCES

1. ANTHONY P.P., ISHAK K.G., NAYAK N.C. *et al* (1977) The morphology of cirrhosis: definition, nomenclature and classification. *Bull. WHO* **55**. 521.
2. BADLEY B.W.D., MURPHY G.M., BOUCHIER I.A.D. *et al* (1969) The role of bile salts in the steatorrhoea of chronic liver disease. *Gastroenterology* **56**, 1136.
3. BERGER J., YANEVA H. & NABARRA B. (1977–8) Glomerular changes in patients with cirrhosis of the liver. *Adv. Nephrology* **7**, 3.
4. BJØRNEBOE M., PRYTZ H. & ØRSKOV F. (1972) Antibodies to intestinal microbes in serum of patients with cirrhosis of the liver. *Lancet* i, 58.
5. BLOODWORTH J.M.B. Jr & SOMMERS S.C. (1959) 'Cirrhotic glomerulosclerosis', a renal lesion associated with hepatic cirrhosis. *Lab. Invest.* **8**, 962.
6. BOUCHIER I.A.D. (1969) Postmortem study of the frequency of gallstones in patients with cirrhosis of the liver. *Gut* **10**, 705.
7. BURACK W.R. & HOLLISTER R.M. (1960) Tuberculous peritonitis: a study of forty-seven proved cases encountered by a general medical unit in twenty-five years. *Am. J. Med.* **28**, 510.
8. BURCH R.E., SACKIN D.A., URSICK J.A. *et al* (1978) Decreased taste and smell acuity in cirrhosis. *Arch. intern. Med.* **138**, 743.
9. EDDLESTON A.L.W.F. & WILLIAMS R. (1978) HLA and liver disease. *Br. med. Bull.* **34**, 295.
10. ELLING P., RANLØV P. & BILDSØE P. (1966) A genetic approach to the pathogenesis of hepatic cirrhosis. A clinical and serological study. *Acta med. Scand.* **179**, 527.
11. EPSTEIN O., AJDUKIEWICZ A.B., DICK R. *et al.* (1979) Hypertrophic hepatic osteoarthropathy. *Am. J. Med.* **67**, 88.
12. GOLDSTEIN M.J., FRANLE W.J. & SHERLOCK P. (1966) Hepatic metastases and portal cirrhosis. *Am. J. med. Sci.* **252**, 26.
13. HOLLANDER D., MEEK J.C. & MANNING R.T. (1967) Free thyroxine in serum of patients with cirrhosis of the liver. *New Engl. J. Med.* **276**, 900.
14. HOWELL W.L. & MANION W.C. (1960) The low incidence of myocardial infarction in patients with portal cirrhosis of the liver: a review of 639 cases of cirrhosis of the liver from 17,731 autopsies. *Am. heart J.* **60**, 341.
15. IBER F.L. (1967) Protein loss into the gastrointestinal tract in cirrhosis of the liver. *Am. J. clin. Nutr.* **19**, 219.
16. JACOB A.I., GOLDBERG P.K., BLOOM N. *et al* (1977) Endotoxin and bacteria in portal blood. *Gastroenterology* **72**, 1268.
17. KERSHENOBICH D., URIBE M., SUAREZ G.I. *et al* (1979) Treatment of cirrhosis with colchicine: a double-blind randomized trial. *Gastroenterology* **77**, 532.
18. KUPFFER C. VON (1878) Ueber Sternzellen der Leber. *Arch. mikr. Anat.* **12**, 355.
19. MCGEE J.O'D. & FALLON A. (1978) Hepatic cirrhosis—a collagen formative disease? *J. clin. Pathol.* **31**, suppl. (Royal Coll. Pathol.) **12**, 150.
20. MACSWEEN R.N.M., ANTHONY P.P. & SCHEUER P.J. (eds) (1979) *Pathology of the Liver.* Churchill Livingstone, Edinburgh.
21. MORGAN M.Y., ROSS M.G.R., NG C.M. *et al* (1980) HLA-B8, immunoglobulins, and antibody responses in alcohol-related liver disease. *J. Clin. Pathol.* **33**, 488.
22. NICHOLAS P., RINAUDO P.A. & CONN H.O. (1972) Increased incidence of cholelithiasis in Laennec's cirrhosis: a postmortem evaluation of pathogenesis. *Gastroenterology* **63**, 112.

23. PLATT D., KIE F.E. & LUBOEINSKI H.P. (1973) Der Einflüss des Atters auf die negative Syntropie zwischen malignen Tum ören, Lebercirrh öse und arteriosklerorischen Umbaurorgangen der Aortawand, Coronar und Cerebral. *Arterien Klin. Wschr.* **51,** 176.

24. POPPER H. (1977) Pathologic aspects of cirrhosis. *Am. J. Pathol.* **87,** 228.

25. ROJKIND M. & DUNN M.A. (1979) Hepatic fibrosis. *Gastroenterology* **76,** 849.

26. RUEBNER B.H., GREEN R., MIYAI K. *et al* (1961) The rarity of intrahepatic metastasis in cirrhosis of the liver. *Am. J. Pathol.* **39,** 739.

27. SCHEUER P.J. (1980) *Liver Biopsy Interpretation.* 3rd edn. Baillière Tindall, London.

28. SHERLOCK S. (1966) Waldenström's chronic active hepatitis. *Acta med. Scand.* **179,** Suppl. 445, p. 426.

29. SUMMERSKILL W.H.J. & MOLNAR G.D. (1962) Eye signs in hepatic cirrhosis. *New Engl. J. Med.* **266,** 1244.

30. THJODLEIFSSON B., BARNES S., CHITRANUKROH A. *et al.* (1977) Assessment of the plasma disappearance of cholyl-1^{14}C-glycine as a test of hepatocellular disease. *Gut* **18,** 697.

31. THOMAS H.C., RYAN C.J., BENJAMIN I.S. *et al.* (1976) The immune response in cirrhotic rats: the induction of tolerance to orally administered protein antigens. *Gastroenterology* **71,** 114.

32. TRIGER D.R., ALP M.H. & WRIGHT R. (1972) Bacterial and dietary antibodies in liver disease. *Lancet* i, 60.

33. TRIGER D.R. & WRIGHT R. (1973) Hyperglobulinaemia in liver disease. *Lancet* i, 1494.

34. VLAHCEVIC Z.R., YOSHIDA T., JUTTIJUDATA P. *et al* (1973) Bile acid metabolism in cirrhosis. III. Biliary lipid secretion. *Gastroenterology* **64,** 298.

Chapter 19
Alcohol and the Liver

The association of alcohol with cirrhosis was recognized by Matthew Baillie in 1793 [4] and later by Addison [1]. In Western countries the incidence of cirrhosis can be directly related to the quantity of alcohol consumed. In France, between 1941 and 1947, rationing of wine from 5 to 1 litre per week led to an 80% reduction in mortality from cirrhosis [40] (fig. 313). Cirrhosis is on the increase. In the United States it is the fourth commonest cause of death in white males. In the United Kingdom, deaths from cirrhosis have increased by approximately 25% in the last decade. The death rate in different communities correlates quite well with alcohol consumption (table 53). The prevalence in various countries depends largely on religious and other customs and on the relation between the cost of alcohol and the weekly wage. In France wine is cheap and cirrhosis is common. The lower the cost of alcohol, the more are lower socio-economic groups affected (fig. 314).

Certain occupations are particularly associated with the risks of alcoholism. They include the liquor trade, 'show business' and those on expense accounts or with ready access to duty-free liquor. In Britain patients with alcoholic

Table 53. Cirrhosis mortality related to alcohol consumption.

	Cirrhosis mortality per 100 000 population over 25 years old	Per capita alcohol consumption/year (litres absolute alcohol)
France	57.2	16.4
Portugal	55.1	14.1
Italy	52.1	14.0
West Germany	39.6	11.3
Spain	38.8	11.7
USA	28.6	5.8
Canada	19.6	6.5
Sweden	15.6	5.7
Holland	7.4	4.8
UK	5.7	6.2

Fig. 313. General mortality and mortality from cirrhosis in Paris from 1935 to 1963. In Paris, drink rationing was much more severe than in France as a whole. Consumption fell to about 3–5 litres of absolute alcohol per adult per year (instead of 35 litres). The fall in the mortality rate from cirrhosis was truly astonishing, going from 35 to six per 100 000 of population from 1941 to 1945, and then generally climbing back to the pre-war figure in 1953 (Pequignot & Cyrulnik 1970).

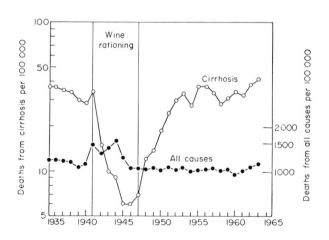

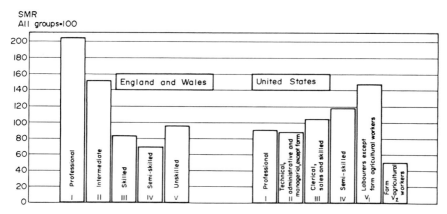

Fig. 314. Cirrhosis of the liver, standardized mortality ratios (SMR), men aged 20–64, by occupational level and social class; United States 1950, England and Wales 1949–53 (Office of Home Economics).

liver disease tend to be executives, Services personnel, physicians and, increasingly all over the world, their lonely wives.

Women seem more susceptible than men [34]. They are less likely to be suspected of alcohol abuse, they present at a later stage and are more likely to relapse after treatment (table 54).

A bottle of spirits contains 240 g alcohol. The 'safe' daily consumption is uncertain: 160 g daily used to be the limit, but now 60 g in men and a mere 20 g in women may suffice [40]. Alcoholics with cirrhosis have usually consumed about 190 g of alcohol daily for 10 years, although there are wide individual variations [25]. Alcoholism of shorter duration may be compensated by a higher daily dose and vice versa.

The liver injury is unrelated to the type of beverage consumed: it is related only to its alcohol content. The non-alcoholic constituents of the drink—congeners—are not particularly hepato-toxic. The steady daily imbiber is much more at risk than the 'spree' drinker whose total alcohol intake may be no less. This may be partly because the intermittent drinker gives his liver a

chance to repair, and partly because his diet suffers less.

GENETICS

Not everyone who drinks excessively develops liver damage. In a group of 526 unselected male alcoholics receiving treatment, liver function tests showed severe liver damage in a quarter, less damage in one-half [25]. Numerous chronic alcoholics with completely normal livers pose an interesting problem. Their hepatic resistance might be genetically determined.

There have been associations between HLA blood groups and susceptibility to chronic liver damage through heavy drinking. This seems to have geographic variations. In the United Kingdom the association is with HLA B8 [3], in Chile with HLA B13 [31], and in Norway with HLA BW40 [6].

METABOLISM OF ALCOHOL (fig. 315) [21, 27]

Alcohol cannot be stored and obligatory oxidation must take place, predominantly in the liver. The healthy individual cannot metabolize more than 160–180 g per day. Alcohol induces enzymes used in its catabolism, and the alcoholic, at least while his liver is relatively unaffected, may be able to metabolize more. One gram of alcohol gives seven calories, and alcoholics literally run on spirit. These 'empty' calories make no contribution to nutrition other than to give energy.

Table 54. Alcoholic liver disease—males: females (Morgan & Sherlock 1977).

Females suspected	38%
Males suspected	77%
Continued to abuse alcohol	
males	71%
females	91%

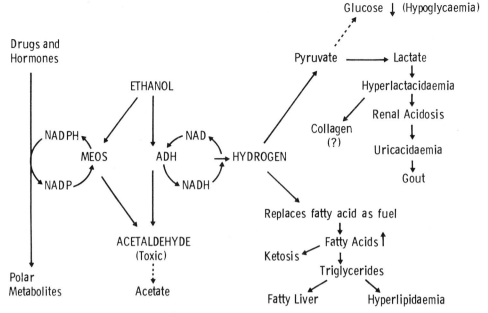

Fig. 315. Oxidation of alcohol in the hepatocyte. The production of acetaldehyde (toxic) is enhanced and conversion to acetate reduced. The hydrogen produced replaces fatty acid as a fuel so that fatty acids accumulate with consequent ketosis, triglyceridaemia, fatty liver and hyperlipidaemia. Unwanted hydrogen is used to convert pyruvate to lactate, which is produced in excess. Hyperlactacidaemia leads to renal acidosis, a rise in serum uric acid and gout. Collagen synthesis may be stimulated. Reduction of the pyruvate to glucose pathway results in hypoglycaemia.

Stimulation of the MEOS drug metabolizing system leads to drug and alcohol tolerance, and increased testosterone metabolism may be related to feminization and to infertility.

Broken lines indicate depressed pathways.

H = excess hydrogen equivalents; ADH = alcohol dehydrogenase; MEOS = microsomal ethanol oxidizing system; NAD = nicotinamide adenine dinucleotide; NADP = nicotinamide adenine dinucleotide phosphate (after Lieber 1978).

The major route of ethanol oxidation is by initial conversion to acetaldehyde catabolized by the enzyme alcohol dehydrogenase (ADH). This takes place in the cytosol. Acetaldehyde in mitochondria and cytosol may be injurious, causing membrane damage and cell necrosis. The acetaldehyde is converted to acetyl CoA with acetaldehyde dehydrogenase acting as a co-enzyme (fig. 315). This can be further broken down to acetate, which may be oxidized to carbon dioxide and water, or converted by the citric acid cycle to other biochemically important compounds including fatty acids. NAD is a co-factor and hydrogen acceptor when alcohol is converted to acetaldehyde and further to acetyl CoA. The NADH generated changes the NADH : NAD ratio and the redox state of the liver. Triglyceride synthesis and lipid peroxidation are increased. The activity of the citric acid cycle is reduced, and this may be responsible for de-

creased fatty acid oxidation. Lipoprotein synthesis is increased by alcohol. The NADH may serve as the hydrogen carrier for the conversion of pyruvate to lactate, and blood lactate and uric acid levels rise after alcohol. Post-alcoholic hypoglycaemia and gout after alcohol ingestion may be explained by this mechanism. The conversion of alcohol to acetaldehyde also leads to inhibition of protein synthesis.

Alcohol is also metabolized by a microsomal ethanol oxidizing system (MEOS). This is inducible by alcohol. This may explain the tolerance of the chronic alcoholic not only to alcohol but to other drugs metabolized by microsomal enzymes. Alcoholics not under the influence of alcohol are unusually resistant to these sedative drugs which are metabolized by microsomal enzymes. Increased testosterone metabolism may be partly responsible for feminization and sterility.

PATHOGENESIS OF LIVER INJURY

Relation to alcohol. The development of alcoholic liver damage is dependent on the duration and dose of alcohol. When volunteers, both normal and alcoholic, were given about 10–20 oz (300–600 dl) of 86 proof alcohol daily for about 8–12 days, liver biopsy sections showed fatty change and EM abnormalities [50]. Alcoholic hepatitis and cirrhosis have been reproduced in baboons fed alcohol isocalorically for carbohydrate. A nutritious diet was not preventative [28, 51].

The deleterious effect of alcohol might be accounted for by the toxicity of acetaldehyde which accumulates in the liver cell or by protein and water retention [5]. There might be a microsomal activation of hepato-toxins and alterations could follow the redox state (fig. 315).

New collagen formation. This is probably the key to the progression of alcoholic hepatitis to cirrhosis. Alcohol stimulates fibrogenesis and collagen synthesis, perhaps by means of 'Ito cells' or lipocytes [49]. Collagenosis may be stimulated by lactic acidosis (fig. 315).

Immunological. Immunological hyper-reactivity may be responsible for the progressive destruction of liver cells and development of cirrhosis [24]. This could explain progression in spite of alcohol abstinence and a good diet. Hyaline might be the antigen concerned for antibodies and cytotoxic lymphocytes against alcoholic hyaline are found in alcoholic hepatitis [23].

Hypermetabolic state. Animals chronically fed alcohol are hypermetabolic and are particularly sensitive to reduced oxygen supply [38]. The increased hepatic oxygen consumption leads to a decrease in oxygen tension in centrizonal areas which are the last to receive oxygen. Hypoxia, necrosis and collagenosis are therefore predominantly centrizonal.

Nutrition and fatty liver. The chronic alcoholic usually eats sparingly and erratically. The diet is particularly poor in protein for such foods are costly. In contrast to other types of cirrhosis, the alcoholic shows many signs of malnutrition.

Increasing evidence that alcohol is itself hepato-toxic has shifted interest away from diet as an aetiological factor. Nevertheless, improvement in liver function does not always follow alcohol abstinence if dietary protein remains low [43]. The alcohol oxidizing enzymes and the integrity of the liver cell depend on a high level of dietary protein and other nutrients. If these are low, the capacity of the liver to metabolize alcohol and its power to synthesize the lipoprotein necessary for the transport of tryglyceride-fat from the liver may be deficient.

Fatty liver is probably of little importance in relation to the development of cirrhosis. The fatty liver of kwashiorkor, for instance, never proceeds to cirrhosis.

The increased liver fat has many sources. Most of it comes from the diet [29] and from adipose tissue. In the liver, alcohol reduces mitochondrial fatty acid oxidation [21] and increases triglyceride formation from fatty acids.

PATHOLOGY [14, 42]

In the early stages the liver is greatly enlarged due to severe fatty change. Every liver cell is laden with fat so that a haematoxylin-eosin stained section resembles Swiss cheese. During decompensation an acute 'hepatitis' is found particularly in central areas. It consists of single cells showing lytic necrosis, the cytoplasm containing an irregular, frequently perinuclear, clump of highly refractile, densely eosinophilic material, the alcoholic hyaline of Mallory (see figs. 316, 317 in colour section). Histochemistry shows it to be a complex glycoprotein with antigenic properties. Hyaline can rarely be found with Wilson's disease, cryptogenic cirrhosis [16], primary biliary cirrhosis and Indian childhood cirrhosis. It is therefore highly suggestive, but not specific, of alcoholism unless it is centrizonal when it is diagnostic [16]. Polymorphs surround the necrosing liver cell (fig. 318). Kupffer cell proliferation is prominent. Cholestasis is noted with jaundice. The portal zones show stellate fibrosis and infiltration with round cells. In severely malnourished alcoholics centrizonal fibrosis may proceed even to obliteration of hepatic venous radicles [12, 13]. Occasionally the picture is of a chronic persistent or active hepatitis [17].

Sclerosing central hyaline necrosis (fig. 317). Fibrous septa, commencing in relation to cell necrosis ('creeping collagenosis') divide the liver up into small, regular, uniformly distributed nodules until a micronodular cirrhosis is produced (fig. 319). In the final stages fat decreases and the liver shrinks so that the aetiology of the cirrhosis cannot be recognized. The stromal collapse and cirrhosis seem to follow the necrosis rather than the fatty change. The two processes of hepatitis

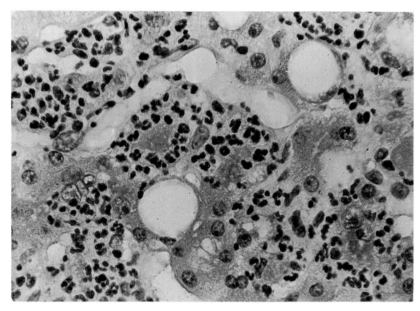

Fig. 318. Acute alcoholic hepatitis. Liver cells undergoing necrosis and containing clumps of Mallory's hyaline are surrounded by cuffs of polymorphonuclear cells. There is fatty change. H & E, × 120.

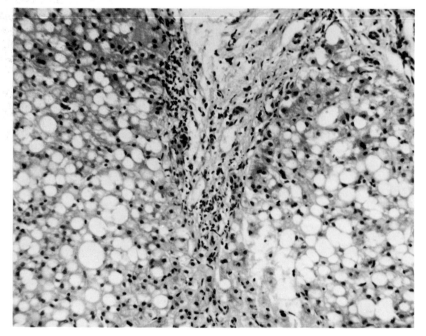

Fig. 319. Cirrhosis of the alcoholic. Fibrous bands divide the liver into small regular nodules. Fatty change is conspicuous. H & E, × 120.

and fat deposition seem to be independent. A macronodular cirrhosis may develop during the years after the patient becomes a total abstainer and active regeneration has become possible [44].

Electron microscopy shows alterations in almost all organelles. Fatty inclusions are seen in the hepatic cells and these elicit a phagocytic response. If jaundice is present, biliary canaliculi are dilated with shortening of their microvilli. Intracellular vacuoles are filled with some component of bile.

Mitochondria are enlarged (megamitochondria) and bizarre. Such giant mitochondria may even be seen under light microscopy as hyaline globular bodies staining pink with eosin and red with trichrome. They always hint at alcoholic liver disease. The mitochondria may not, in fact, be damaged, for mitochondrial marker enzymes are raised, perhaps as an adaptive response to the ethanol load [22].

Mallory bodies represent focal degeneration of many cytoplasmic constituents [45] and especially microtubules. The rough endoplasmic reticulum is packed with vesicles, some agranular but some with ribosomes on the surface. The smooth endoplasmic reticulum increases. The microtubules are shortened and export of protein from the liver cell is reduced [5]. The liver cell contains more water and swells. Protein retention may be partly responsible for hepatomegaly.

Kupffer cells and reactive mesenchymal elements contain lipid which in some instances represents ceroid. The Disse space is collagenized and this correlates with severity of hepatic failure, portal hypertension and centrizonal sclerosis [38].

These ultrastructural changes are very rapid [50]. Within one day of a full dose of alcohol (46% of total calories) mitochondrial alterations and focal cytoplasmic degradation are noted.

CLINICAL FEATURES [9, 42]

Early recognition

This depends on a high index of suspicion on the part of the physician. A patient may present with non-specific digestive symptoms such as anorexia, morning nausea with dry retching, diarrhoea, vague right upper abdominal pain and tenderness, or pyrexia.

The patient may seek medical advice because of the effects of alcoholism such as social disruption, poor work performance, accidents, violent behaviour, fits, tremulousness or depression.

The diagnosis may be made when hepatomegaly, a raised serum transaminase or macrocytosis are discovered at a routine examination, for instance at a Life Insurance check or during investigation of another condition.

Physical signs may be non-contributory, although tender hepatomegaly, prominent vascular spiders and associated features of alcoholism may be helpful. The clinical features do not reflect the hepatic histology and biochemical tests of liver function may be normal [8].

Acute alcoholic hepatitis

This usually appears as severe hepatic decompensation after particularly heavy drinking, perhaps precipitated by vomiting, diarrhoea, an acute infection, or prolonged anorexia. The patient is pyrexial and jaundiced. Neuropsychiatric disturbances are due not only to the alcoholism, but also to hepatic pre-coma (table 55). Subdural haematoma and Wernicke's encephalopathy must also be considered.

Nausea, repeated vomiting and fatty diarrhoea

Table 55. The differences between delirium tremens and hepatic pre-coma (after Davidson & Solomon 1959).

	Delirium tremens	Hepatic pre-coma
Consciousness	Alert	Drowsy
Psychomotor activity	Yes	No
Anxiety	Yes	No
Speech	Rapid	Slurred
Hallucinations	Formed	Unusual
Tremor	Fine	Flapping
Flushing, tachycardia	Present	Absent
Treatment	Chlorpromazine or chlormethiazole	Neomycin and dietary protein abstention

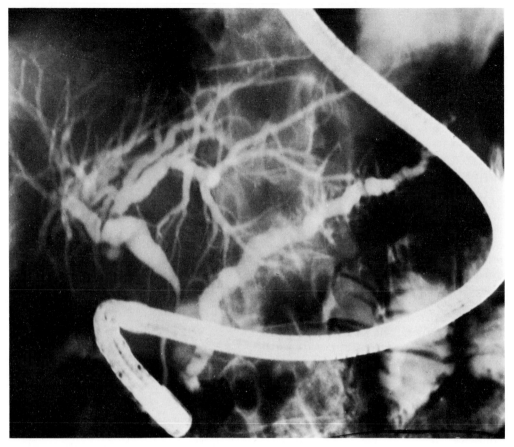

Fig. 320. ERCP in an alcoholic patient with chronic pancreatitis and cholestasis. Showing dilatation and irregularity of the pancreatic duct and smooth constriction of the common bile duct as it passes behind the inflamed pancreas (Scott *et al* 1977).

are frequent. The liver is large and painful and an arterial bruit may be heard over it. The spleen is often impalpable. Ascites may develop rapidly. Faeces are usually pale.

The peripheral blood shows a polymorph leuco-cytosis.

Nutritional changes include peripheral neuritis, sore red tongue, iron deficiency anaemia, scurvy, beri-beri, and ankle oedema. Folic acid deficiency may be related not only to nutritional lack but also to a direct effect of alcohol on the bone-marrow.

Biochemical tests show raised serum alkaline phosphatase and transaminase values. Serum albumin is usually low and gamma-globulin raised; these return to normal as the patient improves.

The serum cholesterol level may be very high, and the serum lipaemic [57]. This may coincide with pancreatitis [47, 57] (*Zieve's syndrome*). Increased lipolysis may play a role as serum lipoprotein lipase is reduced, and a circulating inhibitor of the enzyme is present.

Hypokalaemia may be prominent, especially if there is diarrhoea.

An isotope scan shows virtually no hepatic uptake, the picture simulating an hepatic tumour.

Patients with acute fatty liver may die suddenly in shock, attributable to pulmonary fat emboli. Sudden deaths have also been reported in hypoglycaemia.

Gastro-intestinal haemorrhage is frequently from a local gastric or duodenal lesion, and is secondary to the general bleeding tendency, rather than related to portal hypertension.

Acute alcoholic hepatitis may be confused with acute virus hepatitis. Helpful diagnostic points are the florid vascular spiders, the very large liver and the leucocytosis.

The jaundice may be markedly cholestatic. The pain, occasional pruritus, large liver and fever with leucocytosis and raised serum cholesterol and alkaline phosphatase simulate extra-hepatic biliary obstruction [42]. Surgery must be avoided. The history of alcohol abuse, vascular spiders and, if clotting permits, liver biopsy are diagnostic. Rarely cholangitis with intraductal polymorph inflammation may be found [2].

Cholestasis can occasionally present with severe fatty change and minimal alcoholic hepatitis; it carries a bad prognosis [35].

Cholestasis may also be related to chronic pancreatitis with a stenosis of the intrapancreatic portion of the distal common bile duct [52] (fig. 320). If doubt exists, endoscopic cholangio-pancreatography is mandatory. Liver biopsy showing portal zone fibrosis in the absence of severe alcoholic hepatitis suggests chronic pancreatitis as a possible cause of the cholestasis [36].

Established cirrhosis

This can present without acute alcoholic hepatitis ever having been recognized clinically or histologically. The cirrhosis presumably resulted from alcoholic stimulation of collagen synthesis. The picture resembles other types of end-stage liver disease. Only the history of alcohol abuse, the hepatomegaly and the associated features of alcoholism point to the aetiology.

Splenomegaly is a late feature.

Portal hypertension may be related to nodular regeneration. In addition fatty liver can result in obstruction to portal flow with consequent portal hypertension which subsides as the fat disappears. Portal hypertension may also be post-sinusoidal related to sclerosing hyaline necrosis.

The patient may present with ascites; serum albumin levels are particularly low. Portal systemic encephalopathy has to be distinguished from alcohol withdrawal (table 55).

Associated features

The occasional, bilaterally enlarged parotids may be analogous to those seen with other types of malnutrition [56]. Gynaecomastia often appears after treatment and is a frequent complication of spironolactone therapy. The testes atrophy and infertility may be a feature. Muscle mass wastes.

Dupuytren's contracture of the palmar fascia is related to the alcoholism and not to the cirrhosis [53].

Loss of memory and concentration, insomnia, irritability, hallucinations, convulsions, 'rum-fits' and tremor may be the stigmata of alcoholism. These must be distinguished from early hepatic pre-coma (table 55).

DIAGNOSTIC TESTS

Early diagnosis often depends on the patient's history which is notoriously unreliable. A laboratory test specific for alcoholism would be very helpful.

Elevated blood alcohol values indicate recent ingestion and are useful for follow-up clinics but are otherwise of limited value (fig. 321) [18].

The serum aspartate transaminase (AST, GOT) or alanine transaminase (ALT, GPT) are frequent screening tests indicating liver damage. The AST/ALT ratio may be more useful. Values exceeding 2 are more often found in alcoholic than viral injury. This may be related to alcoholic damage to mitochondria or smooth muscle, with predominant release of AST.

Serum gamma glutamyl transpeptidase (gamma GT) is not specific but is a reliable test for chronic alcoholism. The enzyme is localized to the microsomal fraction of cells and may reflect the proliferation of smooth endoplasmic reticulum

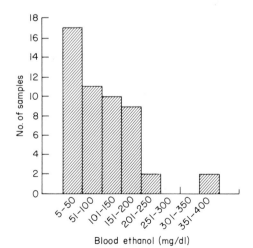

Fig. 321. Alcoholic patients in noon clinic. Histogram of detectable blood ethanol levels. Most values are over the legal driving limit of 80 mg/dl (Hamlyn *et al* 1975).

following chronic alcohol ingestion. Serum glutamate dehydrogenase is another reliable marker of liver cell necrosis in the alcoholic [55].

Serum alkaline phosphatase may be markedly increased (> 4 × normal) especially in those with severe cholestasis and alcoholic hepatitis [41].

Serum IgA values may be very high.

The plasma ratio of alpha amino-N-butyric acid to leucine (A/L) is raised in chronic alcoholics. This appears to be a relatively non-sensitive index of hepato-cellular damage rather than of alcoholism [33].

Non-specific serum changes in acute and chronic alcoholism include elevations in uric acid, lactate, triglyceride and reductions in glucose, phosphate and magnesium. Low serum tri-iodo-thyronine (T3) levels presumably reflect decreased hepatic conversion of T3 to T4. Levels correlate inversely with the severity of alcoholic liver disease.

Even sensitive biochemical methods may fail to reveal alcoholic liver damage, and liver biopsy must be resorted to in cases of doubt.

Needle liver biopsy

This confirms the presence of liver disease and identifies alcohol abuse as the likely cause. The dangers of the liver damage can be emphasized more forcibly to the patient.

Liver biopsy is important prognostically. Fatty change alone is not nearly so serious as perivenular sclerosis, which is probably a precursor of cirrhosis [54]. An established cirrhosis can be confirmed.

Diagnostic difficulties may arise, when the histological picture of alcoholic liver disease is shown in a patient who denies alcohol abuse. Other causes are Indian childhood cirrhosis, gross obesity, post-jejuno-ileal bypass operation, Wilson's disease, diabetes, and long-term glucocorticoid treatment.

PROGNOSIS

The prognosis in alcoholics is much better than with other forms of cirrhosis. Everything depends on whether the alcoholic can overcome his addiction. This in turn is related to family support, financial resources and socio-economic state. In a large group of working-class, often 'skid-row' type alcoholic cirrhotics studied in Boston, the mean life expectancy for men was 33 months compared with 16 months for a non-alcoholic group [15]. In a study at Yale, the patients of a higher socio-economic class, with cirrhosis complicated by ascites, jaundice and haematemesis, showed an overall five-year survival of 50%. If they persisted in alcoholism, this fell to 40%, whereas if they abstained, it was 60% [48]. Very similar figures come from the United Kingdom [9] (fig. 322) and from Australia [48].

The initial response to treatment is important.

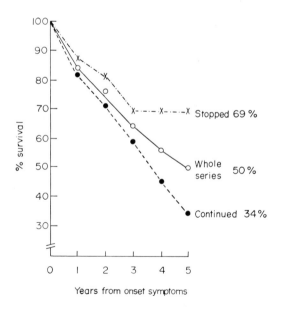

Fig. 322. The probability of survival of patients with established alcoholic liver disease: 50% survived five years, 69% of those who abstained from alcohol were alive at five years, but only 34% of those who continued to imbibe (Brunt *et al* 1974).

Pre-coma, persistent jaundice and azotaemia are bad signs. Such patients are very liable to develop the hepato-renal syndrome. The patient with decompensated cirrhosis improves slowly. Overt jaundice and ascites after three months carry a grave prognosis. Even total abstention may not improve the prognosis when portal hypertension is prominent. In the very late, irreversible stage where cirrhosis has developed to the stage when portal hypertension has necessitated porta-caval shunt, alcohol abstinence cannot be expected to affect the prognosis [39]. The damage has been done and there is no turning back.

Patients with acute alcoholic hepatitis often deteriorate during the first few weeks in hospital. It may take one to six months for resolution, and 20–50% die [19]. Those with a markedly prolonged prothrombin time, unresponsive to intramuscular vitamin K and with a serum bilirubin level greater than 20 mg, have a particularly bad outlook [30]. A depression in serum albumin is also serious.

Mallory bodies in the liver do not necessarily signify a very poor prognosis. Alcoholic hepatitis is slow to resolve even in those who abstain [14]. In those who continue to imbibe, cirrhosis usually follows alcoholic hepatitis, although some continue with the hepatitis alone for many years [14].

Primary liver cancer may develop, particularly in patients who have abstained from alcohol and who have had time to develop a coarsely nodular liver [44].

TREATMENT

EARLY RECOGNITION

Total abstinence from alcohol is essential. A good diet must be taken and supplementary vitamins, especially B complex, supplied. Improvement is usually rapid and the patient is surprised at his well being. After 6–12 months the question of resumption of a modest alcohol intake will be raised. The decision is based on the extent of the patient's previous alcohol dependence, his lifestyle and psychological stability. It also depends on whether the biopsy showed centrizonal collagenosis which is pre-cirrhotic, or simply fatty change which may not be. It is preferable that all patients who have shown an adverse hepatic reaction to alcohol should abstain forever, but in some instances a small social intake may be allowed. Regular medical check-ups are essential.

ESTABLISHED LIVER DISEASE

Those with acute alcoholic hepatitis or cirrhosis should abstain permanently from alcohol. The improvement following this and bed rest may be so striking that it is virtually diagnostic of previous alcoholism. An increased protein intake hastens recovery, but this must be weighed against the possibility of inducing hepatic pre-coma. Calories 25–30 kg and protein 0.5 g/kg are given, the latter increasing as soon as possible to 1 g/kg. Anorexia and vomiting test the dietetic skills of the hospital. Parenteral nutrition may sometimes be helpful. Vitamin B complex is given in large doses, if necessary parenterally. Potassium chloride supplements are usually required, and sometimes additional magnesium and glucose.

Chlormethiazole (Heminevrin) or chlordiazepoxide (Librium) should be given if the patient has recently been drinking heavily in order that the delirium tremens may be prevented.

If the diagnosis is in doubt, management should be conservative and needle biopsy performed as soon as possible. Laparotomy in patients with acute alcoholic hepatitis is dangerous.

The measures recommended for encephalopathy and portal hypertension should be employed. The portal venous pressure may well fall as the alcoholic hepatitis resolves. Surgery for portal hypertension should, if possible, be avoided until the maximum benefit has followed medical treatment.

Renal failure is particularly liable to follow hepato-cellular failure with ascites in alcoholic patients (hepato-renal syndrome) (Chapter 10).

CORTICOSTEROIDS

The high mortality of acute alcoholic hepatitis, about 50% in those with jaundice and encephalopathy, has stimulated the use of corticosteroids. These might decrease inflammation, reduce fibrosis and retard progression to cirrhosis. Controlled trials have shown variable results, sometimes beneficial [20, 26], more usually not [7, 10, 46]. This may be related to selection of patients. If those very ill and in whom liver biopsy is impossible are chosen, the results are poor. In those not so sick, in whom clotting permits biopsy, the results are good. Benefit is more likely in well-nourished employed rural patients, especially women [20, 26], than in under-nourished unemployed men [7, 10].

In the severely ill patient with deep jaundice, fever, markedly prolonged prothrombin time and electrolyte disturbance, a case can be made for 30 mg prednisolone daily for two or three weeks [30]. This seems to decrease early mortality. Long-term corticosteroids increase mortality [11].

OTHER MEASURES

In view of the hypermetabolic state propyl-thiouracil (300 mg per day) has been given short-term to patients with alcoholic hepatitis in a double-blind trial and resulted in functional improvement; hepatic histology was not studied [37]. Patients with inactive cirrhosis were unaffected. Propylthiouracil is worth considering in advanced alcoholic hepatitis soon after alcohol abstention.

D-Penicillamine reduces hepatic collagen pro-line hydroxylase in patients with alcoholic hepatitis and may be beneficial in reducing fibrosis [32]. It is a toxic drug and has not been fully assessed in these patients. Similarly, the use of colchicine, another toxic drug, to reduce fibrosis is only currently being evaluated [23].

REFERENCES

1. ADDISON T. (1836) Observations on fatty degeneration of the liver. *Guy's Hosp. Rep.* **1**, 476.
2. AFSHANI P., LITTENBERG G.D., WOLLMAN J. *et al* (1978) Significance of microscopic cholangitis in alcoholic liver disease. *Gastroenterology* **75**, 1045.
3. BAILEY R.J., KRASNER N., EDDLESTON A.L.W.F. *et al* (1976) Histocompatibility antigens, autoantibodies and immunoglobulins in alcoholic liver disease. *Br. med. J.* ii, 727.
4. BAILLIE M. (1793) *The Morbid Anatomy of Some of the Most Important Parts of the Human Body*, p. 141. J. Johnson, St Paul's Churchyard, and G. Nicol, Pall Mall, London.
5. BARAONA E., LEO M.A., BOROWSKY S.A. *et al* (1977) Pathogenesis of alcohol-induced accumulation of protein in the liver. *J. clin. Invest.* **60**, 546.
6. BELL H. & NORDHAGEN R. (1978) Association between HLA-BW40 and alcoholic liver disease with cirrhosis. *Br. med. J.* i, 822.
7. BLITZER B.L., MUTCHNICK M.G., JOSHI P.H. *et al* (1977) Adrenocorticosteroid therapy in alcoholic hepatitis. A prospective, double blind randomised study. *Am. J. dig. Dis.* **22**, 477.
8. BRUGUERA M., BORDAS J.M. & RODES J. (1977) Asymptomatic liver disease in alcoholics. *Arch. path. lab. Med.* **101**, 644.
9. BRUNT P.W., KEW M.C., SCHEUER P.J. *et al* (1974) Studies in alcoholic liver disease in Britain. 1. Clinical and pathological patterns related to natural history. *Gut* **15**, 52.
10. CAMPRA J.L., HAMLIN E.M. Jr, KIRSHBAUM R.J.

11. COPENHAGEN STUDY GROUP FOR LIVER DISEASES (1969) Effect of prednisone on the survival of patients with cirrhosis of the liver. *Lancet* i, 119.
12. EDMONDSON H.A., PETERS R.L., REYNOLDS T.B. *et al* (1963) Sclerosing hyaline necrosis of the liver in the chronic alcoholic. A recognizable clinical syndrome. *Ann. intern. Med.* **59**, 646.
13. EDMONDSON H.A., PETERS R.L., FRANKEL H.H. *et al* (1967) The early stage of liver injury in the alcoholic. *Medicine (Baltimore)* **46**, 119.
14. GALAMBOS J.T. (1972) Natural history of alcoholic hepatitis. III. Histological changes. *Gastroenterology* **63**, 1026.
15. GARCEAU A.J. & THE BOSTON INTER-HOSPITAL LIVER GROUP (1964) The natural history of cirrhosis. II. The influence of alcohol and prior hepatitis on pathology and prognosis. *New Engl. J. Med.* **271**, 1173.
16. GERBER M.A., ORR W., DENK H. *et al* (1973) Hepatocellular hyalin in cholestasis and cirrhosis: its diagnostic significance. *Gastroenterology* **64**, 89.
17. GOLDBERG S.J., MENDENHALL C.L., CONNELL A.M. *et al* (1977) 'Non-alcoholic' chronic hepatitis in the alcoholic. *Gastroenterology* **72**, 598.
18. HAMLYN A.N., BROWN A.J., SHERLOCK S. *et al* (1975) Casual blood ethanol estimations in patients with chronic liver disease. *Lancet* ii, 345.
19. HARDISON W.G. & LEE F.I. (1966) Prognosis in acute liver disease of the alcoholic patient. *New Engl. J. Med.* **275**, 61.
20. HELMAN R.A., TEMKO M.H., NYE S.W. *et al* (1971) Alcoholic hepatitis: natural history and evaluation of prednisolone therapy. *Ann. intern. Med.* **74**, 311.
21. ISSELBACHER K.J. (1977) Metabolic and hepatic effects of alcohol. *New Engl. J. Med.* **296**, 612.
22. JENKINS W.J. & PETERS T.J. (1978) Mitochondrial enzyme activities in liver biopsies from patients with alcoholic liver disease. *Gut* **19**, 341.
23. KERSHENOBICH E., URIBE M., SUAREZ G.I. *et al* (1979) Treatment of cirrhosis with colchicine: a double-blind randomised trial. *Gastroenterology* **77**, 532.
24. LEEVY C.M. (1966) Abnormalities of hepatic DNA synthesis in man. *Medicine (Baltimore)* **45**, 423.
25. LELBACH W.K. (1975) Cirrhosis in the alcoholic and the relation to the volume of alcohol abuse. *Ann. N.Y. Acad. Sci.* **252**, 85.
26. LESESNE H.R., BOZYMSKI E.M. & FALLON H.J. (1978) Treatment of alcoholic hepatitis with encephalopathy. Comparison of prednisone with caloric supplements. *Gastroenterology* **74**, 169.
27. LIEBER C.S. (1978) Pathogenesis and early diagnosis of alcoholic liver injury. *New Engl. J. Med.* **298**, 888.
28. LIEBER C.S., DE CARLI L.M. & RUBIN E. (1975) Sequential production of fatty liver, hepatitis, and cirrhosis in sub-human primates fed ethanol with adequate diets. *Proc. natl. Acad. Sci. (USA)* **72**, 437.
29. LIEBER C.S. & SPRITZ N. (1966) Effects of prolonged ethanol intake in man: role of dietary, adipose, and endogenously synthesized fatty acids in the pathogenesis of the alcoholic fatty liver. *J. clin. Invest.* **35**, 1400.

et al (1973) Prednisone therapy of acute alcoholic hepatitis. *Ann. intern. Med.* **79**, 625.

30. MADDREY W.C., BOITNOTT J.K., BEDINE M.S. *et al* (1978) Corticosteroid therapy of alcoholic hepatitis. *Gastroenterology* **75**, 193.
31. MELENDEZ M., VARGAS-TANK L., FUENTES C. *et al* (1979) Distribution of HLA histocompatibility antigens, ABO blood groups and Rh antigens in alcoholic liver disease. *Gut* **20**, 288.
32. MEZEY E., POTTER J.J., IBER F.L. & MADDREY W.C. (1979) Hepatic collagen proline hydroxylase activity in alcoholic hepatitis: effect of D-penicillamine. *J. lab. clin. Med.* **93**, 92.
33. MORGAN M.Y., MILSOM J.P. & SHERLOCK S. (1977) Ratio of plasma alpha amino-*n*-butyric acid to leucine as an empirical marker of alcoholism: diagnostic value. *Science* **197**, 1183.
34. MORGAN M.Y. & SHERLOCK S. (1977) Sex-related differences among 100 patients with alcoholic liver disease. *Br. med. J.* i, 939.
35. MORGAN M.Y., SHERLOCK S. & SCHEUER P.J. (1978) Acute cholestasis, hepatic failure and fatty liver in the alcoholic. *Scand. J. Gastroenterol.* **13**, 299.
36. MORGAN M.Y., SHERLOCK S. & SCHEUER P.J. (1978) Portal fibrosis in the livers of alcoholic patients. *Gut* **19**, 1015.
37. ORREGO H., KALANT H., ISRAEL Y. *et al* (1979) Effect of short-term therapy with propylthiouracil in patients with alcoholic liver disease. *Gastroenterology* **76**, 105.
38. ORREGO H., MEDLINE A., BLENDIS L.M. *et al* (1979) Collagenisation of the Disse space in alcoholic liver disease. *Gut* **20**, 673.
39. PANDE N.V., RESNICK R.H., YEE W. *et al* (1978) Cirrhotic portal hypertension: morbidity of continued alcoholism. *Gastroenterology* **74**, 64.
40. PEQUIGNOT G. & CYRULNIK F. (1970) Chronic disease due to overconsumption of alcoholic drinks (excepting neuropsychiatric pathology). In *International Encyclopaedia of Pharmacology and Therapeutics*, vol. II, chapter 14, pp. 375–412. Pergamon Press, Oxford.
41. PERRILLO R.P., GRIFFIN R., DE SCHRYVER-KECSKEMETI K. *et al* (1978) Alcoholic liver disease presenting with marked elevation of serum alkaline phosphatase. A combined clinical and pathological study. *Am. J. dig. Dis.* **23**, 1061.
42. PHILLIPS G.B. & DAVIDSON C.S. (1954) Acute hepatic insufficiency of the chronic alcoholic: clinical and pathological study. *Arch. intern. Med.* **94**, 585.

43. PHILLIPS G.B., GABUZDA G.J. Jr & DAVIDSON C.S. (1952) Comparative effects of a purified and an adequate diet on the course of fatty cirrhosis in the alcoholic. *J. clin. Invest.* **31**, 351.
44. POPPER H., RUBIN E., KRUS S. *et al* (1960) Postnecrotic cirrhosis in alcoholics. *Gastroenterology* **39**, 669.
45. PORTA E.A., BERGMAN B.J. & STEIN A.A. (1965) Acute alcoholic hepatitis. *Am. J. Pathol.* **46**, 657.
46. PORTER H.P., SIMON F.R., POPE C.E. II *et al* (1971) Corticosteroid therapy in severe alcoholic hepatitis. A double-blind drug trial. *New Engl. J. Med.* **284**, 1350.
47. POWELL L.W., ROESER H.P. & HALLIDAY J.W. (1972) Transient intravascular haemolysis associated with alcoholic liver disease and hyperlipidaemia. *Aust. N.Z. J. Med.* **2**, 39.
48. POWELL W.J. Jr & KLATSKIN G. (1968) Duration of survival in patients with Laennec's cirrhosis. *Am. J. Med.* **44**, 406.
49. ROJKIND M. & DUNN M.A. (1979) Hepatic fibrosis. *Gastroenterology* **76**, 849.
50. RUBIN E. & LIEBER C.S. (1968) Alcohol-induced hepatic injury in nonalcoholic volunteers. *New Engl. J. Med.* **278**, 869.
51. RUBIN E. & LIEBER C.S. (1974) Fatty liver, alcoholic hepatitis and cirrhosis produced by alcohol in primates. *New Engl. J. Med.* **290**, 128.
52. SCOTT J., SUMMERFIELD J.A., ELIAS E. *et al* (1977) Chronic pancreatitis: a cause of cholestasis. *Gut* **18**, 196.
53. SU C.-K. & PATEK A.J. Jr (1970) Dupuytren's contracture. Its association with alcoholism and cirrhosis. *Arch. intern. Med.* **126**, 278.
54. VAN WAES L. & LIEBER C.S. (1977) Early perivenular sclerosis in alcoholic fatty liver: and index of progressive liver injury. *Gastroenterology* **73**, 646.
55. VAN WAES L. & LIEBER C.S. (1977) Glutamate dehydrogenase: a reliable marker of liver cell necrosis in the alcoholic. *Br. med. J.* ii, 1508.
56. WOLFE S.J., SUMMERSKILL W.H.J. & DAVIDSON C.S. (1957) Parotid swelling, alcoholism and cirrhosis. *New Engl. J. Med.* **256**, 491.
57. ZIEVE L. (1958) Jaundice, hyperlipemia and hemolytic anemia: a heretofore unrecognized syndrome associated with alcoholic fatty liver and cirrhosis. *Ann. intern. Med.* **48**, 471.

Chapter 20
Iron Overload States

Normal iron metabolism [28, 51]

Dietary iron is absorbed from the intestine in ferrous form to the extent of 1–1.5 mg daily. The amount depends on body stores, more being absorbed the greater the need. In the intestinal cell the iron links on to a gamma-globulin called *transferrin* by which it is carried in serum (fig. 323). The serum iron binding capacity (transferrin) is about 250 μg/100 ml and is one-half to one-third saturated with iron. The absorptive process is an active one capable of transporting iron against a gradient [64].

The morning fasting serum iron is about 125 μg/100 ml. The normal total body content of iron is about 4 g, of which 3 g are present in haemoglobin, myoglobin, catalase and other respiratory pigments or enzymes. Storage iron comprises 0.5 g; of this 0.3 g is in the liver but is not revealed by the usual histological stains for iron. The liver is the predominant site for storage of iron absorbed from the gut. When its capacity is exceeded, iron is deposited in other parenchymal tissues, including the acinar cells of the pancreas, the adrenals, and other secreting tissues throughout the body. The liver, however, contains the bulk of storage iron. The reticulo-endothelial system plays only a limited part in iron storage unless the iron is given intravenously, when it becomes a preferential site for deposition. Iron from erythrocyte breakdown is concentrated in the spleen.

When excess iron is deposited, three pigments may be found in the liver—ferritin, haemosiderin and lipofuscin.

Ferritin is a combination of the protein apoferritin and iron and appears under electron microscopy as particles 50 Å in diameter lying free in the cytoplasm.

Aggregates of ferritin molecules make up *haemosiderin* which stains as blue granules with ferrocyanide. Under the electron microscope the ferritin takes the form of paracrystalline aggregates. The iron-containing nucleus of the molecule consists of six sub-units arranged at the apices of a regular octahedron.

Lipofuscin, or wear and tear pigment, is yellow-brown in colour and does not contain iron. These granules may form the organic basis for iron deposition.

Iron contained in depots as ferritin or haemosiderin is available for mobilization and haemoglobin formation should the demand arise.

IRON OVERLOAD AND LIVER DAMAGE [51]

Fibrosis and hepato-cellular damage are directly related to the iron content of the liver cell. The pattern of damage is similar irrespective of the aetiology, for instance, whether the overload is due to idiopathic haemochromatosis or to multiple transfusions. The severity of fibrosis is proportional to the iron content of the liver, and is maximum in

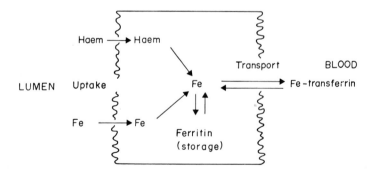

Fig. 323. The transport of dietary iron across the proximal small intestinal mucosal cells as inorganic iron or haem. Storage takes place as ferritin and transport out of the cell is with the transport protein, transferrin.

areas (periportal) where iron is particularly deposited. Cirrhosis has been produced in dogs by massive iron overload [35].

Removal of iron by repeated venesections or by intensive chelation leads to clinical and biochemical improvement and reduction or prevention of hepatic fibrosis [3, 12].

The actual mechanism of liver cell damage is uncertain. Haemosiderin is deposited in peribiliary lysosomes. In idiopathic haemochromatosis these are abnormally fragile with increased enzymes [53]. Lipid peroxidation is increased with subsequent membrane damage. However, electron microscopy of iron loaded rats showed massive lysosomal accumulation of iron, but no other hepato-cellular abnormality [1] so haemochromatosis is not a proven lysosomal disease.

IDIOPATHIC HAEMOCHROMATOSIS

This is a genetically determined metabolic disorder with increased iron absorption over many years [13, 23, 43]. It is a rare disease described in 1886 as *bronzed diabetes* [24]. The tissues contain enormous quantities of iron, of the order of 20–60 g. These large amounts can only have accumulated as a result of increased intestinal absorption over a long period. If 10 mg dietary iron were retained by the tissues daily it would take about 14 years for 50 g to accumulate.

Pathology

A fibrous tissue reaction is found wherever the iron is deposited.

The *liver* in the early stages may show only portal zone fibrosis with deposition of iron in the periportal liver cells and, to a lesser extent, in the Kupffer cells. Fibrous septa then surround groups of lobules and irregularly shaped nodules (*holly-leaf appearance*) [52]. There is partial preservation of the architecture of most lobules although ultimately a macronodular cirrhosis develops (see fig. 324 in colour section). Fatty change is unusual and the glycogen content of the liver cells is normal.

The *pancreas* shows fibrosis and parenchymal degeneration with iron deposition in acinar cells,

macrophages, islets of Langerhans and fibrous tissue.

Iron is found in the enlarged *spleen*, in *gastric* and *intestinal* epithelium and to a lesser extent in the kidneys.

Heart muscle is heavily involved, muscle fibres being replaced by a mass of iron pigment within the sheath. Degeneration of the fibres is rare. Coronary sclerosis, however, is common.

Brain and nervous tissue are usually free of iron.

Epidermal atrophy may reduce the *skin* to a flattened sheet. Hair follicles and sebaceous glands are inconspicuous. Characteristically, pigment is increased in the melanin content of the basal layer. Iron is usually absent from the epidermis but can often be seen deeper, especially in sweat glands, connective tissue, capillary endothelium and in wandering macrophages.

Endocrine glands, including adrenal cortex, anterior lobe of pituitary and thyroid, show varying amounts of iron and fibrosis.

The testes are small and soft with atrophy of the germinal epithelium without iron overload. There is interstitial fibrosis and iron is found in the walls of capillaries.

Aetiology [44, 45]

There is increased, inappropriate, intestinal absorption of iron dating from birth [23]. Absorption only becomes normal when storage iron reaches injurious levels and then increases again after iron stores have been reduced by venesection [66]. This suggests that increased iron absorption is the primary defect.

Control of iron absorption is at the level of the mucosal cell [10]. Under normal circumstances only a proportion of the iron taken up by the mucosal cell is retained in the body; the rest is stored and lost as the intestinal epithelium is exfoliated. In patients with idiopathic haemochromatosis, much more of the absorbed iron is retained in spite of increased body stores. There could be an intrinsic defect in the mucosal cell. For instance this might be in a hitherto unidentified, but genetically determined, enzyme. There might be a defective signal from an extra-mucosal receptor, but the nature of this is not known [46].

Patients with treated idiopathic haemochromatosis show a consistent abnormality in hepatic iron uptake from transferrin [8], suggesting a cellular abnormality of hepatic iron metabolism.

GENETICS

Sheldon [54], in his classical monograph, described idiopathic haemochromatosis as an inborn error of metabolism. Family studies have shown first-degree relatives with raised serum iron levels and/or variable degrees of excess iron deposition in the liver [14, 65]. Overt disease is unusual in two generations. In a group of 40 sufferers, three brothers were found with the disease, 50% of male offspring over 15 years old showed raised serum iron levels, and other relatives had excess pigmentation, diabetes or cirrhosis [65]. Increased hepatic iron has been shown in siblings, even when serum iron values are normal [14, 65]. The nature of the inherited metabolic defect is unknown.

There is an association with HLA 3 [11, 55, 57]. In France there seems to be a further association with HLA B14 and in the United Kingdom, United States and Australia with HLA B7. The abnormal gene or genes may be related to two loci on chromosome 6 close to the HLA loci [11]. The expression of the gene is very variable, and this may be related to other environmental factors operating, such as menstrual loss or alcoholism.

Autosomal recessive inheritance seems likely. The heterozygote shows intermediate increase in transferrin saturation and in hepatic iron but has no clinical manifestation [16]. Serum ferritin, increased in homozygotes but in few heterozygotes, may be a marker of the haemochromatosis allele [9].

RELATION TO ALCOHOLISM AND NUTRITION

Alcoholism is frequent in patients with clinical haemochromatosis, but low among asymptomatic relatives with disordered iron metabolism [65]. Abuse of alcohol may accelerate the accumulation of iron in a subject genetically disposed to disease. High dietary iron intake [41] or liver or pancreatic damage from any other cause may act similarly.

The picture of haemochromatosis has been repeatedly described in patients who are both abstainers from alcohol and well nourished and also in children and in young relatives of sufferers. Idiopathic haemochromatosis must be regarded as a definite entity independent of alcohol excess.

Clinical features

The classical picture (fig. 325) is of a lethargic, middle-aged man with pigmentation, hepatomegaly, diminished sexual activity and loss of body hair; diabetes is common. The full picture is not always seen and attempts should be made at earlier diagnosis.

Haemochromatosis is 10 times as frequent in males as females [23, 54]. The low incidence in females is related to the loss of iron with menstruation and pregnancy. Female patients with haemochromatosis, usually, but not always [36], have absent or scanty menstruation, have had a hysterectomy, or are many years post-menopausal. Families have been reported including two generations of women, two of whom were menstruating [36]. Familial juvenile haemochromatosis is also described [33, 42]. The symptoms appear earlier in males than in females.

Haemochromatosis is rarely diagnosed before the age of 20, and the peak incidence is between 40 and 60. Children developing the disease show a more acute course, presenting with skin pigmentation, endocrine changes and cardiac disease; they may be homozygotes [42].

Profound psychic disturbances are often shown by depression or suicidal tendencies.

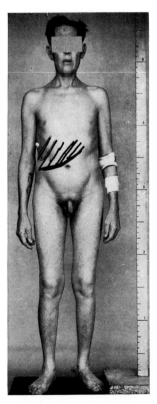

Fig. 325. Pigmented man showing loss of secondary sexual hair, gonadal atrophy and hepatomegaly.

The grey-slatey, pigmentation is maximal in the axillae, groins, genitalia, old scars and exposed parts. It can occur in the mouth. The colour, due to increased melanin in the basal layer, appears through the atrophied, superficial epidermis. The skin is shiny, thin and dry, like that of eunuchs.

HEPATIC CHANGES

The liver is enlarged and firm. Abdominal pain, usually a dull ache with hepatic tenderness, is noted in 37% of patients [23]. The pain may be so severe that an acute abdominal emergency is simulated [38]. Circulatory collapse and sudden death can occur. The mechanism is obscure, although release of ferritin, a vaso-active substance, from the liver has been postulated.

Signs of hepato-cellular failure are usually absent and ascites rare. The signs of portal hypertension are also inconspicuous. The spleen is palpable but rarely large. Oesophageal varices cannot usually be demonstrated and bleeding from them is rare.

Primary liver cancer develops in about 14% [23]. It may be a method of presentation, particularly in the elderly. It should be suspected if the patient shows clinical deterioration with rapid liver enlargement, abdominal pain and ascites. Erythrocytosis can be associated [50]. The serum iron may fall. Serum α-fetoprotein may be positive. Carcinoma can develop after complete removal of iron from the liver by venesection [12].

ENDOCRINE CHANGES

Clinical diabetes is present in about two-thirds [19]. This may be complicated by nephropathy, neuropathy, peripheral vascular disease and proliferative retinopathy [61]. The diabetes may be easy to control or may be resistant to large doses of insulin. It could be related to a family history of diabetes, to cirrhosis of the liver which impairs glucose tolerance or to direct damage to the pancreas by iron deposition.

Pituitary function is impaired to a variable extent in about two-thirds of patients. Failure of trophic hormones can be related to iron deposition in the anterior pituitary, and not to severity of liver disease, or to the degree of abnormality of iron metabolism [59]. Gonadotrophin levels are reduced with little or no response to clomiphene or LH releasing factor [62]. Signs of testicular deficiency such as impotence, loss of libido, testicular atrophy, skin atrophy and loss of secondary sexual hair are frequent and probably related to this. Urinary oestrogens increase following administration of gonadotrophin, suggesting that the testis is capable of responding.

Pan-hypopituitarism with hypothyroidism, and adrenal cortical deficiency are much rarer [62].

CARDIAC CHANGES

Although only 15% of patients with haemochromatosis present with heart failure, about a third subsequently develop cardiac symptoms. They are particularly frequent in the younger subject. The picture is of progressive right-sided heart failure sometimes with sudden death. Constrictive pericarditis or cardiomyopathy may be simulated. The 'iron heart' is a weak one. The heart is globular in shape. Arrhythmias are also seen.

Cardiac complications are presumably related to iron deposits in the myocardium and conducting system [30].

ARTHROPATHY

A specific arthropathy, starting in the metacarpophalangeal joints and also involving larger joints, is present in about two-thirds of patients. Acute episodes often involve the knees and hips and can be disabling. They are related to an acute crystal synovitis with calcium pyrophosphate. Radiologically, chondrocalcinosis is seen in menisci and articular cartilage [20] (fig. 326). This may be an early radiological sign suggesting the diagnosis of haemochromatosis.

Special investigations

Biochemical tests show surprisingly little disturbance. Later the changes are those of cirrhosis of the liver [32].

The *serum iron* is raised to about 220 μg/dl compared with the normal of about 125 μg/dl. The *serum transferrin* is about 90% saturated compared with 30% in the normal.

Chelation tests are no longer performed [2].

Serum ferritin

Ferritin is a large molecule of reticulo-endothelial origin and the major cellular iron-storage protein. Although mainly cellular, sensitive radio-

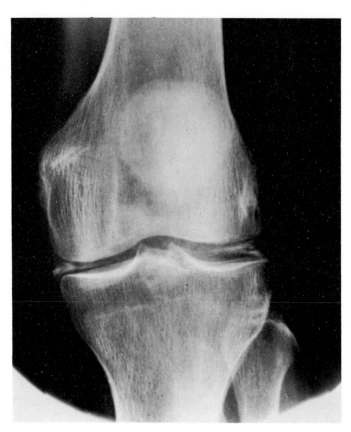

Fig. 326. Idiopathic
haemochromatosis.
Radiograph of the knee joint
shows chondro-calcinosis in
menisci and articular
cartilage. (Courtesy of M.
Barry.)

immunoassays show it to be present in normal
serum. Its function there is uncertain. The concentration is proportional to body iron stores (fig.
327). It has a proven value in uncomplicated iron
overload [46, 48] but can be unreliable in early
diagnosis of the pre-cirrhotic stage [21, 63]. It is
useful in following treatment, but a normal value
does not exclude iron storage disease [7, 48].

With severe hepato-cellular damage serum ferritin levels increase as ferritin, a cytoplasmic protein, is released from damaged liver cells [48].

Needle liver biopsy

This is a most satisfactory method of confirming
the diagnosis. The tough, fibrous liver may cause
technical difficulties, but, if a sample is obtained,
this shows the characteristic pigmentary cirrhosis
(fig. 324).

The amount of iron in the needle biopsy specimen may be quantitated [5]. Results correlate well

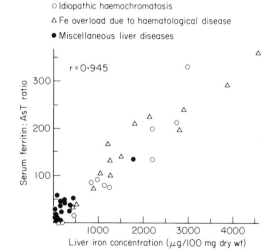

Fig. 327. Relationship between the serum
ferritin : aspartate transaminase (AST) ratio and liver
iron concentration (Prieto *et al* 1975).

with total body storage of iron. If the liver iron is less than 1.5% dry weight in a cirrhotic liver the condition is unlikely to be idiopathic haemochromatosis. Needle liver biopsy also serves as a useful method of following the effect of treatment.

Other biopsies

Skin biopsy should be taken from the pigmented area such as the forearm. Failure to detect iron does not exclude the diagnosis of haemochromatosis.

Iron excess can be shown by biopsy of stomach, synovial membrane or bone-marrow.

CT scan

A uniformly increased absorption coefficient of liver is secondary to excessive iron deposition [39] (fig. 58).

Differential diagnosis

Haemochromatosis may be confused with other forms of cirrhosis, especially in the alcoholic. The association of diabetes mellitus and cirrhosis is not uncommon, and patients with cirrhosis may become impotent, hairless and develop skin pigmentation. Hepato-cellular failure is usually minimal in haemochromatosis. Liver biopsy resolves any doubt, although moderate increases in iron in the liver may be found in cirrhosis, especially in alcoholics. Although hepatic siderosis shown by staining liver biopsies is frequent in alcoholics (57%), significant siderosis is rare (7%) [29].

The serum iron level in cirrhosis may be raised but the iron-binding protein is not saturated. The distinction from other forms of *secondary haemosiderosis* is discussed later.

Prognosis

This is difficult and much depends on early diagnosis and venesection treatment. Evident cardiac failure worsens the outlook and such patients rarely survive longer than one year without treatment. Hepatic failure or bleeding oesophageal varices are terminal features.

The outlook is better than for cirrhosis in alcoholics who stop drinking [46] (fig. 328). The patient with haemochromatosis who continues to consume large quantities of alcohol does worse than the abstinent patient.

Even with improvement after venesection treatment the risk of liver cell carcinoma remains.

Treatment

Iron can be removed by venesection and can be mobilized from tissue stores at rates as high as 130 mg/day [18, 37]. Blood regeneration is extraordinarily rapid, haemoglobin production increasing to six or seven times normal. Large quantities of blood must be removed, for 500 ml removes only 250 mg of iron, whereas the tissues contain up to 200 times this amount. Depending on the initial iron stores, the amount necessary to reduce them effectively varies from 7 to 45 g. Venesections of 500 ml are carried out weekly, or even twice weekly in particularly co-operative patients, and

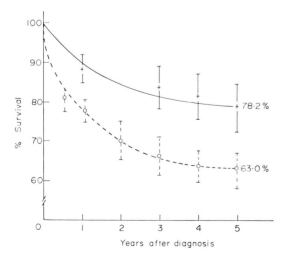

Fig. 328. Cumulative survival after diagnosis in 51 patients with haemochromatosis (solid line) compared with that reported by Powell & Klatskin (1968) for 93 patients with alcoholic cirrhosis who had stopped drinking (interrupted line). The vertical lines at each time interval represent plus or minus one standard error and the differences between the two curves are statistically significant at the fifth year ($P < 0.001$). Both curves were constructed by the same life-table (Powell 1970).

continued for about two years until the haemo-globin and serum iron levels fall. Liver biopsy is a good check that de-ironing is complete. Comparison of a venesection-treated with an untreated group showed a survival of 8.2 compared with 4.9 years and a five-year mortality of 11% compared with 67% [47, 66]. Venesection treatment results in increased well being and gain in weight. Pigmentation and hepato-splenomegaly decrease. Liver function tests improve. Control of diabetes improves in some patients [12]. The arthropathy is unaffected. Cardiac failure may decrease. Testicular function does not improve and the anterior pituitary lesion may be irreversible [66]. In two patients serial hepatic biopsies showed apparent reversal of established cirrhosis [47]. This would agree with the type of fibrosis seen in haemochromatosis, the architecture of most lobules being partly preserved so making reversibility of the liver lesion possible.

Rates of iron accumulation vary between 1.4 and 4.8 mg daily [12] and after de-ironing a 500 ml venesection every three months should prevent iron accumulation.

Primary liver cancer is not prevented by adequate venesection therapy [12].

Siblings with significant iron depositions should also be treated by venesection until liver biopsy shows absence of stainable iron [65].

A low iron diet is impossible to achieve. An alternative is to prescribe large doses of phosphate which prevent iron absorption by forming a precipitate and so increase faecal excretion of dietary iron.

Gonadal atrophy may be treated by substitution therapy with an intramuscular, depot testosterone, or by gonadotrophins.

Diabetes should be treated by diet and, if necessary, insulin. Insulin-resistant cases may be encountered.

The *cardiac complications* respond poorly to the usual measures.

DETECTION OF EARLY HAEMOCHROMATOSIS IN RELATIVES

The screening of first-degree relatives, particularly male siblings, is important so that treatment may be initiated before tissue damage has ensued. Pigmentation and hepatomegaly are helpful, but may not be early signs.

Serum iron, percentage transferrin saturation and serum ferritin should be estimated. The serum ferritin is usually raised but rarely may be normal [63], perhaps because the reticulo-endothelial system is relatively spared in the early stages. If all three values are normal, significantly increased iron stores are very unlikely. If any is abnormal then liver biopsy and measurement of the hepatic iron are indicated. Liver iron content is the most sensitive marker of the disease [22].

The presence of HLA 3 is another marker that a relative may be a sufferer [6, 9, 56].

If significant iron deposition is shown, the relative should be venesected, although there are no controlled trials to confirm the benefit.

OTHER IRON STORAGE DISEASES

TRANSFERRIN DEFICIENCY

Absence of this binding protein has been found in a child with haemochromatosis [25]. The haematological picture was of severe iron deficiency although the tissues were loaded with iron. The parents were heterozygotes and the patient a homozygote.

CANCER INDUCING IRON OVERLOAD

A primary bronchial carcinoma produced an abnormal ferritin that was thought to cause excess iron deposition in the liver and spleen [34].

HEPATIC PORPHYRIA (Chapter 22)

TRANSFUSION SIDEROSIS

More than 100 units must have been transfused before siderosis is clinically recognizable. The iron given with the blood cannot be utilized and is deposited, first in the cells of the reticulo-endothelial system and later in parenchymal cells of the liver, pancreas and other organs. Increased erythropoietic activity is a dominant stimulus for increasing iron absorption and this continues even in the presence of anaemia and of large iron stores.

Transfusion siderosis can therefore be expected in chronic haemolytic states, especially β thalassaemia, sickle cell disease, congenital spherocytosis [4] and hereditary dyserythropoietic anaemia. Patients with chronic aplastic anaemia may also be at risk [58]. The siderosis is enhanced by misdirected iron therapy.

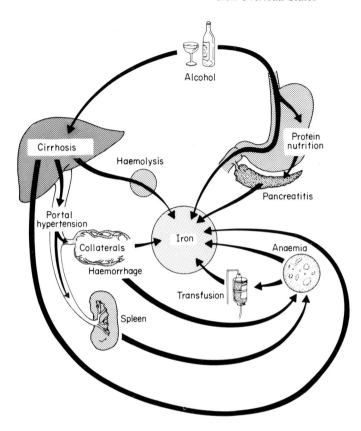

Fig. 329. Factors affecting the hepatic iron deposition in patients with liver disease. These include alcohol intake, pancreatic function, haemorrhage, reduced red cell survival and blood transfusion. Increased intestinal absorption of iron may also be associated with any form of cirrhosis.

The siderosis is recognized clinically by increasing skin pigmentation and by hepatomegaly. Children fail to grow and to have secondary sexual characteristics. Liver failure and frank portal hypertension are rare complications. The fasting blood glucose is raised, but clinical diabetes is excessively rare.

Although the amount of iron deposited in the heart is relatively small, myocardial damage is a major factor determining prognosis especially in younger children [15]. In children, symptoms arise when body iron reaches 20 g (100 units blood transfused); death from heart failure is likely when 60 g is reached [40].

Treatment is difficult. Splenectomy may reduce transfusion needs. A well-balanced low iron diet is virtually impossible. Chelating agents, such as desferrioxamine, given daily intramuscularly, slow up hepatic fibrosis in the thalassaemic child but urinary iron excretion is insufficient to keep pace with iron loading from transfusions [3]. Twelve-hour overnight subcutaneous infusion of 2–4 g desferrioxamine given with a small syringe pump into the anterior abdominal wall is more effective

[27, 49]. Oral ascorbic acid supplements increase the urinary iron excretion. Such measures can only be available to a handful of children with haemo-globinopathies: the cost is prohibitive. Other preparations of desferrioxamine, such as a depot one, are eagerly awaited.

BANTU SIDEROSIS

This condition is seen in South African Bantus whose diet consists of porridge fermented in iron pots at an acid pH [26]. As much as 200 mg iron may be ingested daily. Absorption is facilitated by the acidity of the diet and by malnutrition. Kaffir beers are also rich in iron.

CIRRHOSIS OF THE ALCOHOLIC

Multiple factors contribute to increased hepatic iron deposition (fig. 329). Protein deficiency is frequent. Increased iron absorption is found in cirrhotic patients irrespective of aetiology [67]. Cirrhotic patients with a large portal–systemic collateral circulation may absorb somewhat more.

Table 56. Average alcohol and iron content of common beverages (Jakobovits *et al* 1979).

Beverage	Alcohol (g/100 ml)	Iron (mg/100 ml)
Beers	2.2–6.6	0.01–0.05
Ciders	3.8–10.5	0.3–0.5
Wines—heavy ports, sherry	15.6–16.1	0.3–0.5
Table wines—white	8.8–10.2	0.5–1.2
—red	8.9–10.1	0.65–1.3
Spirits—70% proof	31.5	Trace

Alcoholic beverages, particularly wine, have a high iron content (table 56). Chronic pancreatitis seems to increase iron absorption. Iron medications and haemolysis add to the load of iron, whereas intestinal blood loss diminishes it.

Iron deposition is rarely as great as in the idiopathic disease [29]. Iron deficiency soon follows multiple venesections and body-iron stores are only moderately increased. Hepatic histology shows the features of alcoholism (particularly alcoholic hepatitis) as well as iron deposition. Diagnostic difficulties arise when a patient carrying the gene for idiopathic haemochromatosis is also a heavy drinker.

HAEMOCHROMATOSIS AFTER PORTA-CAVAL SHUNTING

Iron may accumulate rapidly in the liver after porta-caval shunt [67]. It can also develop with a large 'spontaneous' portal–systemic shunt. A prospective controlled study of patients having prophylactic porta-caval shunt showed a significant increase in hepatic iron after the operation. In only nine (20%) of the 46 shunt patients was the hepatic haemosiderosis excessive with iron also present in other organs [17, 67]. In general, the post-shunt siderosis is slight and clinically insignificant [17, 67].

Multiple factors relate to the iron deposition. Iron absorption increases only slightly [67]. The siderosis is probably an exaggeration of that frequently observed in cirrhosis. The porta-caval shunt eliminates the compensatory effect of intestinal blood loss.

RELATION OF THE PANCREAS TO IRON METABOLISM

Increased iron absorption and storage have been found in experimental pancreatic damage and also in patients with calcific pancreatitis and with cystic fibrosis where absorption of inorganic iron but not haemoglobin iron was increased [60]. This suggests that some factor in the exocrine secretion of the pancreas can increase iron absorption. Administration of small doses of pancreatin does in fact reduce iron absorption in haemochromatosis and cirrhosis.

REFERENCES

1. ARBORGH B.A.M., GLAUMANN H. & ERICSSON J.L.E. (1974) Studies on iron loading of rat liver lysosomes. Effect on the liver and distribution and fate of iron. *Lab. Invest.* **30**, 664.
2. BARRY M., CARTEI G.C. & SHERLOCK S. (1970) Measurement of iron stores in cirrhosis using diethylenetriamine penta-acetic acid. *Gut* **11**, 899.
3. BARRY M., FLYNN D.M., LETSKY E.A. *et al* (1974) Long-term chelation therapy in thalassaemia major: effect on liver iron concentration, liver histology, and clinical progress. *Br. med. J.* ii, 16.
4. BARRY M., SCHEUER P.J., SHERLOCK S. *et al* (1968) Hereditary spherocytosis with secondary haemochromatosis. *Lancet* ii, 481.
5. BARRY M. & SHERLOCK S. (1971) Measurement of liver iron concentration in needle biopsy specimens. *Lancet* i, 100.
6. BASSETT M.L., HALLIDAY J.W., POWELL L.W. *et al* (1979) Early detection of idiopathic haemochromatosis: relative value of serum-ferritin and HLA typing. *Lancet* ii, 4.
7. BATEY R.G., HUSSEIN S., SHERLOCK S. *et al* (1978) The role of serum ferrritin in the management of idiopathic haemochromatosis. *Scand. J. Gastroent.* **13**, 953.
8. BATEY R.G., PETTIT J.E., NICHOLAS A.W. *et al* (1978) Hepatic iron clearance from serum in treated hemochromatosis. *Gastroenterology* **75**, 856.
9. BEAUMONT C., SIMON M., FAUCHET R. *et al* (1979) Serum ferritin as a possible marker of the hemochromatosis allele. *New Engl. J. Med.* **301**, 169.
10. BOENDER C.A. & VERLOOP M.C. (1969) Iron absorption, iron loss and iron retention in man; studies after oral administration of a tracer dose of $^{59}Fe\,So_4$ and $^{131}BaSo_4$. *Br. J. Haematol.* **17**, 45.
11. BOMFORD A., EDDLESTON A.L.W.F., KENNEDY L.A. *et al* (1977) Histocompatibility antigens as markers of abnormal iron metabolism in patients with idiopathic haemochromatosis and their relatives. *Lancet* i, 327.
12. BOMFORD A. & WILLIAMS R. (1976) Long term results of venesection therapy in idiopathic haemochromatosis. *Q. J. Med.* **45**, 611.
13. BOTHWELL T.H. & FINCH C.A. (1962) *Iron Metabolism.* Little, Brown & Co., Boston.
14. BRICK I.B. (1961) Liver histology in six asymptomatic siblings in a family with hemochromatosis; genetic implications. *Gastroenterology* **40**, 210.

15. BUJA L.M. & ROBERTS W.C. (1971) Iron in the heart: etiology and clinical significance. *Am. J. Med.* **51**, 209.

16. CARTWRIGHT G.E., EDWARDS C.Q., KRAVITZ K. *et al* (1979) Hereditary hemochromatosis. Phenotypic expression of the disease. *New Engl. J. Med.* **301**, 175.

17. CONN H.O. (1972) Portacaval anastomosis and hepatic hemisiderin disposition: a prospective, controlled investigation. *Gastroenterology* **62**, 61.

18. CROSBY W.H. (1958) Treatment of haemochromatosis by energetic phlebotomy. One patient's response to the letting of 55 litres of blood in 11 months. *Br. J. Haematol.* **4**, 82.

19. DYMOCK I.W., CASSAR J., PYKE D.A. *et al* (1972) Observations on the pathogenesis, complications and treatment of diabetes in 115 cases of haemochromatosis. *Am. J. Med.* **52**, 203.

20. DYMOCK I.W., HAMILTON E.B.D., LAWS J.W. *et al* (1970) Arthropathy of haemochromatosis. Clinical and radiological analysis of 63 patients with iron overload. *Ann. rheum. Dis.* **29**, 469.

21. EDWARDS C.Q., CARROLL M., BRAY P. *et al* (1977) Hereditary hemochromatosis: diagnosis in siblings and children. *New Engl. J. Med.* **297**, 7.

22. FELLER E.R., PONT A., WANDS J.R. *et al* (1977) Familial hemochromatosis. Physiologic studies in the precirrhotic stage of the disease. *New Engl. J. Med.* **296**, 1422.

23. FINCH S.C. & FINCH C.A. (1955) Idiopathic hemochromatosis, an iron storage disease. A. Iron metabolism in hemochromatosis. *Medicine (Baltimore)* **34**, 381.

24. HANOT V. & SCHACHMANN M. (1886) Sur le cirrhose pigmentaire dans le diabète sucré. *Arch. Physiol. norm. path.* **7**, 50.

25. HEILMEYER L., KELLER W., VIVELL O. *et al* (1961) Congenital transferrin deficiency in a seven-year-old girl. *Germ. med. Mth.* **6**, 385.

26. HIGGINSON J., GERRITSEN T. & WALKER A.R.P. (1953) Siderosis in the Bantu of Southern Africa. *Am. J. Path.* **29**, 779.

27. HOFFBRAND A.V., GORMAN A., LAULICHT M. *et al* (1979) Improvement in iron status and liver function in patients with transfusional iron overload with long-term subcutaneous desferrioxamine. *Lancet* i, 947.

28. JACOBS A. (1977) Iron overload—clinical and pathological aspects. *Sem. Hematol.* **14**, 89.

29. JAKOBOVITS A.W., MORGAN M.Y. & SHERLOCK S. (1979) Hepatic siderosis in alcoholics. *Dig. Dis. Sci.* **24**, 305.

30. JAMES T.N. (1964) Pathology of the cardiac conduction system in hemochromatosis. *New Engl. J. Med.* **271**, 92.

31. JENSEN P.S. (1976) Hemochromatosis: a disease often silent but not invisible. *Am. J. Roentgenol.* **126**, 343.

32. KLECKNER M.S. JR, KARK R.M., BAKER L.A. *et al* (1955) Clinical features, pathology and therapy of hemochromatosis. *J. Am. med. Assoc.* **157**, 1471.

33. LAMON J.M., MARYNICK S.P., ROSENBLATT R. *et al* (1979) Idiopathic hemochromatosis in a young female. A case study and review of the syndrome in young people. *Gastroenterology* **76**, 178.

34. LI A.K.C. & BATEY R.G. (1977) A tumour inducing iron overload. *Br. med. J.* ii, 1327.

35. LISBOA P.E. (1971) Experimental hepatic cirrhosis in dogs caused by chronic massive iron overload. *Gut* **12**, 363.

36. LLOYD H.M., POWELL L.W. & THOMAS M.J. (1964) Idiopathic haemochromatosis in menstruating women. *Lancet* ii, 555.

37. MCALLEN P.M., COGHILL N.F. & LUBRAN M. (1957) The treatment of haemochromatosis with particular reference to the removal of iron from the body by repeated venesection. *Q. J. Med.* **36**, 251.

38. MACSWEEN R.N.M. (1966) Acute abdominal crisis, circulatory collapse and sudden death in haemochromatosis. *Q. J. Med.* **35**, 589.

39. MILLS S.R., DOPPMAN J.L. & NIENHUIS A.W. (1977) Computed tomography in the diagnosis of disorders of excessive iron storage of the liver. *J. comp. assist. Tomography* **1**, 101.

40. MODELL C.B. & BECK J. (1974) Long-term desferrioxamine therapy in thalassemia. *Ann. N.Y. Acad. Sci.* **232**, 201.

41. OLSSON K.S., HEEDMAN P.A. & STAUGARD F. (1978) Preclinical hemochromatosis in a population on a high-iron-fortified diet. *J. Am. med. Assoc.* **239**, 1999.

42. PERKINS K.W., MCINNES I.W.S., BLACKBURN C.R.B. *et al* (1965) Idiopathic haemochromatosis in children. *Am. J. Med.* **39**, 118.

43. POWELL L.W. (1970) Changing concepts in haemochromatosis. *Postgrad. med. J.* **46**, 200.

44. POWELL L.W. (ed.) (1978) *Metals and the Liver.* M. Dekker, New York.

45. POWELL L.W., BASSETT M.L. & HALLIDAY J.W. (1980) Haemochromatosis: 1980 update. *Gastroenterology* **78**, 374.

46. POWELL L.W., HALLIDAY J.W. & COWLISHAW J.L. (1978) Relationship between serum ferritin and total body iron stores in idiopathic haemochromatosis. *Gut* **19**, 538.

47. POWELL L.W. & KERR J.F.R. (1970) Reversal of 'cirrhosis' in idiopathic haemochromatosis following long-term intensive venesection therapy. *Aust. Ann. Med.* **19**, 54.

48. PRIETO J., BARRY M. & SHERLOCK S. (1975) Serum-ferritin in patients with iron overload and with acute and chronic liver diseases. *Gastroenterology* **68**, 525.

49. PROPPER R.D., COOPER B., RUFO R.R. *et al* (1977) Continuous subcutaneous administration of desferrioxamine in patients with iron overload. *New Engl. J. Med.* **297**, 418.

50. RAPHAEL B., COOPERBERG A.A. & NILOFF P. (1979) The triad of hemochromatosis, hepatoma and erythrocytosis. *Cancer* **43**, 690.

51. RICHTER G.W. (1978) The iron-loaded cell—the cyto-pathology of iron storage. *Am. J. Path.* **91**, 363.

52. SCHEUER P.J. (1980) Disturbances of iron and copper metabolism. In *Liver Biopsy Interpretation*, 3rd edn. Baillière Tindall, London.

53. SEYMOUR C.A. & PETERS T.J. (1978) Organelle pathology in primary and secondary haemochromatosis with special reference to lysosomal changes. *Br. J. Haematol.* **40**, 239.

54. SHELDON J.H. (1935) *Haemochromatosis.* Oxford University Press.

55. SIMON M., BOUREL M., FAUCHET R. *et al* (1976) Association of HLA-A3 and HLA-B14 antigens with idiopathic haemochromatosis. *Gut* **17**, 332.

56. SIMON M., BOUREL M., GENETET B. *et al* (1977) Idiopathic hemochromatosis. Demonstration of recessive transmission and early detection by family HLA typing. *New Engl. J. Med.* **297**, 1017.

57. SIMON M., FAUCHET R., HESPEL J.P. *et al* (1980) Idiopathic haemochromatosis: a study of biochemical expression in 247 heterozygous members of 63 families: evidence for a single major HLA-linked gene. *Gastroenterology* **78**, 703.

58. STEINHERZ P.G., CANALE V.C. & MILLER D.R. (1976) Hepatocellular carcinoma, transfusion induced hemochromatosis and congenital hypoplastic anemia (Blackfan–Diamond syndrome). *Am. J. Med.* **60**, 1032.

59. STOCKS A.E. & POWELL L.W. (1972) Pituitary function in idiopathic haemochromatosis and cirrhosis of the liver. *Lancet* ii, 298.

60. TØNZ O., WEISS S., STRAHM H.W. *et al* (1965) Iron absorption in cystic fibrosis. *Lancet* ii, 1096.

61. WALSH C.H. & MALINS J.M. (1978) Proliferative retinopathy in a patient with diabetes mellitus and idiopathic haemochromatosis. *Br. med. J.* ii, 16.

62. WALSH C.H., WRIGHT A.D., WILLIAMS J.W. *et al* (1976) A study of pituitary function in patients with idiopathic hemochromatosis. *J. clin. Endocrin. Metab.* **43**, 866.

63. WANDS J.R., ROWE J.A., MEZEY S.E. *et al* (1976) Normal serum ferritin concentration in precirrhotic hemochromatosis. *New Engl. J. Med.* **294**, 302.

64. WHEBY M.S. (1966) Regulation of iron absorption. *Gastroenterology* **50**, 888.

65. WILLIAMS R., SCHEUER P.J. & SHERLOCK S. (1962) The inheritance of idiopathic haemochromatosis: a clinical and liver biopsy study of 16 families. *Q. J. Med.* **31**, 249.

66. WILLIAMS R., SMITH P.M., SPICER E.J.F. *et al* (1969) Venesection therapy in idiopathic haemochromatosis. *Q. J. Med.* **38**, 1.

67. WILLIAMS R., WILLIAMS H.S., SCHEUER P.J. *et al* (1967) Iron absorption and siderosis in chronic liver disease. *Q. J. Med.* **36**, 151.

Chapter 21
Wilson's Disease

This rare disease, predominantly of young people, is characterized by cirrhosis of the liver, bilateral softening and degeneration of the basal ganglia of the brain, and greenish-brown pigmented rings in the periphery of the cornea (Kayser–Fleischer rings). Kinnier Wilson (1912) [41] was the first to define it in an article entitled 'Progressive lenticular degeneration: a familial nervous disease associated with cirrhosis of the liver'.

Aetiology

Increased amounts of copper are deposited in the tissues (fig. 330) [1, 3]. These seem to be responsible for the liver and basal ganglia changes, the Kayser–Fleischer rings in the cornea and the renal tubular lesions.

Biliary copper excretion is low [10]. Urinary copper excretion is increased. The serum copper level, however, is almost invariably reduced. Ceruloplasmin, an α_2 globulin responsible for transfer of copper in the plasma, is reduced [1].

The disease is inherited as an autosomal recessive genetic trait. Both parents must carry the trait (fig. 331). This inheritance is associated with a high consanguinity rate which has been estimated to be as high as 60%. The disease is widespread but is particularly common in Jews of eastern European origin, Arabs, Italians from the south, Japanese, Chinese, Indians, and in any community having a high inter-marriage rate [2].

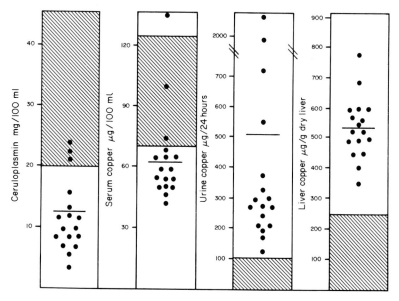

Fig. 330. Copper studies in 17 patients with Wilson's disease presenting as chronic active hepatitis. Horizontal lines indicate mean values. Hatched areas represent the normal ranges for serum ceruloplasmin (20–45 mg/dl) and serum copper (69–125 μg/dl) and delineate the levels above which urine copper concentration (> 250 μg/g dry weight) are compatible with the diagnosis of Wilson's disease (Scott *et al* 1978).

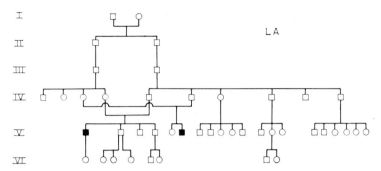

Fig. 331. Pedigree showing two instances of second cousin marriages, each having an affected offspring (Bearn 1953).

A single carrier protein is required to present copper in an appropriate form for incorporation into ceruloplasmin and excretion into bile. Mutation of a structural gene responsible for the synthesis of this hypothetical protein could result in reduction in both biliary copper excretion and ceruloplasmin synthesis [7]. This is unlikely as biliary copper excretion and ceruloplasmin synthesis are independent pathways deriving their copper from separate copper pools [19]. The normal neonate also shows reduced serum ceruloplasmin and greatly elevated hepatic copper concentration. It is possible that Wilson's disease is due to a controller gene mutation resulting in perpetuation of the foetal mode of copper homeostasis into childhood [8]. Failure of synthesis of ceruloplasmin has also been postulated, but it is uncertain whether this is an important abnormality as patients with Wilson's disease are well described with normal ceruloplasmin values. Levels correlate poorly with duration and severity. Moreover, heterozygotes, without clinical symptoms or increased tissue copper, may have no ceruloplasmin in their serum.

A structurally abnormal ceruloplasmin has also been suggested but not proved. Finally, an abnormal tissue copper-binding protein has been considered [37].

Lysosomes are concerned in the biliary excretion of copper and this is reduced in Wilson's disease. A lysosomal defect has therefore been postulated [34]. The lysosomal change, however, is similar to that seen in other copper storage states, such as primary biliary cirrhosis or in the neonate. The lysosomal change in Wilson's disease is probably non-specific. This theory would not account for the abnormalities of ceruloplasmin synthesis.

Pathology

LIVER [24, 25, 36]

The liver shows all grades of change from periportal fibrosis through submassive necrosis to a coarse, macronodular cirrhosis.

Liver cells are ballooned, show multiple nuclei, clumped glycogen and glycogen vacuolation of the nuclei (fig. 332). Fatty change is usual. Kupffer cells are large. In some patients a particularly florid picture is seen simulating acute alcoholic hepatitis, even to the presence of Mallory's hyaline deposits. Inflammatory reaction is inconspicuous. Hepatic histology is not diagnostic, but in a young person with cirrhosis such a picture should always arouse suspicion of Wilson's disease.

Rubeanic acid or rhodanine stains for copper may be unreliable as the metal is patchily distributed, being absent from regenerating nodules. The copper is usually periportal in distribution and associated with atypical lipofuscin deposits.

Electron microscopy [24]

Autophagic vacuoles are seen and mitochondria are large and abnormal even in asymptomatic patients [30]. Fatty change can be related to the mitochondrial alterations. Collagen fibrils infiltrate between cells and light and dark liver cells are seen. Electron probe micro-analysis shows

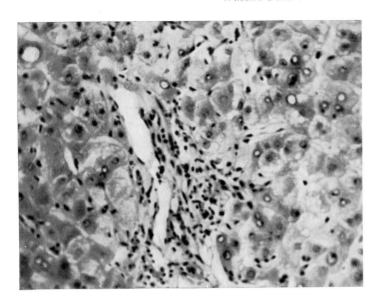

Fig. 332. Hepato-lenticular degeneration (Wilson's disease). Liver cells adjoining a fibrous tissue band show gross vacuolation of their nuclei (glycogenic degeneration) and occasionally fatty change. H & E, ×65 (Sherlock 1962).

copper in lysosomes which are also the site of lipofuscin deposition [14].

OTHER ORGANS

The *kidney* shows fatty and hydropic change with copper deposition in the proximal convoluted tubules.

The *Kayser–Fleischer ring* is due to brownish-green pigment in Descemet's membrane lining the posterior surface of the cornea. The ultrastructure has been described. The presence of copper has been confirmed by analytical electron microscopy [18].

The *brain* shows variable symmetrical changes, maximal in the basal ganglia. These include giant protoplasmic astrocytes (Alzheimer 2 cells), disruption of the spongy tissue and glycogen granules in the brain cells. Disintegration of cortical nerve cells proceeds in some cases to actual cavitation of the basal ganglia. The changes resemble those seen in chronic hepatic encephalopathy.

Clinical picture

The picture is a composite one due to general poisoning of the tissues with copper. The emphasis falls on different parts at different times (fig. 333). In children the liver is chiefly involved (*hepatic form*). As the years advance neuropsychiatric changes become increasingly important (*neurological form*). Patients presenting after age 20 usu-

ally have neurological symptoms [35]. It is unwise to distinguish too rigidly between the two types for in many instances there is considerable overlap. Most patients have developed symptoms or been diagnosed between the ages of five and 30 [35].

The *Kayser–Fleischer ring* (see fig. 334 in colour section) is seen as a greenish-brown ring at the periphery of the cornea on its posterior surface. The upper pole is first affected. Slit-lamp examination by an expert may be necessary for its demonstration.

It is usually present, but can be absent in young children with an acute presentation [26]. It can also rarely be found in patients with prolonged cholestasis and cryptogenic cirrhosis [9, 11]. The Kayser–Fleischer ring is always present with neurological abnormalities. The posterior layer of the capsule of the lens may rarely show greyish-brown 'sunflower' cataracts similar to those due to copper-containing foreign bodies [6].

HEPATIC FORMS

Fulminant hepatitis. This is characterized by progressive jaundice, ascites and hepatic failure, usually in a child or young person [22]. The liver cell necrosis is presumably related to accumulation of copper. Acute intravascular haemolysis may be due to destruction of erythrocytes by a sudden flux of copper from the necrotic hepatocytes [21] (fig. 335). Haemolysis of similar type is reported in

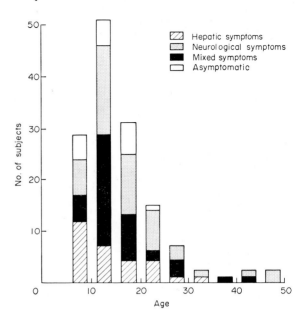

Fig. 333. Type of symptom complex at onset by age in 142 British and Chinese patients with Wilson's disease (Strickland *et al* 1973).

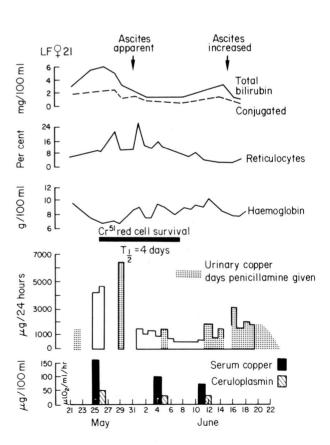

Fig. 335. Haemolytic crisis in Wilson's disease, marked by a rise in serum (mainly unconjugated) bilirubin and followed by reticulocytosis. The haemoglobin fell and red cell survival was reduced. Urinary copper was very high even without the administration of penicillamine. Serum copper was higher than that usually found in Wilson's disease. Ascites developed. The second episode of haemolysis, which was noted in June, was marked by a slight rise in serum bilirubin and a fall in haemoglobin (McIntyre *et al* 1967).

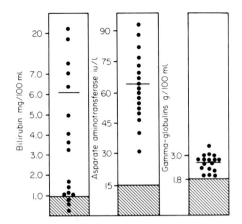

Fig. 336. Biochemical tests in 17 patients with Wilson's disease presenting as chronic active hepatitis. Horizontal lines indicate mean values. Normal ranges are denoted by hatching (serum bilirubin 0.2–0.8 mg/dl; aspartate aminotransferase 4–15 iu/l; gamma-globulins 0.7–1.8 g/dl) (Scott *et al* 1978).

sheep with copper intoxication, and in humans in accidental copper poisoning.

Chronic active hepatitis [26]. The condition presents at 10–30 years of age as an active chronic hepatitis with jaundice, high transaminase values and hypergammaglobulinaemia (fig. 336). Neurological changes appear some two to five years later. The picture may resemble other forms of chronic active hepatitis very closely. This emphasizes the need to screen all such patients for Wilson's disease.

Cirrhosis. The patient may present with insidiously developing cirrhosis. Clinical features include vascular spiders, splenomegaly, ascites and portal hypertension. The disease can exist without any neurological signs. In some patients the cirrhosis is well compensated. Hepatic biopsy may then be necessary for diagnosis. If possible the copper content of the biopsy should be estimated quantitatively.

All young patients with chronic liver disease showing any mental peculiarity, any slurring of the speech, early ascites or haemolysis and especially with a family history of cirrhosis should be screened for Wilson's disease.

NEUROPSYCHIATRIC CHANGES

The neurological condition may be acute and rapidly progressive. Early changes include a flexion–extension tremor of the wrists, grimacing,

difficulty in writing and a slurred speech. The limbs show a fluctuating rigidity. The intellect is fairly well preserved although 61% of patients have some psychiatric disturbance usually presenting as a slow deterioration of the personality.

More usually the neurological changes are chronic: onset is in early adult life with tremor, gross and of a wing-beating type, exaggerated by voluntary movement. Sensory loss and pyramidal tract signs are absent. The expression is fatuous. Dystonia carries a very poor prognosis.

The EEG shows generalized non-specific changes [17]. These appear to follow a familial pattern. The asymptomatic siblings of patients with an abnormal EEG showed similar changes.

RENAL CHANGES

Amino-aciduria, glycosuria, phosphaturia, uricosuria and failure to excrete *p*-amino-hippurate (PAH) reflect renal tubular changes [4]. These are presumably due to copper deposition in the proximal renal tubules.

Renal tubular acidosis is frequent and may be related to stone formation [40].

OTHER CHANGES

Rarely, the lunulae of the nails are blue [5]. Analysis of them has shown increased copper.

Skeletal changes include demineralization, premature osteoarthrosis, sub-articular cysts and fragmentation of bone about the joints of hands, wrists, feet and ankles. Changes in the spine are common [13]. Gall-stones are related to haemolysis [23].

Laboratory tests

Serum ceruloplasmin and copper levels are usually reduced [3, 12]. Distinction must be made from chronic active hepatitis with reduced serum ceruloplasmin due to failure of synthesis [28]. Malnutrition also reduces serum ceruloplasmin. The level may be raised by oestrogen administration, by some oral contraceptive drugs, by biliary obstruction or by pregnancy.

Twenty-four-hour urinary copper excretion is increased. Results may be difficult to evaluate unless strict precautions are taken in collection. In particular, copper-free containers must be used.

In those in whom liver biopsy is contraindicated

and where the serum ceruloplasmin level is normal, incorporation of orally administered radio-copper in ceruloplasmin may be diagnostic [33]. Normally an initial peak is followed by a slow increase as copper is incorporated into ceruloplasmin. In Wilson's disease the initial peak is higher, but the secondary rise is not seen, because incorporation is impaired.

LIVER BIOPSY

This must be done if any suspicion of Wilson's disease is aroused. The copper content must be measured and, before use, the needle must be washed with EDTA and rinsed in 5% dextrose to remove copper. Analysis is made by neutron activation [27]. The normal is less than $55 \mu g/g$ dry liver weight, and concentrations greater than $250 \mu g$ are usual in homozygous Wilson's disease (fig. 337). High values may even be found in those with normal hepatic histology [20]. High values are also found in all forms of longstanding cholestasis (fig. 337).

DETECTION OF SYMPTOM-FREE HOMOZYGOTES

All siblings of sufferers must be carefully screened [20, 32]. A homozygote is suggested by such features as hepatomegaly, splenomegaly, vascular spiders and a slight rise in serum transaminase

values. The Kayser–Fleischer rings may or may not be seen. Serum ceruloplasmin will usually be reduced to below 20 mg/100 ml. Liver biopsy with copper analysis is confirmatory.

Some difficulty may arise in distinguishing the homozygote from the heterozygote, but the distinction is usually clear-cut. The homozygote must be treated with penicillamine, even if symptom-free. The heterozygote does not require treatment. Thirty-six symptom-free homozygotes have been treated and remain well, whereas seven left untreated have all developed the disease and five are dead of Wilson's disease [32].

Treatment

Penicillamine (β,β-dimethyl-cysteine) is the treatment of choice [38]. This chelates copper and increases urinary excretion to as much as 1000–$3000 \mu g$ daily. Treatment is started with 1.2 g D penicillamine hydrochloride by mouth in four doses taken before meals. Improvement is slow and at least six months' continuous therapy should be given. If there is no improvement, dose may then be increased to 1.5 and even to 2 g daily. Improvement is marked by fading and disappearance of the Kayser–Fleischer rings. Speech is clearer, tremor and rigidity lessen. Mentality is more normal. Handwriting is a good test of progress. Liver function improves. Hepatic biopsy shows lessening of activity and reversion to an inactive cir-

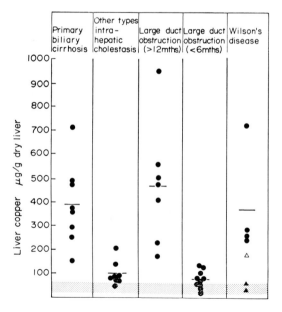

Fig. 337. Liver copper levels in patients with Wilson's disease and various types of cholestasis. Wilson's disease: △ heterozygote, ▲ siblings, probably homozygous normal (these three patients not included in the calculation of the mean) (Smallwood *et al* 1968).

rhosis. Mitochondrial abnormalities are reduced or disappear [31]. Serum ceruloplasmin values fall. Failure to improve implies that irreparable tissue damage was present before treatment started. Failure should not be admitted until two years' massive therapy has been given. This is the usual period for adequate initial therapy. Maintenance dose depends on the individual, usually 900–1200 mg daily.

If renal failure is associated, peritoneal or haemodialysis may be used to remove copper [16].

In contrast to other conditions, reactions to penicillamine are unusual in patients with Wilson's disease. They include rashes, leucopenia, aplastic anaemia [15], proteinuria and an SLE-like syndrome. They are usually solved by stopping the drug and recommencing in increasing doses under prednisolone cover. Clinical pyridoxine deficiency is a theoretical possibility but exceedingly rare. When large doses are being given, pyridoxine supplements can be added.

D-Penicillamine must be continued throughout life. The dose should be monitored at one- to two-year intervals by measuring 24-hour urinary copper excretion off and on therapy, with, if possible, copper estimations on a liver biopsy specimen. Complete de-coppering is unusual even after many years' therapy.

An alternative agent, trilene, can be used, but reactions are more frequent than with penicillamine.

Hepatic transplantation has been successfully performed in patients with Wilson's disease dying in terminal liver failure [29]. This procedure should not be necessary if penicillamine is given early and in adequate doses.

Physiotherapy is of value in the re-education of the patient's gait, writing and movement generally.

Prognosis

In the acute neurological form the prognosis is poor, for cystic changes in the basal ganglia are irreversible. In the more chronic form the outlook depends on early diagnosis, preferably before symptoms have appeared. The final prognosis also depends on the response to six months' continuous penicillamine treatment. In one series, 16 asymptomatic patients were treated and have remained alive and asymptomatic, and three-quarters of 22 symptomatic patients treated for longer than two years are now asymptomatic [35]. Dystonia carries a poor prognosis, being little affected by chelation

therapy. Successful pregnancies have been reported in well-treated cases and penicillamine causes little problem to the foetus [39].

Early acute liver failure is usually fatal despite attempts at copper removal [22].

In chronic active hepatitis, response to treatment can be poor, nine of 17 patients dying in one series [26].

Death is from liver failure, bleeding oesophageal varices or intercurrent infections in those bedridden from neurological disability.

REFERENCES

1. BEARN A.G. (1957) Wilson's disease. An inborn error of metabolism with multiple manifestations. *Am. J. Med.* **22**, 747.
2. BEARN A.G. (1960) A genetical analysis of thirty families with Wilson's disease (hepato-lenticular degeneration). *Ann. hum. Genet.* **24**, 33.
3. BEARN A.G. & KUNKEL H.G. (1952) Biochemical abnormalities in Wilson's disease. *J. clin. Invest.* **31**, 616.
4. BEARN A.G. & KUNKEL H.G. (1954) Abnormalities of copper metabolism in Wilson's disease and their relationship to the amino aciduria. *J. clin. Invest.* **33**, 400.
5. BEARN A.G. & McKUSICK V.A. (1958) Azure lunulae. An unusual change in the finger nails in two patients with hepatolenticular degeneration (Wilson's disease). *J. Am. med. Assoc.* **166**, 904.
6. CAIRNS J.E., WILLIAMS H.P. & WALSHE J.M. (1969) 'Sunflower cataract' in Wilson's disease. *Br. med. J.* iii, 95.
7. COX D.W., FRASER F.C. & SASS-KORTSAK A. (1972) A genetic study of Wilson's disease: evidence for heterogeneity. *Am. J. hum. Genet.* **24**, 646.
8. EPSTEIN O. & SHERLOCK S. (1981) Wilson's disease—evidence for a controller gene defect resulting in failure to adapt from positive copper balance of the foetus to the normal copper balance of the child. *Lancet*. In press.
9. FLEMMING C.R., DICKSON E.R., WAHNER H.W. *et al* (1977) Pigmented corneal rings in non-Wilsonian liver disease. *Ann. intern. Med.* **86**, 285.
10. FROMMER D. (1971) The binding of copper by bile and serum. *Clin. Sci.* **41**, 485.
11. FROMMER D., MORRIS J., SHERLOCK S. *et al* (1977) Kayser–Fleischer-like rings in patients without Wilson's disease. *Gastroenterology* **72**, 1331.
12. GIBBS K. & WALSHE J.M. (1979) A study of the caeruloplasmin concentrations found in 75 patients with Wilson's disease, their kinships and various control groups. *Q. J. Med.* **48**, 447.
13. GOLDING D.N. & WALSHE J.M. (1977) Arthropathy of Wilson's disease. *Ann. rheum. Dis.* **36**, 99.
14. GOLDFISCHER S. & MOSKAL J. (1966) Electron probe microanalysis of liver in Wilson's disease.

Simultaneous assay for copper and for lead deposited by acid phosphatase activity in lysosomes. *Am. J. Pathol.* **48**, 305.

15. GOLLAN J.L., HUSSEIN S., HOFFBRAND A.V. *et al* (1976) Red cell aplasia following prolonged D-penicillamine therapy. *J. clin. Pathol.* **29**, 135.

16. HAMLYN A.N., GOLLAN J.L., DOUGLAS A.P. *et al* (1977) Fulminant Wilson's disease with haemolysis and renal failure: copper studies and assessment of dialysis regimens. *Br. med. J.* ii, 660.

17. HANSOTIA P., HARRIS R. & KENNEDY J. (1969) EEG changes in Wilson's disease. *Electroenceph. clin. Neurophysiol.* **27**, 523.

18. HARRY J. & TRIPATHI R. (1970) Kayser–Fleischer ring. A pathological study. *Br. J. Ophthamol.* **54**, 794.

19. HAZELRIG J.B., OWEN C.A. & ACKERMAN E. (1966) A mathematical model for copper metabolism and its relation to Wilson's disease. *Am. J. Physiol.* **211**, 1075.

20. LEVI A.J., SHERLOCK S., SCHEUER P.J. *et al* (1967) Presymptomatic Wilson's disease. *Lancet* ii, 575.

21. MCINTYRE N., CLINK H.M., LEVI A.J. *et al* (1947) Hemolytic anemia in Wilson's disease. *New Engl. J. Med.* **276**, 439.

22. ROCHE-SICOT J. & BENHAMOU J-P. (1977) Acute intravascular hemolysis and acute liver failure associated as a first manifestation of Wilson's disease. *Ann. intern. Med.* **86**, 301.

23. ROSENFIELD N., GRAND R.J., WATKINS J.B. *et al* (1978) Cholelithiasis and Wilson's disease. *J. Pediatr.* **92**, 210.

24. SCHAFFNER F., STERNLIEB I., BARKA T. *et al* (1962) Hepatocellular changes in Wilson's disease; histochemical and electron microscopic studies. *Am. J. Pathol.* **41**, 315.

25. SCHEUER P.J. (1980) Disturbances of iron and copper metabolism. In *Liver Biopsy Interpretation*, 3rd edn. Baillière Tindall, London.

26. SCOTT J., GOLLAN J.L., SAMOURIAN *et al* (1978) Wilson's disease, presenting as chronic active hepatitis. *Gastroenterology* **74**, 645.

27. SMALLWOOD R.A., WILLIAMS H.A., ROSENOER V.M. *et al* (1968) Liver-copper levels in liver disease. Studies using neutron activation analysis. *Lancet* ii, 1310.

28. SPECHLER S.J. & KOFF R.S. (1980) Wilson's disease: diagnostic difficulties in the patient with chronic hepatitis and hypoceruloplasminemia. *Gastroenterology* **78**, 103.

29. STARZL T.E., KOEP L.J., HALGRIMSON C.G. *et al* (1979) Fifteen years of clinical liver transplantation. *Gastroenterology* **77**, 375.

30. STERNLIEB I. (1968) Mitochondrial and fatty changes in hepatocytes of patients with Wilson's disease. *Gastroenterology* **55**, 354.

31. STERNLIEB I. & FELDMANN G. (1976) Effects of anticopper therapy on hepatocellular mitochondria in patients with Wilson's disease. *Gastroenterology* **71**, 457.

32. STERNLIEB I. & SCHEINBERG I.H. (1967) The prevention of clinical Wilson's disease. *J. clin. Invest.* **46**, 1120.

33. STERNLIEB I. & SCHEINBERG I.H. (1979) The role of radiocopper in the diagnosis of Wilson's disease. *Gastroenterology* **77**, 138.

34. STERNLIEB I., VAN DEN HAMER C.J.A., MORELL A.G. *et al* (1973) Lysosomal defect of hepatic copper excretion in Wilson's disease (hepatolenticular degeneration). *Gastroenterology* **64**, 99.

35. STRICKLAND G.T., FROMMER D., LEU M.-L. *et al* (1973) Wilson's disease in the United Kingdom and Taiwan. I. General characteristics of 142 cases and prognosis. II. A genetic analysis of 88 cases. *Q. J. Med.* **42**, 619.

36. STROMEYER F.W. & ISHAK K.G. (1980) Histology of the liver in Wilson's disease. *Am. J. clin. Pathol.* **73**, 12.

37. UZMAN L.L., IBER F.L., CHALMERS T.C. *et al* (1956) The mechanism of copper deposition in the liver in hepatolenticular degeneration (Wilson's disease). *J. med. Sci.* **231**, 511.

38. WALSHE J.M. (1960) Treatment of Wilson's disease with penicillamine. *Lancet* i, 188.

39. WALSHE J.M. (1977) Pregnancy in Wilson's disease. *Q. J. Med.* **46**, 73.

40. WIEBER D.O., WILSON D.M., McLEOD R.A. *et al* (1979) Renal stones in Wilson's disease. *Am. J. Med.* **67**, 249.

41. WILSON A.K. (1912) Progressive lenticular degeneration: a familial nervous disease associated with cirrhosis of the liver. *Brain* **34**, 295.

Chapter 22
Nutritional and Metabolic
Liver Diseases

CLINICAL NUTRITIONAL LIVER INJURY

Hepatic necrosis and fibrosis can be produced in experimental animals by appropriate diets, particularly those low in protein and essential amino acids [9]. World-wide protein malnutrition is extremely common [26]. All grades are encountered and the liver suffers in common with other organs.

The most clearly defined syndrome is *kwashiorkor*, but this represents only one end of the malnutrition spectrum. The liver is involved in *wasting diseases*, especially with chronic diarrhoea such as ulcerative colitis, and the hepatic changes in the *alcoholic* may be at least in part nutritional.

In *starvation* and hunger oedema, the liver shrinks, increased lipochrome pigment is seen in the liver cells, but there is no fatty change [23]. Microchemical analyses of liver biopsies from malnourished children have shown reduction in liver protein [26]. Liver biopsies from patients with *anorexia nervosa* are essentially normal. Previous malnutrition may 'condition' the liver to toxic and infective agents, but this has not been proved. Increased mortality from virus hepatitis, particularly in pregnancy, may occur in protein-deficient communities.

Kwashiorkor syndrome

People in sub-tropical and tropical areas, under poor economic conditions, eat a low-protein diet; their caloric intake is maintained with carbohydrate. They are therefore in a position to develop nutritional liver disease. This syndrome of protein malnutrition usually affects children and is called kwashiorkor, which, in the Ga language of the Gold Coast means 'Red Boy'. The name varies in different countries. It has a world-wide distribution in under-privileged, over-populated communities [5, 25, 26]. It is rare in Europe although it may appear under such conditions as the siege of Budapest. Very few cases have been noted in the temperate regions of any continent.

PATHOLOGY

Deficiency of dietary protein affects particularly organs concerned with the elaboration of proteins and protein-containing enzymes.

The pancreas shows selective atrophy of acinar cells. Salivary and lacrymal glands and the glands of the small intestinal wall are atrophied and there is muscle wasting. The parotid glands may enlarge during recovery.

The liver shows extensive periportal fatty change. This might be secondary to the pancreatic damage [25] and analogous to the fatty liver of depancreatized dogs. Alternatively, the fatty liver may be due to dietary protein deficiency. The liver loses protein and gains water, sharing in the general oedema [26]. The very fatty liver may be related to mobilization of fat from adipose tissue. Alternatively, the hepatic glucose-6-phosphatase level is reduced. Although hepatic glycogen is increased this suggests failure to handle dietary carbohydrate which may then be converted into fat. Electron microscopy shows surprisingly mild changes [27].

The hepatic change is not specific nor is it the most important feature. In fact it might be a kind of epiphenomenon: the fatty infiltration bears very little relation to clinical severity and causes little disturbance of liver function [26]. Follow-up studies show no evidence of progressive fibrosis or cirrhosis [7].

CLINICAL FEATURES [25]

Children are most commonly affected 6–18 months after weaning when they are fed on an almost pure carbohydrate diet. Even before weaning, the milk of the undernourished mother may have been poor in protein, and this lack is emphasized by the demands of growth. Malaria and hookworm disease may contribute.

The acute breakdown is often initiated by a diminished food intake due to deprivation of mother love or an infection. The child is incredibly miserable with arrested growth, generalized oedema and cold extremities. The hair shows characteristic depigmentation, becoming pale and, losing its crisp black curliness, becomes thin, straight and soft. The characteristic dermatosis starts in the inguinal region and napkin area and spreads to sites of pressure and irritation. The dusky red patches have been likened to crazy paving. The skin desquamates and becomes pallid.

Appetite is decreased and diarrhoea is prominent, especially in the severe case, the stools showing undigested food. The liver may be enlarged or of normal size.

Severe protein malnutrition in adults, resembling kwashiorkor, can be related to ineffective utilization of dietary protein due to pancreatic exocrine deficiency or enteric bacterial colonization [11, 20].

Laboratory findings include reduced haemoglobin and plasma protein concentrations. Pancreatic enzymes are diminished.

Analysis of liver biopsy material shows reduction of pseudo-cholinesterase, D-amino-acid oxidase and xanthine oxidase [15, 26]. Enzymes subserving respiration and oxidative phosphorylation are well preserved.

Serum enzymes are depressed. These enzymes are reduced in keeping with all protein production [26]. Serum transaminase and plasma-free fatty-acid levels are increased [13].

The liver in obesity

In obese subjects the liver becomes fatty in keeping with other organs. Fatty infiltration is in proportion to the increase in body weight. Such fatty change is generally believed benign and not a precirrhotic lesion. However, occasionally the liver shows changes indistinguishable from a mild alcoholic hepatitis [1]. These include centrizonal and peri-sinusoidal fibrosis, polymorph infiltration and Mallory bodies. Such patients are often also diabetic. Liver function tests are abnormal and reflect the underlying histological findings [8]. These changes may be related to protein malnutrition. Any regime used to reduce weight should avoid protein depletion.

Effects of jejuno-ileal bypass

The hepatic changes of obesity are enhanced by this operation and cirrhosis can develop [10, 21]. Serious liver changes develop within two years of operation in 1–17%. The patient may die in hepatic failure [28]. Recovery has followed parenteral nutrition and re-anastomosis [2].

The liver changes probably represent protein–calorie malnutrition [19] and, in addition, conversion of carbohydrate to fat is increased postoperatively [12].

Any treatment causing very rapid weight loss will probably have these side-effects. Newer operations such as gastric bypass will probably not have such severe hepatic side-effects.

Obese subjects are prone to supersaturated bile and hence to cholesterol gall-stone formation. During weight reduction, bile acid pool size falls and biliary cholesterol saturation may increase. Chenodeoxycholic acid may protect against gallstones in these patients [17].

Hepatic granulomas have been reported after jejuno-ileal bypass [3].

Parenteral hypernutrition

Cholestasis has developed in infants given long-term hyper-alimentation for neonatal intestinal obstruction [6]. In adults, increases in serum transaminases, alk. phosphatase and bilirubin values follow fat-free total parenteral nutrition for two weeks or longer [14]. Liver biopsies show fatty change and mild periportal cholestasis. Abnormal biochemical tests also complicate enteral elemental diets in adults [24, 29].

Vitamins

The fat-soluble vitamins A, D and K are not absorbed if biliary bile acid excretion is inadequate. Deficiencies therefore complicate cholestasis (Chapter 15).

Hypervitaminosis A leads to peri-sinusoidal fibrosis, central vein sclerosis and focal congestion with peri-sinusoidal lipid storage cells. Vitamin A fluorescence may be shown in frozen sections [22]. Portal hypertension and ascites are consequences.

Vitamin C deficiency is seen in alcoholics with or without liver disease and is related to low intake. It is also seen in primary biliary cirrhosis perhaps related to cholestyramine binding of the vitamin [4].

Alcoholics may show thiamine deficiency. Clinical evidence of this in non-alcoholic patients with liver disease is very rare [18]. Similarly folic acid may be reduced in alcoholics.

Low circulating levels of PLP, the active form of vitamin B_6 compounds, in cirrhosis is probably due to increased degradation [16].

REFERENCES

1. ADLER M. & SCHAFFNER F. (1979) Fatty liver hepatitis and cirrhosis in obese patients. *Am. J. Med.* **67**, 811.
2. BAKER A.L., ELSON C.O., JASPAN J. *et al* (1979) Liver failure with steatonecrosis after jejunoileal bypass: recovery with parenteral nutrition and reanastomosis. *Arch. intern Med.* **139**, 289.
3. BANNER B.F. & BANNER A.S. (1978) Hepatic granulomas following ileal bypass for obesity. *Arch. Pathol.* **102**, 655.
4. BEATTIE A.D. & SHERLOCK S. (1976) Ascorbic acid deficiency in liver disease. *Gut* **17**, 571.
5. BROCK J.F. (1954) Survey of the world situation on kwashiorkor. *Ann. N.Y. Acad. Sci.* **57**, 696.
6. BROWN M.R. & PUTNAM T.C. (1978) Cholestasis associated with central intravenous nutrition in infants. *N.Y. State J. Med.* **78**, 27.
7. COOK G.C. & HUTT M.S.R. (1967) The liver after kwashiorkor. *Br. med. J.* iii, 454.
8. GALAMBOS J.T. & WILLS C.E. (1978) Relationship between 505 paired liver tests and biopsies in 242 obese patients. *Gastroenterology* **74**, 1191.
9. HIMSWORTH H.P. & GLYNN L.E. (1944) Massive hepatic necrosis and diffuse hepatic fibrosis (acute yellow atrophy and portal cirrhosis): their production by means of diet. *Clin. Sci.*, **5**, 93.
10. HOLZBACH R.T., WEILAND R.G., LEIBER C.S. *et al* (1974) Hepatic lipid in morbid obesity. *New Engl. J. Med.* **290**, 296.
11. JONES E.A., CRAIGIE A., TAVILL A.S. *et al* (1968) Protein metabolism in the intestinal stagnant loop syndrome. *Gut* **9**, 466.
12. KESSLER J.I., NIRMEL K., MACLEAN L.D. *et al* (1979) Alteration of hepatic triglyceride in patients before and after jejunoileal bypass for morbid obesity. *Gastroenterology* **76**, 159.
13. LEWIS B., HANSEN J.D.L., WITTMAN W. *et al* (1964) Plasma free fatty acids in kwashiorkor and the pathogenesis of the fatty liver. *Am. J. clin. Nutr.* **15**, 161.
14. LINDOR K.D., FLEMING C.R., ABRAMS A. *et al* (1979) Liver function values in adults receiving total parenteral nutrition. *J. Am. med. Assoc.* **241**, 2398.
15. MCLEAN A.E.M. (1966) Enzyme activity in the liver and serum of malnourished children in Jamaica. *Clin. Sci.* **30**, 129.
16. MEZEY E. (1978) Liver disease and nutrition. *Gastroenterology* **74**, 770.
17. MOK H.Y.I., VON BERGMANN K., CROUSE J.R. *et al* (1979) Biliary lipid metabolism in obesity: effects of bile acid feeding before and during weight reduction. *Gastroenterology* **76**, 556.
18. MORGAN A.G., KELLEHER J., WALKER B.E. *et al* (1976) Nutrition in cryptogenic cirrhosis and chronic aggressive hepatitis. *Gut* **17**, 113.
19. MOXLEY R.T., POZEFSKY T. & LOCKWOOD D.H. (1974) Protein nutrition and liver disease after jejunoileal bypass for morbid obesity. *New Engl. J. Med.* **290**, 921.
20. NEALE G., ANTCLIFF A.C., WELBOURN R.B. *et al* (1967) Protein malnutrition after partial gastrectomy. *Q. J. Med.* **36**, 469.
21. PETERS R.L. (1977) Patterns of hepatic morphology in jejunoileal bypass patients. *Am. J. clin. Nutr.* **30**, 53.
22. RUSSELL R.M., BOYER J.L., BHAGERI S.A. *et al* (1974) Hepatic injury from chronic hypervitaminosis A resulting in portal hypertension and ascites. *New Engl. J. Med.* **291**, 435.
23. SHERLOCK S. & WALSHE V.M. (1951) Hepatic structure and function. In *Studies of Undernutrition, Wuppertal, 1946–9*. Medical Research Council Special Report, Series No. 275, p. 111.
24. SKIDMORE F.D., TWEEDLE D.E.F., GLEAVE E.N. *et al* (1979) Abnormal liver function during nutritional support in postoperative cancer patients. *Ann. R. Coll. Surg. Engl.* **61**, 183.
25. TROWELL H.C., DAVIES J.N.P. & DEAN R.F.A. (1954) *Kwashiorkor*. Edward Arnold, London.
26. WATERLOW J.C., CRAVIOTO J. & STEPHEN J.M.L. (1960) Protein malnutrition in man. *Adv. Protein. Chem.* **15**, 131.
27. WEBBER B.L. & FREIMAN I. (1974) The liver in kwashiorkor. *Arch. Pathol.* **98**, 400.
28. WEISMANN R.E. & JOHNSON R.E. (1977) Fatal hepatic failure after jejunoileal bypass: clinical and laboratory evidence of prognostic significance. *Am. J. Surg.* **134**, 253.
29. ZARCHY T.M., LIPMAN T.O. & FINKELSTEIN J.D. (1978) Elevated transaminases associated with an elemental diet. *Ann. intern. Med.* **89**, 221.

CARBOHYDRATE METABOLISM IN LIVER DISEASE

HYPOGLYCAEMIA

This is usually due to reduction in hepatic glucose release. The hepatectomized dog rapidly develops hypoglycaemia [1] and this is seen in acute liver failure (Chapter 9). In fulminant hepatitis it may be intractable [2]. Hypoglycaemia is rare in chronic liver disease even terminally. Very rarely it is found in cirrhotic patients after a porta-caval anastomosis. Reactive hypoglycaemia, $1\frac{1}{2}$–2 hours after glucose, has been seen in two patients with active chronic hepatitis; blood insulin levels were high. Alcohol can also induce hypoglycaemia, especially in cirrhotic patients.

Hypoglycaemia may complicate Reye's syndrome in children (page 394), primary hepatic carcinoma (page 461), glycogen storage disease (page 371) and hereditary fructose intolerance (p. 374).

REFERENCES

1. MANN F.C. & MAGATH T.B. (1922) Studies on the physiology of the liver. II. The effect of the removal of the liver on the blood sugar level. *Arch. intern. Med.* **30**, 73.
2. SAMSON R.I., TREY G., TIMME A.H. *et al* (1967) Fulminating hepatitis with recurrent hypoglycemia and hemorrhage. *Gastroenterology* **53**, 291.

THE LIVER IN DIABETES MELLITUS

The hyperglycaemia of diabetes mellitus results from over-production of glucose by the liver and diminished tissue utilization. In the fasting diabetic state, blood glucose is steady at a hyperglycaemic value, hepatic glucose output is normal, and the peripheral utilization of glucose must also be normal. The normal peripheral disposal of glucose can occur when the arterial glucose level is high.

Insulin and the liver

Insulin in small doses decreases hepatic glucose output in man [3]. The human liver takes up insulin [16]. Peripheral tissues also take up insulin but to a lesser extent. Glucagon is taken up. Hyperinsulinaemia is a characteristic association of cirrhosis. This is due to failure of degradation and not to hypersecretion or portal–systemic bypassing [10, 11, 18].

In chronic active hepatitis peripheral insulin levels may be reduced, probably related to a concomitant auto-immune pancreatitis.

In diabetes, glucose-6-phosphatase increases in the liver, facilitating glucose release into the blood. The opposing enzymes which phosphorylate glucose, are hexokinase, which is unaffected by insulin, and glucokinase, which decreases in diabetes. As a result the liver continues to produce glucose even with severe hyperglycaemia. Under these circumstances the normal liver would shut off and deposit glycogen [5]. Fructose-1-6 phosphate activity is also increased in diabetes. Gluconeogenesis is thus favoured.

Substances released from the pancreas into the portal blood are known to increase hepatic regeneration (*hepato-trophic substances*) [19]. Insulin is the main hepato-trophic substance although glucagon may also be important. Blood glucagon is increased in liver disease, probably due to pancreatic over-secretion.

Liver changes

A low liver glycogen is unusual even in autopsy material. Needle biopsy shows normal or increased amounts of glycogen in the livers of severe untreated diabetes [9]. Even higher values follow the administration of insulin, provided hypoglycaemia is prevented.

Histologically the zonal structure is normal. The granular appearance of the glycogen is a fixation effect for, in life, the glycogen is in solution in the cells. In sections stained H and E, the glycogen-filled cells appear pale and fluffy. The periportal cells always contain less than the central ones and this is accentuated by glycogenolysis. In the insulin-sensitive, ketotic diabetic, the liver cells appear bloated and oedematous; glycogen is maintained or even increased [9].

Glycogenic infiltration of the liver cell nuclei (fig. 338) [20] is shown as a vacuolization, the nature of which is confirmed by glycogen stains. It is not specific for diabetes mellitus but is found in about two-thirds of diabetics.

Fatty change in the liver is common in the obese, insulin-resistant diabetic, but is minimal in the

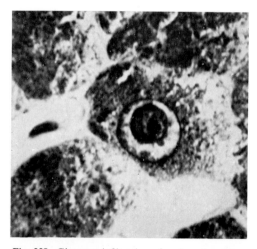

Fig. 338. Glycogen infiltration of an hepatic nucleus. Cells contain much glycogen. Best's carmine for glycogen, × 1150.

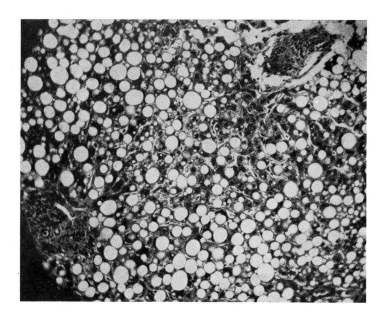

Fig. 339. Diabetes mellitus. Liver biopsy sections show great increase in fat in the liver cells. H & E, × 145 (Sherlock *et al* 1951).

thin, insulin-sensitive subject [6]. It is mainly periportal (fig. 339). There is no fibrosis.

A picture resembling alcoholic hepatitis can also be seen, particularly in the obese diabetic [7, 14].

Liver changes in the various types of diabetes mellitus

THE INSULIN-SENSITIVE TYPE (JUVENILE, ACUTE)

There are usually no clinical features referable to the liver. Occasionally, however, the liver is greatly enlarged, firm and with a smooth, tender edge. Some of the nausea, abdominal pain and vomiting of diabetic ketosis may be due to hepatomegaly [8]. Hepatic enlargement is found particularly in young people and children with severe, uncontrolled diabetes. In adults, hepatomegaly occurs with prolonged acidosis. In one large series, hepatomegaly was noted in only 9% of well-controlled diabetics, in 60% of uncontrolled diabetics and in 100% of patients in ketosis [8]. The liver returns to a normal size when the diabetes is brought under complete control. The enlargement is due to increased glycogen. Insulin therapy in the presence of a very high blood sugar level augments still further the glycogen content of the liver and in the initial stages of treatment, hepatomegaly may increase. The liver cells in severe acidosis may contain more water than usual; it is probably retained to keep the glycogen in solution.

The blood glucose level and hepatic glucose output fall promptly with insulin [2]. In ketosis, hepatic insulin sensitivity is lost [17].

THE INSULIN-INSENSITIVE (MATURITY-ONSET) TYPE

The liver may be enlarged, with a firm, smooth, non-tender edge. Enlargement is due to increased deposition of liver fat, largely related to the obesity.

The blood glucose level and the hepatic glucose output respond poorly to a small dose of insulin [2, 17].

Diabetes in childhood

The liver may be enlarged and this enlargement has been attributed both to fatty infiltration and to increased amounts of glycogen. Aspiration biopsy studies show that the fatty change is slight but that the liver does contain an excess of glycogen. The hepatic changes are similar to those already described in the adult insulin-sensitive diabetic.

Sometimes a huge liver is associated with retarded growth, obesity, florid facies and hypercholesterolaemia (*Mauriac syndrome*) [12].

Splenomegaly, portal hypertension and hepato-
cellular failure do not occur.

Liver function tests

In well-controlled diabetics routine tests are usually normal and any change is due to a cause other
than diabetes. Acidosis may produce mild changes
including hyperglobulinaemia, urobilinuria and a
slightly raised serum bilirubin level. These return
to normal with diabetic control.

Hepatomegaly, whether due to increased
amounts of glycogen in the sensitive group or to
fatty change in the insulin-sensitive type, does not
correlate with the results of the liver function tests.

Association between cirrhosis and diabetes

Cirrhotic patients often have an impaired oral and
intravenous glucose tolerance test and increased
resistance to exogenous insulin [13] (fig. 340). In
contrast to diabetes mellitus, however, the fasting blood sugar is usually normal and blood insulin levels are increased. Clinical features of diabetes are not seen. The impaired glucose tolerance
may be particularly marked after porta-caval
shunt. Insulin therapy is not required. High carbohydrate feeding may be necessary in the management of cirrhosis, especially if there is encephalopathy. This always takes precedence over any
impairment of glucose tolerance whether genuine
diabetes or secondary to the liver disease.

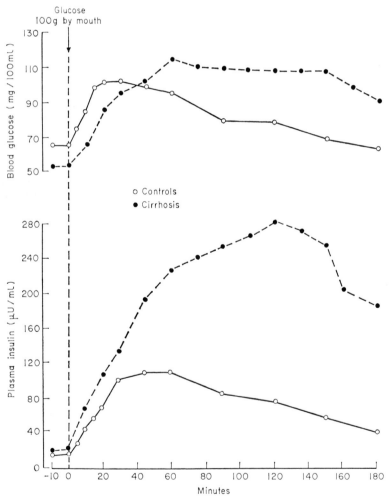

Fig. 340. The oral glucose tolerance test in cirrhosis.
The cirrhotic patients showed a normal fasting
blood glucose but some impaired tolerance. Plasma
insulin levels rose slowly in controls and there was
insulin resistance (Megyesi *et al* 1967).

An association between genuine, maturity onset diabetes and cirrhosis has been suggested [4]. Cirrhotics are twice as likely as the general population to have diabetes [15]. The cirrhosis may have unmasked a genetically determined diabetic trait.

Any real increased incidence of cirrhosis in diabetics seems unlikely. In most instances the cirrhosis is diagnosed first, before impaired glucose tolerance is recognized.

Diagnosis of cirrhosis in the presence of diabetes is usually easy, for diabetes alone does not cause vascular spiders, jaundice, hepato-splenomegaly and ascites. If necessary liver biopsy is diagnostic.

REFERENCES

1. ALBERTI K.G.M.M., RECORD C.O., WILLIAMSON D.H. *et al* (1972) Metabolic changes in active chronic hepatitis. *Clin. Sci.* **42**, 591.
2. BEARN A.G., BILLING B.H. & SHERLOCK S. (1951) Hepatic glucose output and hepatic insulin sensitivity in diabetes mellitus. *Lancet* ii, 698.
3. BEARN A.G., BILLING B.H. & SHERLOCK S. (1952) The response of the liver to insulin in normal subjects and in diabetes mellitus: hepatic vein catheterization studies. *Clin. Sci.* **11**, 151.
4. BLOODWORTH J.M.B. (1961) Diabetes mellitus and cirrhosis of the liver. *Arch. intern. Med.* **108**, 695.
5. CAHILL G.F. Jr, ASHMORE J., RENOLD A.E. *et al* (1959) Blood glucose and the liver. *Am. J. Med.* **26**, 264.
6. CREUTZFELDT W., FRERICHS H. & SICKINGER K. (1970) Liver diseases and diabetes mellitus. In *Progress in Liver Disease*, vol. 3, p. 371, eds H. Popper & F. Schaffner. Grune and Stratton, New York.
7. FALCHUK K.R., FISKE S.C., HAGGITT R.C. *et al* (1980) Pericentral hepatic fibrosis and intracellular hyalin in diabetes mellitus. *Gastroenterology* **78**, 535.
8. GOODMAN J.I. (1953) Hepatomegaly and diabetes mellitus. *Ann. intern. Med.* **39**, 1077.
9. HILDES J.A., SHERLOCK S. & WALSH V. (1949) Liver and muscle glycogen in normal subjects, in diabetes mellitus and in acute hepatitis. *Clin. Sci.* **7**, 287.
10. JOHNSTON D.G., ALBERTI K.G.M.M., FABER O.K. *et al* (1977) Hyperinsulinism of hepatic cirrhosis: diminished degradation or hypersecretion? *Lancet* i, 10.
11. JOHNSTON D.G., ALBERTI G.M.M., GEORGE K. *et al* (1978) C-peptide and insulin in liver disease. *Diabetes* **27**, 201.
12. MAURIAC P. (1946) Hépatomégalie, nanisme, obésité dans le diabète infantile: pathogénie du syndrome. *Presse méd.* **54**, 826.
13. MEGYESI C., SAMOLS E. & MARKS V. (1967) Glucose tolerance and diabetes in chronic liver disease. *Lancet* ii, 1051.
14. MILLER D.J., ISHIMARU H. & KLATSKIN G. (1979) Non-alcoholic liver disease mimicking alcoholic hepatitis and cirrhosis. *Gastroenterology* **77**, A27.
15. MÜTING D., LACKAS N., REIKOWSKI H. *et al* (1966) Cirrhosis of the liver and diabetes mellitus. A study of 140 combined cases. *Dtsch. med. Monatsschr.* **11.**, 385.
16. SAMOLS E. & RYDER J.A. (1961) Studies on tissue uptake of insulin in man using a differential immunoassay for endogenous and exogenous insulin. *J. clin. Invest.* **40**, 2092.
17. SHERLOCK S., BEARN A.G. & BILLING B. (1951) The effect of insulin on the liver in normal and diabetic man. *Trans. 10th Conf. Liver Injury.* Josiah Macy Jr Foundation, New York.
18. SMITH-LAING G., SHERLOCK S. & FABER O.K. (1979) Effects of spontaneous portal–systemic shunting on insulin metabolism. *Gastroenterology* **76**, 685.
19. STARZL T.E., WATANABE K., PORTER K.A. *et al* (1976) Effects of insulin, glucagon, and insulin/glucagon infusions on liver morphology and cell division after complete portacaval shunt in dogs. *Lancet* i, 821.
20. ZIMMERMAN H.J., MacMURRAY F.G., RAPPAPORT H. *et al* (1950) Studies of the liver in diabetes mellitus. I. Structural and functional abnormalities. *J. lab. clin. Med.* **36**, 912.

THE GLYCOGENOSES

These are diseases with excessive and/or abnormal glycogen in the tissues [8]. Various forms have different enzymatic or structural defects. Enzyme analysis of liver needle biopsy material is essential to categorize the type [11] (table 57). All forms seem to be inherited, usually as an autosomal recessive except type VI which is sex-linked. The types vary greatly in their severity and in their clinical picture. The critical abnormality is usually insufficient glucose production by the liver, which results in hypoglycaemia when the blood glucose level is not supported by an inflow of glucose from the intestinal tract. The other abnormalities follow this defect and from the metabolic reactions to hypoglycaemia.

Type I (Von Gierke's disease)

This type involves liver and kidney but not muscle and heart. The inheritance is autosomal recessive. Siblings may be involved, but transmission through successive generations has not been shown.

HEPATIC CHANGES

The liver is enlarged, smooth and brown. Hepatic biopsy shows a very high glycogen content; this

Table 57. The hepatic glycogen storage diseases.

Type	Enzyme defect	Tissues involved
I	Glucose 6-phosphatase	Liver, kidney, intestines
II	Lysosomal alpha-1,4 glucosidase (acid maltase)	Generalized
III	Amylo-1,6 glucosidase (debranching enzyme)	Liver, muscle, WBC
IV	Alpha-1,4 glucan-6 glucosyl transferase (branching enzyme)	Generalized
IV	Liver phosphorylase	Liver, WBC
VIII	Phosphorylase activation	Liver
IXa, IXb	Phosphorylase kinase	Liver, WBC, RBC

is not diagnostic. The liver cells and their nuclei are laden with glycogen. In formol-fixed material, glycogen is washed out leaving an appearance of clear, plant-like cells. Excess fat is usually present. The glycogen is usually stable, persisting many days *post mortem* and despite severe ketosis or prolonged anaesthesia. Cirrhosis does not develop. Hepato-cellular adenomas and, rarely, carcinomas are late developments [6].

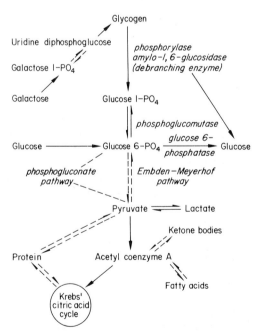

Fig. 341. Metabolic pathways in glycogen breakdown (Sokal 1962).

CLINICAL FEATURES

In early infancy the symptoms include irritability, pallor, cyanosis, feeding difficulties and seizures usually associated with hypoglycaemia. Episodes of diarrhoea and vomiting are frequent.

Presentation is by massive hepatomegaly about two years old. The spleen is not enlarged, a point of distinction from the lipoidoses, the cirrhoses and congenital hepatic fibrosis.

Hypoglycaemic episodes and fasting ketosis are usual.

The child is short and fat with particularly fat cheeks. Mental development is usually normal.

INVESTIGATIONS

Routine liver functions tests are usually normal. Occasionally transaminases are raised.

The fasting blood glucose level is low. Ketosis is related to defective glucose metabolism. Hyperlipaemia, hypercholesterolaemia and a fatty liver are common. Plasma uric acid levels are raised and gout develops after puberty. There is chronic lactic acidosis.

Diagnosis depends on showing that the blood glucose fails to rise adequately when hepatic glycogenolysis is stimulated. *Glucagon* (20 µg/kg body weight) is given intramuscularly after a fast of 10–12 hours, or 3–4 hours if hypoglycaemia is severe. Results are classified according to the blood glucose response. Normals show a rise of 35 mg/100 ml, subnormals 15–35 mg/100 ml, and absent or minimal less than 15 mg/100 ml. Lactic acid changes are classified as normal with increases of less than 10 mg/100 ml or abnormal with increases of more than 10 mg/100 ml.

These patients cannot utilize galactose or fructose as a source of blood glucose and intravenous lactose and fructose tests may also be performed.

The erythrocyte glycogen level is increased.

If the test is positive, biopsy of liver should be taken for histology, including histochemistry and quantitative glycogen analysis. A specimen should also be sent, appropriately preserved, to a centre where *in vitro* study of the enzymes present and of the glycogen structure can be done. Classification into the actual type can then be attempted. Fibrosis or cirrhosis may develop.

A *bleeding disorder* is similar to thrombasthenia.

TREATMENT

Repeated glucose feeds are needed to prevent fasting hypoglycaemia [4]. Parenteral hyper-alimentation may be useful [2]. Dietary protein is normal and the fat content low. Allopurinol may be given for the high serum uric acid.

End-to-side porta-caval shunt diverts glucose absorbed from the digestive tract away from the liver for utilization in peripheral tissues. This operation has resulted in improved growth and bone mineralization. Hypoglycaemia, hyperlipaemia and metabolic acidosis were relieved [13], liver size lessened, but hepatic glycogen was unaffected.

PROGNOSIS

Many patients die in early childhood, often with infections. There are great variations in severity. The disease tends to become milder after puberty so that the liver becomes impalpable. Later deaths are due to gouty nephropathy or to hepato-cellular tumours. The adaptive mechanisms associated with survival are unknown.

Type II (Pompe's disease)

This primary lysosomal disease is due to deficiency of lysosomal acid alpha-1,4 glucosidase which prevents degradation of glycogen within lysosomes.

There is weakness of skeletal muscle, cardiomegaly, hepatomegaly and macroglossia. Mental development is normal. Infantile, childhood and adult onset forms exist. The infantile is the most

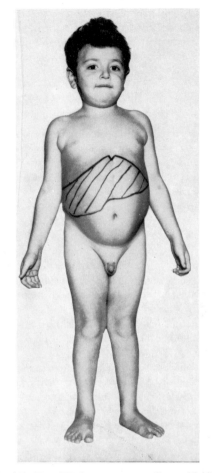

Fig. 342. Type III glycogen storage disease (Cori's disease). A boy of four years with enormous hepatomegaly but without splenomegaly.

severe. Glucagon and adrenalin tests are normal and hypoglycaemia does not occur. Hyperlipidaemia is conspicuous.

All organs show vacuolated cells due to the enlarged lysosomes which contain the glycogen [10]. Vacuolated lymphocytes are found in peripheral blood and marrow. The liver cells at autopsy show particularly prominent vacuoles.

Type III (Cori's disease)

Clinically this resembles type I glycogenosis. Acidosis, hypoglycaemia and hyperlipaemia may be present. Blood glucose does not rise after glucagon, but galactose and fructose tolerance are normal. Serum transaminases are usually increased. Symptoms may be mild and by adult life only the hepatomegaly may remain [1]. The prognosis is fair to good. Periportal fibrosis can develop.

Glycogen is increased in muscle and liver and the debranching enzyme, amylo-1,6 glucosidase, is absent.

Type IV (Andersen's disease)

This very rare form of generalized glycogenosis is associated with low normal tissue levels of glycogen. The glycogen structure is abnormal due to deficiency of the branching enzyme amylo-1,4,1,6 transglucosidase.

A cirrhosis develops which may be associated with many giant cells. It can resemble that of the alcoholic. The chief distinction is the presence of intracellular deposits of abnormal glycogen partially removed by diastase digestion. This may show abnormal staining properties turning purplish with iodine instead of the usual reddish-brown. It stains strongly with PAS. The cirrhosis is presumably due to a reaction to this abnormal glycogen. This abnormal material is found in every organ examined [12].

The child develops hepatosplenomegaly, ascites and finally liver failure. Enzyme deficiencies in skin fibroblasts have been shown and may allow diagnosis and detection of heterozygotes [5]. The features of cirrhosis are present. Death is in early childhood.

Type VI (Hers' disease)

This involves only the liver and is marked by deficiency of phosphorylase. Growth retardation and hepatomegaly are marked. Hypoglycaemia and acidosis are usually found. Mental function is normal. Survival into adult life is usual.

Variants have been described as type VIII and type XI glycogenosis [7]. Here, although phosphorylase is reduced it can be increased to normal by glucagon or adrenaline, or *in vitro* by substitution of an activation system. In these patients the low hepatic phosphorylase activity is not the result of deficiency of the enzyme.

Low molecular weight glycogen [9]

This very rare condition is associated with cirrhosis, early death and a widespread deposition in tissues, including the liver, of a polysaccharide material of low molecular weight.

Hepatic glycogen synthetase deficiency [3]

This very rare condition is associated with glucose intolerance, hypoglycaemia and mental retardation. Analysis of liver biopsy material shows complete absence of the enzyme glycogen synthetase.

REFERENCES

1. BRANDT I.K. & DE LUCA V.A. Jr (1966) Type III glycogenosis. A family with an unusual tissue distribution of the enzyme lesion. *Am. J. Med.* **40**, 779.
2. BURR I.M., O'NEILL J.A., KARZON D.T. *et al* (1974) Comparison of the effects of total parenteral nutrition, continuous intragastric feeding and portacaval shunt on a patient with type I glycogen storage disease. *J. Pediatr.* **85**, 792.
3. DYKES J.R.W. & SPENCER-PEET J. (1972) Hepatic glycogen synthetase deficiency. Further studies on a family. *Arch. Dis. Childh.* **47**, 558.
4. GREENE H.L., SLONIM A.E., O'NEILL J.A. *et al* (1976) Continuous nocturnal intragastric feeding for management of type I glycogen-storage disease. *New Engl. J. Med*, **294**, 423.
5. HOWELL R.R., KABACK M.M. & BROWN B.I. (1971) Type IV glycogen storage disease: branching enzyme deficiency in skin fibroblasts and possible heterozygote detection. *J. Pediatr.* **78**, 638.
6. HOWELL R.R., STEVENSON R.E., BEN-MENACHEM Y. *et al* (1976) Hepatic adenomata with type I glycogen storage disease. *J. Am. med. Assoc.* **236**, 1481.
7. HUG G., SCHUBERT W.K., CHUCK G. *et al* (1967) Liver phosphorylase. Deactivation in a child with progressive brain disease, increased hepatic glycogen storage disease. *J. Am. med. Assoc.* **236**, **42**, 139.
8. HUIJING F. (1975) Glycogen metabolism and glycogen-storage diseases. *Physiol. Rev.* **55**, 609.
9. KRIVIT W., SHARP H.L. & LEE J.C. (1973) Low molecular weight glycogen as a cause of generalised glycogen storage disease. *Am. J. Med.* **54**, 88.
10. MCADAMS A.J., HUG G. & BOVE K.E. (1974) Glycogen storage disease, types I to X: criteria for morphologic diagnosis. *Hum. Pathol.* **5**, 463.
11. RYMAN B.E. (1975) The glycogen storage diseases. *J. clin. Pathol.* **27**, (suppl.), vol. 8, 106.
12. SCHOCHET S.S. Jr, MCCORMICK W.F. & ZELLWEGER H. (1970) Type IV glycogenosis (amylopectinosis): light and electron microscopic observations. *Arch. Pathol.* **90**, 354.
13. STARZL T.E., PUTNAM D.W., PORTER K.A. *et al* (1973) Portal diversion for the treatment of glycogen storage in humans. *Ann. Surg.* **178**, 939.

HEREDITARY FRUCTOSE INTOLERANCE

This autosomal recessive disease is usually due to a deficiency of hepatic fructose-1-phosphate aldolase [1] and rarely to hepatic fructose-1,6-diphos-phatase deficiency [2].

It is marked by jaundice, ascites, albuminuria and amino-aciduria. Fructosaemia, fructosuria and hypophosphataemia are features. Hypogly-caemia follows fructose administration. Hepatic histology shows similar findings to a galacto-saemia with the ultimate development of cirrhosis. Treatment is by a low carbohydrate diet without sucrose and fructose.

REFERENCES

1. FROESCH E.R., WOLF H.P., BAITSCH H. *et al* (1963) Hereditary fructose intolerance: inborn defect of hepatic fructose-1-phosphate splitting aldolase. *Am. J. Med.* **34**, 151.
2. PAGLIARI A.S., KARL I.E., KEATING J.P. *et al* (1972) Hepatic fructose-1,6-diaphosphatase deficiency. *J. clin. Invest.* **51**, 2115.

GLUTARIC ACIDURIA TYPE II

This disturbance of organic acid metabolism presents in infants or adults as recurrent hypogly-caemia with elevated serum free fatty acid [1]. The liver shows fatty change, glycogen depletion and patchy necrosis.

REFERENCE

1. DUSHEIKO G., KEW M.C., JOFFE B.I. *et al* (1979) Recurrent hypoglycaemia associated with glutaric aciduria type II in an adult. *New Engl. J. Med.* **301**, 1405.

GALACTOSAEMIA

The liver and red blood cells lack the specific enzyme, galactose-1-phosphate-uridyl transferase, essential for galactose metabolism [1]. Toxic effects are related to the accumulation in the tissues of galactose-1-phosphate. The mechanism of toxicity is uncertain.

Transferase deficiency is inherited in an auto-somal, recessive manner. A significant reduction of the uridyl transferase is found in heterozygotes.

CLINICAL PICTURE

The disease starts *in utero*. The infant presents with feeding difficulties, with vomiting, diarrhoea and malnutrition, often with jaundice. Ascites and hepatosplenomegaly are noted. Cataracts de-velop. Death may result in the first few weeks, but survivors become mentally retarded and finally show the features of cirrhosis, portal hypertension and, later, ascites.

HEPATIC CHANGES [5]

Those dying in the first few weeks show diffuse hepato-cellular fatty change. In the next few months the liver shows pseudoglandular or ductular structures around the canaliculi which may contain bile. Regeneration is conspicuous, necrosis scanty and a macronodular cirrhosis results. Giant cells may be numerous.

DIAGNOSIS [4]

The biochemical changes [1] include galacto-saemia, galactosuria, hyperchloraemic acidosis, albuminuria and aminoaciduria. Diagnosis is made by finding a urinary reducing substance which is glucose oxidase negative. Definite diag-nosis comes from determining galactose-1-phos-phate uridyl transferase levels in the erythrocytes.

The condition should be considered in all young patients with cirrhosis and even in the adult if there are suggestive features such as cataract. Galacto-saemia has been diagnosed as late as 63 years [3]. A survey of a group of juvenile cirrhotics with this disease, however, failed to reveal a single case and this must be a rare cause of adult cirrhosis [2].

PROGNOSIS AND TREATMENT

Great improvement results from withdrawal of dietary milk and milk products from the diet. If the child survives to five years of age recovery may be complete apart from persistent cataracts or cir-rhosis. Those living into childhood and adult life without treatment may be only partially enzyme-deficient. Alternatively they may have developed another pathway for handling galactose [1]. The consumption of galactose-containing foods also decreases with age.

REFERENCES

1. COHN R.M. & SEGAL S. (1973) Galactose metabol-ism and its regulation. *Metabolism* **22**, 627.

2. FISHER M.M., SPEAR S., SAMOLS E. *et al* (1964)
   Erythrocytic galactose-1-phosphate uridyl transferase levels in hepatic cirrhosis. *Gut* **5**, 170.
3. HSIA D.Y.-Y. & WALKER F.A. (1961) Variability
   in the clinical manifestations of galactosaemia. *J.
   Pediatr.* **59**, 872.
4. MONK A.M., MITCHELL A.J.H., MILLIGAN
   D.W.A. *et al* (1977) The diagnosis of classical
   galactosaemia. *Arch. Dis. Childh.* **52**, 943.
5. SMETANA H.F. & OLEN E. (1962) Hereditary galactose disease. *Am. J. clin. Pathol.* **93**, 3.

MUCOPOLYSACCHARIDOSES

There are several different disorders in which various mucopolysaccharides accumulate in the
tissues.

Hurler's syndrome (gargoylism) (MPU) is the
most important. It is inherited as an autosomal
recessive and is characterized by deficiency of the
lysosomal degrading enzyme, alpha-L-iduronidase
in liver, cultured skin fibroblasts and leucocytes.
It is characterized by coarse facial features, dwarf-
ism, limitation of joint movement, deafness, abdominal hernias, hepatosplenomegaly, cardiac abnormalities and mental retardation.

The liver in the mucopolysaccharidoses is large
and firm. Fibrosis and cirrhosis may be present.
Microscopically, liver cells and Kupffer cells are
swollen, empty or vacuolated [1]. The vacuoles
consist of lysosomes containing mucopolysac-
charide. The material is demonstrated by a colloidal iron stain.

Diagnosis may be made by finding increased
urinary or WBC mucopolysaccharides. Culture of
skin biopsies shows fibroblasts containing mucopolysaccharides.

REFERENCE

1. VAN HOOF F. (1974) Mucopolysaccharidoses and
   mucolipidoses. *J. clin. Pathol.* **27** (suppl. 8), 64.

HEPATIC AMYLOIDOSIS

This waxy infiltration of the organs was termed
amyloidosis because it resembled starch in its
staining [8]. The term encompasses a number of
diseases having in common extracellular deposition of fibrillar material with typical staining properties [2]. All forms are related to over-production of a protein that can assume a fibrillar form;

Table 58. Classification of the amyloid diseases.

Type	Pathology	Protein
Primary	Pericollagen	AL
With multiple myeloma	Pericollagen	AL
Secondary	Perireticulin	AA
With familial Mediterranean fever	Perireticulin	AA

they can be termed β-fibrilloses [3]. At least six different proteins can be concerned.

The amyloidosis may be classified according to
the protein deposited (table 58). In the case of primary amyloidosis and the amyloidosis accompanying multiple myeloma the protein consists of
immunoglobulin light chains and is termed AL [3].
In the case of secondary amyloidosis and the
amyloidosis complicating familial Mediterranean
fever (FMF) the protein shares antigenicity and
structure with the acute phase protein of human
serum and is termed AA. Some of this protein
comes from polymorphs.

The mechanism of the protein over-production
is unknown. An antigenic stimulus must be concerned. If this can be removed the amyloid fibrils
may resolve. This emphasizes the importance of
searching for all chronic diseases in every patient
with amyloidosis.

The amyloid fibrils are deposited along pre-
existing fibres which may be reticulin, giving peri-
reticulin amyloidosis, or collagen, giving peri-
collagen amyloidosis [4].

Peri-reticulin amyloidosis is primarily a disease
of small blood vessels, capillaries (including
sinusoids) and small veins. Parenchymal tissue is
replaced only secondarily to the spill-over of
amyloid beyond affected capillary structures.

Peri-collagen amyloidosis affects vessels, connective tissue round vessels, the stroma of various
organs, sarcolemma and neurilemma.

Primary amyloidosis (*peri-collagen 'atypical'*). This is rare and occurs without pre-existing
disease. The liver is rarely involved by deposits in
the walls of the small hepatic arterioles in the
portal tracts. The deposits may stain poorly with
Congo red.

Amyloidosis complicating myeloma (*peri-collagen*). This occurs in about 15% of patients. The

deposits are usually in the atypical ('primary') distribution.

Familial Mediterranean fever (FMF) [4]. Although of peri-reticulin type, the hepatic sinusoids, surprisingly, are spared. Hepatic involvement is seen only in the arterioles. The glomeruli, spleen and pulmonary alveoli bear the brunt of the disease. Renal failure is fatal.

Secondary (acquired, peri-reticular). This is the commonest form, involving spleen, kidneys, liver and adrenal glands, in that order of frequency. It follows chronic diseases such as tuberculosis, pleuro-pulmonary suppuration, longstanding rheumatoid arthritis, ulcerative colitis, Crohn's disease, leprosy, some neoplasms and Hodgkin's disease. Affected organs have a firm waxy consistency and develop a deep red-brown colour on the addition of dilute iodine.

CLINICAL FEATURES OF HEPATIC INVOLVEMENT

Hepato-cellular failure and portal hypertension are rare. Jaundice is present in only about 5%. Biochemical tests are usually normal apart from a slight rise in alk. phosphatase [5]. Amyloidosis is suspected when an enlarged, smooth, non-tender liver is detected in a patient with a predisposing cause; however, occasionally the liver may not be enlarged. An enlarged spleen, infiltrated with amyloid, may be found. Intra-hepatic cholestasis may rarely complicate primary amyloidosis [7]. It is presumably due to the intense amyloid deposition interfering with bile passage into canaliculi and small bile ducts. The prognosis is very poor for the cholestatic type.

There may be a nephrotic syndrome, albuminuria or progressive renal failure.

DIAGNOSTIC METHODS

Dye absorption tests using Evans' blue and Congo red have been abandoned.

Aspiration liver biopsy is the most satisfactory technique for diagnosis. Hepatic amyloidosis is diffuse and the sampling error is negligible. The procedure is said to be dangerous, but this has been over-emphasized.

Histologically, the amyloid is shown as homogeneous, amorphous, eosinophilic material (fig. 343). It stains red with Congo red or methyl violet and reddish brown with iodine. All these reactions are transient and remain for only a few weeks.

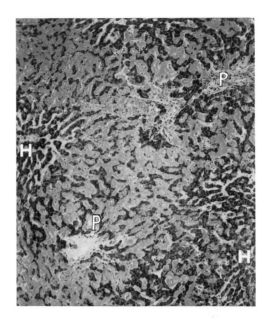

Fig. 343. Amlyoid material is deposited in the sinusoidal wall, especially in the periportal zones. The liver cell trabeculae are narrowed. H = central hepatic veins; P = portal tracts. Best's carmine, × 70.

Polarization microscopy of Congo red stained sections shows the amyloid as green birefringent fibrils [4]. Amyloid may also be shown by fluorescent microscopy.

The amyloid is deposited between the columns of liver cells and the sinusoidal wall in the space of Disse. The liver cells themselves are not involved but are compressed to a variable extent. The mid-zonal and portal areas are most heavily infiltrated.

Occasionally, in primary amyloidosis or complicating multiple myeloma, the amyloid is found only in the portal tracts in the walls of hepatic arterioles, around the interlobular arteries and lying free in clumps.

Percutaneous renal biopsy is used for the diagnosis of renal involvement.

Rectal biopsy [5] is safe and useful. The amyloid is deposited in the walls of arterioles.

Hepatic scan. Multiple filling defects simulate metastases.

PROGNOSIS

This depends on the causative condition and on the extent of the kidney involvement. Ninety per cent of patients with secondary amyloid disease are dead within two years of diagnosis, usually from the toxaemia of their chronic infection. In the few patients who live long enough, death occurs from secondarily contracted amyloid kidneys. These patients never die of liver failure.

TREATMENT

Amyloidosis is potentially a reversible condition and, if the underlying disease is controlled, amyloid may regress. If tuberculosis is cured then amyloid may disappear [9]. Similarly, clinical improvement in rheumatoid arthritis may be paralleled by disappearance of clinical signs of amyloidosis. There is no specific treatment.

The amyloid complicating multiple myeloma may remit with alkylating agents [1]. Colchicine, which blocks amyloid induction, is of value in the amyloidosis complicating FMF [6, 10].

REFERENCES

1. BUXBAUM J.N., HURLEY M.E., CHUBA J. *et al* (1979) Amyloidosis of the AL type: clinical, morphologic and biochemical aspects of the response to therapy with alkylating agents and prednisone. *Am. J. Med.* **67**, 867.
2. FRANKLIN E.C. (1979) Some unsolved problems in the amyloid diseases. *Am. J. Med.* **66**, 365.
3. GLENNER G.G. (1980) Medical progress: amyloid deposits and amyloidosis. The β-fibrilloses. *New Engl. J. Med.* **302**, 1283.
4. HELLER H., MISSMAHL H.-P., SOHAR E. *et al* (1964) Amyloidosis: its differentiation into perireticulin and peri-collagen types. *J. Path. Bact.* **88**, 15.
5. KYLE R.A. & BAYRD E.D. (1975) Amyloidosis: review of 236 cases. *Medicine (Baltimore)* **54**, 271.
6. RAVID M., ROBSON M. & KEDAR I. (1977) Prolonged colchicine treatment in four patients with amyloidosis. *Ann. intern. Med.* **87**, 568.
7. RUBINOW A., KOFF R.S. & COHEN A.S. (1978) Severe intrahepatic cholestasis in primary amyloidosis: a report of four cases and a review of the literature. *Am. J. Med.* **64**, 937.
8. VIRCHOW R. (1855) Über den Gang der Amyloiden Degeneration. *Virchows Archiv.* **8**, 364.
9. WALDENSTRÖM H. (1928) On the formation and disappearance of amyloid in man. *Acta chir. Scand.* **63**, 479.
10. ZEMER D., REVACH M., PRAS M. *et al* (1974) A controlled trial of colchicine in preventing attacks of familial Mediterranean fever. *New Engl. J. Med.* **291**, 932.

α_1 ANTI-TRYPSIN DEFICIENCY [7]

α_1 anti-trypsin is synthesized in the rough endoplasmic reticulum of the liver. It comprises 80–90% of the serum α_1 globulin and is an inhibitor of trypsin and other proteases *in vitro*.

Its genetic control is by a single autosomal dominant gene responsible for 24 different alleles distinguished by starch gel electrophoresis. These are labelled alphabetically. Pi (protease inhibitor) M is the predominant normal type and the serum α_1 anti-trypsin value is 200–400 mg/dl. Genetic deficiency with liver disease is seen in the PiZZ and Pi-nul phenotypes and their serum α_1 anti-trypsin value is 20–160 mg/dl or even 0 in the Pi-nul phenotype. Intermediate phenotypes PiSZ, PiMZ, and PiMS exist.

PATHOGENESIS OF LIVER DISEASE

This is uncertain. The glycoprotein may have a protective function in tissues, inhibiting many proteolytic enzymes. When α_1 trypsin is deficient, these enzymes may produce more tissue damage. The liver damage, however, is unrelated to the deposition of α_1 trypsin in the liver. An additional factor has been postulated in those suffering liver damage. This might control protease/antiprotease balance in tissues.

CLINICAL PICTURE

Patients with only 10% of serum α_1 anti-trypsin may remain well throughout life, or can develop pulmonary emphysema.

Many present with hepatitic-cholestatic jaundice of variable severity in the first four months of life [9]. This may be fatal, but usually subsides by about the age of six or seven months, leaving hepatomegaly. A period of relative well being is followed, in childhood and early adult life, by cirrhosis and its complications [5]. The patient may present as a problem of portal hypertension or ascites. Cirrhosis may remain compensated for many years.

The condition is rare in adults. In an adult liver clinic, only five homozygotes (ZZ phenotype), α_1 anti-trypsin deficient patients, were found in 469 patients with chronic liver disease and all five gave a history of neonatal jaundice [3].

Rarely, both pulmonary and hepatic disease affect the same patient [1, 4, 5, 7].

Cirrhosis has also been reported in adults with partial α_1 anti-trypsin deficiency of SZ phenotype [2, 10].

Primary liver cancer may be a complication [8].

The acute picture is of neonatal hepatitis except that giant cells are not prominent. After 12 weeks, intracellular inclusions staining brilliantly with PAS are seen in periportal liver cells (see fig. 344 in colour section) [6]. The liver contains increased amounts of copper.

Electron microscopy discloses clumps of protein in dilated rough endoplasmic reticulum. These fluoresce when exposed to an antibody against α_1 anti-trypsin [1].

DIAGNOSIS

The condition should be suspected with neonatal jaundice. It should also be considered in any patient with cirrhosis, whatever the age, particularly with a past history of infantile liver disease or with associated chest infections.

It may be suggested by absence of α_1 globulin on serum protein electrophoresis. Confirmation comes by measuring serum α_1 anti-trypsin. The exact phenotype should be determined by starch gel electrophoresis.

TREATMENT

Unfortunately there is no specific treatment. Phenobarbital and corticosteroids have no effect. Ultimately liver transplantation may be the treatment of choice.

REFERENCES

1. COHEN K.L., RUBIN P.E., ECHEVARRIA R.E. *et al* (1973) Alpha$_1$-antitrypsin deficiency, emphysema and cirrhosis in an adult. *Ann. intern. Med.* **78**, 227.
2. CRAIG J.R., DUNN A.E.G. & PETERS R.L. (1975) Cirrhosis associated with partial deficiency of alpha-1-antitrypsin: a clinical and autopsy study. *Hum. Pathol.* **6**, 113.
3. FISHER R.L., TAYLOR L. & SHERLOCK S. (1976) α-1-antitrypsin deficiency in liver disease: the extent of the problem. *Gastroenterology* **71**, 646.
4. GANROT P.O., LAURELL C.-B. & ERIKSSON S. (1967) Obstructive lung disease and trypsin inhibitors in alpha-1-antitrypsin deficiency. *Scand. J. clin. lab. Invest.* **19**, 205.
5. GLASGOW J.F.T., LYNCH M.J., HERCZ A. *et al* (1973) Alpha$_1$ antitrypsin deficiency in association with both cirrhosis and chronic obstructive lung disease in two sibs. *Am. J. Med.* **54**, 181.
6. JEPPSSON J-O., LARSSON C. & ERIKSSON S. (1975) Characterisation of α_1-antitrypsin in the inclusion bodies from the liver in α_1-antitrypsin deficiency. *New Engl. J. Med.* **293**, 576.
7. SHARP H.L. (1976) The current status of α-1-antitrypsin, a protease inhibitor, in gastrointestinal disease. *Gastroenterology* **70**, 611.
8. SHARP H.L., BRIDGES R.A., KRIVIT W. *et al* (1969) Cirrhosis associated with alpha-1-antitrypsin deficiency: a previously unrecognised inherited disorder. *J. lab. clin. Med.* **73**, 934.
9. SVEGER T. (1976) Liver disease in alpha$_1$-antitrypsin deficiency detected by screening of 200,000 infants. *New Engl. J. Med.* **294**, 1316.
10. TRIGER D.R., MILLWARD-SADLER G.H., CZAYKOWSKI A.A. *et al* (1976) Alpha-1-antitrypsin deficiency and liver disease in adults. *Q. J. Med.* **451**, 351.

HEREDITARY TYROSINAEMIA

This autosomal recessive disorder is due to lack of the enzyme *p*-hydroxyphenyl pyruvate hydroxylase, but this is probably not the only defect [1].

It is characterized by cirrhosis, severe hypophosphataemic rickets, renal tubular defects and a derangement of tyrosine metabolism with hyperaminoacidaemia. Patients with the acute type usually die in spite of restricting dietary tyrosine; the chronic will respond to this treatment.

REFERENCE

1. CARSON N.A.J., BIGGART J.D., BITTLES A.H. *et al* (1976) Hereditary tyrosinaemia: clinical, enzymatic and pathological study of an infant with the acute form of the disease. *Arch. Dis. Childh.* **51**, 106.

CYSTIC FIBROSIS OF THE PANCREAS

Fatty change is the commonest abnormality associated with this generalized disorder of mucus secretion. This is analogous to the steatosis reported in experimental or human pancreatectomy.

In about half the patients a more characteristic liver lesion is seen. Dilated intra-hepatic bile ducts are obstructed by eosinophilic material producing a focal biliary fibrosis [1]. This may rarely increase so that many hepatic lobules are stranded in fibrous tissue and a coarse cirrhosis is found. The biliary obstruction is presumably produced in similar fashion to that in the pancreatic ducts. Cholestasis varies from place to place. Gall bladder abnormalities include atrophy and gall-stones.

Post-natal jaundice is often associated with meconium ileus.

Clinical features of cirrhosis rarely become apparent until the pulmonary and pancreatic diseases have been overt for many years.

The cirrhosis is usually clinically silent but may cause portal hypertension requiring surgical treatment.

Portal systemic shunting is generally well tolerated [2, 3]. The prognosis seems to be determined by the respiratory state rather than the liver.

REFERENCES

1. BODIAN M. (1952) *Fibrocytic Disease of the Pancreas*, p. 104. Heinemann, London.
2. SCHUSTER S.R., SHWACHMAN H., TOYAMA W.M. *et al* (1977) The management of portal hypertension in cystic fibrosis. *J. pediatr. Surg.* **12**, 201.
3. STERN R.C., STEVENS D.P., BOAT T.F. *et al* (1976) Symptomatic hepatic disease in cystic fibrosis: incidence, course and outcome of portal systemic shunting. *Gastroenterology* **70**, 654.

LIVER AND THYROID

The liver metabolizes thyroxine by oxidative deamination, deiodination, conjugation and finally biliary excretion. There is an entero-hepatic circulation, but only about 3% thyroxine is reabsorbed [6].

The liver contains 35% of the body's exchangeable thyroxine (T4), and 5% of the triiodothyronine (T3)—there is a ready exchange with the bound hormone in plasma. The liver converts T4 to T3. Reversed T3 (rT3) is probably produced in extra-hepatic tissues [9]. The liver also produces thyroxine-binding globulin.

Thyrotoxicosis

Jaundice in thyrotoxic patients may be due to heart failure. Thyrotoxicosis may also aggravate an underlying defect in serum bilirubin metabolism, such as Gilbert's syndrome. This may account for some instances of jaundice in thyrotoxics who are not in heart failure and who have a normal liver biopsy [3].

Hepatic blood flow in hyperthyroidism is little

if at all increased in spite of an increased cardiac output [7]. The increased hepatic metabolism, however, is reflected in an increased hepatic oxygen consumption which is elevated even more than the general metabolic rate.

CHANGES IN HEPATO-CELLULAR DISEASE

Most patients with liver disease are clinically euthyroid although standard function tests may give misleading results [2]. The radio-iodine uptake may be abnormally low. Serum total T4 may be raised or decreased in association with varying levels of thyroid hormone binding proteins. Estimation of the free thyroxine index is usually normal.

In *alcoholic liver disease* raised serum levels of thyrotrophin (TSH) and free T4 are associated with normal or low T3 values [9]. The conversion of T4 to T3 is reduced. This suggests a compensatory increase in TSH in response to relative T3 deficiency. The total and free T3 levels are reduced in proportion to the degree of liver damage [2]. Plasma rT3 levels are high.

In *primary biliary cirrhosis and chronic active hepatitis* thyroxine-binding globulins are increased and these may be markers of inflammatory activity [10]. Although average total T4 and T3 would be increased, the corresponding free hormone concentrations are reduced probably because of decreased thyroid function associated with the high incidence of auto-immune thyroiditis in these patients.

Liver biopsy is normal in those not in congestive failure [5]. Electron microscopy [4] shows enlarged mitochondria, hypertrophied smooth endoplasmic reticulum and decreased glycogen.

Analysis of the biopsy shows reduced cell protein and an increased phosphoglycerate reflecting increased glycolysis [8].

There is no evidence that thyroid excess produces significant hepatic functional and structural changes in an otherwise normal liver.

Myxoedema

Ascites without congestive heart failure in patients with myxoedema has been attributed to centrizonal congestion and fibrosis [1]. The pathogenesis is unknown. It disappears on giving thyroid.

Jaundice may be related to neonatal thyroid deficiency.

REFERENCES

1. BAKER A., KAPLAN M. & WOLFE H. (1972) Central congestive fibrosis of the liver in myxedema ascites. *Ann. intern. Med.* **77**, 927.
2. CHOPRA I.J., SOLOMON D.H., CHOPRA U. *et al* (1974 Alterations in circulating thyroid hormones and thyrotropin in hepatic cirrhosis: evidence for euthyroidism despite subnormal serum triiodothyronine. *J. clin. Endocrinol. Metabol.* **39**, 501.
3. GREENBERGER N.J., MILLIGAN F.D., DEE GROOT L.J. *et al* (1964) Jaundice and thyrotoxicosis in the absence of congestive heart failure. *Am. J. Med.* **36**, 840.
4. KLION F.M., SEGAL R. & SCHAFFNER F. (1971) The effect of altered thyroid function on the ultrastructure of the human liver. *Am. J. Med.* **50**, 317.
5. MOVITT E.R., GERSTL B. & DAVIS A.E. (1953) Needle liver biopsy in thyrotoxicosis. *Arch. intern. Med.* **91**, 729.
6. MYANT N.B. (1956) Enterohepatic circulation of thyroxine in humans. *Clin. Sci.* **15**, 550.
7. MYERS J.D., BRANNON E.S. & HOLLAND B.C. (1950) A correlative study of the cardiac output and the hepatic circulation in hyperthyroidism. *J. clin. Invest.* **29**, 1069.
8. NIKKILÄ E.A. & PITKÄNEN E. (1959) Liver enzyme pattern in thyrotoxicosis. Determination of 14 enzymes in samples removed by needle biopsy. *Acta endocrinol. (Kbh)* **31**, 573.
9. NOMURA S., PITTMAN C.S., CHAMBERS J.B. Jr *et al* (1975) Reduced peripheral conversion of thyroxine to triiodothyronine in patients with hepatic cirrhosis. *J. clin. Invest.* **56**, 643.
10. SCHUSSLER G.C., SCHAFFNER F. & KORN F. (1978) Increased serum thyroid hormone binding and decreased free hormone in chronic active liver disease. *New Engl. J. Med.* **299**, 510.

LIVER AND GROWTH HORMONE

The liver and kidneys degrade growth hormone. Patients with cirrhosis have raised peripheral growth hormone levels [3]. Serum somatomedins are produced by the liver and values are low in cirrhosis [2]. In spite of the chronic elevation of peripheral growth hormones acromegaly does not develop.

In acromegaly the liver enlarges in line with other viscera. The splanchnic blood flow is normal so that tissue perfusion must be reduced relative to the increment in hepatic mass [1].

REFERENCES

1. PREISIG R., MORRIS T.Q., SHAVER J.C. *et al* (1966) Volumetric, hemodynamic and excretory characteristics of the liver in acromegaly. *J. clin. Invest.* **65**, 1379.
2. TAKANO K., HIZUKA N., SHIZUME K. *et al* (1977) Serum somatomedin peptides measured by somatomedin A radioreceptor assay in chronic liver disease. *J. clin. Endocrinol. Metabol.* **45**, 828.
3. ZANOBONI A. & ZANOBONI-MUCIACCIA W. (1977) Elevated basal growth hormone levels and growth hormone response to TRH in alcoholic patients with cirrhosis. *J. clin. Endocrinol. Metabol.* **45**, 576.

HEPATIC PORPHYRIAS

Hepatic porphyrias are disorders associated with abnormalities in the biosynthesis of haem (fig. 345) [1, 3, 8]. Three are inherited as dominants: acute intermittent porphyria, hereditary coproporphyria and variegate porphyria. All are marked by neuropsychiatric attacks with vomiting, abdominal colic, constipation and peripheral neuropathy. All are exacerbated by drugs such as barbiturates, sulphonamides, oestrogens, oral contraceptives, griseofulvin, chloroquine and possibly alcohol. These induce the enzymes concerned in haem biosynthesis. During the attacks, large amounts of the colourless porphyrin precursors, porphobilinogen and delta aminolaevulinic acid (ALA), are

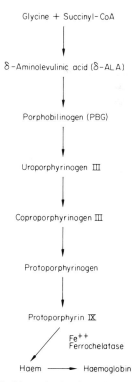

Fig. 345. The biosynthesis of porphyrins.

excreted in the urine. In all three, an acute attack is treated by glucose loading. Infusions of haematin which regress or inhibit hepatic ALA synthetase may be valuable in the acute attack [2].

The fourth type, porphyria cutanea tarda, is probably hereditary and may be associated with actual hepato-cellular disease. It is not exacerbated by barbiturates and acute attacks are not seen.

ACUTE INTERMITTENT PORPHYRIA

The basic deficiency is in hepatic uroporphyrinogen I synthetase. A diagnostic deficiency may be shown in red cells. The enzyme delta aminolaevulinic acid-synthetase (ALA-S) is secondarily induced in the liver through a negative-feedback mechanism by haem.

Photosensitivity is absent. The urine darkens on standing and gives a positive Ehrlich test. It contains slight increases in ALA-S and porphobilinogen. Latent cases develop acute attacks on various drugs and in later stages of pregnancy.

HEREDITARY COPROPORPHYRIA

The deficiency is in coproporphyrinogen oxidase. Attacks are similar to those of other hepatic porphyrias. ALA-S activity is increased in the liver. Faecal and urinary coproporphyrin are increased with a corresponding increase in protoporphyrin.

PORPHYRIA VARIEGATA

The defect is in protoporphyrinogen oxidase. ALA-S is increased in the liver. This variant is frequently encountered in South Africa. The features are intermediate between acute intermittent porphyria and hereditary coproporphyria. Protoporphyrin is increased in the stools at all times.

PORPHYRIA CUTANEA TARDA

The deficiency is in uroporphyrinogen decarboxylase [7]. Alcoholism is a common association and a precipitating factor and so is sex hormone treatment. It may be a toxic effect of chlorinated hydrocarbons. Sensitivity to drugs such as barbiturates is absent.

It is characterized clinically by photosensitive skin, blistering and scarring, pigmentation and hypertrichosis. Acute attacks are absent. There is usually evidence of liver dysfunction. Uroporphyrin is increased in the urine.

Liver biopsy shows sub-acute hepatitis or cirrhosis and iron overload. Uroporphyrin can be shown by red fluorescence in ultraviolet light.

Exacerbation of symptoms accompanies deterioration of liver function. At this time, porphyrins which would normally be excreted into the bile may be directed via the kidneys to the urine. Where the liver is healthy, the porphyrin is excreted harmlessly into the bile; when it is diseased, it is retained in the blood. The porphyria itself may be hepato-toxic.

Chloroquine causes an exacerbation which may be followed by a remission of a few months [4].

Venesection has a good effect probably related to removal of excess iron. About six months is taken to clinical remission and 13 months to biochemical remission [5].

ERYTHROPOIETIC PROTOPORPHYRIA

The defect is in haem synthetase. The inheritance is dominant. Protoporphyrin is increased in tissues and urine.

This type is characterized by skin photosensitivity. Protoporphyrin is increased in tissues and urine, perhaps secondary to abnormalities in haem synthesis.

The liver may be the major site of the protoporphyrin. Liver biopsies examined by fluorescent microscopy or phase microscopy [6] show focal deposits of pigment containing protoporphyrin. Complications include gall-stones containing protoporphyrin.

Deaths have been reported in liver failure [9, 10]. These are presumably related to accumulation of the protoporphyrin within the liver cell.

SECONDARY COPROPORPHYRIAS

Heavy metal intoxication, especially with lead, causes porphyria with ALA-S and coproporphyrin in the urine. Erythrocyte protoporphyrins are increased. Coproporphyrin may also be seen with sideroblastic anaemia, various liver diseases, the Dubin–Johnson syndrome and the complications of drug therapy.

A patient has been described with an *hepatic adenoma* who developed photosensitivity with skin blisters and showed uroporphyrin and coproporphyrin in the urine [11]. Family history was negative. The tumour was removed and contained con-

siderable quantities of proto-, copro- and uroporphyrin. Post-operatively the skin lesions disappeared and the urinary excretion of porphyrins
returned to normal.

REFERENCES

1. BLOOMER J.R. (1976) The hepatic porphyrias:
   pathogenesis, manifestations and management.
   Gastroenterology **71**, 689.
2. DHAR G.J., BOSSENMAIER I., PETRYKA Z.J. *et al*
   (1975) Effects of hematin in hepatic porphyria:
   further studies. *Ann. intern. Med.* **83**, 20.
3. DOSS M. (ed.) (1977) *Diagnosis and Therapy of Porphyrin and Lead Intoxication.* Springer, Berlin.
4. FELSHER B.F. & REDEKER A.G. (1966) Effect of
   chloroquine on hepatic uroporphyrin metabolism
   in patients with porphyria cutanea tarda. *Medicine
   (Baltimore)* **45**, 575.
5. GROSSMAN M.E., BICKERS D.R., POH-FITZPATRICK
   M.B. *et al* (1979) Porphyria cutanea tarda: clinical
   features and laboratory findings in 20 patients. *Am.
   J. Med.* **67**, 277.
6. KLATSKIN G. & BLOOMER J.R. (1974) Birefringence
   of hepatic pigment deposits in erythropoietic protoporphyria. Specificity of polarization microscopy in the identification of hepatic protoporphyrin deposits. *Gastroenterology* **67**, 294.
7. KUSHNER J.P., BARBUTO A.J. & LEE G.R. (1976)
   An inherited enzymatic defect in porphyria
   cutanea tarda: decreased uroporphyrinogen decarboxylase activity. *J. clin. Invest.* **58**, 1089.
8. MEYER U.A. & SCHMID R. (1978) The porphyrias.
   In *The Metabolic Basis of Interited Disease*, 4th
   edn, p. 1166, eds J.B. Stanbury, J.B. Wyngarden
   & D.S. Frederickson. McGraw-Hill, New York.
9. SCOTT A.J., ANSFORD A.J., WEBSTER B.H. *et al*
   (1973) Erythropoietic protoporphyria with
   features of a sideroblastic anaemia terminating in
   liver failure. *Am. J. Med.* **54**, 251.
10. SINGER J.A., PLAUT A.G. & KAPLAN M.M. (1978)
    Hepatic failure and death from erythropoietic pro-
    toporphyria. *Gastroenterology* **74**, 588.
11. TIO TIONG HOO, LEIJNSE B., JARRETT A. *et al* (1957)
    Acquired porphyria from a liver tumour. *Clin. Sci.*
    16, 517.

HEREDITARY HAEMORRHAGIC
TELANGIECTASIA

Hepatomegaly is a common feature of this disease.
The liver may show telangiectasia and cirrhosis.
Bands of fibrous tissue surrounding the regenerative nodules contain numerous thin-walled telangiectases (see fig. 346 in colour section) [2]. Benign
fibro-vascular lesions are always suggestive [1]. It
has been suggested that the telangiectases interfere
with the nutrition of liver cells [2].

Occasionally large intra-hepatic arteriovenous
aneurysms lead to portal hypertension, haemorrhage from varices and high output heart failure.

REFERENCES

1. DALY J.J. & SCHILLER A.L. (1976) The liver in
   hereditary haemorrhagic telangiectasia (Osler–
   Weber–Rendu disease). *Am. J. Med.* **60**, 723.
2. MARTIN G.A. (1955) Lebercirrhöse bei Morbus
   Osler, Cirrhosis hepatis teleangiectatica. *Gastroen-
   terologia, Basel* **73**, 157.

Chapter 23
The Liver in Infancy and Childhood

Biochemical tests in infancy

Serum bilirubin levels are a guide to the development of kernicterus. Serial levels are useful in the assessment of prolonged jaundice. Fractionation allows the important differentiation into unconjugated and conjugated hyperbilirubinaemia. This is particularly important in the neonatal period [62, 93].

Serum cholesterol. Extremely high levels may be recorded in prolonged cholestasis, particularly intra-hepatic.

Serum alkaline phosphatase levels are influenced by bone metabolism as well as by cholestasis. Levels are increased in the first month of life as well as around puberty.

Serum 5 nucleotidase or gamma glutamyl transpeptidase levels may be estimated if there is doubt concerning the origin of a raised serum alkaline phosphatase level.

Serum transaminase values are about twice the normal adult level during the first month of life.

Bile acid metabolism. Bile acid secretion appears to be an evolving immature function during the final trimester of pregnancy and in the early neonatal period [58]. In the newborn, pool size, synthesis rate and duodenal concentration are at levels below those of the adult, especially in low-birth-weight infants [96]. Plasma bile acid concentrations are higher than in adults [89]. Newborns therefore seem to be subject to 'physiological' cholestasis related to immaturity of bile acid metabolism and turnover. This is somewhat analogous to physiological hyperbilirubinaemia. Certain syndromes of neonatal cholestasis may be an exaggeration of normal developmental deficiencies [55].

Circulatory factors and hepatic necrosis

At the time of birth, the left lobe of the liver, deprived of its highly oxygenated placental blood supply, receives instead poorly oxygenated portal blood [29]. This can lead to atrophy of the left lobe.

Right-sided hepatic necrosis may be seen in post-mature infants dying about the time of birth [18]. This is related to poor placental blood supply and anoxia at the time of delivery.

Disseminated mid-zonal necrosis is found with congenital cardiac defects [86]. This may be due to decrease in total hepatic blood flow. In others the centrizonal changes of congestive heart failure may be seen.

Localized necrosis of the liver may be due to trapping in defects of the anterior abdominal wall.

NEONATAL JAUNDICE

A simple classification is made into those cases where the increase in serum bilirubin is predominantly unconjugated (total serum bilirubin > 3.0 mg with less than 30% direct reacting), and those where the increase is in the conjugated fraction [62, 93] (tables 59, 60).

Unconjugated hyperbilirubinaemia (table 59)

This is common in the newborn [99]. The development of hepatic conjugating and transport systems for bilirubin is delayed in the neonate. Factors which further depress hepatic function or add to the load of bilirubin on the liver lead to marked hyperbilirubinaemia. In the neonatal period this is complicated by the development of bilirubin encephalopathy (*kernicterus*).

'Physiological' and prematurity jaundice

Jaundice, reaching its peak within two to five days of delivery and disappearing in two weeks, is common in normal infants. It is more serious in prematures when it is liable to be complicated by kernicterus. The urine contains both urobilin and bilirubin and the stools are paler than normal. Serum

Table 59. Unconjugated hyperbilirubinaemia in neonates related to onset.

Birth to 2 days
  haemolytic disease

3–7 days
  physiological ± prematurity
                hypoxia
                acidosis

1–8 weeks
  congenital haemolytic disorders
  breast milk jaundice
  Lucey–Driscoll
  Crigler–Najjar
  hypothyroidism
  perinatal complications: haemorrhage, sepsis
  upper gastro-intestinal obstruction

unconjugated bilirubin is moderately or markedly raised.

The cause is multi-factorial. Haemolysis of surplus erythrocytes, relative deficiency of hepatic bilirubin conjugating enzymes and increased absorption of bilirubin from the intestines [76] are important. The hyperbilirubinaemia is enhanced by hypoxia and hypoglycaemia. Drugs such as water-soluble vitamin K analogues add to the jaundice [60]. Induction of labour with oxytocin increases unconjugated serum bilirubin levels slightly. This may be due to the oxytocin affecting the erythrocyte so that it is more rapidly destroyed [12]. The increase in bilirubin is insignificant if low doses of oxytocin are used [99].

MANAGEMENT

Phototherapy. Hyperbilirubinaemia may be prevented or controlled by exposure of the infant to light of wavelength near 450 nm [74]. This is probably due to the light converting bilirubin IX alpha photochemically to a relatively stable geometric isomer [100]. Side-effects include increased insensible water loss, haemolysis and bronzing of the skin [53]. The eyes must be protected.

Light exposure is not necessary as a routine for all neonatal units, but is of value in selected cases [15]. It is also useful in the Crigler–Najjar syndrome.

Exchange transfusion is given if the serum bilirubin level is 340 mmol/l (20 mg/dl). It is rarely necessary with the advent of phototherapy.

Enzyme induction, using phenobarbitone, is effective when given to the mother [64]. Anti-

pyrine similarly reduces infantile serum bilirubin levels but without causing drowsiness [56].

Haemolytic disease of the newborn

Antigens in foetal red cells may provoke the development of maternal antibodies which, passing into the foetal circulation, lead to haemolysis of foetal red blood corpuscles. The incompatibility usually concerns the rhesus blood factors and rarely the ABO or other blood groups.

Characteristically, the firstborn escapes the disease unless the mother's blood has been sensitized by a previous transfusion of Rh-positive blood. A normal first pregnancy sensitizes the mother's blood sufficiently to provoke haemolytic disease in subsequent infants. The clinical forms of the disease vary in severity, but the underlying pathological lesions are essentially similar.

The infant is jaundiced during the first two days of life. Serum unconjugated bilirubin is increased. Urine contains bilirubin and urobilinogen. The critical period occurs in the first few days when the more deeply jaundiced infants may develop *kernicterus*.

Diagnosis may be suspected by antenatal examination of the mother's blood for specific antibodies and confirmed by a positive Coombs' test in the infant and by blood-typing on mother and child.

KERNICTERUS (BILIRUBIN
ENCEPHALOPATHY) [21]

This grave condition is a complication of prematurity jaundice and of haemolytic disease. It can complicate neonatal hepatitis.

Within the first five days of life, the jaundiced infant becomes restless or lethargic and febrile, developing a stiff neck and head retraction which proceeds to opisthotonus. There is stiffness of the limbs with pronated arms, eye squinting, lid retraction, twitching or convulsions and a high-pitched cry.

Death may supervene rapidly in 12 hours and 70% of affected infants die within seven days of the onset. The remaining 30% may survive, but are maimed by mental defect, cerebral palsy or athetosis, unless they eventually die from intercurrent infections.

Autopsy reveals yellow staining of the basal ganglia predominantly and also of other areas of the brain and spinal cord with unconjugated bilirubin which, being lipid-soluble, has an affinity for nervous tissue. Unconjugated bilirubin is able to disturb cerebral metabolism.

The development of kernicterus is related to circulating unbound bilirubin crossing the blood–brain barrier. Bilirubin is bound by serum albumin, a reduction of which potentiates kernicterus by allowing more unbound bilirubin to enter the brain. Infusions of albumin have been used therapeutically. These lower cerebral bilirubin concentrations although the serum levels rise [22]. Any organic anion which competes for bilirubin binding sites on albumin will increase kernicterus although the serum bilirubin level falls [43]. Such anions include salicylates, sulphonamides, free fatty acids and haematin. Kernicterus is seen in the neonate but not in the adult. This has led to the concept of immaturity of the blood–brain barrier but this has never been proved [21].

CONGENITAL HAEMOLYTIC DISORDERS

These can all lead to unconjugated hyperbilirubinaemia in the first two days of life. They include the red cell enzyme deficiencies—glucose 6PD and pyruvate kinase, congenital spherocytosis and pyknocytosis.

Glucose-6-phosphate dehydrogenase. Infants having a deficit of this enzyme in their erythrocytes may develop jaundice, usually on the second or third day of life. The precipitating haemolytic agent may be a drug such as salicylate, phenacetin, or sulphonamides transmitted in the maternal breast milk. This condition is frequent in the Mediterranean area [25], in the Far East and in Nigeria [13].

BREAST MILK JAUNDICE

This form of unconjugated neonatal hyperbilirubinaemia affects about 1% of breast-fed babies on the sixth to eighth day and to a varying degree. The condition lasts from two weeks to more than two months after delivery. It disappears when breast feeding is stopped and resumption increases the jaundice. Kernicterus does not develop. Not every sibling is affected.

It has been attributed to a substance in breast milk which inhibits bilirubin conjugation [6, 36]. Increased free fatty acids in breast milk inhibiting

bilirubin conjugation has also been suggested [41].

TRANSIENT FAMILIAL HYPERBILIRUBINAEMIA (Lucey–Driscoll type) [7, 59]

This appears in the first few days of life and persists to the second or third week. It affects every sibling. It is believed to be due to an inhibitor of bilirubin conjugation present in maternal and infantile serum.

CRIGLER–NAJJAR HYPERBILIRUBINAEMIA (Chapter 13)

This may present in the first few days of life.

HYPOTHYROIDISM [61]

This is three times more common in girls than boys. Mild anaemia is common and the infant is sluggish. The diagnosis is confirmed by finding low serum thyroxine and triiodothyronine levels with high thyroid stimulating hormone and by observing the effects of therapy. The mechanism of the jaundice is unknown.

PERINATAL COMPLICATIONS

Haemorrhage with release of blood into the tissues provides a bilirubin load which may exacerbate jaundice, particularly in the premature. Anaemia depresses hepato-cellular function. Cephalohaematoma is a common association. The prothrombin time should be measured and vitamin K given.

Sepsis, whether umbilical or elsewhere, leads to unconjugated hyperbilirubinaemia in the first few days of life. Blood, urine and, if necessary, cerebro-spinal fluid are cultured and appropriate antibodies given.

UPPER GASTRO-INTESTINAL OBSTRUCTION [32]

About 10% of infants with congenital pyloric stenosis are jaundiced due to unconjugated bilirubin. The mechanism may be similar to that postulated for the increase in jaundice when patients with Gilbert's syndrome are fasted (fig. 180).

HEPATITIS AND CHOLESTATIC SYNDROMES (CONJUGATED HYPERBILIRUBINAEMIA)

The reaction of the neonatal liver to different insults is similar. Proliferation of giant cells is always a part and this reflects an increased regenerative ability. In some instances the condition may be the so-called 'idiopathic' hepatitis formerly called giant cell hepatitis. In others a specific virus such as type B hepatitis or another infection can be identified. Metabolic disturbances, such as galactosaemia, can cause a giant cell reaction. Cholestatic syndromes are also seen which may be associated with hepatitis and, in these, hepatic histology may include a giant cell reaction. In all these conditions the conjugated 'direct reacting' bilirubin is more than 30% of the total (table 60).

It is extremely important to recognize those that are immediately treatable, such as congenital syphilis or bacterial infections—which will respond to antibiotics, and galactosaemia or tyrosinosis—which will require exclusion diets. Later the main bile duct atresias, which might benefit from surgical treatment, must be recognized.

Diagnosis of the hepatitic–cholestatic syndromes

Family history is important in diagnosing galactosaemia, α_1 anti-trypsin deficiency, tyrosinosis, cystic fibrosis and hereditary fructose intolerance.

Virus infections in the mother during pregnancy, such as rubella, hepatitis, or genital herpes, must be recorded.

At the onset it is valuable to test the blood of mother, father and other siblings by appropriate methods and to store the sera for later use. The *routine biochemical tests* of the adult are of little value in the diagnosis of jaundice in infancy and childhood. A serum alkaline phosphatase level three times normal and a serum cholesterol value exceeding 250 mg/100 ml suggest intra-hepatic biliary atresia. A direct reacting bilirubin value exceeding 4 mg (68 mmol) suggests extra-hepatic biliary obstruction.

Serum tyrosine is measured if tyrosinosis is suspected and serum α_1 anti-trypsin values noted for the diagnosis of α_1 anti-trypsin deficiency.

The use of *biliary isotopic scanning agents* (HIDA, Pipida) establishes patency of the main bile passages. These techniques have replaced the use of ^{131}I Rose Bengal for this purpose.

Table 60. Conjugated hyperbilirubinaemia in neonates.

Infection
  viruses (CMV rubella, coxsackie, herpes, hepatitis B) (Chapter 15)
  syphilis
  bacteria (*E. coli*)

Metabolic (Chapter 22)
  galactosaemia
  α_1 anti-trypsin deficiency
  tyrosinosis
  cystic fibrosis
  hereditary fructose intolerance
  total parenteral nutrition

Idiopathic
  'neonatal' hepatitis
  congenital hepatic fibrosis
  Byler's disease

Biliary atresia
  intra-hepatic
  extra-heptatic
Erythroblastosis with cholestasis

Serological methods. The serum is tested for HBsAg and for syphilis. Antibodies to herpes simplex, rubella, toxoplasma, cytomegala and adenovirus and Coxsackie viruses are estimated in both baby and mother. There are clinical manifestations of disseminated disease. Blood cultures are performed if *E. coli* infection is suspected.

Urine tests. Cultures are taken for Gram-negative organisms and for cytomegala infection. Amino-aciduria is noted. Reducing substances are sought if galactosaemia is suspected.

Liver biopsy. This is usually delayed until the age of three months so that some of the immediate neonatal changes in the liver, such as giant cells and extramedullary erythropoiesis, will have subsided.

Needle biopsy of the liver is easy and well tolerated in neonates, infants and in children. Interpretation of the histological appearances is always difficult due to the overlap between hepatitis and cholestatic syndromes, both of intra-hepatic and extra-hepatic origin.

Portal zone duct proliferation [11] and a biliary type of fibrosis are helpful in diagnosing extra-hepatic atresia. A relative paucity of portal zone bile ducts supports the diagnosis of intra-hepatic cholestasis but is not constant.

The PAS positive bodies of α_1 anti-trypsin deficiency may be seen after 12 weeks.

Ultrasonography. This is of special value in the diagnosis of choledochal cyst.

Percutaneous and endoscopic cholangiography. The percutaneous technique is of great value when liver biopsy findings are equivocal and the HIDA test suggests biliary atresia [35, 46]. Endoscopic cholangiography is rarely employed, largely due to the lack of suitably sized instruments.

Virus hepatitis

In the neonatal period, immunity, particularly cell-based, is reduced and virus hepatitis is frequent. The infection is very liable to persist and chronic hepatitis and cirrhosis ensue. Similarly, older children with immunological deficits such as agammaglobulinaemia or those receiving treatment with immuno-suppressive drugs for such conditions as leukaemia or nephritis may develop a virus infection which tends to persist.

HEPATITIS B

This disease develops in babies of mothers who suffer the acute disease during the later part of pregnancy, within two months of delivery, or, rarely, who are asymptomatic carriers [72, 85]. The mother is usually hepatitis B, 'e' antigen positive [37, 71]. Maternal anti 'e' may favour HBsAg clearance and recovery in neonatally acquired infections. Antigenaemia is usually found between six weeks and six months of birth, suggesting transmission from the mother's blood during delivery or later during her care of the infant. The condition is possibly spread by breast milk. Successive children may be affected [65].

Umbilical cord sera may occasionally be positive for HBsAg and Dane particles, and placental transmission is possible. Positivity does not necessarily imply infectivity by this route, for the umbilical cord sera may have been contaminated by maternal blood [37]. Disease can also be contracted in the neonatal period by blood products such as through exchange transfusions.

The baby may be asymptomatic although antigenaemia persists with increased serum transaminase levels. It may suffer a mild hepatitis with bilirubinuria and failure to thrive. The picture can be a severe and even fatal viral hepatitis [27]. Chronic hepatitis and cirrhosis and even probably primary liver cancer are late sequelae. The antigenaemia tends to persist for many months or

years, and the baby is often 'e' antigen positive, confirming its infectivity [87].

By light microscopy, the liver may show an unresolved hepatitis, a chronic hepatitis or even cirrhosis. In the acute stage, a giant cell hepatitis is seen (fig. 347).

Prophylaxis by hepatitis B immune globulin given at birth is controversial. Certainly, large doses do seem to be effective [24], and 0.5 ml/kg given within 48 hours of birth, and subsequently in a dose of 0.6 ml/kg every month for six months, prevented neonatal hepatitis B, compared with a controlled group [79].

The cost-effectiveness of screening all prospective mothers for hepatitis B depends on the carrier rate in that particular community [20].

CYTOMEGALOVIRUS

This is a very common virus infection (Chapter 27). The incidence in small children is 5–10% in those living in good hygienic conditions rising to 80% in the under-privileged.

It is usually acquired placentally from an asymptomatic mother. It can also be transmitted via exchange blood transfusion. Many congenital infections are asymptomatic. The disease may, however, be fulminant with intense jaundice, purpura, hepatosplenomegaly and neurological and pulmonary defects. Survivors may run a prolonged course with persistent jaundice and hepatomegaly.

HERPES SIMPLEX

The liver may be involved in the course of a fulminating viraemia, contracted at birth from herpes simplex infection of the maternal birth canal. Jaundice is due to viral involvement of the liver, which shows white nodules. Histologically, these represent necrosis with little or no inflammatory reaction. Giant cells are absent, but inclusion bodies may be found.

CONGENITAL RUBELLA SYNDROME

This disease, if contracted in the first trimester of pregnancy, may cause foetal malformations. The infection may also persist through the neonatal period and on into later life. The liver with the brain, lung, heart and other organs can be involved in the generalized virus infection [66].

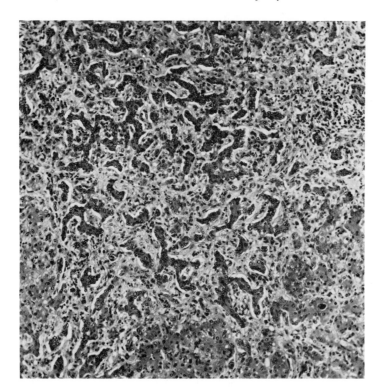

Fig. 347. Virus hepatitis in an infant of three months. Necrosis of liver cells and multinucleated giant liver cells are seen. Bile thrombi stained very darkly. H & E, ×115.

The hepatitis is marked by jaundice commencing within the first one to two days and by hepatosplenomegaly. A cholestatic picture may sometimes be seen. Serum transaminase levels are slightly elevated.

Hepatic histology shows bile in swollen Kupffer cells and ductules with a focal hepato-cellular necrosis and portal fibrosis. Erythroid haematopoietic tissue is relatively increased and may persist. A typical giant cell hepatitis can be seen [90]. The virus can be identified from the liver at necropsy or by biopsy.

The hepatitis may resolve completely with restitution of a normal liver structure. Alternatively it may pursue a chronic undulant course culminating in death at three to eight weeks. At autopsy a cirrhosis has been seen and rubella may be one cause of childhood cirrhosis.

ADENOVIRUSES

These may disseminate in babies with decreased resistance due to thymic alymphoplasia and agammaglobulinaemia [98]. A marked coagulative necrosis with inclusion bearing cells may be seen in the liver. Under similar circumstances this lesion can also complicate *varicella*.

Non-viral causes of hepatitis

CONGENITAL SYPHILIS

This condition is very rare. Visceral involvement is late in acquired syphilis but common in foetal infection. Tremendous numbers of treponemata can be found in the liver. Such involvement leads to a fine pericellular cirrhosis with a marked connective tissue reaction. Jaundice is usual.

CONGENITAL TOXOPLASMOSIS

This protozoon is transmitted to the foetus from an inapparent maternal infection. Jaundice develops within a few hours of birth with hepatomegaly, encephalo-myelitis, hydrocephalus, microcephaly, choroido-retinitis and intracerebral calcification.

The liver shows infiltration of portal zones with mononuclear cells. Extramedullary haemopoiesis with increased stainable iron is conspicuous. Histiocytes containing toxoplasma may be present. The jaundice is difficult to relate to the extent of liver damage and haemolysis may be contributory.

PYOGENIC INFECTION

The upsurgence of Gram-negative infections, particularly *E. coli* in nurseries, has led to an increase in jaundice due to this cause.

The origins include umbilical sepsis, exchange blood transfusion, pneumonia, otitis media or even gastro-enteritis [39]. Diagnosis may be difficult as focal signs are minimal or absent. Jaundice appears suddenly in a child who does not look ill. Hepatomegaly need not be present and splenomegaly is never great. The leucocyte count exceeds 12000. A blood culture is usually positive. The umbilical stump should be cultured. Liver functions tests are of little value.

Hepatic histology is non-contributory. The jaundice seems to be due to a combination of haemolysis, hepato-cellular dysfunction and even cholestasis.

Prognosis depends on early treatment and age of onset, the mortality being 80% below the age of one week and 25% later. Antibiotics are given, depending on the nature of the infection.

Portal vein occlusion may be diagnosed years later.

Liver abscesses in older children are associated with blood-spread organisms. A third have acute blastic leukaemia [19].

Hepatic histology shows non-specific changes with Kupffer cell hypertrophy and portal zone infiltrate. Culture of liver biopsies is usually negative.

URINARY TRACT INFECTIONS

Jaundice may be associated with urinary tract infections both in infants and children. The infants fail to thrive, show fever, jaundice and moderate hepatomegaly. Bilinuria is found. Liver biopsy shows a non-specific hepatitis. Urine culture is an essential investigation in any jaundiced child or infant [69].

'Idiopathic' neonatal hepatitis

AETIOLOGY

When identifiable causes of neonatal and infantile hepatitis, such as hepatitis B or galactosaemia,

have been excluded, there remain about 75% of patients in whom, after thorough investigation, the aetiology remains unknown. These are sometimes called 'idiopathic' giant cell hepatitis, or neonatal hepato-cellular cholestasis. The condition is often familial, the inheritance being autosomal recessive. It is possible that the familial incidence reflects common exposure to a toxic agent.

CLINICAL FEATURES

This may be a cause of stillbirth or the infant may die soon after or before jaundice has had time to develop. More usually a fluctuant jaundice appears during the first two weeks or even up to four months. The liver and sometimes the spleen are enlarged and the stools pale. The child may appear well and continue to gain weight or may fail to thrive. Serum transaminase is usually above 800 units/100 ml. Hypoprothrombinaemia may be profound. Stools are pale and urine contains bilirubin.

HEPATIC HISTOLOGY [23, 84]

The normal zonal architecture is lost. The most prominent feature is the large multinucleated cell containing 20–40 nuclei in a cytoplasmic mass. Liver cells may be aggregated into acini, simulating bile ducts. Necrosis is not conspicuous and, if present, focal. Haemosiderosis is constant and foci of erythropoiesis are obvious. Fibrosis is periportal and also extends between groups of liver cells. Cholestasis is seen both in small proliferated ductules in the portal zone and between necrotic liver cells.

PROGNOSIS AND TREATMENT

Prognosis is variable. About 10–33% die, usually from liver failure. Progressive liver disease and cirrhosis develop in 5–20%.

Treatment is purely symptomatic. Medium chain triglycerides may be useful to promote nutrition. The haemorrhagic diathesis must be controlled. Corticosteroid therapy is useless.

CHOLESTATIC SYNDROMES

This is a confused subject. The cholestatic syndromes may be divided into two broad groups: the atresias, which are defined as inability to excrete bile associated with malformation of the biliary tract, and the intra-hepatic cholestases where the difficulty may be functional or associated with destruction of intra-hepatic bile ducts perhaps secondary to a hepatitis. There is an overlap, for apparently congenital abnormalities of the extra-hepatic bile ducts may be acquired as intra-uterine infections. Moreover, intra- and extra-hepatic cholestasis can be present together in one infant. The distinction between intra- and extra-hepatic is, however, important for the atresias have a much worse prognosis than the intra-hepatic cholestatic syndromes.

Multiple defects are common in both types and other congenital lesions may be present, for instance, heart defects and eye or skeletal abnormalities. A chromosomal abnormality, namely trisomy 17–18, and Down's syndrome have been associated with neonatal hepatitis and atresia [4], but these are rare.

Further diagnostic confusion arises because intra-hepatic cholestasis leads to reduction of bile flow through extra-hepatic bile ducts and hence to their functional hypoplasia.

Biliary atresia

This is defined as the inability to excrete bile associated with malformations of the biliary tree. The abnormality may be in any part of the biliary system. Multiple defects are common and other congenital lesions may be present.

DEVELOPMENTAL ASPECTS

The biliary passages may fail to develop from the primitive foregut bud. The gall bladder may also be absent or the biliary tract represented only by a gall bladder connecting directly with the duodenum. The more usual defect is failure of vacuolation of the solid biliary bud. This is usually partial and rarely extends throughout the biliary tree. The cystic duct only may be involved, the gall bladder becoming a mucous cyst. This has no clinical significance. Involvement of the common bile duct or hepatic duct gives rise to the characteristic syndrome of biliary atresia with deep cholestatic jaundice.

PATHOLOGY

The ducts may be absent or replaced by fibrous strands. The site and extent of the atresia are variable. Bile is absent in the extra-hepatic biliary system including the gall bladder.

Hepatic histology shows the features of cholestatic jaundice with a variable number of giant cells, making the differentiation from a neonatal hepatitis difficult. Proliferated bile ductules are conspicuous.

CLINICAL FEATURES

Cholestatic jaundice starts soon after birth. The baby becomes icteric by the first week and the icterus continues unremittingly. When deeply jaundiced the infant even cries yellow tears. Pruritus is severe and the child suffers increasingly from it as the months pass. The urine is dark. The stools are pale, although some pigment may reach the intestine, presumably through the intestinal secretions. Serum transaminase values rarely exceed 300 units. Nutrition is well maintained for the first two months and then falls off, the child usually dying before three years. The serum cholesterol level may rise very high and skin xanthomas appear (fig. 348). The prolonged steatorrhoea can result in osteomalacia (*biliary rickets*). Death is usually due to intercurrent infection, to liver cell failure, or to bleeding related to vitamin K deficiency or to oesophageal varices. Ascites is a late and terminal event.

PROGNOSIS

Prognosis is poor unless the cystic duct only is involved or the bile ducts are hypoplastic and not entirely obliterated. Where surgical relief is possible recovery may be complete, but very few patients are amenable to surgical treatment.

SURGERY [57]

If the proximal bile ducts are patent but end blindly before the duodenum the condition is *correctable* by Roux en Y jejunal anastomosis to the common hepatic duct. This is an exceedingly rare circumstance.

In the vast majority of infants the atresia is *noncorrectable* because extra-hepatic ducts are not patent. In these circumstances the Kasai operation (hepatic porto-enterostomy) must be considered [50]. The entire ductal system is resected in the porta hepatis and the proximal transected common hepatic duct anastomosed to the intestine. The basis for subsequent biliary drainage is the

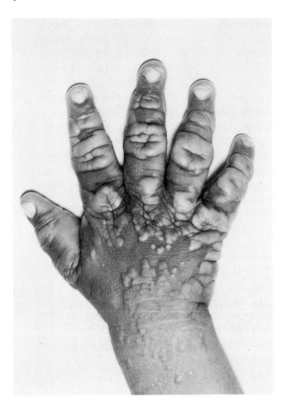

Fig. 348. Intra-hepatic biliary atresia in a child of four years. Cholesterol deposits are noted on the hands, particularly on the extensor surfaces. Note also skin pigmentation and white nailbeds.

presence of minuscule biliary ductules in the scarred 'non-patent' extra-hepatic bile ducts. These communicate with the intra-hepatic biliary system and when surgically transected may drain bile from the liver into the interposed intestine. The operation has to be done early (at less than four months of age) as the small ducts disappear with time. About 30–40% of patients survive free of jaundice and with stable liver function. Post-operative cholangitis and progressive portal hypertension are serious post-operative complications [5]. This operation is based on very uncertain grounds. The physician has to be quite sure that the baby is not, in fact, suffering from the biliary hypoplasia syndrome when the prognosis is relatively good and jaundice will lessen without porto-enterostomy. At three to four months of age it is very difficult to make a distinction between this and large duct, extra-hepatic, atresia.

The intra-hepatic atresia (biliary hypoplasia) syndrome

Intra-hepatic cholestasis in early life may be related to a known cause such as α_1 anti-trypsin

deficiency. In the majority, however, no clear aetiology is evident. The early histological appearances may resemble 'giant cell hepatitis'. This neonatal hepatitis progresses histologically to bile duct disappearance and biliary cirrhosis. This suggests that hepatitis, often viral, in the neonatal period or even *in utero* may be the first change, ultimately leading to biliary hypoplasia [44]. In most instances the causative virus cannot be identified, although occasionally an association with congenital cardiac defects, nerve deafness or rising titres of rubella antibody suggests that this virus is at fault.

Some conditions are familial and 16 cases of neonatal cholestasis have been described in seven sibships in the same family in south-west Norway [1].

Adverse effects of bile acids on the liver have been postulated. Atypical bile acids not normally found in the adult, and similar to those found in cholestatic states, have been identified in meconium [8]. Unsaturated mono-hydroxy bile acids, synthesized by the developing liver and combined with defective sulphation, might damage the biliary tract from the hepatocyte to the ampulla [49].

Trihydroxycoprostanic acid, an abnormal bile acid, has been found in the bile of infants with intra-hepatic bile duct anomalies [40]. It is uncertain to what extent these bile acid abnormalities are the cause or the effect of the intra-hepatic cholestasis.

Association with hormones administered in pregnancy has been noted [44].

CLINICAL PRESENTATION

Jaundice usually appears within three days of birth, but may be delayed to three to four weeks, or even up to six years.

BIOCHEMICAL CHANGES

The findings are those of chronic cholestasis with very high serum 'biliary' alkaline phosphatase levels. Serum cholesterol levels are very high and xanthomas appear after about the first year of life (fig. 348). Serum bile acids are increased. Hepatic copper concentrations increase markedly and urinary copper is also elevated [30].

HEPATIC HISTOLOGY [44]

The early changes are those of cholestasis, inflammation and fibrosis. 'Giant cells' may be conspicuous. Later the picture is of hypoplasia of intra-hepatic bile ducts, increasing portal fibrosis and eventually cirrhosis.

SYMPTOMATIC MEASURES

Steatorrhoea can be attributed to a reduction in duodenal bile salt concentration to below the critical micellar level. Calcium and vitamin D are not absorbed and *biliary rickets* is a consequence [52]. Vitamin A (50 000 units), vitamin D (50 000 units) and vitamin K_1 (5 mg) must be given by intramuscular injections (not by mouth) every four weeks. The child is encouraged to drink skimmed milk.

Medium chain triglyceride (coconut oil) is added to puréed fruit and vegetables and used in cooking. Portagen (Mead–Johnson) is a valuable food but is costly and not always available.

The tendency to bone thinning absolutely contraindicates the use of corticosteroids, which also stunt growth. In any case they are not of permanent value. In partial cholestasis cholestyramine (Questran) is given to the limit of tolerance levels. It may be flavoured with apple purée, tomato juice or chocolate syrup. It is valuable in

controlling pruritus and in reducing skin xanthomas. Serum lipids, bile salts and bilirubin are reduced.

Penicillamine has been used to remove excess liver copper but without noticeable benefit [31].

Arterio-hepatic dysplasia (Watson-Alagille syndrome) [2, 82, 97]

Chronic intra-hepatic cholestasis presents in the neonatal period and decreases with age. Inheritance is autosomal dominant with variable expressivity.

Peripheral pulmonary stenosis is usually associated.

The facies is triangular with a prominent broad forehead and a pointed mandible. Some of the changes may be secondary to vitamin D deficiency.

Skeletal changes include short distal phalanges (fig. 348) and butterfly vertebral bodies. The eyes show various abnormalities including retinal pigmentation and posterior embryotoxon.

Patients survive into adult life with varying degrees of physical and mental impairment (fig. 349).

Post-haemolytic cholestasis

Occasionally, infants with neonatal jaundice, due to such conditions as hepatic prematurity or haemolytic disease, develop the picture of cholestasis [42]. The conjugated serum bilirubin levels rise, and this reflects hepato-cellular damage in severe erythroblastosis. The bile accumulations in the liver are secondary rather than causal.

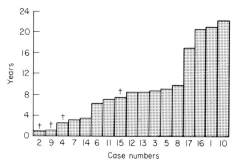

Fig. 349. Histogram showing the ages to date of 17 children with chronic intra-hepatic cholestasis (Heathcote *et al* 1976).

INTRA-HEPATIC CHOLESTASIS RELATED TO PARENTERAL NUTRITION

Premature infants, after about 42 days on parenteral nutrition, develop intra-hepatic cholestasis. This continues as long as the parenteral nutrition. Eventually serum bilirubin returns to normal [10]. The cause is probably hepatic excretory immaturity [89].

IDIOPATHIC HYPOPITUITARISM

This is associated with severe hypoglycaemia, hepatomegaly and hyperbilirubinaemia (direct and indirect) during the neonatal period [26].

SPONTANEOUS PERFORATION OF THE BILE DUCTS [34]

This occurs between birth and three months, usually in the anterior wall of the common bile duct, close to the junction with the cystic duct. The child seems relatively well, but then develops non-bile-stained vomiting and acholic stools. Jaundice is mild, intermittent and variable. Abdominal hernias develop and the scrotum becomes green. Percutaneous cholangiography shows the blocked cystic duct with the hepatic duct leak. The results of surgery are good.

REYE'S SYNDROME

In 1963 Reye and associates described this syndrome of acute encephalopathy and fatty change in the viscera [80].

AETIOLOGY AND EPIDEMIOLOGY

The syndrome has followed almost any known viral disease and can be encountered in epidemic form. Large outbreaks have been particularly associated with influenza B [16]. Other viruses include chickenpox, particularly in young children, and all upper respiratory viruses at every age.

Postulated toxic factors include aflatoxin [73]. A virus in association with a toxic factor, perhaps an insecticide, is possible [17]. The factors determining why an individual child, suffering from a viral infection, should develop this syndrome are unknown.

Epidemics usually develop during winter and early spring.

Metabolic changes include an increase in blood ammonia and reduction in citrulline levels. This indicates an abnormality in the Krebs' cycle. Changes are similar to those seen in inherited ornithine transcarbamylase deficiency. Indeed there is a reduced activity of this enzyme in the liver early in the disease [88, 92]. Various agents (viral or toxic) probably cause widespread mitochondrial dysfunction with transient abnormalities of the intramitochondrial urea cycle enzymes in the liver.

CLINICAL FEATURES [75]

Sexes are equally affected, usually below 14 years old; young adults [95] and even up to 34-year-olds have been affected. It has been described in siblings [45]. Three to seven days after a viral-type illness the child develops intractable vomiting and progressive, neurological deterioration. The encephalopathy is marked by erratic behaviour, irritability and listlessness progressing through lethargy to stupor and coma. The liver enlarges rapidly and then shrinks. Mortality is 30–60%.

LIVER BIOPSY

This shows small droplet, triglyceride accumulation in the hepatocytes, probably due to failure of export of triglyceride from the liver. Plasma very low density lipoprotein values fall, then recover [75]. The picture is similar to fatty liver of pregnancy or tetracycline toxicity.

Liver electron microscopy [47] shows swelling and polymorphic distortion of the mitochondria. The severity of the mitochondrial changes does not correlate with clinical severity. The changes in the mitochondria disappear, to be followed by showers of peroxisomes.

Changes in other organs. The kidney shows proximal tubular fat. The myocardium is fatty. There is marked cerebral oedema. Electron microscopy of the neurones reveals similar mitochondrial changes to those seen in the liver [75].

LABORATORY FINDINGS

Characteristic features are an increase in blood ammonia and serum transaminase levels with usually an increased prothrombin time. Hypoglycaemia is found in about 50%. The cerebro-spinal fluid is normal.

TREATMENT

The patient presents as a problem in liver disease, but it is the cerebral oedema that is lethal. Treatment is directed towards this, combined with intense supportive care. There is no specific treatment.

Cirrhosis in infancy and childhood

The cirrhosis of infants and children has many aetiologies. As in the older age group, many are cryptogenic.

In some, the disease seems to follow a typical *acute virus hepatitis*. An increasing number, presenting in later childhood and at puberty, show the picture of *chronic active 'lupoid' hepatitis*.

Neonatal 'giant cell' hepatitis may be followed by cirrhosis and this may also apply to some of the neonatal virus hepatites such as chronic rubella, hepatitis B, or non-A, non-B.

Wilson's disease, galactosaemia, Fanconi's disease, type IV glycogen disease and *fibro-cystic disease* may be followed by cirrhosis.

In the tropics the Kwashiorkor syndrome is not followed by cirrhosis whereas *veno-occlusive disease* is followed by centrizonal fibrosis and finally a cirrhosis.

Congenital hepatic fibrosis may cause portal hypertension but the hepatic lesion is not a cirrhosis.

Cholestatic syndromes are followed by biliary cirrhosis and also α_1 anti-trypsin deficiency (Chapter 22).

Cardiac cirrhosis is unusual in childhood except complicating constrictive pericarditis.

CLINICAL FEATURES

Portal hypertension is usually prominent. The spleen tends to be larger than in the adult. Presentation with splenomegaly and hepatomegaly at a school medical examination or while in hospital for another condition is not unusual. Vascular spiders are conspicuous. Growth is uninterrupted; indeed the adolescent growth spurt may be particularly great so that the child is above normal in height (fig. 350).

At puberty, both sexes may show acne and facial mooning with cutaneous striae, girls amenorrhoea and boys gynaecomastia.

This relatively inactive stage can continue for years. Decompensation is followed by deepening jaundice and very high serum globulin and transaminase values. When pre-coma appears it is accompanied by mania, screaming, fits and psychic outbursts. Ascites is usual at this late stage (fig. 351).

The prognosis is very variable depending on the aetiology. The outlook is better than for an adult with an equivalent degree of clinical decompensation.

Indian childhood cirrhosis

This condition affects both sexes aged one to three years [14]. The familial incidence suggests genetic factors although it may indicate a common environmental origin. Death is usually due to liver failure and occurs within a year of diagnosis.

Hepatic histology shows profound injury to individual liver cells which may contain Mallory's hyaline bodies [68] and which are surrounded by polymorph accumulations. A fine, micronodular cirrhosis results. The picture resembles acute alcoholic hepatitis, but without the fatty change.

Hepatic copper is markedly increased, and this

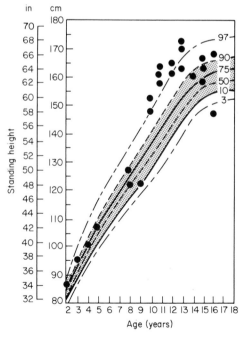

Fig. 350. Cirrhosis in female children. The age and height are in agreement. Note that children between 10 and 13 years are taller than 90% of the population (Sherlock 1958).

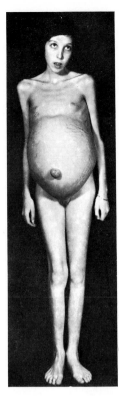

Fig. 351. Girl of 12 years. Never well after virus hepatitis three years before. Ascites for one year. Died two weeks later. Note height 5 ft 3 in (160 cm).

is largely located in the cytoplasm [77, 91]. The distribution is not that of Wilson's disease or cholestasis. Whether this represents a primary metabolic defect or a secondary event, perhaps related to excess copper ingestion, remains uncertain. The therapeutic use of copper-chelating agents has not been evaluated.

Peliosis hepatis

This is a rare, ill-defined lesion in which the liver appears mottled blue, and on section shows numerous blue-black dots less than 0.2 mm in diameter. These consist of blood-filled lacunar spaces distributed at random like the holes in Swiss cheese. They may be without an endothelial lining or may represent distended sinusoids, portal or central veins. Rupture with haemorrhage may be fatal.

The condition is of unknown aetiology. It may be a chance finding at autopsy, especially in patients dying of tuberculosis. It has also been reported after androgen and anabolic hormones [9] such as norethandrolone [38] or oral contraceptives (Chapter 17) (fig. 302).

Hamartomas

These benign, congenital lesions present as an abdominal mass in the first two years of life. They may be an incidental finding at autopsy. They must be distinguished from malignant tumours [81]. They are not true neoplasms. They consist of abnormal arrangements of all the cells of the normal liver, particularly bile ducts and fibroblasts. They contain central veins. They are nearly always cystic. They require no treatment.

Tumours of the liver [28, 70]

Primary tumours in infants and children are rare. Two-thirds are diagnosed before the second year of life. They may arise from liver cells and/or from supporting structures. Secondary tumours are extremely rare and are usually associated with a neuroblastoma of the adrenals.

HEPATO-CELLULAR

These are the commonest. They range from simple, benign-looking adenoma to the highly malignant, embryonic hepatoblastoma of infancy [67]. There is usually no accompanying cirrhosis although in older children primary carcinoma may complicate giant cell hepatitis, post-hepatitis cirrhosis, particularly with a positive HBsAg test, biliary atresia or even congenital hepatic fibrosis [51].

The patients present with weight loss, abdominal swelling usually in the right upper quadrant, pain, ascites and jaundice. Calcification in the tumour may be noted.

HAEMANGIO-ENDOTHELIOMA

This is a benign, vascular tumour of infancy. It consists of endothelium-lined channels of capillary size. It may be associated with skin haemangiomas. Anaemia is usual. Cardiac failure may be related to arteriovenous shunts within the tumour. These may cause severe intractable high output heart failure in the newborn [54]. A systolic bruit may be heard in the epigastrium [94]. Rupture can cause haemoperitoneum [70]. Associated congenital defects are frequent.

Severe anaemia has been attributed to micro-angiopathic haemolysis related to the abnormal, tortuous narrow anastomotic vessels within the tumour [3]. Thrombocytopenia may also be seen.

Diagnosis

Biochemical tests may be normal. The most usual abnormality is an increase in serum 5′-nucleotidase and α_2 globulin levels. Serum α_1-fetoprotein may be present.

The site and extent of the tumour must be defined by splenic venography, coeliac angiography and scanning. Haemangio-endotheliomas show a blush in the liver on selective coeliac angiography [48].

Needle hepatic biopsy is usually a safe method of confirming the diagnosis.

TREATMENT

The only procedure offering hope of cure in the primary carcinoma group is resection [78]. This will cure the benign lesions. Cure may even follow in the malignant group for the tumour is usually single, often large and metastasizes late [33]. In any case palliation is usual. Subsequent growth and development are normal after hepatic lobectomy.

The prognosis is very poor if resection is impossible.

Hepatic haemangio-endotheliomas are treated by resection and this may have to be done as an emergency if congestive heart failure is life-threatening [63]. If the hepatic haemangiomas are extensive, administration of corticosteroids may be useful [48]. Ligation or embolization of the hepatic artery may give good results. Radiotherapy may be useful in the presence of cardiac failure [83].

REFERENCES

1. AAGENAES Ø., VAN DE HOGEN C.B. & REFSUM S. (1968) Hereditary recurrent intrahepatic cholestasis from birth. *Arch. Dis. Childh.* **43**, 646.
2. ALAGILLE D., ODIÈVRE M., GAUTIER M. *et al* (1975) Hepatic ductular hypoplasia associated with characteristic facies, vertebral malformations, retarded physical, mental and sexual development and cardiac murmur. *J. Pediatr.* **86**, 63.
3. ALPERT L.I. & BENISCH B. (1970) Hemangioendothelioma of the liver associated with microangiopathic hemolytic anemia. Report of four cases. *Am. J. Med.* **48**, 624.
4. ALPERT L.I., STRAUSS L. & HIRSCHHORN K. (1969) Neonatal hepatitis and biliary atresia associated with trisomy 17–18 syndrome. *New Engl. J. Med.* **270**, 16.
5. ALTMAN R.P. (1978) The portoenterostomy procedure for biliary atresia: a five year experience. *Ann. Surg.* **188**, 351.
6. ARIAS I.M., GARTNER L.M., SEIFTER S. *et al* (1964) Prolonged neonatal unconjugated hyperbilirubinemia associated with breast feeding and a steroid, pregnane-3-(alpha), 20(beta)-diol, in maternal milk that inhibits glucuronide formation *in vitro*. *J. clin. Invest.* **43**, 2037.
7. ARIAS I.M., WOLFSON S., LUCEY J.F. *et al* (1965) Transient familial neonatal hyperbilirubinemia. *J. clin. Invest.* **44**, 1442.
8. BACK P. & WALTER K. (1980) Developmental pattern of bile acid metabolism as revealed by bile acid analysis of meconium. *Gastroenterology* **78**, 671.
9. BAGHERI S.A. & BOYER J.L. (1974) Peliosis hepatis associated with androgenic–anabolic steroid therapy. A severe form of hepatic injury. *Ann. intern. Med.* **81**, 610.
10. BEALE E.F., NELSON R.M., BUCCIARELLI R.L. *et al* (1979) Intrahepatic cholestasis associated with parenteral nutrition in premature infants. *Pediatrics* **64**, 342.
11. BROUGH A.J. & BERNSTEIN J. (1969) Liver biopsy in the diagnosis of infantile obstructive jaundice. *Pediatrics* **43**, 319.
12. BUCHAN P.C. (1979) Pathogenesis of neonatal hyperbilirubinaemia after induction of labour with oxytocin. *Br. med. J.* ii, 1255.
13. CAPPS F.P.A., GILLES H.M., JOLLY H. *et al* (1963) Glucose-6-phosphate dehydrogenase deficiency and neonatal jaundice in Nigeria. Their relation to the use of prophylactic vitamin K. *Lancet* ii, 379.
14. CHANDRA R.K. (1974) Indian childhood cirrhosis. *Med Chir. Dig.* **3**, 63.
15. COCKINGTON R.A. (1979) A guide to the use of phototherapy in the management of neonatal hyperbilirubinemia. *J. Pediatr.* **95**, 281.
16. COREY L., RUBIN R.J., HATTWICK M.A.W. *et al* (1976) A nationwide outbreak of Reye's syndrome: its epidemiologic relationship to influenza B. *Am. J. Med.* **61**, 615.
17. CROCKER J.F.S., ROZEE K.R., OZERE R.L. *et al* (1974) Insecticide as a cause of fatty visceral changes and encephalopathy in the mouse. *Lancet* ii, 22.
18. DAAMEN C.B.F. & SCHABERG A. (1969) Hemilateral liver degeneration in perinatal death. *J. Pathol.* **97**, 29.
19. DEHNER L.P. & KISSANE L.M. (1969) Pyogenic hepatic abscesses in infancy and childhood. *J. Pediatr.* **74**, 763.
20. DERSO A., BOXALL E.H., TARLOW M.J. *et al* (1978) Transmission of HBsAg from mother to infant in four ethnic groups. *Br. med. J.* i, 949.
21. DIAMOND I. (1966) Kernicterus: revised concepts of pathogenesis and management. *Pediatrics* **38**, 539.
22. DIAMOND I. & SCHMID R. (1966) Experimental bilirubin encephalopathy. The mode of entry of

bilirubin-^{14}C into the central nervous system. *J. clin. Invest.* **45**, 678.

23. DIBLE J.H., HUNT W.E., PUGH V.W. *et al* (1954) Foetal and neonatal hepatitis and its sequelae. *J. Pathol. Bact.* **67**, 195.

24. DOSIK H. & JHAVERI R. (1978) Prevention of neonatal hepatitis B infection by high-dose hepatitis B immune globulin. *New Engl. J. Med.* **298**, 602.

25. DOXIADIS S.A. & VALAES T. (1964) The clinical picture of glucose 6-phosphate dehydrogenase deficiency in early infancy. *Arch. Dis. Childh.* **39**, 545.

26. DROP S.L.S., COLLE E. & GUYDA H.J. (1979) Hyperbilirubinaemia and idiopathic hypopituitarism in the newborn period. *Acta. Paediat. Scand.* **68**, 277.

27. DUPUY J.M., FROMMEL D. & ALAGILLE D. (1975) Severe viral hepatitis type B in infancy. *Lancet* i, 191.

28. EDMONDSON H.A. (1956) Differential diagnosis of tumors and tumor-like lesions of liver in infancy and childhood. *Am. J. Dis. Child.* **91**, 168.

29. EMERY J.L. (1952) Degenerative changes in the left lobe of the liver in the newborn. *Arch. Dis. Childh.* **27**, 558.

30. EVANS J., NEWMAN S. & SHERLOCK S. (1978) Liver copper levels in intrahepatic cholestasis of childhood. *Gastroenterology* **75**, 875.

31. EVANS J., NEWMAN S.P. & SHERLOCK S. (1980) Observations on copper associated protein in childhood liver disease. *Gut* **21**, 970.

32. FELSHER B.F., CARPIO N.M., WOOLLEY M.M. *et al* (1974) Hepatic bilirubin glucuronidation in neonates with unconjugated hyperbilirubinaemia and congenital gastrointestinal obstruction. *J. lab. clin. Med.* **83**, 90.

33. FISH J.C. & McGARY R.G. (1966) Primary cancer of the liver in childhood. *Arch. Surg.* **93**, 355.

34. FITZGERALD R.J., PARBHOO K. & GUINEY E.J. (1978) Spontaneous perforation of bile ducts in neonates. *Surgery* **83**, 303.

35. FRANKEN E.A. Jr, SMITH W.L., SMITH J.A. *et al* (1978) Percutaneous cholangiography in infants. *Am. J. Roentgenol.* **130**, 1057.

36. GARTNER L.M. & ARIAS I.M. (1966) Studies of prolonged neonatal jaundice in the breast-fed infant. *J. Pediatr.* **68**, 54.

37. GERETY R.J. & SCHWEITZER I.L. (1977) Viral hepatitis type B during pregnancy, the neonatal period, and infancy. *J. Pediatr.* **90**, 368.

38. GORDON B.S., WOLF J., KRAUSE T. *et al* (1960) Peliosis hepatis and cholestasis following administration of norethandrolone. *Amer. J. clin. Pathol.* **33**, 156.

39. HAMILTON J.R. & SASS-KORTSAK A. (1963) Jaundice associated with severe bacterial infection in young infants. *J. Pediatr.* **63**, 121.

40. HANSEN R.F., ISENBERG J.N., WILLIAMS G.C. *et al* (1975) The metabolism of 3α,7α,12α-trihydroxy-5β-cholestan-26-oic acid in two siblings with cholestasis due to intrahepatic bile duct anomalies. *J. clin. Invest.* **56**, 577.

41. HARGREAVES T. (1973) Effect of fatty acids on bilirubin conjugation. *Arch. Dis. Childh.* **48**, 446.

42. HARRIS R.C., ANDERSEN D.H. & DAY R.L. (1954) Obstructive jaundice in infants with normal biliary tree. *Pediatrics* **13**, 293.

43. HARRIS R.C., LUCEY J.F. & MACLEAN J.R. (1958) Kernicterus in premature infants associated with low concentrations of bilirubin in the plasma. *Pediatrics* **21**, 375.

44. HEATHCOTE J., DEODHAR K.P., SCHEUER P.J. *et al* (1976) Intrahepatic cholestasis in childhood. *New. Engl. J. Med.* **295**, 801.

45. HILTY M.D., McCLUNG H.J., HAYNES R.E. *et al* (1979) Reye's syndrome in siblings. *J. Pediatr.* **94**, 576.

46. HOWARD E.R. & NUNNERLEY H.B. (1979) Percutaneous cholangiography in prolonged jaundice of childhood. *J. R. Soc. Med.* **72**, 495.

47. IANCCU T.C., MASON W.H. & NEUSTEIN H.B. (1977) Ultrastructural abnormalities of liver cells in Reye's syndrome. *Human Pathol.* **8**, 421.

48. JACKSON C., GREENE H.L., O'NEILL J. *et al* (1977) Hepatic hemangio-endothelioma: angiographic appearance and apparent prednisone responsiveness. *Am. J. Dis. Childh.* **131**, 74.

49. JENNER R.E. & HOWARD E.R. (1975) Unsaturated monohydroxy bile acids as a cause of idiopathic obstructive cholangiopathy. *Lancet* ii, 1073.

50. KASAI M., WATANABE I. & OHI R. (1975) Follow-up studies of long-term survivors after hepatic porto-enterostomy for 'non-correctable' biliary atresia. *J. Pediatr. Surg.* **10**, 173.

51. KEELING J.W. (1971) Liver tumours in infancy and childhood. *J. Pathol.* **103**, 69.

52. KOOH S.W., JONES G., REILLY B.J. *et al* (1979) Pathogenesis of rickets in chronic hepatobiliary disease in children. *J. Pediatr.* **94**, 870.

53. KOPELMAN A.E., BROWN R.S. & ODELL G.B. (1972) The 'bronze' baby syndrome: a complication of phototherapy. *J Pediatr.* **81**, 466.

54. LEONIDAS J.C., STRAUSS L. & BECK A.R. (1973) Vascular tumors of the liver in newborns. *Am. J. Dis. Child.* **125**, 507.

55. LESTER R. (1980) Physiologic cholestasis. *Gastroenterology* **78**, 864.

56. LEWIS P.J. & FRIEDMAN L.A. (1979) Prophylaxis of neonatal jaundice with maternal antipyrine treatment. *Lancet* i, 300.

57. LILLY J.R. (1977) Surgical jaundice in infancy. *Ann. Surg.* **186**, 549.

58. LITTLE J.M., SMALLWOOD R.A., LESTER R. *et al* (1975) Bile salt metabolism in the primate fetus. *Gastroenterology* **69**, 1315.

59. LUCEY J.F., ARIAS I.M. & McKAY R.J. Jr (1960) Transient familial neonatal hyperbilirubinemia. *Am. J. Dis. Child.* **100**, 787.

60. LUCEY J.F. & DOLAN R.G. (1959) Hyperbilirubinemia of newborn infants associated with the parenteral administration of a vitamin K analogue to the mothers. *Pediatrics* **23**, 553.

61. MACGILLIVRAY M.H., CRAWFORD J.D. & ROBEY J.S. (1967) Congenital hypothyroidism and prolonged neonatal hyperbilirubinemia. *Pediatrics* **40**, 283.

62. MATHIS R.K., ANDRES J.M. & WALKER W.A. (1977) Liver disease in infants. II. Hepatic disease states. *J. Pediatr.* **90**, 864.

63. MATOLO N.M. & JOHNSON D.G. (1973) Surgical treatment of hepatic hemangioma in the newborn. *Arch. Surg.* **106**, 725.

64. MAURER H.M., WOLFF J.A., FINSTER M. *et al* (1968) Reduction in concentration of total serum-bilirubin in offspring of women treated with phenobarbitone during pregnancy. *Lancet* ii, 122.

65. MOLLICA F., MUSUMECI S., FISCHER A. *et al* (1977) Neonatal hepatitis in five children of a hepatitis B surface antigen carrier woman. *J. Pediatr.* **90**, 949.

66. MONIF G.R.G., ASOFSKY R. & SEVER J.L. (1966) Hepatic dysfunction in the congenital rubella syndrome. *Br. med. J.* i, 1086.

67. NAPOLI V.M. & CAMPBELL W.G. Jr (1977) Hepatoblastoma in infant sister and brother. *Cancer* **39**, 2647.

68. NAYAK N.C. & ROY S. (1976) Morphological types of hepatocellular hyalin in Indian childhood cirrhosis. *Gut* **17**, 791.

69. NG S.H. & RAWSTRON J.R. (1971) Urinary tract infections presenting with jaundice. *Arch. Dis. Childh.* **46**, 173.

70. NIKAIDOH H., BOOGS J. & SWENSON O. (1970) Liver tumors in infants and children: clinical and pathological analysis of 22 cases. *Arch. Surg.* **101**, 245.

71. OKADA K., KAMIYAMA I., INOMATA M. *et al* (1976) 'e' antigen and anti-'e' in the serum of asymptomatic carrier mothers as indicators of positive and negative transmission of hepatitis B virus to their infants. *New Engl. J. Med.* **294**, 746.

72. OKADA K., YAMADA T., MIYAKAWA Y. *et al* (1975) Hepatitis B surface antigen in the serum of infants after delivery from asymptomatic carrier mothers. *J. Pediatr.* **87**, 360.

73. OLSON L.C., BOURGEOIS C.H. Jr, COTTON R.B. *et al* (1971) Encephalopathy and fatty degeneration of the viscera in north-eastern Thailand. Clinical syndrome and epidemiology. *Pediatrics* **47**, 707.

74. OSTROW J.D. (1971) Photocatabolism of labelled bilirubin in the congenitally jaundiced Gunn rat. *J. clin. Invest.* **50**, 707.

75. PARTIN J.C. (1975) Reye's syndrome (encephalopathy and fatty liver): diagnosis and treatment. *Gastroenterology* **69**, 511.

76. POLAND R.L. & ODELL G.B. (1971) Physiologic jaundice: the enterohepatic circulation of bilirubin. *New Engl. J. Med.* **284**, 1.

77. POPPER H., GOLDFISCHER S., STERNLIEB I. *et al* (1979) Cytoplasmic copper and its toxic effects; studies in Indian childhood cirrhosis. *Lancet* i, 1205.

78. RANDOLPH J.G., ALTMAN R.P., ARENSMAN R.M. *et al* (1978) Liver resection in children with hepatic neoplasms. *Ann. Surg.* **187**, 599.

79. REESINK H.W., REERINK-BRONGER S., LAFEBER-SCHUT B.J.Th. *et al* (1979) Prevention of chronic HBsAg carrier state in infants of HBsAg-positive mothers by hepatitis B immunoglobulin. *Lancet* ii, 436.

80. REYE R.D.K., MORGAN G. & BARAL J. (1963) Encephalopathy and fatty degeneration of the viscera. A disease entity in childhood. *Lancet* ii, 749.

81. RHODES R.H., MARCHILDON M.B., LUEBKE D.C. *et al* (1978) A mixed haematoma of the liver; light and electron microscopy. *Hum. Pathol.* **9**, 211.

82. RIELY C.A., COTLIER E., JENSEN P.S. *et al* (1979) Arteriohepatic dysplasia: a benign syndrome of intrahepatic cholestasis with multiple organ involvement. *Ann. intern. Med.* **91**, 520.

83. ROTMAN M., JOHN M., STONE S. *et al* (1980) Radiation treatment of pediatric hepatic hemangiomatosis and coexisting cardiac failure. *New Engl. J. Med.* **302**, 852.

84. SCHEUER P.J. (1980) Liver disease in childhood and heredofamilial disorders. In *Liver Biopsy*. Baillière Tindall, London.

85. SCHWEITZER I.L., MOSLEY J.W., ASHCAVAI M. *et al* (1973) Factors influencing neonatal infection by hepatitis B virus. *Gastroenterology* **655**, 277.

86. SHIRAKI K. (1970) Hepatic cell necrosis in the newborn: a pathogenic study of 147 cases with particular reference to congenital heart disease. *Am. J. Dis. Child.* **119**, 395.

87. SKINHOJ P. (1978) Infection with hepatitis B virus in infancy: a longitudinal study of 8 cases. *Arch. Dis. Childh.* **53**, 746.

88. SNODGRASS P.J. & DE LONG G.R. (1976) Urea-cycle enzyme deficiencies and an increased nitrogen load producing hyperammonemia in Reye's syndrome. *New Engl. J. Med.* **294**, 855.

89. SONDHEIMER J.M., BRYAN H., ANDREWS W. *et al* (1978) Cholestatic tendencies in premature infants on and off parenteral nutrition. *Pediatrics* **62**, 984.

90. STERN H. & WILLIAMS B.M. (1966) Isolation of rubella virus in a case of neonatal giant-cell hepatitis. *Lancet* i, 293.

91. TANNER M.S., PORTMANN B., MOWAT A.P. *et al* (1979) Increased hepatic copper concentration in Indian childhood cirrhosis. *Lancet* i, 1203.

92. THALER M.M. (1976) Metabolic mechanisms in Reye's syndrome. *Am. J. Dis. Child.* **130**, 241.

93. THALER M.M. (1977) Jaundice in the newborn: algorithmic diagnosis of conjugated and unconjugated hyperbilirubinemia. *J. Am. med. Assoc.* **237**, 58.

94. TOULOUKIAN R.J. (1970) Hepatic hemangioendothelioma during infancy: pathology, diagnosis and treatment with prednisone. *Pediatrics* **45**, 71.

95. VARMA R.R., REIDEL D.R., KOMOROWSKI R.A. *et al* (1979) Reye's syndrome in non-pediatric age groups. *J. Am. med. Assoc.* **242**, 1373.

96. WATKINS J.B., INGALL D., SZCZEPANIK P. *et al* (1973) Bile-salt metabolism in the new born. Measurement of pool size and synthesis by stable isotope technique. *New Engl. J. Med.* **288**, 431.

97. WATSON G.H. & MILLER V. (1973) Arteriohepatic dysplasia: familial pulmonary arterial stenosis with neonatal liver disease. *Arch. Dis. Childh.* **48**, 459.

98. WIGGER H.J. & BLANC W.A. (1966) Fatal hepatic and bronchial necrosis in adenovirus infection with thymic alymphoplasia. *New Engl. J. Med.* **275**, 870.

99. WOOD B., CULLEY P., ROGINSKI C. *et al* (1979) Factors affecting neonatal jaundice. *Arch. Dis. Childh.* **54**, 111.

100. ZENONE E.A., STOLL M.S. & OSTROW J.D. (1977) Mechanism of excretion of unconjugated bilirubin (UCB) during phototherapy. *Gastroenterology* **72**, 1180.

Chapter 24
The Liver in Pregnancy

Liver function

In normal pregnancy hepatic function is not impaired. Vascular spiders and palmar erythema may be related to increases in circulating oestrogens.

Biochemical tests show a rise in the serum alkaline phosphatase level in the ninth month [31]. This is mainly due to placental alkaline phosphatase and can be distinguished from the hepatic enzyme by electrophoresis or immunochemistry. Serum gammaglutamyltranspeptidase remains normal. Serum total cholesterol is raised but esterification is normal. Serum albumin is reduced and globulins rise prior to delivery. Transaminases are normal just prior to delivery and post-partum.

The bromsulphalein (BSP) test shows occasional slight impairment in the last trimester of pregnancy. Storage [S] rises 122% during the last half of pregnancy, returning towards normal during the first week post-partum. In contrast, the Tm decreases 27% in the last half of pregnancy and rapidly increases to normal levels after delivery [7].

Needle liver biopsy in normal pregnancy gives virtually normal histological appearances [12]. Minor non-specific changes include difference in size of liver cells, increase in nuclear size, some increase in binucleate cells and occasionally very mild lymphocytic infiltration in the portal zones. Electron microscopy shows some increase in endoplasmic reticulum.

Liver blood flow is within the normal range [24]. This is important because, in pregnancy, blood volume and cardiac output increase. The liver blood flow comprises 35% of the cardiac output in non-pregnant females and only 28% of the cardiac output in pregnancy. The excess blood volume is shunted through the placenta.

Rupture of the liver

This rare, frequently fatal condition presents spontaneously near term as toxaemia, right upper quadrant pain and sudden hypotension [25]. A large haematoma bursts into the peritoneal cavity.

Adenomas may also rupture in pregnancy.

Hepatic pregnancy

Placental hepatic attachment is very rare and presents as slow intra-abdominal haemorrhage [15]. The placenta is usually attached to the inferior surface of the right lobe of the liver.

JAUNDICE IN PREGNANCY

The jaundice may be peculiar to pregnancy such as acute fatty liver of pregnancy, cholestatic jaundice in pregnancy, or jaundice complicating the toxaemias. The jaundice may be an intercurrent one affecting the pregnant woman such as virus hepatitis or gall-stones. Finally, the effect of pregnancy on underlying chronic liver disease must be considered (table 61).

Jaundice occurs in about one out of every 1500 gestations, an incidence of 0.067% [10]. At least 41% of all cases with jaundice are due to viral hepatitis and about 21% to intra-hepatic cholestasis of pregnancy. Common bile duct obstruction accounts for less than 6% of all cases. These results are reported from Switzerland and different statistics can be expected from other parts of the world.

Acute fatty liver

Sheehan [32] described a specific type of severe jaundice in pregnancy which is now termed 'acute fatty liver of pregnancy' [8].

This condition largely affects the young prima gravida in the last trimester. The cause is unknown. There is a resemblance to experimental liver injury due to protein or amino acid deficiency. There is an association between massive intravenous tetracycline given in the last trimester and acute fatty liver. This drug is known to inhibit protein metabolism and should not be given in pregnancy. This condition has also been reported in a pregnant woman who was in a very poor nutritional state [8]. It somewhat resembles Reye's syndrome.

Table 61. Jaundice in pregnancy.

Peculiar to pregnancy	
Acute fatty liver	Poor prognosis. Note relation to tetracycline therapy
Toxaemias	Rare cause of jaundice but can be deep if associated DIC. Rupture of liver may occur
Recurrent cholestasis	Good prognosis. Develop jaundice and pruritus if given oral contraceptives
Hyperemesis gravidarum	Rare cause of jaundice
Intercurrent jaundice	
Viral hepatitis	Prognosis same as in non-pregnant. High incidence of stillbirths. Type B can be related to neonatal hepatitis
Gall-stones	Surprisingly rare as a cause of jaundice in pregnancy
Hepato-toxic drugs	Chlorpromazine may cause prolonged cholestasis. Prognosis otherwise as for non-pregnant
Underlying cirrhosis	Rare to become pregnant. No indication for premature termination. Prognosis variable

The association with toxaemia of pregnancy puts the condition into the spectrum of pregnancy toxaemia [13].

Clinical features [27]

Presentation is as acute liver failure, often with renal failure. The pregnancy has been relatively uneventful until the 32nd–38th week when the patient develops vomiting, epigastric distress, haematemesis, jaundice and encephalopathy and oliguria proceeding to anuria. Toxaemia may be associated.

Presentation may be a few days before or after delivery of a stillborn foetus.

The patient is questioned concerning drug therapy, particularly with tetracyclines, but this is usually non-contributory.

Disseminated intravascular coagulation may develop [5].

Special investigations

Serum bilirubin and transaminase levels are only slightly increased. Serum uric acid values are very high, perhaps due to massive protein catabolism and to renal failure. Hypoglycaemia is frequent. Blood urea is raised and serum albumin and cholesterol levels are low. The thrombotest is markedly reduced. There is a leucocytosis.

Needle biopsy of the liver may have to be postponed until the recovery stage, because of impairment in blood coagulation. Histology shows multiple intracellular fat droplets in centrizonal areas without significant necrosis or inflammation. Electron microscopy shows a striking honeycomb appearance in the smooth endoplasmic reticulum [8].

Diagnosis from fulminant viral hepatitis

This is difficult but is suggested by the presentation with vomiting and epigastric distress in late pregnancy. Serum bilirubin and transaminase levels are relatively low and blood uric acid values and blood urea levels high. Liver biopsy, if blood clotting permits, is diagnostic.

Prognosis

In a series of 81 patients collected between 1934 and 1976 the maternal mortality was 77% and foetal mortality 76% [22]. Better recognition is allowing milder cases to be diagnosed and many of these will survive. The prognosis for the survivors is good.

Treatment

The routine for acute liver and kidney failure is adopted (Chapter 9). Special attention must be given to the correction of hypoglycaemia [3].

Obstetric management is controversial. The mode of delivery does not seem to influence the outcome, but early Caesarean section under epidural anaesthesia may be useful, particularly if

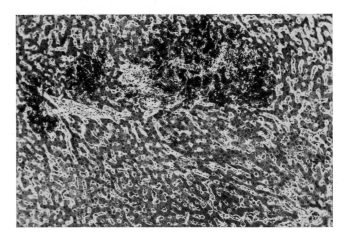

Fig. 352. The liver in eclampsia. Focal periportal necrosis of liver cells; the lesion contains fibrin. Mallory's phosphotungstic acid, × 80.

toxaemia is associated. Labour should certainly be induced once intra-uterine death has occurred.

Further pregnancies are not contraindicated. It has been reported without recurrence and with resulting healthy babies [4, 19].

Pregnancy toxaemias

Raised serum alkaline phosphatase and transaminase are common in toxaemia, but jaundice is rare [33]. The jaundice is mainly haemolytic. Occasionally, however, jaundice is deep, and secondary to disseminated intravascular coagulation with haemolysis and hepatic necrosis [14, 18]. Failure of renal bilirubin excretion may contribute. It is a grave sign, often being terminal. It may be associated with acute fatty liver of pregnancy.

Hepatic histology shows periportal, fibrin deposition in the sinusoids with haemorrhages (fig. 352). Centrizonal necrosis and haemorrhage represent shock. An inflammatory reaction is characteristically absent.

Recurrent intra-hepatic cholestatic jaundice [23]

This usually appears in the last trimester of pregnancy [34]. It has been termed hépatite bénigne de la grossesse [6] and is now called cholestatic jaundice of pregnancy [10].

Aetiology

This is unknown. It probably represents an unusual cholestatic reaction to a steroid produced in pregnancy. Whether this is an abnormal response to a natural steroid or to the production of an un-

known cholestatic one remains uncertain. Normal women in the last trimester show increased difficulty in the transfer of BSP to the biliary canaliculi [7]. The response in recurrent cholestatic jaundice of pregnancy may be an exaggeration of the normal one. Moreover, natural oestrogens, in large doses, also cause abnormalities in the handling of BSP. Oestriol metabolism is undoubtedly abnormal, but this seems to be secondary to the cholestasis rather than a primary event. The abnormality in these women probably resides in the liver rather than in the type of steroid synthesized [7, 16].

There is a relationship between this condition and jaundice following some oral contraceptive drugs. Twenty-seven of 40 patients developing cholestasis after oral contraceptives had suffered either jaundice or late pruritus during pregnancy [26]. This suggests an abnormal reaction to steroid hormones whether given therapeutically or naturally produced in pregnancy.

There is a genetic incidence both in cholestasis of pregnancy and cholestasis after oral contraceptives. An incidence has been shown in family members [9, 11, 30]. Reports of jaundice following oral contraceptives come from countries where current intra-hepatic cholestasis of pregnancy is frequent, such as Chile and Scandinavia [26, 29].

Clinical features

In the mildest form, jaundice is absent and the only abnormality is pruritus. Many patients experiencing generalized itching in the last weeks of pregnancy may be suffering from this condition. Jaundice is rarely deep, the urine is dark and the stools pale. General health is preserved and there is no pain. The liver and spleen are impalpable. After delivery, within one to two weeks pruritus ceases and the jaundice disappears. The condition recurs with subsequent pregnancies.

Biochemical changes

Serum shows an increase in conjugated bilirubin, usually less than 6 mg/100 ml, alkaline phosphatase and bile acid values. Serum transaminases are normal or slightly increased although occasionally very high values are found.

Hepatic histology

Histology, obtained by needle biopsy, shows centrizonal, often patchy, cholestasis. Hepato-cellular necrosis and cellular reaction are absent. Electron microscopy shows the dilatation, blunting and swelling of the microvilli which is constantly found in all forms of cholestasis. At operation, in one case, bile viscosity and secretion pressure were normal [2].

Prognosis

This is good. However, mothers may develop postpartum haemorrhage due to vitamin K deficiency [28]. Intra-uterine deaths and premature births are increased [28], particularly when cholestasis is severe [17].

The diagnosis, however, must be distinguished from more serious forms of cholestasis, such as primary biliary cirrhosis, which may present during pregnancy.

Treatment

Mild pruritus may respond simply to antihistaminics. Otherwise, cholestyramine should be given in full dosage. Vitamin K is given intramuscularly.

Viral hepatitis

This is the commonest cause of jaundice in pregnant women. Numerous needle punctures during the antenatal period are a possible source of infection. Moreover, women of child-bearing age are in close contact with the excreta of their children. Hepatitis is most frequent between the ages of

three and 10. Family contacts with young children expose them to type A infection. Pregnant women are not more susceptible to hepatitis than the general population. The incidence of hepatitis in epidemics is the same in the pregnant and non-pregnant [21]. It is equal in all trimesters of pregnancy. The clinical course, liver function tests and hepatic histology are the same as in the disease in the general population. A favourable outcome may usually be anticipated for the mother with hepatitis [1]. It is often stated that virus hepatitis is particularly lethal to the pregnant woman. In Europe and the United States this is certainly not so [1, 10, 21]. High mortality rates are reported from areas where protein malnutrition is frequent. A high mortality rate has for instance been reported from under-nourished women in India [20]. Such reports have led the World Health Organization to recommend that, when supplies of prophylactic γ-globulin are limited, these should be used preferentially for pregnant women exposed to the disease.

Management is similar in the pregnant and the non-pregnant. If necessary, diagnosis may be confirmed by needle biopsy, using the Menghini technique. Termination of pregnancy in fulminant hepatitis should be avoided because it adds the strain of operation upon an already failing liver.

There are variable reports concerning the effects on the foetus. Hepatitis is said to induce a tendency towards abortion or premature delivery [21], the survival depending on the stage of maturity at birth and not on the mother's disease [10]. Others have not observed an increased foetal wastage in pregnancies complicated by hepatitis [1].

Transmission of virus hepatitis (type B) to the foetus is discussed in Chapter 23.

Gall-stones

At all ages gall-stones are more frequent in women than men and especially so below the age of 50. Gall-stones are also associated with obesity and parity (Chapter 29). Stones in the common bile duct may therefore coincide with pregnancy and cause jaundice. The association is, however, surprisingly rare. In one combined series it comprised only 27 of 456 patients with jaundice in pregnancy [10]. The clinical picture does not differ from that in the non-pregnant and the management should be the same. In the jaundiced, liver biopsy, ultrasound and ERCP may be necessary.

Hepato-toxic drugs and the pregnant woman

The pregnant woman can react to drugs causing jaundice in similar fashion to the non-pregnant. Increased sensitivity to tetracycline has already been discussed and this would apply to any drug which decreases hepatic synthetic processes. Sensitivity to chlorpromazine with consequent cholestatic jaundice is infrequent. When it does affect the pregnant, however, it may be particularly prolonged, lasting for up to three and a half years.

The effect of drugs in potentiation of jaundice or kernicterus in the newborn must be considered (Chapter 17). In particular, drugs such as sulphonamides, which displace bilirubin from its binding to serum bilirubin, or novobiocin, which inhibits conjugation in the liver, should be avoided. Drugs such as phenacetin, given to the mother, may precipitate jaundice in an infant with glucose-6-phosphate dehydrogenase deficiency.

Effect of pregnancy on pre-existing liver disease

The mild jaundice associated with the benign, familial hyperbilirubinaemias (Dubin–Johnson, Rotor types) is reported both to increase and decrease with pregnancy. In the Gilbert type, where the hyperbilirubinaemia is unconjugated, jaundice is decreased by hepatic glucuronyl transferase induction due to increased amounts of sex hormones in pregnancy.

Pregnancy is uncommon in women with cirrhosis of the liver. This may in general be due to the age incidence of the cirrhotic women and to reduced fertility. In a comprehensive review, Haemmerli [10] could cite only 35 published cases. Patients with chronic active hepatitis or Wilson's disease [35] tend to be younger and to be physically attractive. It is not surprising that they marry and

that those whose disease has become relatively inactive become pregnant. Eight such patients became pregnant and five went to term [36]. Four of these had normal deliveries (one patient twice) and one a Caesarean section. Four deteriorated during pregnancy, two developing toxaemia, one bleeding from varices and having a porta-caval anastomosis (fig. 353) and one ascites. Within two months of delivery all five were in their pre-pregnancy state. Five of the babies were normal; one was malformed and subsequently died. Another patient died at 30 weeks, having been delivered of a stillborn baby. Three others had abortions, two spontaneous, one therapeutic. It can be concluded that if patients with chronic active hepatitis become pregnant they will not suffer permanent deterioration of liver function. The coincidence of liver disease and pregnancy should not *per se* indicate termination. Special care must be taken during the pregnancy. A specialist obstetric unit is essential. Spontaneous delivery should be anticipated.

Primary biliary cirrhosis may present as a cholestatic jaundice in or shortly after pregnancy.

REFERENCES

1. ADAMS R.H. & COMBES B. (1965) Viral hepatitis during pregnancy. *J. Am. med. Assoc.* **192,** 195.
2. ADLERCREUTZ H., SVANBORG A. & ÄNBERG Ä. (1967) Recurrent jaundice in pregnancy. I. clinical and ultrastructural study. *Am. J. Med.* **42,** 335.
3. BREEN K.J., PERKINS K.W., MISTILIS S.P. *et al* (1970) Idiopathic acute fatty liver of pregnancy. *Gut* **11,** 822.
4. BREEN K.J., PERKINS K.W., SHENKER S. *et al* (1972) Uncomplicated subsequent pregnancy after idiopathic fatty liver of pregnancy. *Obstet. Gynecol.* **40,** 813.

Fig. 353. Serial serum bilirubin levels during pregnancy in a patient with chronic active hepatitis. One haematemesis before and three during pregnancy were followed by an end-to-end porta-caval shunt in the fifth month. Oedema developed in the last trimester and a live baby was delivered normally at term. This woman was alive and well six years later (Whelton & Sherlock 1968).

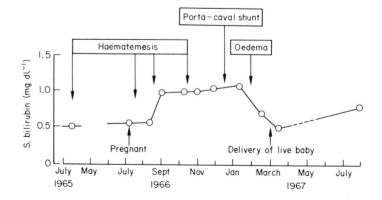

5. CANO R.I., DELMAN M.R., PITCHUMONI C.S. *et al* (1975) Acute fatty liver of pregnancy. Complication by disseminated intravascular coagulation. *J. Am. med. Assoc.* **231**, 159.

6. CAROLI J., PUYO G. & RAMPON (1954) Remarques sur les hépatites ictérigènes de la grossesse. *Sem. Hôp. Paris* **30**, 1692.

7. COMBES B., SHIBATA H., ADAMS R. *et al* (1963) Alterations in sulfobromophthalein sodium-removal mechanisms from blood during normal pregnancy. *J. clin. Invest.* **42**, 1431.

8. DUMA R.J., DOWLING E.A., ALEXANDER H.C. *et al* (1965) Acute fatty liver of pregnancy. Report of a surviving patient studied with serial liver biopsies. *Ann. intern. Med.* **63**, 851.

9. FURHOFF A.-K. & HELLSTRÖM J. (1973) Jaundice in pregnancy. A follow-up study of the series of women originally reported by L. Thorling. *Acta med. Scand.* **193**, 259.

10. HAEMMERLI U.P. (1966) Jaundice during pregnancy with special emphasis on recurrent jaundice during pregnancy and its differential diagnosis. *Acta med. Scand.* **179** (suppl.), 444.

11. HOLZBACH R.T. & SANDERS J.H. (1965) Recurrent intrahepatic cholestasis of pregnancy. Observations on pathogenesis. *J. Am. med. Assoc.* **193**, 542.

12. INGERSLEV M. & TEILUM G. (1951) Jaundice during pregnancy. *Acta obstet. gynecol. Scand.* **31**, 74.

13. JOSKE R.A., McCULLLY D.J. & MASTAGLIA F.L. (1968) Acute fatty liver of pregnancy. *Gut* **9**, 489.

14. KILLAM A.P., DILLARD S.H., PATTON R.C. *et al* (1975) Pregnancy-induced hypertension complicated by acute liver disease and disseminated intravascular coagulation. *Am. J. Obstet. Gynecol.* **123**, 823.

15. KIRBY N.G. (1969) Primary hepatic pregnancy. *Br. med. J.* i, 296.

16. KREEK M.J., SLEISENGER M.H. & JERRRIES G.H. (1967) Recurrent cholestatic jaundice of pregnancy with demonstrated estrogen sensitivity. *Am. J. Med.* **43**, 795.

17. LAATIKAINEN T. & IKONEN E. (1977) Serum bile acids in cholestasis of pregnancy. *Obstet. Gynecol.* **50**, 313.

18. LONG R.G., SCHEUER P.J. & SHERLOCK S. (1977) Pre-eclampsia presenting with deep jaundice. *J. clin. Pathol.* **30**, 212.

19. MACKENNA J., PUPKIN M., CRENSHAW C. Jr *et al* (1977) Acute fatty metamorphosis of the liver. A report of two patients who survived. *Am. J. Obstet. Gynecol.* **127**, 400.

20. MALKANI P.K. & GREWAL A.K. (1957) Observations on infectious hepatitis in pregnancy. *Indian J. med. Res.* **45** (suppl.), 77.

21. MARTINI G.A. (1953) Hepatitis und Schwangerschaft. *Schweiz. Z. allg. Pathol.* **16**, 475.

22. MILLER J.P. (1977) Diseases of the liver and alimentary tract. *Clin. Obstet. Gynaecol.* **4**, 297.

23. MISTILIS S.P. (1968) Liver disease in pregnancy, with particular emphasis on the cholestatic syndromes. *Aust. Ann. Med.* **17**, 248.

24. MUNNELL E.W. & TAYLOR H.C. Jr (1947) Liver blood flow in pregnancy—hepatic vein catheterization. *J. clin. Invest.* **26**, 952.

25. NELSON E.W., ARCHIBALD L. & ALBO D. Jr (1977) Spontaneous hepatic rupture in pregnancy. *Am. J. Surg.* **134**, 817.

26. ORELLANA-ALCALDE J.M. & DOMINGUEZ J.P. (1966) Jaundice and oral contraceptive drugs. *Lancet* ii, 1278.

27. PARBHOO S.P., OWENS D., SCHEUER P.J. *et al* (1972) Acute fatty liver of pregnancy. *Gut* **13**, 319.

28. REID R., IVEY K.J., RENCORET R.H. (1976) Fetal complications of obstetric cholestasis. *Br. med. J.* i, 870.

29. REYES H., GONZALES M.C., RIBALTA J. *et al* (1978) Prevalence of intrahepatic cholestasis of pregnancy in Chile. *Ann. intern. Med.* **88**, 487.

30. REYES H., RIBALTA J. & GONZÁLES-CERÓN, M. (1976) Idiopathic cholestasis of pregnancy in a large kindred. *Gut* **17**, 709.

31. ROMSLO I., SAGEN N. & HARAM K. (1975) Serum alkaline phosphatase in pregnancy. I. A comparative study of total, L-phenylalanine-sensitive and heat-stable alkaline phosphatase at 56°C and at 65°C in normal and pregnancy. *Acta Obstet. Gynecol. Scand.* **54**, 437.

32. SHEEHAN H.L. (1940) The pathology of acute yellow atrophy and delayed chloroform poisoning. *J. Obstet. Gynaecol. Br. Emp.* **47**, 49.

33. SHEEHAN H.L. (1961) Jaundice in pregnancy. *Am. J. Obstet. Gynecol.* **81**, 427.

34. SVANBORG A. & OHLSSON S. (1959) Recurrent jaundice of pregnancy: a clinical study of twenty-two cases. *Am. J. Med.* **27**, 40.

35. WALSHE J.M. (1977) Pregnancy in Wilson's disease. *Q. J. Med.* **46**, 73.

36. WHELTON M.J. & SHERLOCK S. (1968) Pregnancy in patients with hepatic cirrhosis. Management and outcome. *Lancet* ii, 995.

FIBROPOLYCYSTIC DISEASE

This large group of diseases is mostly inherited [4, 7, 23]. They range from those in which cysts are predominant, such as adult fibropolycystic disease, to congenital hepatic fibrosis, where fibrosis is the major abnormality (table 62) (fig. 354). They all have a genetic basis and are associated with various defects in the kidney. This suggests a primary developmental defect of parenchymatous origin. In addition, there is the condition of congenital intra-hepatic biliary dilatation (Caroli's syndrome), where the kidneys are not usually involved and which is apparently not familial. The various types may be combined.

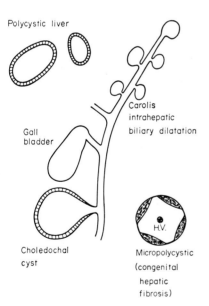

Fig. 354. The fibropolycystic diseases. The family includes congenital intra-hepatic biliary dilatation (Caroli's syndrome) and choledochal cyst; these communicate with the biliary tree. Polycystic disease is large cysts independent of the biliary tract. In congenital hepatic fibrosis microscopic cysts are found in the portal zones. Members of the family may be independent of one another or associated.

Choledochal cysts may be associated with any of them. Malignant change may complicate hepatic fibrosis, hepatic duct cysts and Caroli's syndrome [3].

The importance of the renal problem relative to the hepatic one varies from patient to patient [28].

These conditions are best regarded as a family of inherited hepato-biliary abnormalities and should be termed fibropolycystic disease of the liver and biliary tract [7].

Adult fibropolycystic disease

The liver may be involved by cysts which are probably developmental and similar to and frequently associated with polycystic kidneys.

The cysts may arise from defective development of the intra-hepatic bile ducts in the portal tracts. This may occur at about the 23 mm stage of foetal life, when the original segment of blind bile ducts is being replaced by a second generation of highly active, proliferating bile ducts. The original group may become distorted and degenerate into cysts. These, frequently localized, cystic areas are accompanied by normal second generation bile ducts elsewhere, so there is no biliary dysfunction. The situation is comparable to polycystic kidneys.

PATHOLOGY

Depending on the number and size of the cysts, the liver may be normal or greatly enlarged. Cysts may be scattered diffusely or restricted to one lobe, usually the left. The outer surface may be considerably deformed. A cyst may vary in size from a pin's head to a child's head, the largest having a capacity of over a litre. They are rarely greater than 10 cm in diameter. The larger ones are probably derived by rupture of septa between adjacent cysts, and the cut liver may display a honeycomb appearance. The cavities are thin walled and contain clear or brown fluid due to altered blood. They never contain bile.

Table 62. Hepatic fibropolycystic disease.

Subtype	Inheritance	Presentation	Hepatic	Portal hypertension	Renal
Adult fibropolycystic	Dominant	Adult	Cysts	Rare	Cysts
Childhood fibropolycystic					
Perinatal	Recessive	Birth	Fibrosis ± Ducts dilated +	–	90% tubules
Neonatal	Recessive	1 month	Fibrosis + + Ducts dilated +	–	60% tubules
Infantile	Recessive	3–6 months	Fibrosis + + Ducts dilated +	Common	25% tubules
Hepatic fibrosis	Recessive	Child or adult	Fibrosis + + + Ducts dilated +	Usual	0–10% tubules
Intra-hepatic biliary dilatation	?	Cholangitis any age	Dilated ducts only	–	–

Histologically (fig. 355) the lobular architecture is unchanged and the liver cells are normal. The cystic areas are related to the bile ducts in the portal areas. They are surrounded by a fibrous tissue capsule and lined by columnar epithelium, unless they are very large when the epithelium becomes flattened or even absent.

Frequently, there is cystic disease of other organs, including kidneys, spleen, pancreas, ovary and lungs. About half the patients with polycystic disease of the liver also have polycystic kidneys, but the reverse is less frequent and variously reported in up to a third of cases of polycystic kidney.

Other congenital anomalies are common and include spina bifida and polydactyly.

CLINICAL FEATURES

In many patients the liver lesion is only discovered at autopsy. In other instances, the patient presents with some other disease or perhaps with polycystic kidneys and the liver cysts are discovered incidentally.

Patients with symptoms and signs pointing to the liver are usually in the fourth or fifth decade. The patient complains of a gradual swelling of the upper abdomen. Pressure on the stomach and duo-

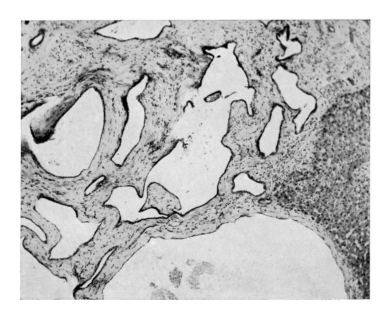

Fig. 355. Polycystic disease of the liver. The cysts vary in size and are lined by flattened epithelium. H & E, ×63.

denum causes epigastric discomfort, nausea, flatulence and occasional vomiting. Rarely, severe pain simulates biliary colic [10].

The symptoms are more often due to associated polycystic kidney disease.

On examination the liver may be impalpable or so large that it seems to fill the whole abdomen. The edge is firm and nodules can be palpated. The cystic character of the nodule is not always easy to define and there may be difficulty in diagnosing cysts from other types of liver nodule.

Bilaterally enlarged irregular *kidneys* may suggest the associated renal cysts.

Hepatic function is excellent for the liver cells are uninvolved.

Portal venous obstruction is usually absent. Oesophageal varices are rare [11]. The spleen is not enlarged. *Needle biopsy* has proved safe and a portion of cyst wall may be obtained for section [10].

Radiological diagnosis. A plain radiograph of the abdomen confirms the hepatomegaly, and a barium meal may show displacement of stomach and duodenum.

Scintiscanning and *ultrasound* show multiple filling defects in the liver [35] (fig. 53). *Hepatic arteriography* shows the branches of the hepatic artery stretched around the cysts which are avascular.

DIFFERENTIAL DIAGNOSIS

Polycystic liver may be suspected in an apparently fit person often over 30 years of age, with nodular hepatomegaly, but no evidence of hepatic dysfunction, associated with polycystic kidney or a family history of this condition.

The condition may be confused with *hydatid disease* (Chapter 27). The liver is not usually diffusely nodular, and hepatic calcification, eosinophilia and the hydatid complement fixation test are diagnostically helpful.

Metastases are accompanied by failure in health, rapid increase in size of the liver, a raised sedimentation rate, and, possibly, evidence of a primary neoplasm.

Cirrhosis may have accompanying signs of hepato-cellular disease.

PROGNOSIS AND TREATMENT

Polycystic disease of the liver is compatible with long life. In one series in no instance had polycystic disease of the liver contributed to the death or ill-health of the patient [10].

The prognosis of polycystic disease of the liver is determined by the extent of associated renal cystic disease. Malignant change is rare [3].

Exploratory laparotomy is rarely indicated for diagnosis. Active surgical treatment is usually unnecessary. Cysts containing pus or blood must be drained externally. Large cysts (greater than 10 cm) may be excised if causing symptoms and if accessible.

Congenital hepatic fibrosis [21]

This condition consists, histologically, of broad, densely collagenous fibrous bands surrounding otherwise normal hepatic lobules (fig. 357; see colour section for fig. 358) [21]. The bands contain large numbers of microscopic, well-formed bile ducts, some containing bile. Rarely the intrahepatic ducts are dilated and contain concretions [8]. Caroli's syndrome may be associated [25], also choledochal cyst.

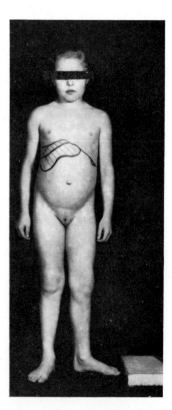

Fig. 356. Girl of eight years. Hepatosplenomegaly discovered at routine examination. Liver biopsy showed congenital fibrosis. Note normal development.

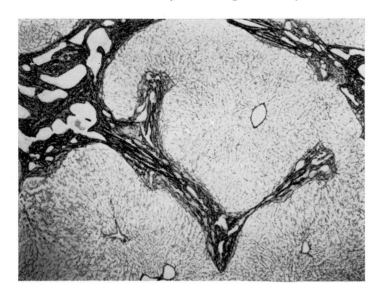

Fig. 357. Congenital hepatic fibrosis. Broad bands of fibrous tissue containing bile ducts separate and surround liver lobules. Silver impregnation, × 36. (Kerr *et al* 1961.)

The disease appears both sporadically and in a familial form. It is probably inherited as an autosomal recessive.

Portal hypertension is common. Occasionally this may be due to defects in the main portal veins. More often it is caused by hypoplasia or fibrous compression of portal vein radicles in the fibrous bands surrounding the nodules.

Associated renal conditions include renal tubular ectasia, adult type polycystic kidneys and nephrophthisis [5].

CLINICAL FEATURES

The condition is usually misdiagnosed as cirrhosis. The patient is usually diagnosed between the ages of three and 10 years but recognition may be delayed until adult life. The patient presents with haemorrhage from oesophageal varices, a symptomless, large, very hard liver or splenomegaly (table 63) (fig. 356).

Occasionally a large cyst may obstruct a bile duct causing cholestatic jaundice. Other congenital anomalies, especially of the biliary system, may be present. Pulmonary fibrosis has been associated.

Carcinoma, both hepato-cellular and cholangiolar, may be a complication [26, 34].

INVESTIGATIONS

Serum protein, bilirubin and transaminase levels are usually normal, but serum alkaline phosphatase values are sometimes increased.

Liver biopsy is essential for diagnosis. Because of the tough consistency of the liver this may fail, and a wedge, operative sample may be necessary.

Portal venography reveals the collateral circulation and a normal or distorted intra-hepatic portal tree [21].

Intravenous pyelography may show cystic changes or medullary sponge 'kidney'.

PROGNOSIS AND TREATMENT

Congenital hepatic fibrosis must be distinguished from cirrhosis since hepato-cellular function is preserved and the prognosis is considerably better.

Following haemorrhage these patients are excellent candidates for porta-caval anastomosis.

Death can be due to renal failure.

Table 63. The presentation of sixteen patients with congenital hepatic fibrosis.

Presentation	No.	Age (yr)
Large abdomen	9	$2\frac{1}{2}$–9
Haematemesis or melaena	5	3–6
Jaundice	1	10
Anaemia	1	16

Congenital intra-hepatic biliary dilatation (Caroli's disease) [8]

This rare syndrome is characterized by congenital, segmental saccular dilatations of the intra-hepatic bile ducts. The dilated ducts connect with the main duct system and are liable to become infected and contain stones.

The liver also shows the features of congenital hepatic fibrosis [7, 25, 29].

Caroli's disease is not familial. Kidney lesions are usually absent, but renal tubular ectasia [25] and larger cysts have been associated.

CLINICAL FEATURES [17]

The condition presents at any age, but usually in childhood or early adult life, as abdominal pain and fever with Gram-negative septicaemia [10, 29].

Jaundice is mild or absent but may increase dur-ing the episodes of cholangitis. Malabsorption is frequent [22]. Portal hypertension is absent.

Ultrasound shows dilated intra-hepatic ducts. *Percutaneous endoscopic operative cholangiography* shows sacculation of dilated ducts. The common bile duct may also be dilated (fig. 359). Only one lobe may be affected. *Intravenous cholangiography*, even with tomography, usually fails.

In one patient biliary drainage through a T tube was grossly excessive and flow was further increased by an infusion of secretin which increases ductular flow. It is likely that the high resting flow rate arose from the cysts [37].

Cholangiocarcinoma may be a complication [3].

TREATMENT

Antibiotics are given to treat the cholangitis as it appears, and drainage of the common bile duct is required to remove calculi.

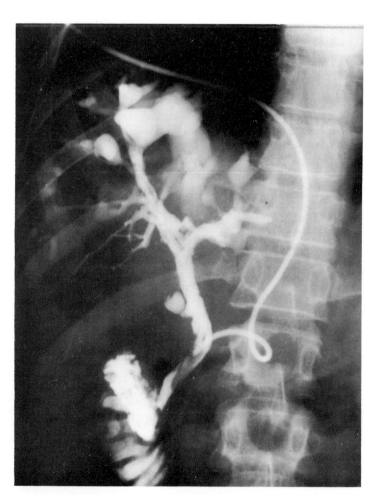

Fig. 359. Congenital intra-hepatic biliary dilatation. Operative cholangiography through a tube in the common bile duct shows a common bile duct of normal size. The intra-hepatic biliary tree is marked by saccular dilatations (Turnberg *et al* 1968).

The prognosis is poor but episodes of cholangitis can extend over many years.

Death from renal failure is very unusual.

Choledochal cyst

This is an aneurysmal dilatation of the common bile duct [36]. It arises in embryonic life from localized proliferation with subsequent vacuolization. The gall bladder, cystic duct and hepatic ducts above the cyst are not dilated. Multiple cysts may be present.

The lesion presents as a partially retroperitoneal, cystic tumour varying from 2–3 cm in size, to a capacity of 8 litres. The cyst contains thin, dark brown fluid. It is sterile but may become secondarily infected. The cyst can burst.

In the adult, recurrent pancreatitis can be associated [12], and gall-stones may form in the gall bladder [27].

There is an association with malignant tumours in the cyst or in bile ducts [20].

Histologically, the cyst wall consists of fibrous tissue lacking epithelium or smooth muscle.

CLINICAL FEATURES

The patient is usually female and under 10 years old. It may present in the newborn. Occasionally the lesion is latent and survivals up to 79 years have been recorded. There is a preponderance in the Japanese.

The characteristic triad of symptoms is intermittent jaundice, pain and abdominal tumour. In the infant the presentation is as obstructive jaundice [15].

The jaundice is intermittent, of cholestatic type, and associated with fever. The pain is colicky and mainly experienced in the right upper abdomen. The tumour is cystic and in the right upper quadrant of the abdomen. It characteristically varies in size and in tenseness.

Choledochal cysts may be associated with congenital hepatic fibrosis or with dilatation of the intra-hepatic bile ducts.

In infancy the cyst may perforate, causing bile peritonitis. Portal hypertension may be due to obstruction of the portal vein by the cyst.

Plain X-ray of the abdomen may show a soft tissue mass.

Barium meal shows displacement of the stomach and duodenum to the left and anteriorly and the hepatic flexure of the colon downwards.

Cholecystography often fails, but may show the gall bladder to be displaced to the right and flattened.

Intravenous cholangiography sometimes visualizes the cyst.

Percutaneous or *retrograde cholangiography* are diagnostic.

Ultrasound or *CT scanning* may be helpful.

TREATMENT

Surgical excision of the cyst is the treatment of choice, the continuity of the biliary tract being maintained by choledochojejunostomy [24]. In many instances this is technically impossible, and surgical excision of the duodenal portion of the cyst wall is performed [12]. Anastomosis of the cyst to the intestinal tract, usually jejunum or duodenum, is simpler to perform, but post-operative cholangitis necessitating re-operation is frequent [24].

Solitary non-parasitic liver cyst

This extremely rare condition might be a variant of polycystic disease.

The lining wall has partitions, which suggest an origin from conglomerate polycystic disease. The fibrous capsule contains aberrant bile ducts and blood vessels. The contents vary from colourless to brown altered blood. It appears as a smooth, glistening, greyish-blue cyst usually on the antero-inferior aspect of the right lobe. The tension is low in contrast to the high pressure of hydatid cysts.

Symptoms are related to abdominal distension, or pressure effects on adjacent organs including the bile ducts, causing intermittent jaundice [32].

Rarely, severe symptoms of shock follow rupture or haemorrhage into the cyst. Surgical excision is indicated only for complications.

Other cysts

These are all very rare, small and superficial. Their contents vary with the cause. Bile cysts may follow prolonged extra-hepatic biliary obstruction of all types. Mucous cysts arise from mucous glands in the walls of the biliary passages. Blood cysts follow haemorrhage into a simple cyst. They can also follow trauma to the liver. Small cystic spaces containing blood may follow needle biopsy. They are seen when autopsy follows within a short time of the biopsy. Lymphatic cysts are due to obstruction or congenital dilatation of liver lymphatics. They are usually on the surface of the liver.

Malignant pseudocysts result from degeneration and softening of secondary malignant growths.

CONGENITAL ANOMALIES OF THE BILIARY TRACT

The liver and biliary tract develop from a bud-like outpouching of the ventral wall of the primitive foregut just cranial to the yolk sac. Two solid buds of cells form the right and left lobes of the liver while the original elongated diverticulum forms the hepatic and common bile ducts. The gall bladder arises as a smaller bud of cells from this same diverticulum. The biliary tract is patent in early intra-uterine life but becomes solid later by epithelial proliferation within the lumen. Eventually revacuolization takes place, starting simultaneously in different parts of the solid gall bladder bud and spreading until the whole system is recanalized. At five weeks the ductal communications of gall bladder, cystic duct and hepatic ducts are completed and at three months the foetal liver begins to secrete bile [19].

The majority of the congenital anomalies can be related to alterations in the original budding from the foregut or to failure of vacuolization of the solid gall bladder and bile diverticulum [14] (table 64).

These congenital defects are usually of no importance and cannot be related to symptoms [2]. Occasionally they may predispose to bile stasis, inflammation and gall-stones. They are of importance to the radiologist and to the biliary surgeon.

Anomalies of the biliary tree and liver may be associated with congenital lesions elsewhere, including cardiac defects, polydactyly and polycystic kidneys. They can also be related to maternal virus infections, such as rubella.

Absence of the gall bladder

This is a rare congenital anomaly [16]. Multiple congenital defects are usually present [16]. Two types can be recognized.

Type I is the failure of the gall bladder and cystic duct to develop as an outgrowth from the hepatic diverticulum of the foregut. This type is often found with other anomalies of the biliary passages.

Type II is the failure of the gall bladder to vacuolize from its solid state. This is usually associated with atresia of the extra-hepatic ducts. The gall bladder is not absent but *rudimentary*. This type is therefore found in infants who present the picture of congenital biliary atresia.

Failure to identify the gall bladder at operation is not proof of its absence. The gall bladder may be intra-hepatic, buried in extensive adhesions, or atrophied following previous cholecystitis. Cholangiography is useful in confirming absence of the gall bladder. There are no specific symptoms.

Double gall bladder

Double gall bladder is very rare [9]. In embryonic life, little pockets often arise from the hepatic or common bile ducts. Occasionally these persist and form a second gall bladder having its own cystic duct (fig. 360). This may enter the hepatic sub-

Table 64. Classification of congenital anomalies of the biliary tract.

Anomalies of the primitive foregut bud
Failure of bud
  Absent bile ducts
  Absent gall bladder
Accessory buds or splitting of bud
  Accessory gall bladder
  Bilobed gall bladder
  Accessory bile ducts
Bud migrates to left instead of right
  Left-sided gall bladder

Anomalies of vacuolization of the solid biliary bud
Defective bile duct vacuolization
Congenital obliteration of bile ducts
Congenital obliteration of cystic duct
Choledochal cyst
Defective gall bladder vacuolization
  Rudimentary gall bladder
Fundal diverticulum
Serosal type of Phrygian cap
Hour-glass gall bladder

Persistent cysto-hepatic duct
Diverticulum of body or neck of gall bladder

Persistence of intra-hepatic gall bladder

Aberrant folding of gall bladder anlage
Retroserosal type of Phrygian cap

Accessory peritoneal folds
Congenital adhesions
Floating gall bladder

Anomalies of hepatic and cystic arteries
Accessory arteries
Abnormal relation of hepatic artery to cystic duct

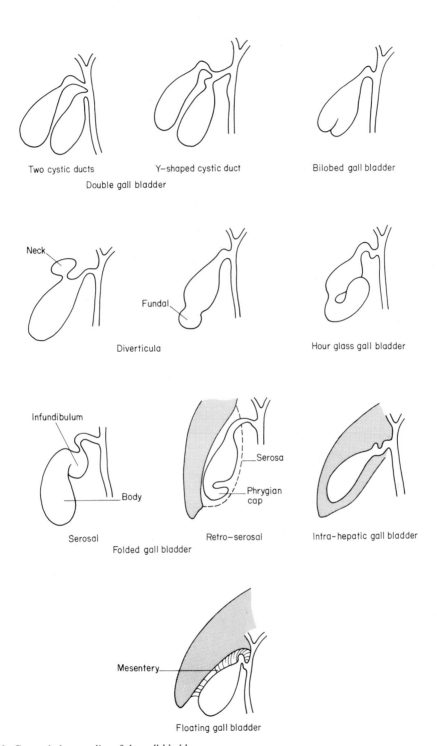

Fig. 360. Congenital anomalies of the gall bladder.

stance directly. If the pouch forms from the cystic duct the two gall bladders share a cystic duct (Y-shaped cystic duct) (fig. 360).

Double gall bladder can be recognized by cholecystography. The accessory organ is frequently diseased.

Bilobed gall bladder [18] is an extremely rare congenital anomaly, there being only about 10 recorded cases. Embryologically, the single bud forming the gall bladder becomes paired but primary connection is maintained, thus forming two separate and distinct fundi with a single cystic duct.

The anomaly is of no clinical significance.

Accessory bile ducts

These are rare. The extra duct is usually the right hepatic and joins the common hepatic duct somewhere between the junction of the right and left hepatic ducts and the entry of the cystic duct. It may, however, join the cystic duct, the gall bladder or the common bile duct.

Cholecysto-hepatic ducts are due to persistence of foetal connections between the gall bladder and the liver parenchyma with failure of recanalization of the right and left hepatic ducts [19]. Continuity is maintained by the cystic duct entering a remaining hepatic duct or common hepatic duct or the duodenum directly.

Accessory ducts are of importance to the biliary surgeon as they may be inadvertently ligated or cut with resultant biliary stricture or fistula.

Left-sided gall bladder

In this rare anomaly the gall bladder lies under the left lobe of the liver to the left of the falciform ligament [30]. The embryonic bud from the hepatic diverticulum migrates to the left instead of to the right. Alternatively, it may be due to independent development of a second gall bladder from the left hepatic duct with failure of development or regression of the normal structure on the right side.

In transposition of the viscera, the gall bladder bears its normal relationship to the liver but lies on the left side of the abdomen.

A left-sided gall bladder is of little clinical significance; it is recognized by cholecystography.

Rokitansky–Aschoff sinuses of the gall bladder

These consist of hernia-like protrusions of the gall bladder mucosa through the muscular layer (intra-mural diverticulosis) [31]. Although potentially congenital they are particularly prominent with chronic cholecystitis when intra-luminar pressure rises. They may be seen in an oral cholecystogram as a halo-like stippling surrounding the gall bladder.

Folded gall bladder

The gall bladder is deformed so that the fundus appears folded 'bent down to the breaking point after the manner of a *Phrygian cap*' [6]. A Phrygian cap is defined as a conical cap or bonnet, with the peak bent or turned over in front, worn by the ancient Phrygians, and identified with the Cap of Liberty (*Oxford English Dictionary*).

Two varieties are recognized:

Kinking between body and fundus (retroserosal; Phrygian cap) (fig. 360). This is due to aberrant folding of the gall bladder within the embryonic fossa.

Kinking between body and infundibulum (serosal) (fig. 360). This is due to aberrant folding of the fossa itself in the early stages of development. The bend in the gall bladder is fixed by development of foetal ligaments, vestigial septa or constrictions of the lumen following delayed vacuolization of the solid epithelial anlage.

These kinked gall bladders empty at a normal rate and are of no clinical significance [6]. The importance lies in the correct interpretation of cholecystograms.

Hour-glass gall bladder. This probably represents an exaggerated form of Phrygian cap, presumably of the serosal type. The constancy of position of the fundus during contraction and the small size of the opening between the two parts indicate that this is probably a fixed, congenital malformation.

Diverticula of the gall bladder and ducts

Diverticula of body and neck may arise from persistent cysto-hepatic ducts which run in embryonic life between the gall bladder and the liver.

The *fundal variety* arises from incomplete vacuolization of the solid gall bladder of embryonic life. An incomplete septum pinches off a small cavity at the tip of the gall bladder (fig. 360).

These diverticula are rare and of no clinical significance. The congenital variety should be distinguished from *pseudo-diverticula* usually containing a large stone developing in the diseased gall bladder as a result of partial perforation; the pseudo-diverticulum in these cases usually contains a large gallstone.

Intra-hepatic gall bladder

The gall bladder is included and buried in hepatic tissue up to the second month of intra-uterine life, thereafter assuming an extra-hepatic position. In some instances the intra-hepatic condition may persist. The gall bladder is higher than normal and more or less buried but never entirely covered by liver tissue. It is frequently diseased, for the embedded organ has difficulty in contracting and so becomes infected, with subsequent gall-stone formation.

Congenital adhesions to the gall bladder

These are very frequent. Developmentally these peritoneal sheets are due to an extension of the anterior mesentery, which forms the lesser omentum. The sheet may run from the common bile duct laterally over the gall bladder down to the duodenum, to the hepatic flexure of the colon and even to the right lobe of the liver, perhaps closing the foramen of Winslow. In a milder form a band of tissue runs from the lesser omentum across to the cystic duct and anterior to the gall bladder; or a loose veil forms a mesentery to the gall bladder ('floating gall bladder').

These adhesions are of no clinical importance. Surgically, their presence should be remembered, so that they are not mistaken for inflammatory adhesions.

Floating gall bladder and torsion of the gall bladder

The gall bladder possesses a supporting membrane in 4–5% of specimens. The peritoneal coat surrounding the gall bladder continues as two approximated leaves to form a fold or mesentery to support the gall bladder from under the surface of the liver. This fold may allow the gall bladder to hang for as much as 2–3 cm below the inferior hepatic surface.

The mobile gall bladder is apt to twist, and *torsion* results. The blood supply is impaired in the small pedicle and infarction follows.

The condition usually occurs in thin, elderly women. With ageing, omental fat lessens and visceroptosis increases. The gall bladder with mesentery becomes more pendulous and can twist. It can affect all ages, including children.

Torsion is followed by sudden, severe, constant epigastric and right costal margin pain passing through to the back with vomiting and collapse. Characteristically a palpable tumour appears, having the features of an enlarged gall bladder. Within a few hours it may disappear. The treatment is cholecystectomy.

Recurrent partial torsion leads to acute episodes [1]. Cholecystogram shows a normally functioning gall bladder situated low in the abdomen and even in the pelvis. It is suspended by a very long, down-curved cystic duct. Early cholecystectomy is indicated.

Anomalies of the cystic duct and cystic artery [14]

In 20% of subjects the cystic duct does not join the common hepatic duct directly but first runs parallel to it, lying in the same sheath of connective tissue. Occasionally it makes a spiral turn around the duct.

These variations are extremely important to the surgeon. Unless the cystic duct is carefully dissected and its union with the common hepatic duct identified, the common hepatic duct may be ligated, with disastrous consequences.

The *cystic artery* can arise not, as normally, from the right hepatic artery but from the left hepatic artery or even from the gastro-duodenal artery. Accessory cystic arteries usually arise from the right hepatic artery. Again, the surgeon must be careful during cholecystectomy to identify the cystic artery precisely.

REFERENCES

1. ASHBY B.S. (1965) Acute and recurrent torsion of the gall-bladder. *Br. J. Surg.* **52**, 182.
2. BARTEL J. (1918) Uber eine Formanomalie der Gallenblase und ihre biologischen Beziehungen. *Wien. klin. Wochenschr.* **31**, 605.
3. BLOUSTEIN P.A. (1977) Association of carcinoma with congenital cystic conditions of the liver and bile ducts. *Am. J. Gastroenterol.* **67**, 40.
4. BLYTH H. & OCKENDEN B.G. (1971) Polycystic disease of kidneys and liver presenting in childhood. *J. med. Genet.* **8**, 257.
5. BOICHIS H., PASSWELL J., DAVID R. *et al* (1973) Congenital hepatic fibrosis and nephrophthisis. A family study. *Q. J. Med.* **42**, 221.
6. BOYDEN E.A. (1935) The 'Phrygian cap' in cholecystography. A congenital anomaly of the gall bladder. *Am. J. Roentgenol.* **33**, 589.

7. BRUNT P.W. (1973) Genetics of liver disease. *Clin. Gastroenterol.* **2**, 615.

8. CAROLI J. & CORCOS V. (1964) La dilatation congénitale des voies biliaries intrahépatiques. *Rev. méd.-chir. Mal. Foie* **39**, 1.

9. CLOT M., THIERRÉE R.A. & TOD R. (1972) Vesicule biliare double. Une observation. *Presse méd.* **1**, 2313.

10. COMFORT M.W., GRAY H.K., DAHLIN D.C. *et al* (1952) Polycystic disease of the liver: a study of 24 cases. *Gastroenterology* **20**, 60.

11. DEL GUERCIO E., GRECO J., KIM K.E. *et al* (1973) Esophageal varices with polycystic kidney and liver disease. *New Engl. J. Med.* **289**, 678.

12. GOLDBERG P.B., LONG W.B., OLEAGA J.A. *et al* (1980) Choledochocele as a cause of recurrent pancreatitis. *Gastroenterology* **78**, 1041.

13. HADAD A.R., WESTBROOK K.C., GRAHAM G.G. *et al* (1977) Symptomatic non-parasitic liver cysts. *Am. J. Surg.* **134**, 739.

14. HAND B.H. (1973) Anatomy and function of the extrahepatic biliary system. Diseases of the biliary tract, ed. I.A.D. Bouchier. *Clin. Gastroenterol.* **2**, 1.

15. HARRIS V.J. & KAHLER J. (1978) Choledochal cyst: delayed diagnosis in a jaundiced infant. *Pediatrics* **62**, 235.

16. HAUGHTON V. & LEWICKI A.W. (1973) Agenesis of the gallbladder. Is preoperative diagnosis possible? *Radiology* **106**, 305.

17. HERMANSEN M.C., STARSHAK R.J. & WERLIN S.L. (1979) Caroli disease: the diagnostic approach. *J. Pediatr.* **94**, 879.

18. HOBBY J.A.E. (1970) Bilobed gall-bladder. *Br. J. Surg.* **57**, 870.

19. JACKSON J.B. & KELLY T.R. (1964) Cholecystohepatic ducts: case report. *Ann. Surg.* **159**, 581.

20. KAGAWA Y., KASHIHARA S., KURAMOTO S. *et al* (1978) Carcinoma arising in a congenitally dilated biliary tract. *Gastroenterology* **74**, 1286.

21. KERR D.N.S., HARRISON C.V., SHERLOCK S. *et al* (1961) Congenital hepatic fibrosis. *Q. J. Med.* **30**, 91.

22. KOCOSHIS S.A., RIELY C.A., BURRELL M. *et al* (1980) Cholangitis in a child due to biliary tract anomalies. *Dig. Dis. Sci.* **25**, 59.

23. LIEBERMAN E., SALINAS-MADRIGAL L., GWINN J.L. *et al* (1971) Infantile polycystic disease of the kidneys and liver. *Medicine (Baltimore)* **50**, 277.

24. LILLY J.R. (1979) The surgical treatment of choledochal cyst. *Surg. Gynecol. Obstet.* **149**, 36.

25. MALL J.C., GHAHREMANI G.G. & BOYER J.L. (1974) Caroli's disease associated with congenital hepatic fibrosis and renal tubular ectasia. A case report. *Gastroenterology* **46**, 1029.

26. MANES J.L., KISSANE J.M. & VALDES A.J. (1977) Congenital hepatic fibrosis, liver cell carcinoma and adult polycystic kidneys. *Cancer* **39**, 2619.

27. MATSUMOTO Y., UCHIDA K., NAKASE A. *et al* (1977) Congenital cystic dilatation of the common bile duct as a cause of primary bile duct stone. *Am. J. Surg.* **134**, 346.

28. MILUTINOVIC J., FIALKOW P.J., RUDD T.G. *et al* (1980) Liver cysts in patients with autosomal dominant kidney disease. *Am. J. Med.* **68**, 741.

29. MURRAY-LYON I.M., SHILKIN K.B., LAWS J.W. *et al* (1972) Non-obstructive dilatation of the intrahepatic biliary tree with cholangitis. *Q. J. Med.* **41**, 477.

30. NEWCOMBE J.F. & HENLEY F.A. (1964) Left-sided gallbladder. *Arch. Surg.* **88**, 494.

31. ROSS W.D., FINBY N. & EVANS J.A. (1955) Intramural diverticulosis of the gallbladder. *Radiology* **64**, 366.

32. SANTMAN F.W., THIJS L.E., VAN DER VEEN E.A. *et al* (1977) Intermittent jaundice: a rare complication of a solitary non-parasitic liver cyst. *Gastroenterology* **72**, 325.

33. SCHOLZ F.J., CARRERA G.F. & LARSEN C.R. (1976) The choledochocele: correlation of radiological, clinical and pathological findings. *Radiology* **118**, 25.

34. SCOTT J., SHOUSHA S., THOMAS H.C. *et al* (1980) Bile duct carcinoma: a late complication of congenital hepatic fibrosis. Case report and review of literature. *Am. J. Gastroenterol.* **73**, 113.

35. SPIEGEL R.M., KING D.L. & GREEN W.M. (1978) Ultrasonography of primary cysts of the liver. *Am. J. Roentgenol.* **131**, 235.

36. SPITZ L. (1978) Choledochal cyst. *Surg. Gynecol. Obstet.* **147**, 444.

37. TURNBERG L.A., JONES E.A. & SHERLOCK S. (1968) Biliary secretion in a patient with cystic dilation of the intrahepatic biliary tree. *Gastroenterology* **54**, 1155.

Chapter 26
The Liver in Systemic Disease;
Hepatic Trauma

THE LIVER IN THE COLLAGEN DISEASES

The liver has no significant role in aetiology. If hepatomegaly is present, it is probably due to amyloidosis in chronic rheumatoid arthritis, or to cardiac failure with rheumatic fever or systemic lupus erythematosus. Splenomegaly reflects reticulo-endothelial hyperplasia rather than portal hypertension.

There is an increased prevalence of HLA-B8 in many collagen diseases and in chronic active hepatitis.

Primary biliary cirrhosis is associated with collagen diseases (Chapter 14).

BIOCHEMISTRY

Serum α- and β-globulins may be elevated and serum albumin values slightly depressed. Serum bilirubin, transaminase and alkaline phosphatase levels are normal or mildly disturbed.

In *polyarteritis nodosa*, the hepatic arterioles may show characteristic lesions with, occasionally, small hepatic infarcts. Needle biopsy may be useful in diagnosis. Hepatic arterial aneurysms are sometimes found.

Hepatitis B carriage may be associated with polyarteritis nodosa [2], with migrating arthralgias, or with polymyositis [7]. Immune complexes containing HBsAg can be shown in the tissues.

Giant cell arteritis can be found with granulomatous liver disease [5].

In *rheumatoid arthritis*, the liver shows non-specific changes, such as mild fatty infiltration, focal necroses, or complicating amyloidosis [9].

In *Felty's syndrome*, lymphocytic infiltration of the sinusoids with nodular regenerative hyperplasia of normal appearing liver cells may lead to oesophageal variceal bleeding [1].

In *systemic lupus erythematosus*, hepatomegaly and jaundice, usually haemolytic, are occasionally found. Liver histology either shows no significant

change, lymphoid infiltration or chronic hepatitis [8]. Rarely a severe hepatic arteritis is present. Rupture of the liver has been reported [4].

In *polymyalgia rheumatica*, changes include a granulomatous hepatitis and lymphocytic infiltration [6]. These usually remit with corticosteroid treatment.

In *Weber–Christian disease* (relapsing febrile nodular non-suppurative panniculitis) severe fatty change may be seen with Mallory's hyaline. These changes are related to reduced lipoprotein synthesis in the deformed rough endoplasmic reticulum [3].

REFERENCES

1. BLENDIS L.M., LOVELL D., BARNES C.G. *et al* (1978) Oesophageal variceal bleeding in Felty's syndrome associated with nodular regenerative hyperplasia. *Ann. rheum. Dis.* **37**, 183.
2. DRUËKE T., BARBANEL C., JUNGERS P. *et al* (1980) Hepatitis B antigen-associated periarteritis nodosa in patients undergoing long-term hemodialysis. *Am. J. Med.* **68**, 86.
3. KIMURA H., KAKO M., YO K. *et al* (1980) Alcoholic hyalins (Mallory bodies) in a case of Weber–Christian disease; electron microscopic observations of liver involvement. *Gastroenterology* **78**, 807.
4. LEVITIN P.M., SWEET D., BRUNNER C.M. *et al* (1977) Spontaneous rupture of the liver; an unusual complication of SLE. *Arthritis Rheum.* **20**, 748.
5. LITWACK K.D., BOHAN A. & SILVERMAN L. (1977) Granulomatous liver disease and giant cell arteritis: case report and literature review. *J. Rheumatol.* **4**, 307.
6. LONG R. & JAMES O. (1974) Polymyalgia rheumatica and liver disease. *Lancet* i, 77.
7. MIHAS A.A., KIRBY D. & KENTS P. (1978) Hepatitis B antigen and polymyositis. *J. Am. med. Assoc.* **239**, 221.
8. RUNYON B.A., LA BRECQUE D.R. & ANURAS S. (1980) The spectrum of liver disease in systemic lupus erythematosus. *Am. J. Med.* **69**, 187.
9. WHALEY K. & WEBB J. (1977) Liver and kidney disease in rheumatoid arthritis. *Clin. rheum. Dis.* **3**, 527.

LIVER CHANGES IN ORGAN TRANSPLANT RECIPIENTS

Virus hepatitis. There is an increased prevalence of persistent carriage of hepatitis B in patients on long-term haemodialysis for end-stage kidney disease, and in those having renal transplants. Immunosuppression facilitates the viraemia [7, 11]. Such patients provide a potential reservoir of spread of hepatitis B to the general population [5].

Other types of virus hepatitis, such as non-A, non-B, herpes and cytomegala are also frequent in these patients [10, 11].

Hepatitis B-associated polyarteritis nodosa has been described in patients having long-term haemodialysis [4].

Vascular changes. These are probably related to prolonged administration of such drugs as 6-mercaptopurine or azathioprine. They include idiopathic portal hypertension due to peri-sinusoidal fibrosis [8] and veno-occlusive disease [6]. Peliosis hepatis is associated with sub-endothelial thickening at the junction of the sinusoid and centrizonal vein [3].

Cholestasis is also related to azathioprine therapy [1].

Nodular transformation of normal hepatocytes may be shown by reticulin stains of a liver biopsy; it is of unknown aetiology.

Hepatic changes after bone-marrow transplantation. A graft-versus-host reaction may involve skin, gut and liver [9]. Veno-occlusion can also be seen [2, 12].

REFERENCES

1. ANURAS S., PIROS J., BONNEY W.W. *et al* (1977) Liver disease in renal transplant recipients. *Arch. intern. Med.* **137**, 42.
2. BERK P.D., POPPER H., KRUEGER G.R.F. *et al* (1979) Veno-occlusive disease of the liver after allogeneic bone marrow transplantation. *Ann. intern. Med.* **90**, 158.
3. DEGOTT C., RUEFF B., KREIS H. *et al* (1978) Peliosis hepatis in recipients of renal transplants. *Gut* **19**, 748.
4. DRÜEKE T., BARBANEL C., JUNGERS P. *et al* (1980) Hepatitis B antigen-associated periarteritis nodosa in patients undergoing long term haemodialysis. *Am. J. Med.* **68**, 86.
5. FINE R.N., MALEKZADEH M.H., PENNISI A.J. *et al* (1977) HBs antigenemia in renal allograft recipients. *Ann. Surg.* **185**, 411.
6. MARUBBIO A.T. & DANIELSON B. (1975) Hepatic veno-occlusive disease in a renal transplant patient receiving azathioprine. *Gastroenterology* **69**, 739.
7. MAYOR G.H., KELLY T.J., HOURANI M.R. *et al* (1980) Intermittent hepatitis B surface antigenuria in a renal transplant recipient. *Am. J. Med.* **68**, 305.
8. NATAF C., FELDMANN G., LEBREC D. *et al* (1979) Idiopathic portal hypertension (perisinusoidal fibrosis) after renal transplantation. *Gut* **20**, 531.
9. SHULMAN H.M., SULLIVAN K.M., WEIDEN P.L. *et al* (1980) Chronic graft-versus-host syndrome in man. A long-term clinicopathologic study of 20 Seattle patients. *Am. J. Med.* **69**, 204.
10. SOPKO J. & ANURAS S. (1978) Liver disease in renal transplant recipients. *Am. J. Med.* **64**, 139.
11. WARE A.J., LUBY J.P., HOLLINGER B. *et al* (1979) Etiology of liver disease in renal-transplant patients. *Ann. intern. Med.* **91**, 364.
12. WOODS W.G., DEHNER L.P., NESBIT M.E. *et al* (1980) Fatal veno-occlusive disease of the liver following high dose chemotherapy, irradiation and bone marrow transplantation. *Am. J. Med.* **68**, 285.

HEPATIC GRANULOMAS

Hepatic granulomatous lesions, having a common histological pattern but sometimes differing in detail, are found in a number of diseases (table 65). The lesions are reticulo-endothelial in origin. Although seen anywhere in the liver they are most frequent near the portal tracts. They are sharply defined and do not disturb the normal pattern of the liver. They consist basically of pale-staining, epithelioid cells with surrounding lymphocytes. Giant cells, central caseation and necrosis may be present. Older lesions may be surrounded by a fibrous capsule, and healing is accompanied by hyaline change (fig. 362). In general they reflect a disturbance of cellular immunity. They cause little hepatic functional disturbance. The term *granulomatous hepatitis* which has been used for them [19] is, with a few exceptions, a misnomer, for the lesion is not a hepatitis and hepato-cellular dysfunction is rare.

The importance of granulomata is not in the hepatic functional disturbance they may cause, but as a means of diagnosing the causative condition. Hepatic biopsy can be used to obtain histological confirmation of the diagnosis. The percentage of granulomata obtained is surprisingly high considering the random scattering of lesions and the small size of the biopsy sample. Serial sections of the biopsy may need to be examined. In this way, the percentage of success can be increased by one-third.

Aetiology

Hepatic granulomas are found in 4–10% of needle liver biopsy specimens. They are associated with a multitude of diseases [5, 8]. Sarcoidosis and tuberculosis account for 50–65% and others include brucellosis and other bacterial infections, histoplasmosis and other fungal infections. Syphilis, leprosy, cytomegalovirus infection, infectious mononucleosis, schistosomiasis and other parasitic infestations, berylliosis, Hodgkin's disease, Crohn's disease [4], primary biliary cirrhosis, and rarely drug reactions such as to the sulphonamides, allopurinol [18, 21] or phenyl butazone [6].

Even after the fullest possible investigation in some 20–26% the cause remains unknown. In some the granulomas may have been found by chance in a needle biopsy specimen. The interpretation is difficult. Many of these patients may, in fact, be suffering from sarcoidosis or tubercu-

losis with minimal clinical evidence. In these symptomless patients the granuloma must be ignored but the patient should be observed over the next year or so, perhaps with a further chest X-ray and needle biopsy of the liver if circumstances permit it.

GRANULOMATOUS HEPATITIS

Hepatic granulomas may be associated with a severe, prolonged, febrile syndrome [12, 19]. Some are eventually diagnosed as Hodgkin's disease, others defy aetiological diagnosis. The granulomas are not widespread and pulmonary involvement is unusual. Biochemical tests of liver function are moderately impaired with increase in serum alkaline phosphatase, and slight increases in serum transaminases and globulins. Serum bilirubin is normal. A trial of antituberculous chemotherapy may be justified in these patients. Prednisone

Table 65. Differential diagnosis of hepatic granulomas.

Disease	Clinical accompaniments	Diagnostic aids
Sarcoidosis	Lung changes, uveitis, skin lesions, splenomegaly, lymphadenopathy	Chest X-ray. Kveim and tuberculin tests. Serum angiotensin converting enzyme
Tuberculosis	Pulmonary disease. Choroidal tubercles. Meningitis	Chest X-ray. Tuberculin test. Isolation of organism
Erythema nodosum	Sarcoidosis, primary tuberculosis, streptococcal infection, drug sensitivity	Chest X-ray. Kveim and tuberculin tests. Antistreptolysin titre
Brucellosis	Fever. Lassitude. Hepatosplenomegaly	Blood culture. Complement fixation test.
Berylliosis	Industrial exposure. Loss of weight. Skin lesions	Chest X-ray. Urinary beryllium. Beryllium skin patch test
Syphilis	Skin lesions. Cerebral involvement	Treponema test
Leprosy	Skin and nerve lesions	Lepromin skin test
Histoplasmosis	Non-specific	Complement fixation test. Histoplasmin skin test. Chest X-ray
Ascariasis	Gastro-intestinal and pulmonary symptoms	Faeces examination. Eosinophilia
Infectious mononucleosis	See Chapter 27	Blood film. Heterophile antibodies. E.B. antibodies
Tularaemia	Septicaemic and pulmonary features	Complement fixation test. Isolation of causal organism
Hodgkin's	Pyrexia, weight loss, splenomegaly, lymphadenopathy	Chest X-rays. Lymph node biopsy. CAT scan
Primary biliary cirrhosis	See Chapter 18	Mitochondrial antibodies
Hypogamma-globulinaemia	Recurrent bacterial infections	Serum immunoglobulins
Granulomatous disease of childhood	Skin granulomas. Recurrent bacterial infections	Chest X-ray, nitroblue tetrazolium test

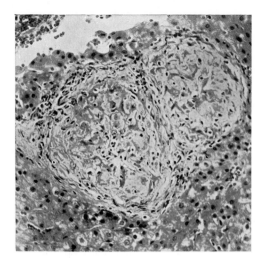

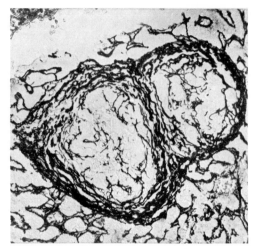

Fig. 362. Healing hepatic sarcoid. Two adjacent lesions are acquiring a structureless hyaline appearance and are surrounded by a connective tissue capsule. H & E, ×90.

Fig. 363. Same section stained to show reticulin formation around the granulomas. Stained modified silver, ×90.

treatment may be beneficial but clearly this should not be given without the fullest possible investigation.

SARCOIDOSIS

Sarcoidosis is a disease of unknown aetiology, characterized by widespread granulomatous lesions involving most organs. Involvement of lungs, lymph nodes, eyes, skin and of the neurological system may be associated with well-recognized clinical features, although this is not always so.

The liver is frequently affected although granulomas are often asymptomatic [10]. Overt evidences of hepatic insufficiency are rare. The liver is palpable in only 20% of patients [14]. Occasionally the picture is of active liver disease with marked hepatic functional abnormalities and liver cell destruction, and fibrosis on liver biopsy [10]. In general, however, the evidence of hepatic involvement arises not by the clinical picture but from the result of liver biopsy. This technique confirms sarcoidosis in about 60%. This agrees with autopsy figures showing hepatic involvement in about two-thirds [14]. Serial sections may be needed to reveal the granulomas.

Liver biopsy is indicated when another more accessible tissue, such as lymph gland or skin, is not available for biopsy [17].

Hepatic histology

Rounded, well-demarcated lesions can occur anywhere, but most often in the portal zones. The distinction is particularly striking in sections stained for glycogen, although the pallor makes them distinctive even in haematoxylin–eosin-stained sections.

The granuloma (see fig. 361 in colour section) contains a central area of eosinophilic necrosis, often containing nuclear debris. There is no caseation. The delicate reticulin framework is maintained, whereas this is destroyed in tuberculous lesions. Surrounding are the clusters of basophilic epithelioid cells. Also conspicuous are giant cells in which the nuclei may be peripheral or scattered through the cell. The cytoplasm may be vacuolated, or may contain non-specific inclusions of various types. A thin, peripheral ring of lymphocytes surrounds the lesion. Acid-fast bacilli are not seen.

Proliferation of Kupffer cells, even in areas remote from granulomas, demonstrates the widespread reticulo-endothelial activity.

Healing is by sclerosis. The granuloma is converted into an acellular mass of hyaline material with a fibrous capsule (figs. 362, 363); many disappear.

Since the hepatic lesions are focal, and fibrosis is restricted to healing lesions, sarcoidosis does not produce the diffuse fibrosis and nodular regeneration of cirrhosis. It is, therefore, difficult to accept the occasional reports of cirrhosis following sarcoidosis, and a fortuitous combination seems more likely. The association with jaundice and hepatic failure is very rare and unexpected.

Corticosteroid therapy seems to have little effect on the liver biopsy appearances.

Biochemical changes

The reticulo-endothelial involvement causes a rise in serum IgG. The alkaline phosphatase may be slightly raised. Serum bilirubin level is normal. Serum angiotensin converting enzyme is increased [20].

Portal hypertension

Occasionally the portal hypertension is presinusoidal related to massive granulomatous deposits in the liver [11]. However, the wedged hepatic venous pressure is often raised [10] and obstruction at sinusoidal or hepatic venous level must also be present. In others thrombotic occlusion of a portal or splenic vein may be found. Rarely, oesophageal bleeding is a real problem. These patients tolerate surgical shunts well.

TUBERCULOSIS

Miliary dissemination is a well recognized accompaniment of the primary complex, and is also common with chronic adult tuberculosis. Aspiration liver biopsies on patients with tuberculosis have shown positive results in about 25%. In another series 24 of 30 patients with extrapulmonary tuberculosis showed granulomas by liver biopsy [9].

Aspiration biopsy has been used in the diagnosis of tuberculous meningitis when other methods have failed, and also in miliary tuberculosis at the stage of an indeterminate pyrexia. In such cases, Ziehl–Neelsen stains should be performed, and an unfixed portion of the biopsy cultured for tubercle bacilli.

The distinction between these granulomas and those of sarcoidosis may be impossible. Distinctive features of tuberculosis are the presence of acid-fast bacilli and caseation with destruction of the reticulin framework. Irregularity of the contour with a particularly dense cuff of lymphocytes and less numerous lesions with a tendency to coalesce also suggest tuberculosis.

Miliary granulomas are found after BCG vaccination, especially in the immuno-suppressed [2].

BRUCELLOSIS

Hepatic granulomas complicate *Br. abortus* infection. *Br. suis* is more invasive with hepatic suppuration sometimes followed by calcification in the liver and spleen.

Although there are no specific clinical features and slight hepatomegaly is inconstant, focal granulomas may be widespread throughout the liver. Aspiration hepatic biopsy usually gives positive results. The hepatic lesions bear no relation to the severity of the infection nor to the clinical status.

Hepatic histology

The granulomatous lesions are not specific for brucellosis and cannot be distinguished from those of sarcoidosis, although they tend to be smaller and

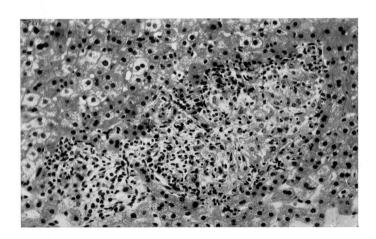

Fig. 364. Brucellosis. Granulomas in the liver. The smaller is little more than a collection of round cells. H & E, × 170.

less clearly demarcated (fig. 364). Healing results in scarring.

Focal accumulations of lymphocytes in the portal tract or scattered throughout the lobule, without the characteristic granulomas, are suggestive of brucellosis.

In *Br. melitensis*, the picture may be of scattered inflammatory cells and necrotic hepatocytes without granulomas [22].

A small portion of the unfixed biopsy specimen should be cultured and is occasionally positive for *Br. abortus* or *melitensis*.

It seems unlikely that brucellosis, a miliary liver lesion, could be followed by sufficiently diffuse fibrosis to justify the term cirrhosis. Cirrhosis has not been produced in experimental brucella infection.

INDUSTRIAL CAUSES

Beryllium poisoning may lead to pulmonary granulomas. There may also be hepatic involvement consisting of miliary granulomas, as in sarcoidosis. Aspiration liver biopsy material is, therefore, valueless in differential diagnosis.

Pulmonary and hepatic granulomas may be due to inhalation of *cement* and *mica dust* [16] and in vineyard sprayers to *copper* [15].

OTHER CONDITIONS WITH HEPATIC GRANULOMAS

Similar granulomas are found in the liver of patients suffering from acquired secondary *syphilis*.

In lepromatous *leprosy*, hepatic granulomas indistinguishable from sarcoidosis may be found in 62% compared with the tuberculoid form when only 21% are positive [7]. Lepra bacilli are sometimes present [7].

Histoplasmosis. The liver is second only to the spleen in frequency of involvement. In the granulomatous form, the lesions are histologically identical with those of sarcoidosis, except for the presence of the intracellular fungus in the Kupffer cells. Liver biopsy can be used in the diagnosis of histoplasmosis. Sections should be stained for *Histoplasma capsulatum* and an unfixed portion of the biopsy should be cultured. Histoplasmosis leads to discrete hepatic calcification [13].

Coccidioidomycosis and *blastomycosis* also produce sarcoid-like hepatic granulomas and the organism may be demonstrated.

Hepatic granulomas can be due to migrating larvae of *Ascaris lumbricoides*. Hepatic granulomas may also be found in children suffering from *Toxocara canis*.

Acute *cytomegalovirus* infection produces a mononucleosis syndrome. Transient well-formed hepatic granulomas may be associated [1].

Hepatic granulomas may also be seen in *schistosomiasis*, but the presence of ova usually makes the diagnosis easy.

In the early stages of *primary biliary cirrhosis* the liver may show widespread hepatic granulomas (fig. 218). This histological picture may be indistinguishable from sarcoidosis (table 31).

NON-SPECIFIC RETICULO-ENDOTHELIAL PROLIFERATIONS

Focal accumulations of mononuclear and epithelioid cells are found in a great variety of diseases. They are perhaps most frequent in virus infections, including infectious mononucleosis, during the recovery phase of hepatitis, especially non-A, non-B, when they contain iron, and in influenza. Occasionally, they are noted in pyogenic infections and septicaemias where polymorphonuclear leucocytes are also present.

Their distinction from small sarcoid granulomas may be difficult, especially since they may also be seen in sarcoidosis. If such an accumulation of cells is found in a liver biopsy section, the whole block should be sectioned serially to identify typical granulomas.

Generalized proliferation of Kupffer cells is another frequent histological finding of doubtful diagnostic value. As well as occurring in primary reticulo-endothelial conditions, it occurs in infections and in malignant disease arising in any part of the body. Generalized Kupffer cell proliferation is also seen in a liver containing local lesions—such as malignant deposits or an amoebic abscess.

REFERENCES

1. BONKOWSKY H.L., LEE R.V. & KLATSKIN G. (1975) Acute granulomatous hepatitis: occurrence in cytomegalovirus mononucleosis. *J. Am. med. Assoc.* **233**, 1284.
2. CASE RECORDS OF THE MASSACHUSETTS GENERAL HOSPITAL (1975) *New Engl. J. Med.* **293**, 443.
3. CHEN T.S.N., DRUTZ D.J. & WHELAN G.E. (1976) Hepatic granulomas in leprosy: their relation to bacteremia. *Arch. Pathol. lab. Med.* **100**, 182.

4. EADE M.N., COOKE W.T., BROOKE B.N. *et al* (1971) Liver disease in Crohn's colitis: a study of 21 consecutive patients having colectomy. *Ann. intern. Med.* **74**, 518.

5. IRANI S.K. & DOBBINS W.O. III (1979) Hepatic granulomas: a review of 73 patients from one hospital and survey of the literature. *J. clin. Gastroenterol.* **1**, 131.

6. ISHAK K.G., KIRCHNER J.P. & DHAR J.K. (1977) Granulomas and cholestatic-hepatocellular injury associated with phenylbutazone: report of two cases. *Am. J. dig. Dis.* **22**, 611.

7. KARAT A.B.A., JOB C.K. & RAO P.S.S. (1971) Liver in leprosy: histological and biochemical findings. *Br. med. J.* i, 307.

8. KLATSKIN G. (1977) Hepatic granulomata: problems in interpretation. *Mount Sinai J. Med. (N.Y.)* **44**, 798.

9. KORN R.J., KELLOW W.F., HELLER P. *et al* (1965) Hepatic involvement in extrapulmonary tuberculosis. *Am. J. Med.* **27**, 60.

10. MADDREY W.C., JOHNS C.J., BOITNOTH J.K. *et al* (1970) Sarcoidosis and chronic hepatic disease: a clinical and pathological study of 20 patients. *Medicine (Baltimore)* **49**, 375.

11. MISTILIS S.P., GREEN J.R. & SCHIFF L. (1964) Hepatic sarcoidosis with portal hypertension. *Am. J. Med.* **36**, 470.

12. NEVILLE E., PIYASENA K.H.G. & JAMES D.G. (1975) Granulomas of the liver. *Postgrad. med. J.* **51**, 361.

13. OKUDAIRA M., STRAUB M. & SCHWARZ J. (1961) The etiology of discrete splenic and hepatic calcifications in an endemic area of histoplasmosis. *Am. J. Pathol.* **39**, 599.

14. PORTER G.H. (1961) Hepatic sarcoidosis. A cause of portal hypertension and liver failure; review. *Arch. intern. Med.* **108**, 483.

15. PIMENTEL J.C. & MENEZES A.P. (1975) Liver granulomas containing copper in vineyard sprayer's lung. *Ann. Rev. resp. Dis.* **111**, 189.

16. PIMENTEL J.C. & MENEZES A.P. (1978) Pulmonary and hepatic granulomatous disorders due to the inhalation of cement and mica dusts. *Thorax* **33**, 219.

17. SCADDING J.G. & SHERLOCK S. (1948) Liver biopsy in sarcoidosis. *Thorax* **3**, 79.

18. SIMMONS F., FELDMAN B. & GERETY D. (1972) Granulomatous hepatitis in a patient receiving allopurinol. *Gastroenterology* **62**, 101.

19. SIMON H.B. & WOLFF S.M. (1973) Granulomatous hepatitis and prolonged fever of unknown origin: a study of 13 patients. *Medicine (Baltimore)* **52**, 1.

20. STUDDY P., BIRD R., JAMES D.G. *et al* (1978) Serum angiotensin-converting enzyme (SACE) in sarcoidosis and other granulomatous disorders. *Lancet* ii, 1331.

21. SWANK L.A., CHEJFEC G. & NEMCHAUSKY B.A. (1978) Allopurinol-induced granulomatous hepatitis with cholangitis and a sarcoid-like reaction. *Arch. intern. Med.* **138**, 997.

22. YOUNG E.J. (1979) *Brucella melitensis* hepatitis: the absence of granulomas. *Ann. intern. Med.* **91**, 414.

HEPATO-BILIARY ASSOCIATIONS OF INFLAMMATORY BOWEL DISEASE

The liver is involved in many ways in the patient with longstanding ulcerative colitis and other forms of chronic intestinal disease such as granulomatous enterocolitis (Crohn's disease) [1, 5]. In one large clinic over half the patients with ulcerative colitis showed liver function abnormalities [6]. The surgeon sees acute fatty liver when operating on patients with fulminant colitis, biliary strictures in those with sclerosing cholangitis, or gall-stones in patients with ileal resection. In treating ulcerative colitis the physician sees chronic active (lupoid) hepatitis or chronic cholestasis in those with pericholangitis and sclerosing cholangitis. The pathologist may encounter hepatic granulomas or amyloidosis in a liver biopsy from a patient with inflammatory bowel disease. Involvement of the liver in patients with malabsorption has been discussed in Chapter 22.

Sclerosing cholangitis (Chapter 14) [3] presents in many forms and is being increasingly diagnosed as more endoscopic and trans-hepatic cholangiograms are being done. *Gall-stones* are present in up to a third of patients with Crohn's disease of the terminal ileum [2].

Fatty change

This is very frequent. As with other types of fatty infiltration, the incidence is higher when autopsy rather than biopsy material is used for diagnosis. It may be focal but usually starts at the periphery of the lobule and spreads centrally. Cirrhosis is not a sequel.

This change is related to the anorexia, anaemia, faecal protein loss and malnutrition of severe colitis.

Carcinoma of the bile ducts (Chapter 32)

This has been reported in ulcerative colitis with or without accompanying biliary disease [8, 9]. The ulcerative colitis is usually of long standing. The bile duct carcinoma develops independently of the extent and severity of the colitis. It may develop many years after proctocolectomy [8]. It must be considered in any patient with ulcerative colitis developing deep, persistent cholestatic jaundice. Differentiation from sclerosing colitis is often impossible without surgical exploration.

Prognosis

This is considerably better than originally thought. If the large duct obstruction can be relieved, liver cell function can be preserved and the patients may remain asymptomatic for periods of more than five years. The prognosis is probably better than for primary biliary cirrhosis and resembles that of a partial traumatic (post-operative) biliary stricture.

Chronic active hepatitis and macronodular cirrhosis

Five per cent of cirrhotic patients have ulcerative colitis, a greater incidence than in the general population. In some the cirrhosis is of chronic active hepatitic type. The colitis is then part of the general spectrum of this multi-system disease. In these patients, and in contrast to sclerosing cholangitis, the colitis tends to present with the cirrhosis and to severe but often not subsequently relapsing [4]. The recognition of the cirrhosis may precede the diarrhoea.

In others the cirrhosis is of inactive type and diagnosed after many years of chronic relapsing colitis. Initially the colitis is predominant and the cirrhosis mild but as the years pass the positions reverse.

The aetiology of the cirrhosis is in doubt. In part is can be related to the long course of the illness, many hospital attendances, injections, infusions, blood transfusions, all carrying the hazard of viral hepatitis. This cannot be the whole answer for the cirrhosis may precede the colitis. The position of disturbed immunity in relation to chronic active hepatitis is uncertain.

The latter stages of pericholangitis and sclerosing cholangitis may be associated with piecemeal necrosis of liver cells and scar formation. This could proceed to a biliary cirrhosis [7]. If only the late stages in the liver are seen, the sequence by which the cirrhosis arose is difficult to determine.

REFERENCES

1. ATKINSON A.J. & CARROLL W.W. (1964) Sclerosing cholangitis. Association with regional enteritis. *J. Am. med. Assoc.* **188**, 183.
2. BAKER A.L., KAPLAN M.M., NORTON R.A. *et al* (1974) Gallstones in inflammatory bowel disease. *Am. J. dig. Dis.* **19**, 109.
3. CHAPMAN R.W.G., ARBORGH B.A.M., RHODES J.M. *et al* (1980) Primary sclerosing cholangitis: a review of its clinical features, cholangiography, and hepatic histology. *Gut* **21**, 870.
4. HOLDSWORTH C.D., HALL E.W., DAWSON A.M. *et al* (1965) Ulcerative colitis in chronic liver disease. *Q. J. Med.* **34**, 211.
5. KLECKNER M.S., STAUFFER M.H., BARGEN J.A. (1952) Hepatic lesions in the living patient with chronic ulcerative colitis as demonstrated by needle biopsy. *Gastroenterology* **22**, 13.
6. LUPINETTI M., MEHIGAN D. & CAMERON J.L. (1980) Hepatobiliary complications of ulcerative colitis. *Am. J. Surg.* **139**, 113.
7. MISTILIS S.P. (1965) Pericholangitis and ulcerative colitis. I. Pathology, aetiology, and pathogenesis. *Ann. intern. Med.* **63**, 1.
8. ROBERTS-THOMPSON I.C., STRICKLAND R.G. & MACKAY I.G. (1973) Bile duct carcinoma in chronic ulcerative colitis. *Aust. N.Z. J. Med.* **3**, 264.
9. THORPE M.E.C., SCHEUER P.J. & SHERLOCK S. (1967) Primary sclerosing cholangitis, the biliary tract and ulcerative colitis. *Gut* **8**, 435.

HEPATIC TRAUMA

CAUSES

Hepatic trauma is usually due to road traffic accidents, to penetrating wounds from stabbing or to gun-shots. It may be a sequel of birth injury. Spontaneous rupture may occur in the last trimester of pregnancy, usually complicated by toxaemia [9].

Non-penetrating injuries may be due to deceleration (leading to splits and tears from shearing) or to direct violence causing contusion or disruption of the liver substance [10].

DIAGNOSIS

This can be difficult as the physical signs may be minimal. Pattern bruising of the abdominal wall indicates severe abdominal compression.

Diagnostic peritoneal aspiration can be misleading. Ultrasonography may be useful. There should be no hesitation in performing laparotomy if any suspicion of liver trauma is aroused.

The possibility of other organs being damaged, such as spleen, intestines, kidneys, or the coincidence of head injuries and fractures, must be remembered [1].

MANAGEMENT

This is usually surgical [10, 12]. Transfusion facilities must be adequate. Classification into mild, moderate and severe hepatic injury is useful in determining surgical management [1].

Mild injuries such as splits and lacerations, without serious haemorrhage, are treated by suture and simple drainage.

Moderate injury with deeper lacerations and tearing of intra-hepatic vessels and bile ducts is treated by ligating the bleeding vessels and repairing the liver with deep sutures.

Severe injury consists of major disruption of the liver with tearing of the hepatic vein or inferior vena cava. Bleeding is controlled by digital compression of the hepatic artery and portal vein in the lesser omentum. Occasionally bleeding may be controlled by selective hepatic arterial ligation [11], but this may be followed by extensive liver necrosis [6]. Such ligation is usually a 'last ditch' procedure when bleeding cannot be controlled by other means [12]. Emergency hepatic arterial branch embolectomy with gelfoam, after selective hepatic arteriography, must also be considered [5].

At the time of emergency laparotomy definitive surgical treatment is often impossible. In such circumstances, haemorrhage in the damaged area may be controlled by primary packing, and the patient transferred immediately to a specialized unit where definitive operative treatment can be carried out [2].

In the majority of cases hepatic trauma can be managed by local pressure and aggressive debridement with hepatic segmentectomy, not necessarily following the anatomists' neat lines [12]. With damaged liver exposed, ragged areas of questionable viability can be excised, local haemostasis obtained and efficient drainage established. Excellent results have been noted after resection of as much as 400 g of liver tissue. Hepatic resection and lobectomy are required only in a small number of cases.

Repair of major venous injuries requires adequate exposure. The mid-line abdominal incision is extended, cephaled, and a median sternal split made. This allows control of the hepatic vein and any tear of the sub-diaphragmatic inferior vena cava. Repairs of the inferior vena cava or hepatic vein are sutured or side-clamped. Portal vein injuries are rare and treated by suture, end-to-side anastomosis or, if necessary, acute portal vein ligation [8].

T tube drainage of the common bile duct is not necessary unless the extra-hepatic bile ducts have been damaged.

Coagulopathy is a frequent and serious complication of severe liver trauma [3]. Other post-operative complications include jaundice, infection of a haematoma and hypoproteinaemia.

PROGNOSIS [7]

The overall mortality is about 11%. Deaths are due to uncontrolled intra-operative haemorrhage or to post-operative complications. The prognosis obviously depends on the extent of the hepatic injury [1] and the number of organs involved [12]. Injuries to the hepatic veins or retro-hepatic inferior vena cava are highly lethal. Shot-gun injuries are most serious, followed by blunt trauma, gun-shot wounds and lastly stab wounds [12].

RUPTURE OF THE GALL BLADDER

Rupture of the gall bladder can follow blunt abdominal trauma [4]. It is rare because the gall bladder is cushioned by surrounding bony and visceral structures. The gall bladder is usually distended at the time of rupture. Early diagnosis is difficult. The condition is recognized by fever, jaundice, increasing distension and ascites. Paracentesis shows bile-stained fluid. The perforation is confirmed by percutaneous or endoscopic cholangiography.

Treatment is by cholecystectomy.

REFERENCES

1. ALDRETE J.S., HALPERN N.B., WARD S. *et al* (1978) Factors determining the mortality and morbidity in hepatic injuries. *Ann. Surg.* **189**, 466.
2. CALNE R.Y., MCMASTER P. & PENTLOW B.D. (1979) The treatment of major liver trauma by primary packing with transfer of the patient for definitive treatment. *Br. J. Surg.* **66**, 338.
3. CLAGETT G.P. & OLSEN W.R. (1978) Non-mechanical hemorrhage in severe liver injury. *Ann. Surg.* **187**, 369.
4. FRANK D.J., PEREIRAS R. Jr, LIMA M.S.S. *et al* (1978) Traumatic rupture of the gallbladder with massive biliary ascites. *J. Am. med. Assoc.* **240**, 252.
5. JANDER H.P., LAWS H.L., KOGUTT M.S. *et al* (1977) Emergency embolization in blunt hepatic trauma. *Am. J. Roentgenol.* **129**, 249.
6. LUCAS C.E. & LEDGERWOOD A.M. (1978) Liver necrosis following hepatic artery transection due to trauma. *Arch. Surg.* **113**, 1107.
7. MCINNIS W.D., RICHARDSON J.D. & AUST J.B. (1977) Hepatic trauma. *Arch. Surg.* **112**, 157.

8. PACHTER H.L., DRAGER S., GODFREY N. *et al* (1979) Traumatic injuries of the portal vein. *Ann. Surg.* **189,** 383.

9. PAVLIC R.S. & TOWNSEND D.E. (1962) Spontaneous rupture liver in pregnancy. *Am. J. Obstet. Gynecol.* **83,** 1373.

10. SMITH Lord (1978) Injuries of the liver, biliary tree and pancreas. *Br. J. Surg.* **65,** 673.

11. TANPHIPHAT C. (1976) Lobar dearterialization in liver trauma. *Br. J. Surg.* **63,** 213.

12. WALT A.J. (1978) The mythology of hepatic trauma—or Babel revisited. *Am. J. Surg.* **135,** 12.

Chapter 27
The Liver in Infections

PYOGENIC LIVER ABSCESS

Pyogenic liver abscess used most often to be due to portal infection, often in young people secondary to acute appendicitis. This is now less frequent, probably because of earlier diagnosis and treatment. Abscesses secondary to obstruction and infection of the biliary tree, and affecting an older age group, have, however, continued to increase. Earlier diagnosis should have followed increased use of scanning and cholangiographic techniques, but failures are usually due to the clinician not considering the diagnosis.

Portal pyaemia

Pelvic or gastro-intestinal infection may result in portal pylephlebitis or septic emboli. This may follow appendicitis, empyema of the gall bladder, diverticulitis, perforated simple or malignant gastric or colonic ulcers, leaking anastomoses, pancreatitis, infected haemorrhoids or pelvic suppuration.

Neonatal umbilical vein sepsis may spread to the portal vein with the production of hepatic abscesses.

Cholangitic

Cholangitis related to gall-stones, cancer, sclerosing cholangitis, congenital biliary anomalies, or biliary strictures is the most common antecedent of hepatic abscess [11]. The abscesses are commonly multiple.

Direct infection

A solitary liver abscess may follow a penetrating wound or direct spread from an adjacent septic focus such as a perinephric abscess. It may be secondary to pyogenic contamination of an amoebic abscess or an intra-hepatic haematoma, for instance, following automobile accidents. Carcinomatous deposits can also become infected.

Cryptogenic

In about one-half of instances there is no obvious predisposing cause. Such abscesses are termed 'cryptogenic'. The abscess is usually single.

BACTERIOLOGY

The commonest infecting organisms are Gram-negative. *E. coli* is found in two-thirds. *Str. faecalis* and *Pr. vulgaris* are also frequent. Recurrent pyogenic cholangitis may be due to *Salmonella typhi*.

Anaerobic organisms have become increasingly important, and include bacteroides, aerobacteria, actinomyces and anaerobic and microaerophilic streptococci [12]. This emphasizes the need to culture all possibly infective material, including blood, pus, bile and swabs, under strictly anaerobic as well as aerobic conditions.

Staphylococci are found in nearly a half, especially in those who have received chemotherapy, when they are usually resistant. Friedländer's bacillus, pseudomonas and *Cl. welchii* may also be found.

Infection is often mixed.

The abscess may be sterile, but this is usually due to lack of adequate, particularly anaerobic, culture techniques or previous antibiotics.

PATHOLOGY

The enlarged liver may contain multiple yellow abscesses, 1 cm in diameter, or a single abscess encased in fibrous tissue.

When there is an associated pylephlebitis, the portal vein and its branches show inflamed, dilated walls and may contain pus and blood clot. The abscesses are particularly in the right lobe (fig. 365). If there has been subserous inflammatory change there may be perihepatitis or even adhesion formation.

In bacteroides infections, the pus has a foul odour and the abscess wall is ill defined.

When infection is spread by the bile ducts, multiple foci correspond to the bile duct system.

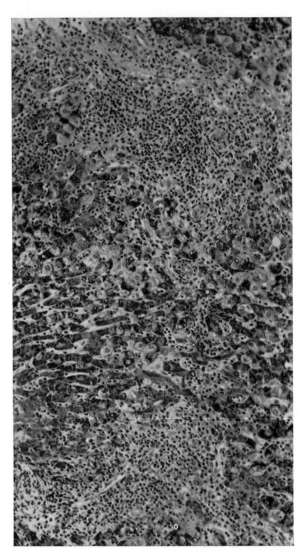

Fig. 365. Pylephlebitis complicating acute appendicitis. The portal tracts show an acute inflammatory exudate in which polymorphonuclear leucocytes are conspicuous. The walls of the portal vein radicles are thickened and the lining epithelium is desquamating. The inflammatory cells are invading the adjoining liver parenchyma and the periportal liver cells are necrosing. Culture of this biopsy grew *E. coli*. Best's carmine, × 145.

A chronic solitary liver abscess may persist for as long as two years before death or diagnosis.

There may be small pyaemic abscesses elsewhere, such as lungs, kidneys, brain and spleen. Direct extension from the liver may lead to subphrenic or pleuro-pulmonary suppuration. Extension to the peritoneum or rupture of a sinus pointing under the skin are rare. A small amount of ascites is present in about a third of patients.

CLINICAL FEATURES

When suppuration involves the liver, the clinical features of the original septic focus are supplanted by rigors, sweating, spiking fever, weakness and other manifestations of a severe constitutional upset. Prostration and shock are prominent with the Gram-negative bacteraemias.

In many instances the picture is non-specific and marked only by pyrexia, hepatic tenderness, leucocytosis and evidences of a bacteraemia [5, 12].

The patient appears toxic and complains of a dull ache in the right hypochondrium. If there is subdiaphragmatic irritation or pleuro-pulmonary spread of infection, he may complain of right shoulder pain and an irritating cough. The liver is enlarged and tender, and pain may be accentuated by percussion over the lower rib cage.

The spleen is palpable in chronic cases. Ascites is rare. Jaundice is late unless there is suppurative cholangitis when it is early and conspicuous.

Recovery may be followed by portal hypertension due to thrombosis of the portal vein.

INVESTIGATIONS

General

Jaundice is usually mild, but may be marked in the cholangitic types. It is more common than with amoebic abscess. The combination of a raised serum alkaline phosphatase, low albumin with an ESR exceeding 100 in one hour suggests liver abscess. A raised serum B_1 level supports active liver infection rather than a non-specific reactive hepatitis due to infection elsewhere [8].

Repeated blood cultures may show the causative infection or infections.

Fluoroscopic examination

This may show a high, immobile, right diaphragm with alterations in contour and a pleural effusion. A penetrating film may show a fluid level, indicating gas-producing organisms [3]. In a barium meal a left lobe abscess displaces the cardia, lesser curvature and duodenal cap.

Localization of the abscess

Scanning is valuable in diagnosis, determining the site for a liver biopsy, and in localizing a drainage procedure. The technetium scan is 'negative', but the abscess cavity is 'positive' with gallium. Scanning results in 25% false-negative results. Ultrasonic scanning distinguishes a solid tumour from a fluid-filled abscess. CT scanning is particularly valuable in localization.

Coeliac axis arteriography in the hepatogram phase may show abscess cavities as rounded filling defects.

Cholangitic abscesses may be diagnosed by percutaneous trans-hepatic *cholangiography* [4]. Endoscopic cholangiography may also be useful in localizing an abscess and is particularly valuable when the percutaneous method is contraindicated by sepsis or bleeding [1, 6] (fig. 366). With both these procedures material may be obtained for culture.

Needle liver biopsy

In areas remote from the abscess the picture may be of infection in the portal tracts surrounding disintegrated liver cells being infiltrated by polymorphonuclear leucocytes (fig. 365). If the abscess has been localized, the needle may be directed towards the lesion so that material for culture may be obtained.

TREATMENT

Prevention is by early treatment of acute abdominal infections and the adequate drainage of intra-abdominal purulent collections under adequate antibiotic cover.

Antibiotics are rarely effective alone, and should not be continued where drainage is mandatory. The course should be intensive and the choice of antibiotic depends on the causative organism. When the abscess has been localized it has to be drained. Percutaneous catheter drainage with installation of antibiotics into the cavity is often successful [2]. This can be repeated. Surgical drainage may not be necessary. There may be difficulties in localization at surgery. Large bore needling to find pus with methylene blue injections may be helpful. Peroperative real-time ultrasonography, using a hand-held probe, may be valuable [7].

PROGNOSIS

The high mortality is largely due to failure to diagnose and to drain the abscess [10]. Overall about 50% die, and this includes those in whom the diagnosis is only made at autopsy [5]. The prognosis is better for a unilocular abscess in the right lobe. If adequately treated the survival is 90%. The outcome for multiple abscesses throughout the liver is very poor; only one-fifth survive [5, 9]. When there is delay in diagnosis of jaundice, continued fever, multiple infections shown by blood culture and old age, the prognosis is worse.

REFERENCES

1. ASCIONE A., ELIAS E., SCOTT J. *et al* (1978) Endoscopic retrograde cholangiography (ERC) in non-amebic liver abscesses. *Am. J. dig. Dis.* **23,** 39.
2. DOOLEY J.S., DICK R., OLNEY J. *et al* (1979) Non-surgical treatment of biliary obstruction. *Lancet* ii, 1040.

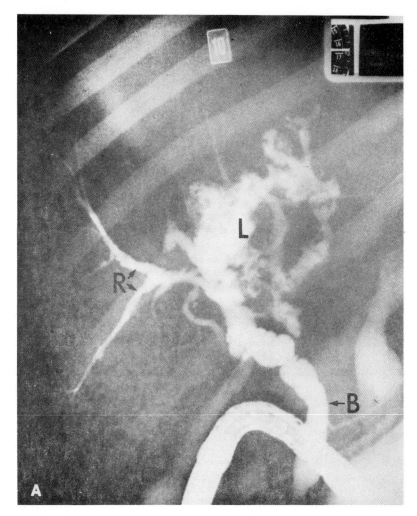

Fig. 366. Retrograde cholangiogram in pyogenic liver abscess. The common bile duct (B) is dilated. The main divisions of the right hepatic duct (R) are seen to be irregular in calibre. The left main hepatic duct (L) is grossly disorganized and surrounded by areas of extravasation of dye into the liver substance. This is shown in greater detail in B (*facing*) (Ascione *et al* 1978).

3. FOSTER S.C., SCHNEIDER B. & SEAMAN W.B. (1970) Gas-containing pyogenic intrahepatic abscesses. *Radiology* **94**, 613.

4. GROSSMAN R.I., RING E.J., OLEAGA J.A. *et al* (1979) Diagnosis of pyogenic hepatic abscesses by percutaneous transhepatic cholangiography. *Am. J. Roentgenol.* **132**, 919.

5. HEYMANN A.D. (1979) Clinical aspects of grave pyogenic abscesses of the liver. *Surg. Gynecol. Obstet.* **149**, 209.

6. LAM S.K., WONG K.P., CHAN P.K.W. *et al* (1978) Recurrent pyogenic cholangitis: a study by endoscopic retrograde cholangiography. *Gastroenterology* **74**, 1196.

7. LYTTON B. & COOK J. (1979) Intraoperative ultrasound. In *Ultrasound in Urology* p. 340, eds. M.I. Resnick & R.C. Saunders. Williams and Wilkins, Baltimore.

8. NEALE G., CAUGHEY D.E., MOLLIN D.L. *et al* (1966) Effects of intrahepatic and extrahepatic infection on liver function. *Br. med. J.* i, 382.

9. PITT H.A. & ZUIDEMA G.D. (1975) Factors influencing mortality in the treatment of pyogenic hepatic abscess. *Surg. Gynecol. Obstet.* **140**, 228.

10. SATIANI B. & DAVIDSON E.D. (1978) Hepatic abscesses: improvement in mortality with early diagnosis and treatment. *Am. J. Surg.* **135**, 647.

11. SHERMAN J.D. & ROBBINS S.L. (1960) Changing trends in the casuistics of hepatic abscess. *Am. J. Med.* **28**, 943.

12. SILVER S., WEINSTEIN A. & COOPERMAN A. (1979) Changes in the pathogenesis and detection of intrahepatic abscess. *Am. J. Surg.* **137**, 608.

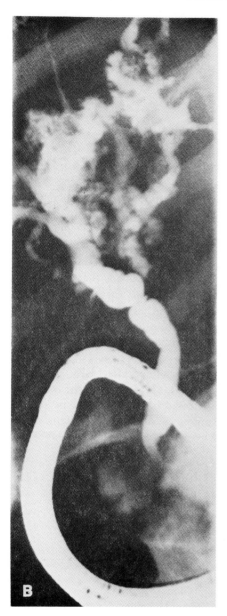

and small intestine and changes into the vegetative, trophozoite form in the colon. Here, it invades the mucosa, forming typical flask-shaped ulcers. Amoebae are carried to the liver in the portal venous system. Occasionally, they pass through the hepatic sinusoids into the systemic circulation with the production of abscesses in lungs and brain.

Amoebae multiply and block small intrahepatic portal radicles with consequent focal infarction of liver cells. They contain a proteolytic enzyme which destroys the liver parenchyma. The lesions produced are single or multiple and of variable size. They rarely develop in the cirrhotic liver [2].

The amoebic abscess is usually about the size of an orange. The most frequent site is in the right lobe, often supero-anteriorly, just below the diaphragm. The centre consists of a large necrotic area which has liquefied into thick, reddish- brown pus. This has been likened to anchovy or chocolate sauce. Although it is referred to as amoebic pus, it is not strictly so because it is produced by lysis of liver cells. Fragments of liver tissue may be recognized in it. Initially, the abscess has no well-defined wall, but merely shreds of shaggy, necrotic liver tissue. Histologically, the necrotic areas consist of degenerate liver cells, leucocytes, red blood cells, connective tissue strands and debris. Amoebae may be identified in scrapings from the wall.

Small lesions heal with scars, but larger abscesses show a chronic wall of connective tissue of varying age. Amoebiasis never leads to cirrhosis.

There seems to be no pathological justification for retaining the term 'acute amoebic hepatitis' [7]. Histologically, the liver remote from the isolated abscesses or micro-abscesses is normal. The amoebic lesion from the outset is not diffuse but focal. These hepatolytic areas remain silent and evoke clinical attention only when they have progressed to a larger abscess [7].

Many factors determine the balance between healing or progression. The virulence of infection and resistance of the host must play a part. Another factor is secondary bacterial infection, which occurs in about 20%. The pus then becomes green or yellow and foul smelling.

HEPATIC AMOEBIASIS

Entamoeba histolytica exists in a free-living vegetative form and as cysts which, because they can survive outside the body, are highly infective. This cystic form passes unharmed through the stomach

EPIDEMIOLOGY [5]

Colonic amoebae have a world-wide distribution, but the actual disease, however, is essentially one of the tropics and sub-tropics. In temperate climates, symptomless carriers of toxic strains are found, but colonic ulcers are not seen. Various factors might explain the change in virulence in the tropics.

In the tropics there is a high carrier rate so that a new arrival is heavily exposed. Spread of infection by faeces is easier when sanitation is poor. Locals are less prone to hepatic amoebiasis than Europeans, presumably because of partial immunity induced by repeated contact. There is a striking predominance in adult males.

The latent period between the intestinal infection and hepatic involvement has not been explained.

Liver abscesses may be induced in hamsters by intraperitoneal inoculation of amoebae and by direct inoculation of human, sterile pus containing amoebae [12].

CLINICAL FEATURES

Note must be made of any residence or illness suffered in tropical or sub-tropical areas. Amoebic dysentery is present in only a very small number. A past history of dysentery is rare. Hepatic amoebiasis has been recorded as long as 30 years after the primary bowel infection. It is most frequent in young males aged 30–50 [1].

The onset is usually gradual but, rarely, may be sudden with rigors and sweating. Fever is variously intermittent, remittent or even absent unless an abscess becomes secondarily infected; it rarely exceeds 40 °C. Jaundice is unusual and, if present, is mild [1]. The patient looks ill, with a peculiar sallowness of the skin, like faded suntan.

Pain in the liver area may commence as a dull ache, later becoming sharp and stabbing. If the abscess is near the diaphragm, there may be referred shoulder pain and this may be accentuated by deep breathing or coughing. Alcohol makes the pain worse, as do postural changes. The patient tends to lean to the left side; this opens up the right intercostal spaces and diminishes the tension on the liver capsule. The pain increases at night. Pain and tenderness are greatest when the lesion is expanding rapidly.

The liver is enlarged upwards, downwards or horizontally. A swelling may be visible in the epigastrium or bulging the intercostal spaces. Hepatic tenderness is virtually constant. It may be elicited over a palpable liver edge or by percussion over the lower right chest wall [7]. The spleen is not enlarged.

Examination of the lungs may show consolidation of the right lower zone, signs of pleurisy or an effusion. Pleural fluid may be blood stained.

Hepatic function tests are usually normal. Sometimes the serum alkaline phosphatase level is moderately raised.

Examination of faeces. Cysts and vegetative forms should be sought in several fresh stool specimens. Positive results are rare and usually in the early stages.

Sigmoidoscopy may show healed scars and any lesions should be biopsied.

SEROLOGICAL TESTS [6]

Numerous tests are now available. They are useful, but may remain positive for a long time after clinical cure.

The amoebic complement fixation test has had limited use because of the non-specific results obtained.

A simple latex agglutination test is now available commercially [9]. The haemagglutination inhibition test is sensitive and particularly valuable in community surveys [8].

Counter-immunoelectrophoresis using cellulose acetate is useful for rapid screening for amoebic liver abscess [11].

An enzyme-linked immuno-sorbent assay (ELISA) will add great sensitivity for serum diagnosis and may be useful for stool and aspirates from liver abscesses [6].

Haematological findings

The leucocyte count is moderately raised, compared with the high values associated with pyogenic liver abscess. The count is usually of the order of 13 000–16 000/mm³, with 70–80% polymorphonuclear leucocytes. Higher levels suggest secondary infection of the abscess. There is often mild anaemia in the chronic case.

Radiological features

A plain, penetrating radiograph of the upper abdomen may demonstrate an enlarged liver shadow, with a raised right diaphragm which may, on screening, be immobile (fig. 367). Lateral radiographs may be useful (fig. 368). The abscess is commonly situated supero-anteriorly, causing a bulge

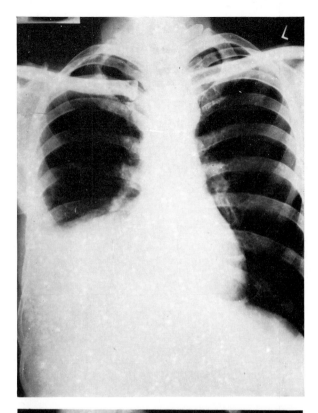

Fig. 367. Amoebic abscess of liver. Note the elevated right diaphragm with overlying reaction in the chest.

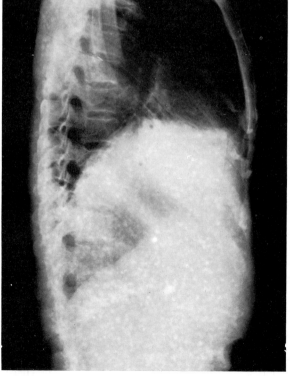

Fig. 368. Amoebic abscess. Lateral view confirms the elevation of the diaphragm.

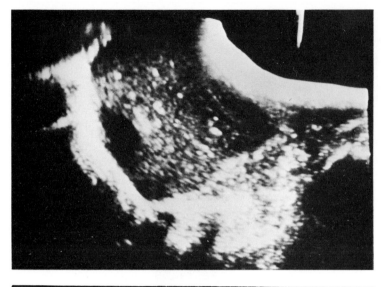

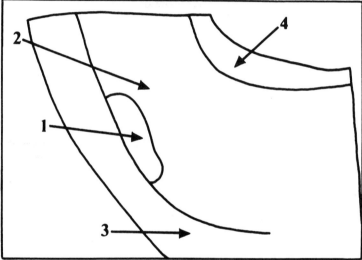

Fig. 369. Amoebic liver abscess. Ultrasound
demonstrates an amoebic abscess (1) in the liver (2)
lying posteriorly against the diaphragm (3). The
anterior abdominal wall (4) is also shown.

in the antero-medial part of the right diaphragm,
with obliteration of the cardio-phrenic angle
anteriorly and of the anterior costo-phrenic angle
laterally. This is in contradistinction to subphrenic
abscess, where the obliteration is more commonly
noted in the posterior costo-phrenic space laterally.

A right lateral abscess may cause widening of
the intercostal spaces.

A central or inferior abscess may show few signs.

An abscess in the left lobe of the liver may show
a crescentic deformity of the lesser curve of the
stomach.

Chest radiographs may show a high right diaphragm, obliteration of the costo-phrenic and cardio-phrenic angles by adhesion, pleural effusions
or right basal pneumonia. Perpendicular string-
like adhesions may pass from the diaphragm to the
lung-base.

Scintiscanning is essential for accurate diagnosis

and to assess the effects of treatment. A filling defect is shown in the liver. Multiple abscesses are frequent in such areas as Mexico and Taiwan. Ultrasound shows that the lesion contains fluid (fig. 369).

Arteriography shows an avascular mass with distortion of the normal vascular architecture.

Diagnostic aspiration

The characteristic odourless anchovy sauce (pus) can be aspirated, unless secondary infection has already converted it into thick yellow or even foul-smelling pus.

Needle biopsy can be combined with diagnostic aspiration.

DIAGNOSIS

Certain criteria are of value in reaching a diagnosis of hepatic amoebiasis [7].

1. An enlarged tender liver in a young male.
2. Response to metronidazole.
3. Leucocytosis without anaemia in those with a short history, and less marked leucocytosis and anaemia in those with a long history.
4. Suggestive radiological findings particularly in the postero-anterior and lateral chest X-ray.
5. Demonstration of amoebic pus possibly containing trophozoites by aspiration or because of rupture into an adjacent viscous or serous cavity.
6. Scintiscanning showing a filling defect.
7. A positive amoebic haemagglutination test.

COMPLICATIONS

The commonest site of rupture is into the lungs or pleura causing empyema, hepatobronchial fistula or pulmonary abscess. The patient coughs up pus, develops pneumonitis or lung abscess or a pleural effusion.

Rupture into the pericardium is a complication of amoebic abscess in the left lobe [4].

Intraperitoneal rupture results in acute peritonitis. If the patient survives the intial effect, long-term results are good. Abscesses of the left lobe may perforate into the lesser sac [1].

Rupture into the portal vein, bile ducts or gastro-intestinal tract is rare.

Secondary infection is suspected if prostration is particularly great, and fever and leucocytosis particularly high. Aspiration reveals yellowish, often foetid, pus and culture reveals the causative organism.

TREATMENT

Metronidazole (Flagyl) 750 mg three times a day for 10 days is the treatment of choice for amoebic dysentery or liver abscess. An intravenous (costly) preparation is available for those unable to take the drug orally. Complications of metronidazole include nausea, diarrhoea, metallic taste, dizziness and discoloration of the urine. Alcohol should not be permitted during treatment. Failures are very few, and may be related to persistence of intestinal amoebiasis [3], drug resistance or inadequate absorption.

Dehydroemetine with chloroquine is used only in the rare, resistant case.

Aspiration is rarely required. It may be necessary with very large abscesses or where there is lack of response to four days' metronidazole treatment. The site is chosen by the presence of bulging intercostal spaces or abdominal wall, by tenderness, radiology or scanning. The needle should be at least 10 cm long, of 1–2 cm diameter, and with a fitted stilette. If pus is not encountered at the first needling, the direction of the needle can be changed and further efforts made at aspiration. If this is still unsuccessful, a different site in the skin can be selected and further attempts made.

Open drainage is reserved for those with secondary infection of the abscess cavity.

CHRONIC AMOEBIC HEPATITIS

A chronic disease with mild symptoms has been attributed to *Entamoeba histolytica* and called chronic amoebic hepatitis. The patient is generally unwell with fatigue, poor appetite and right upper abdominal discomfort. The liver may or may not be palpable and tender. There is no fever or leucocytosis, and amoebic cysts are not found in the stools. Many doubt the existence of chronic amoebic hepatitis. In some ways the condition resembles the post-hepatitis syndrome (Chapter 15).

Treatment. If the patient has a clear-cut past history of amoebiasis or has lived in areas where this disease is endemic, it is worthwhile giving a course of treatment with metronidazole and noting the response.

REFERENCES

1. BARBOUR G.L. & JUNIPER K. Jr (1972) A clinical comparison of amebic and pyogenic abscess of the liver in sixty-six patients. *Am. J. Med.* **53**, 323.
2. FALAIYE J.M., OKEKE G.C.E. & FREGENE A.O. (1980) Amoebic abscess in the cirrhotic liver. *Gut* **21**, 161.
3. GREGORY P.B. (1976) A refractory case of hepatic amoebiasis. *Gastroenterology* **70**, 585.
4. IBARRA-PEREZ C., GREEN S.L., CALVILLO-JUÁREZ M. *et al* (1972) Diagnosis and treatment of rupture of amebic abscess of the liver into the pericardium. *J. thorac. cardiovasc. Surg.* **64**, 11.
5. KNIGHT R. & WRIGHT S.G. (1978) Progress report. Intestinal protozoa. *Gut* **19**, 940.
6. KROGSTAD D.J., SPENCER H.C. Jr & HEALY G.R. (1978) Current concepts in parasitology: amebiasis. *New Engl. J. Med.* **298**, 262.
7. LAMONT N.McE. & POOLER N.R. (1958) Hepatic amoebiasis. A study of 250 cases. *Q. J. Med.* **27**, 389.
8. MILGRAM E.A., HEALY G.R. & KAGAN I.G. (1966) Studies on the use of the indirect hemagglutination test in the diagnosis of amebiasis. *Gastroenterology* **50**, 645.
9. MORRIS M.N., POWELL S.J. & ELSDON-DEW R. (1970) Latex agglutination test for invasive amoebiasis. *Lancet* i, 1362.
10. SHABOT J.M. & PATTERSON M. (1978) Amebic liver abscess: 1966–1976. *Am. J. dig. Dis.* **23**, 110.
11. TOSSWILL J.H.C., RIDLEY D.S. & WARHURST D.C. (1980) Counter immunoelectrophoresis as a rapid screening test for amoebic liver abscess. *J. clin. Pathol.* **33**, 33.
12. WILES H.L., MADDISON S.E., POWELL S.J. *et al* (1963) The passage of bacteriologically sterile *Entamoeba histolytica* in hamster livers. *Ann. trop. Med. Parasitol.* **57**, 71.

TUBERCULOSIS OF THE LIVER

Although the liver is frequently involved by haematogenous spread of the tubercle bacillus, the lesions tend to heal spontaneously. Hepatic tuberculosis is therefore seldom of clinical importance and rarely diagnosed during life.

The basic lesion is the *granuloma* which is very frequent in the liver of a patient with both pulmonary and extra-pulmonary tuberculosis (Chapter 26). The lesions usually heal without scarring but sometimes with focal fibrosis and calcification.

Tuberculomata are rare. There are 90 published cases [2]. They may be multiple, consisting of white, irregular, caseous abscesses surrounded by a fibrous capsule. Their naked eye distinction from Hodgkin's disease, secondary carcinoma or actinomycosis may be difficult. The focal fibrosis

around the lesion is never sufficient to merit the term 'cirrhosis'. Occasionally, the necrotic area calcifies.

Tuberculous cholangitis is extremely rare, resulting from spread of caseous material from the portal tracts into the bile ducts. The caseous central areas become bile stained.

Tuberculous pylephlebitis results from rupture of caseous material, often in portal lymph nodes, into the portal vein. It is rapidly fatal.

CLINICAL FEATURES

These may be few or absent. An associated pyrexia is usually due to concomitant, active tuberculosis elsewhere rather than to hepatic disease. The condition may present as a pyrexia of unknown origin. Jaundice may appear in overwhelming miliary tuberculosis, particularly in the racially susceptible. The liver is not usually enlarged except in some instances of miliary tuberculosis.

BIOCHEMICAL TESTS [4]

Serum alkaline phosphatase levels may be raised. Hyperglobulinaemia reflects a chronic infection and hepatic granulomas.

DIAGNOSIS

This is difficult. Liver biopsy is essential [1, 3]. The main indications are fever of unknown origin or hepatomegaly. A small portion of the tissue obtained should be cultured and positives are obtained in about 50%. A small portion should also be cultured.

A plain X-ray of the abdomen may reveal hepatic calcification.

Extra-hepatic features of tuberculosis may not be obvious.

Treatment is that of haematogenous tuberculosis. No specific treatment of the liver is indicated.

THE EFFECT ON THE LIVER OF TUBERCULOSIS ELSEWHERE

Amyloidosis may complicate chronic tuberculosis. Fatty change in the liver in terminal disease is due to wasting and toxaemia.

Sufferers may contract type B hepatitis because of their poor resistance and the frequency of their therapeutic injections. Drug jaundice may follow therapy, especially with isoniazid.

REFERENCES

1. BRUNNER K. & HAEMMERLI U.P. (1964) Die blinde Leberbiopsie als zuverlassiges Mittel zur Fruh diagnose der Miliartuberkulose. *Dtsch. Med. Wochenschr.* **89,** 657.
2. GRACEY L. (1965) Tuberculous abscess of the liver. *Br. J. Surg.* **52,** 442.
3. HERSCH C. (1964) Tuberculosis of the liver. A study of 200 cases. *S.A. med. J.* **39,** 587.
4. KORN R.J., KELLOW W.F., HELLER P. *et al* (1959) Hepatic involvement in extra-pulmonary tuberculosis. *Am. J. Med.* **27,** 60.

HEPATIC ACTINOMYCOSIS

This disease is due to the fungus *Actinomyces israelii*.

Hepatic involvement is a sequel to intestinal actinomycosis, especially of the caecum and appendix. It spreads by direct extension or, more often, by the portal vein. Large greyish-white masses, superficially resembling malignant metastases, soften and form collections of pus, separated by fibrous tissue bands, simulating a honeycomb. The liver becomes adherent to adjacent viscera and to the abdominal wall, with the formation of sinuses. These lesions contain the characteristic 'sulphur granules', which consist of branching filaments with eosinophilic, clubbed ends.

Clinically, the patient is toxic, febrile, sweating, wasted and anaemic. There is local, sometimes irregular, enlargement with tenderness of one or both lobes of the liver. The overlying skin may have the livid, dusky hue seen over a taut abscess which is about to rupture. Multiple irregular sinus tracks develop, from which bile may exude. Similar sinuses may develop from the ileo-caecal site or from the chest wall if there is pleuro-pulmonary extension.

The *diagnosis* is obvious at the stage of sinus tracks, because the organism can be isolated from the characteristic pus. If actinomycosis is suspected before this stage, aspiration liver biopsy should be avoided, because of the danger of developing a persistent sinus. In the early stages, the condition presents as pyrexia with hepatosplenomegaly, anaemia and non-specific hepatic cellular infiltrates [1]. It may be months before minuscule abscesses are detected. Laparotomy may be necessary for diagnosis.

Treatment. Penicillin should be given in massive doses for six weeks. Because of the thick fibrous capsule surrounding the abscess, parenterally administered penicillin may reach the area with difficulty. It should be supplemented by local instillation of penicillin wherever possible.

REFERENCE

1. MEADE R.H. III (1980) Primary hepatic actinomycosis. *Gastroenterology* **78,** 355.

SYPHILIS OF THE LIVER

CONGENITAL

The liver bears the brunt of any transplacental infection. It is firm, enlarged and swarming with spirochaetes. Initially, there is a diffuse hepatitis, but gradually fibrous tissue is laid down between the liver cells and in the portal tracts, and this leads to a true pericellular cirrhosis.

Since hepatic involvement is but an incident in a widespread spirochaetal septicaemia, the clinical features are seldom those of the liver disease. The foetus may be still born or die soon after birth. If the infant survives, other manifestations of congenital syphilis are obvious, apart from the hepatosplenomegaly and mild jaundice. Syphilis nowadays is a very rare cause of neonatal jaundice.

In older children who have survived without this florid neonatal picture, the hepatic lesion may be a gumma.

Diagnosis can be confirmed by blood serology which is always positive. Needle liver biopsy has been used for diagnosis and to assess the effects of treatment. Electron microscopy confirms the presence of spirochaetes [1].

SECONDARY

In the secondary septicaemic stage, spirochaetes invade the liver with the production of miliary granulomas.

Rarely, jaundice and hepatitis are seen, apparently *not* due to a coincidental virus hepatitis.

Serology is positive. Serum alkaline phosphatase levels are very high [3]. Liver biopsy shows non-specific changes with moderate infiltration with polymorphs and lymphocytes, some hepatocellular disarray, but no cholestasis (fig. 370).

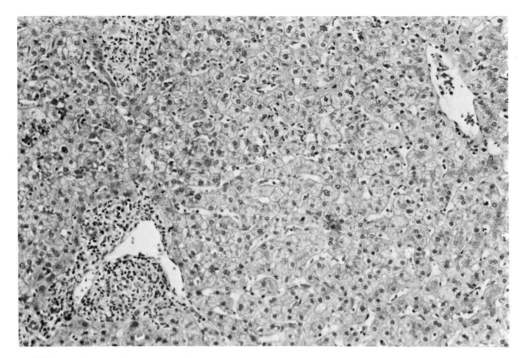

Fig. 370. Liver in secondary syphilis. Mononuclear cell infiltration can be seen in portal zones and in the sinusoids. H & E, × 160.

Portal-to-central zonal necrosis can be seen. Spirochaetes are not usually detected.

The response to treatment is rapid [2].

TERTIARY

Gummas may be single or multiple. They are usually situated in the right lobe. They consist of a caseous mass, circumscribed by a fibrous capsule, from which fibrous tissue spreads out interstitially. Healing occurs with the production of deep scars and coarse lobulation (*hepar lobatum*) [4]. Despite this distortion, the liver architecture is not disturbed and the lesion is not a true cirrhosis. Syphilis and cirrhosis are not related.

Hepatic gummas are usually discovered incidentally at laparotomy or autopsy. Occasionally, the enlarged nodular liver may be confused with cirrhosis or hepatic metastases. Liver function tests are unhelpful and the presence of positive serology is insufficient evidence of hepatic syphilis. Aspiration liver biopsy of an accessible nodule provides histological confirmation. The response to adequate penicillin may be diminution in size of a gumma over prolonged periods of time.

Jaundice complicating penicillin treatment

Rarely, the patient shows an idiosyncrasy to treatment with penicillin. Jaundice, chills and fever, often with a rash (*erythema of Milian*), occur about nine days after starting therapy. This forms part of the Herxheimer reaction. The mechanism of the jaundice is unclear.

REFERENCES

1. BROOKS S.E.H. & AUDRETSCH J.J. (1978) Hepatic ultrastructure in congenital syphilis. *Arch. Pathol. lab. Med.* **102**, 502.
2. CAMPISI D. & WHITCOMB C. (1979) Liver disease in early syphilis. *Arch. intern. Med.* **139**, 365.
3. PAREEK S.S. (1979) Liver involvement in secondary syphilis. *Am. J. dig. Dis.* **24**, 41.
4. SYMMERS D. & SPAIN D.M. (1946) Hepar lobatum. *Arch. Pathol.* **42**, 64.

WEIL'S DISEASE (LEPTOSPIROSIS)

In 1886, Weil [6] described a disease characterized by intense prostration, fever, jaundice, renal injury and a haemorrhagic tendency. This was later shown to be due to a leptospira, *L. icterohaemor-rhagiae*, and to be transmitted by rats. Later various other leptospira were related to human disease. These do not cause a distinct clinical pattern and the whole group should be designated leptospirosis and Weil's disease applied only to infections with *L. icterohaemorrhagiae*. There are at least 22 sera types, most of them causing disease in man.

MODE OF INFECTION

The renal tubules of rats form the principal reservoir of infection for man. Living leptospira are continually excreted and are capable of surviving for months in pools, canals or damp soil. The portal of entry in man is thought to be the respiratory or gastro-intestinal canal, or through abrasions in the skin. The highest incidence is therefore in adult males, particularly agricultural workers, sewer workers, coalminers, ditch diggers and fish cutters.

PATHOLOGY

Liver [1, 2]. Necrosis is minimal and focal. Dissociation of the cells one from another is prominent but is probably mainly a post-mortem phenomenon. The centrizonal necrosis of acute virus hepatitis is absent. Active hepato-cellular regeneration, shown by mitoses and nuclear polyploidy, is out of proportion to cell damage. Kupffer cells proliferate.

Periportal infiltration with leucocytes is constant and centrizonal bile thrombi are prominent if the patient is deeply jaundiced. The histological changes do not parallel the severity of icterus. Cirrhosis is not a sequel.

Kidney shows tubular necrosis.

Skeletal muscles show punctate haemorrhages and focal necrosis of muscle fibres.

Heart may show haemorrhages in all layers. Pericarditis may complicate the uraemia.

Haemorrhage into tissues, especially skin and lungs, is apparently due to capillary injury and thrombocytopenia.

The jaundice is complex. Hepato-cellular dysfunction is probably important, although serious, even fatal, deeply jaundiced, patients may show minimal changes in the liver. Jaundice is magnified by the concomitant renal failure, preventing urinary bilirubin excretion. Tissue haemorrhage

and intravascular haemolysis increase the bilirubin load on the liver. Hypotension with diminished hepatic blood flow is contributory.

The uraemia is related to pigment in the tubules, a direct effect of the spirochaetes on the kidney and lowered renal blood flow.

CLINICAL FEATURES [2] (fig. 371)

The disease is most prevalent in late summer and autumn. The incubation period is 6–15 days. The course may be divided into three stages: the first or septicaemic phase lasts about seven days, the second or toxic stage for a similar period, and the third or convalescent period begins in the third week.

The first or septicaemic stage is marked by the presence of the spirochaete in the circulating blood.

The onset is abrupt, with prostration, high fever, even rigors. The temperature rises rapidly to 39·5–40·5 °C and falls by lysis within 3–10 days.

Abdominal pain, nausea and vomiting may simulate an acute abdominal emergency, and severe muscular pains especially in the back or calves are common.

Central nervous system involvement is shown by severe headache, mental confusion and sometimes meningism. The cerebro-spinal fluid confirms the meningeal infection, there being an increase in protein, with a leucocytosis. If jaundice is present, there is xanthochromia, the infection increasing the permeability of the meninges to bile pigments.

The eyes show a characteristic suffusion.

There is a haemorrhagic tendency usually in those with a severe attack. Bleeding may occur from nose, gut or lung, with skin petechiae or ecchymoses.

Pneumonitis with cough, sore throat and rhonchi occurs in 40% of sufferers.

Jaundice appears between the fourth and seventh day in 80% of patients [2, 3]. It is a grave sign, for the disease is never fatal in the absence of icterus. The liver is enlarged, but not the spleen.

The urine shows albumin, urobilin and bile pigment. The stools are well coloured.

There is a leucocytosis of 10 000–30 000/mm³ with a relative increase in polymorphs. Thrombocytopenia may be profound.

The second or immune stage in the second week is characterized by a normal temperature but without clinical improvement. This is the stage of

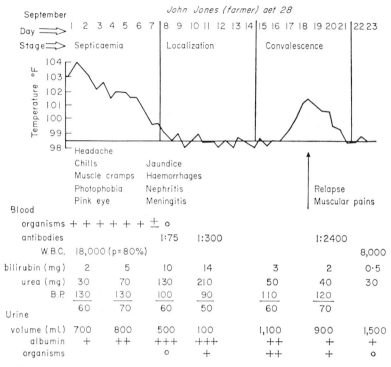

Fig. 371. The clinical course of a patient with Weil's disease.

deepening jaundice, with increasing renal and myocardial damage. Albuminuria persists, there is a rising blood urea, and oliguria may proceed to anuria. Death may be due to renal failure.

Severe prostration is accompanied by a low blood pressure and a dilated heart. There may be transient cardiac arrhythmias and electrocardiographic evidence of a prolonged P–R or Q–T interval, with T wave changes. Death may be due to circulatory failure.

During this stage, the leptospira can be found in the urine, and rising antibody titres demonstrated in the serum.

The third or convalescent stage starts at the beginning of the third week. Clinical improvement is shown by a brightening of the mental state, fading of the jaundice, a rise in blood pressure and an increased urinary volume, with a drop in the blood urea concentration. Albuminuria is slow to disappear. Permanent renal and hepatic damage has not been reported.

Temperature may rise during the third week (fig. 371), associated with muscle pains. Such relapses occur in 20% of cases.

There is great variation in the clinical course, ranging from a mild illness, clinically indistinguishable from influenza, to a prostrating, fatal disease with anuria.

INVESTIGATIONS [5]

In the first week, the spirochaetes are found in the blood, becoming less evident with the development of antibodies at the end of the first week. Thereafter, they may be isolated from the urine.

Diagnosis in the first week

1. Thick, dry, blood films are used for staining for spirochaetes and for dark field examination.
2. Blood culture is performed in a semi-solid medium such as Fletcher's.
3. Acute-phase serological antibodies are measured as a base line for subsequent rising titres.
4. The leucocyte count is raised—a point of distinction from viral hepatitis.

5. Blood is injected intraperitoneally into guinea-pigs, who develop jaundice and fever within a few days. Spirochaetes are demonstrated in liver and other tissues.

Diagnosis after the first week

From the 10th to the 20th day, leptospira may be shown in the urine. Injection into a guinea-pig may be positive, but the organisms are not often viable from urine.

Serological antibodies appear after the first week and usually reach a peak in the fourth week. They may persist for years.

The leptospiral agglutination test is usually positive in a titre of at least 1 in 300 and a rising titre can be demonstrated. Cross-agglutination occurs between the various serotypes and the infecting type may not be ascertained without actual isolation of the leptospira.

Aspiration liver biopsy. In spite of the bleeding tendency, biopsies have been performed. The histological picture is not specific for leptospirosis, because the dissociation of liver cells, histiocytic proliferation and periportal changes are seen in other severe infections. The histological picture, however, is quite distinct from acute virus hepatitis. A portion of the liver biopsy may be used for culture of the leptospira, and positive results were obtained in eight of the nine biopsies in one series.

Spinal fluid shows increased protein and leucocytes. It is often xanthochromic.

Liver function tests are non-contributory. The serum bilirubin level is raised and the alkaline phosphatase and transaminases slightly increased.

DIFFERENTIAL DIAGNOSIS

In the early stages, Weil's disease is confused with septicaemic bacterial infections or typhus fever. When jaundice is evident, there may be difficulty in excluding acute virus hepatitis (table 66). Important distinguishing points are the sudden onset and albuminuria of Weil's disease.

Spirochaetal jaundice would be diagnosed more often if blood samples for agglutinins were taken from patients with obscure icterus and fever.

PROGNOSIS

There is a mortality of about 16%. This depends on the degree of jaundice, renal and myocardial involvement, and the extent of haemorrhages. Death is usually due to renal failure. The mortality is negligible in non-icteric patients, and is lower under 30 years old. Since many mild infections are probably unrecognized, the overall mortality may well be considerably less.

Although transient relapses in the third and fourth weeks are common, final recovery is complete.

PREVENTION

Specific immune serum has proved preventative in exposed laboratory workers.

Protective clothing, such as rubber boots and

Table 66. The diagnosis of Weil's disease from virus hepatitis during the first week of illness.

	Weil's disease	Virus hepatitis
Onset	Sudden	Gradual
Headache	Constant	Occasional
Muscle pains	Severe	Mild
Jaundice	74%	Virtually constant
Conjunctival infection	Present	Absent
Prostration	Great	Mild
Disorientation	Common	Rare
Haemorrhagic diathesis	Common	Rare
Nausea and vomiting	Present	Present
Abdominal discomfort	Common	Common
Bronchitis	Common	Rare
Albuminuria	Present	Absent
Leucocyte count	Polymorph leucocytosis	Leucopenia with lymphocytosis
Inoculation of blood into guinea-pig	Spirochaetes present	Spirochaetes absent

gloves, should be provided for workers in indus-
tries with a high incidence of Weil's disease, and
adequate measures taken to control rodents. Bath-
ing in stagnant water should be avoided.

TREATMENT

Large doses of penicillin may be given in human
disease. There is, however, no conclusive evidence
of its value in man [2, 4]. It would certainly be ineffective and useless after the first four days, i.e.
at the time when the diagnosis is usually made.

The diet should contain little protein but abundant calories. Facilities should be available for the
treatment of acute circulatory and renal failure.

OTHER TYPES OF LEPTOSPIROSIS

There are many species of leptospira pathogenic
to man, varying in antigenic constitution and geographic distribution [2, 3]. In general these infections are less severe than those due to *L. icterohaemorrhagiae*. *L. canicola* infection, for instance, is
characterized by headache, meningitis and con-
junctival infection. Albuminuria is only found in
40%, and jaundice in only 18% of patients. Its frequent presentation is that of 'benign aseptic
meningitis'. The disease affects young adults who
have usually been in close contact with an infected
dog. Fatalities in man are virtually unknown.

Diagnosis is confirmed in a similar way to Weil's
disease. A convenient method is the demonstration of rising antibody titres. The spinal fluid
shows a lymphocytic fluid in most cases, even in
the absence of meningitis.

REFERENCES

1. AREAN V.M. (1962) The pathologic anatomy and
   pathogenesis of fatal human leptospirosis (Weil's
   disease). *Am. J. Pathol.* **40**, 393.
2. EDWARDS G.A. & DOMM B.M. (1960) Human leptospirosis. *Medicine (Baltimore)* **39**, 117.
3. HEATH C.W. Jr, ALEXANDER A.D. & GALTON
   M.M. (1965) Leptospirosis in the United States.
   Analysis of 483 cases in man. 1949–1961. *New Engl.
   J. Med.* **273**, 857.
4. KOCEN R.S. (1962) Leptospirosis. A comparison of
   symptomatic and penicillin therapy. *Br. med. J.*
   i, 1181.
5. TURNER L.H. (1970) Leptospirosis III: Maintenance, isolation and demonstration of leptospiras.
   Trans. R. Soc. trop. Med. Hyg. **64**, 623.
6. WEIL A. (1886) Über eine eigenthumliche mit Milz-
   tumor, Icterus und Nephritis einhergehene, acute
   Infektion skrankheit. *Dtsch. Arch. klin. Med.* **39**,
   209.

RELAPSING FEVER

This arthropod-borne infection is caused by spirochaetes of the genus *Borrelia recurrentis*. It is
encountered throughout the world except in New
Zealand, Australia, and some parts of the West
Pacific.

The borrelia multiply in the liver, invading liver
cells and causing focal necrosis. Just before the
crisis the borrelia roll up and are ingested by reticulo-endothelial cells. This effect is related to
immunologically competent lymphocytes. Surviving borrelia remain in the liver, spleen, brain and
bone-marrow until the next relapse [2].

CLINICAL FEATURES [1]

The incubation period is from three to 15 days.
The onset is acute with chills, a continuous high
temperature, headache, muscle pains and profound prostration. The patient is flushed, sometimes with injected conjunctivae, and epistaxes. In
severe attacks, tender hepatosplenomegaly and
jaundice develop. The jaundice is similar to that
seen in Weil's disease. Sometimes a rash develops
on the trunk. There may be bronchitis.

These symptoms continue for four to nine days
and then the temperature falls, often with collapse
of the patient. This peripheral collapse may be
fatal, but more usually the symptoms and signs
then rapidly abate. The patient remains afebrile
for about a week, when there is a relapse. There
may be a second or even a third milder relapse
before the disease ends.

DIAGNOSIS

Spirochaetes can rarely be found in thick blood
films. Agglutination and complement fixation tests
are available [2]. Organisms may be identified by
lymph node aspiration, or from the bite site.

TREATMENT

Tetracyclines and streptomycin are more effective
than penicillin. Mortality is 5%.

REFERENCES

1. BRYCESON A.D.M., PARRY E.H.O., PERINE P.L. *et al* (1970) Louse-borne relapsing fever: a clinical and laboratory study of 62 cases in Ethiopia and a reconsideration of the literature. *Q. J. Med.* **39**, 129.
2. FELSENFELD O. & WOLF R.H. (1969) Immunoglobulins and antibodies in borrelia turicetae infections. *Acta Trop.* **26**, 156.

Q FEVER [1]

This rickettsial disease has predominantly pulmonary manifestations. Occasionally hepatitis may be prominent and clinical features may mimic anicteric virus hepatitis. The liver shows so-called hepato-cellular necrosis with lymphocytic and eosinophil infiltration. In some, necrosis is widespread and granulomas are seen. Rickettsia may be demonstrated by direct fluorescent antibody microscopy. Hepatic changes may be present without jaundice.

REFERENCE

1. DUPONT H.L., HORNICK R.B., LEVIN H.S. *et al* (1971) Q fever hepatitis. *Ann. intern. Med.* **74**, 198.

SCHISTOSOMIASIS (BILHARZIASIS)

Hepatic schistosomiasis is usually a complication of the intestinal disease, since emboli of schistosoma ova reach the liver from the intestines via the mesenteric veins. *S. mansoni* and *S. japonicum* affect the liver. *S. haematobium* can sometimes involve the liver.

Schistosomiasis is prevalent in Japan, China and the Philippines and *S. mansoni* in Africa, Egypt, the West Indies, Puerto Rico and northern parts of South America.

PATHOGENESIS

Eggs, excreted in the faeces, hatch out in water to free-swimming embryos which enter appropriate snails and develop into fork-tailed cercariae. These re-enter human skin in contact with infested water. They burrow down to the capillary bed, whence there is widespread haematogenous dissemination. Those reaching the mesenteric capillaries enter the intra-hepatic portal system, where they grow rapidly.

In the liver, the ova penetrate and obstruct the portal branches and are deposited either in the large radicles, producing the coarser type of bilharzial hepatic fibrosis, or in the small portal tracts, producing the fine diffuse form.

The granulomatous reaction to the schistosoma ovum is an immunological one of delayed hypersensitivity type [10]. The granulomas seem to be related to antigen released by the egg. Gamma-globulin increases in the mesenchymal cells of liver and spleen in proportion to granuloma formation. Serum of patients binds antigenic material in the worm or ova.

Portal fibrosis is related to the adult worm load [5]. The classic, clay-pipe stem cirrhosis is due to fibrotic bands originating from the granulomas.

Wide, irregular, thin-walled vascular spaces are found in 85% of cases and form a characteristic feature in the thickened portal tracts [1]. These angiomatoids are useful in distinguishing the bilharzial liver from other forms of hepatic fibrosis. Remnants of ova are also diagnostic. There is little or no bile duct proliferation. The extent of nodular regeneration and disturbance of the hepatic architecture is not sufficient to justify the term 'cirrhosis'. If cirrhosis is present it can usually be attributed to other aetiological factors such as past virus hepatitis. The hepatic lesion may predispose to primary liver cancer.

Splenic enlargement is mainly due to the resulting portal venous hypertension, although there is also reticulo-endothelial hyperplasia. Very few ova are found in the spleen. Portal–systemic collateral channels are numerous.

There are associated bilharzial lesions in the intestines and elsewhere. Fifty per cent of patients with rectal schistosomiasis have granulomata in the liver.

CLINICAL FEATURES

Schistosomiasis shows three stages of infection. Itching follows the entry of the cercariae through the skin. This is followed by a stage of fever, urticaria and eosinophilia. Finally the third stage of deposition of ova results in intestinal, urinary and hepatic involvement.

Initially there is merely hepatosplenomegaly. Both liver and spleen are firm, smooth and easily

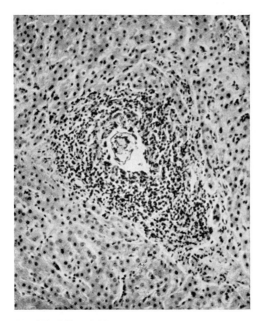

Fig. 372. Bilharzial liver. An ovum of *S. mansoni* has lodged in a portal tract which shows a granulomatous reaction. H & E, × 220

palpable. This is followed by hepatic fibrosis and eventually portal hypertension which may appear years after the original infection.

The general health of the patient suffers. The liver shrinks in size and the spleen becomes much larger. Haematemeses, dilated abdominal wall veins and a venous hum over the liver are indications of the portal venous obstruction. Ascites and oedema may develop. The blood shows a leucopenia and anaemia. The faeces at this stage contain few, if any, parasites, but scrapings taken during sigmoidoscopy may reveal them.

Patients tolerate blood loss well and hepatic encephalopathy is unusual [12]. This is because hepato-cellular function remains good although there is a large portal–systemic collateral circulation.

Aspiration liver biopsy (fig. 372). A 'squash' preparation in glycerol may be made of a portion of the biopsy. Eggs or their remnants are seen in 94% of livers from those with faecal eggs and this method is of diagnostic value. The incidence is less in the more chronic forms where eggs cannot be found in the faeces or rectal biopsy. Sections are essential to determine the extent of hepatic damage in those with an established diagnosis.

Rectal biopsy is a useful diagnostic method but

bleeding may be a complication in those with marked portal hypertension.

Serological tests [11]

The complement fixation test detects exposure to schistosomal antigen [11] but tends to be nonspecific. The fluorescent antibody method may be useful.

A radio-immunoassay method, using *S. mansoni* egg antigen, can detect human schistosomiasis [8].

Patients with schistosomiasis are more likely to be carriers of HBsAg than a control population [7].

Portal hypertension

The intra-splenic pressure is raised, while the wedged hepatic vein pressure is normal. The portal hypertension is therefore pre-sinusoidal and presumably related to the portal zone reaction [3]. In advanced schistosomiasis, hepatic arterial hypertension contributes to increased sinusoidal pressure [2]. Retrograde flow develops in the portal vein [4]. Hepatic blood flow is not significantly reduced [9].

At the stage when haemorrhage occurs from varices the granulomatous reaction may have subsided and the picture is predominantly that of fibrosis. Bleeding is associated with a very high intra-splenic pressure.

Splenic venography shows an enormous collateral circulation.

Biochemical changes

Serum alkaline phosphatase may be raised. Hypoalbuminaemia can be related to the poor nutrition and to the effects of repeated gastro-intestinal haemorrhages. Serum transaminases are virtually normal.

TREATMENT

Antimony compounds were the traditional therapy but have been replaced by newer drugs. Niridazole can be effective but has marked sideeffects in those with hepatic involvement.

Oxamniquine is one of the drugs of choice for treating patients with *S. mansoni* infections with or without advanced decompensated bilharzial hepatosplenomegaly. It is given orally in a dose of

20–30 mg/kg for three consecutive days. The main side-effect is fever with eosinophilia which develops two to three days after completing treatment.

Praziquantel is given in a single oral dose of 30–45 mg/kg, and is effective against all three species of schistosomal infection [6]. Side-effects are few; they include spasmodic abdominal pain lasting one to a few hours which responds to antispasmodic drugs, headache and occasional vomiting. It is safe to use in patients with schistosomal hepatic fibrosis.

Control is by mass education on hygiene and on the avoidance of infected water. Immunological control must also be considered. The developing worms produce an antigenic stimulus which prevents re-infection. Knowledge of its nature and its practical application to man remains for the future [10].

In the later stages haemorrhage from oesophageal varices may raise the question of portacaval anastomosis. In spite of good pre-operative liver function, the patients often develop encephalopathy after the shunt [12] and, on the whole, these patients are not such good candidates for surgery as might be anticipated.

REFERENCES

1. AIDAROS S.M. & SOLIMAN L.A.M. (1961) Portal vascular changes in human bilharzial cirrhosis. *J. Pathol. Bact.* **82**, 19.
2. ALVES C.A.P., ALVES A.R., ABREU I.O.N. *et al* (1977) Hepatic artery hypertrophy and sinusoidal hypertension in advanced schistosomiasis. *Gastroenterology* **72**, 126.
3. COUTINHO A. (1968) Hemodynamic studies of portal hypertension in schistosomiasis. *Am. J. Med.* **44**, 547.
4. EL-GENDI M.A. (1979) Radiographic and haemodynamic patterns of portal hypertension in hepatosplenic schistosomiasis: selection of surgical procedure. *Gut* **20**, 177.
5. KAMEL I.AA., ELWI A.M., CHEEVER A.W. *et al* (1978) *Schistosoma mansoni* and *S. haematobium* infections in Egypt. IV Hepatic lesions. *Am. J. trop. Med. Hyg.* **27**, 939.
6. LEADER (1980) Praziquantel: a new hope for schistosomiasis. *Lancet* i, 635.
7. LYRA L.G., REBOUCA S. & ANDRADE Z.A. (1976) Hepatitis B surface antigen carrier state in hepatosplenic schistosomiasis. *Gastroenterology* **71**, 641.
8. PELLEY R.P., WARREN K.S. & JORDAN P. (1977) Purified antigen radioimmunoassay in serological diagnosis of *Schistosomiasis mansoni*. *Lancet* ii, 781.
9. RAMOS O.L., SAAD F. & LESER W.P. (1964) Portal hemodynamics and liver cell function in hepatic schistosomiasis. *Gastroenterology* **47**, 241.
10. WARREN K.S. (1973) Regulation of the prevalence and intensity of schistosomiasis in man: immunology or ecology? *J. infect. Dis.* **127**, 595.
11. WARREN K.S., KELLERMEYER R.W., JORDAN P. *et al* (1973) Immunologic diagnosis of schistosomiasis. I. *Am. J. trop. Med. Hyg.* **22**, 189.
12. WARREN K.S., REBOUCAS G. & BAPTISTA A.G. (1965) Ammonia metabolism and hepatic coma in hepatosplenic schistosomiasis. *Ann. intern. Med.* **62**, 1113.

MALARIA

In the *erythrocytic stage*, the parasite is engulfed by reticulo-endothelial cells. The liver suffers from the general effects of the toxaemia and pyrexia.

The *pre-erythrocytic stage* (exo-erythrocytic) schizogony takes place in the liver without obvious effect on its function. The hepatocyte is invaded by the sporozoite which grows to accommodate the schizont. The nucleus of the parasite divides many times and, at last (in 6–12 days according to the species), a spherical or irregular body containing thousands of ripe merozoites is formed. This pre-erythrocytic schizont bursts and the merozoites are discharged into the sinusoids and invade red blood corpuscles. In quartan or benign tertian malaria a few merozoites return to the liver cells to initiate the exo-erythrocytic or relapse cycle. In malignant tertian this does not happen and there are no true relapses. So far only *P. falciparum* and *P. vivax* have been found in the liver of man. The tissue stage of human malaria is confined to the liver cells.

PATHOLOGICAL CHANGES

Macroscopically there is little change apart from some enlargement.

Liver biopsy studies show reticulo-endothelial proliferation, both of Kupffer cells and in the portal tracts [1]. Focal accumulations of histiocytes, forming non-specific granulomatous lesions, may be seen in the sinusoids. Brown 'malarial' pigmentation, representing iron and haemofuscin, is seen in the Kupffer cells. Malarial parasites are not demonstrable. Hepato-cellular change is slight. The cells may be swollen, with nuclei of variable size and shape and increased mitoses.

The centrizonal necrosis described in malignant (*P. falciparum*) malaria is probably a post-mortem phenomenon. Sinusoids may contain parasitized clumped erythrocytes [1].

The reaction of the liver to the malarial parasite is reticulo-endothelial, with minor effects on the liver cells. Fibrosis does not follow and malaria is not precirrhotic. The high incidence of cirrhosis in malarial areas may be attributed to other factors operating in the region concerned.

Electron microscopy [3] shows destruction of the plasma membrane and mitochondrial damage. Malarial pigment is shown as rectangular and trapezoidal bodies.

CLINICAL FEATURES

There are usually no clinical features specific for the liver. Occasionally, in acute malignant malaria, there may be mild jaundice, hepatomegaly and tenderness over the liver [2].

HEPATIC FUNCTION CHANGES

The haemolysis and mild liver cell damage are associated with increases of the serum bilirubin concentration, but rarely above 3 mg/dl. Serum transaminases increase slightly.

Reticulo-endothelial proliferation is associated with a rise in the serum globulin concentration.

REFERENCES

1. DE BRITO T., BARONE A.A. & FARIA R.M. (1969) Human liver biopsy in *P. falciparum* and *P. vivax*. *Virchows Arch.* **348,** 220.
2. RAMACHANDRAN S. & PERERA M.V.F. (1976) Jaundice and hepatomegaly in primary malaria. *J. trop. Med. Hyg.* **79,** 207.
3. ROSEN S., ROYCROFT D.W., HANO J.E. *et al* (1967) The liver in malaria. Electron microscopic observations on a hepatic biopsy obtained 15 minutes post mortem. *Arch. Pathol.* **83,** 271.

KALA AZAR

Leishmaniasis is a reticulo-endothelial disease. Periportal cellular infiltrations and macrophage accumulations are scattered throughout the liver and within them the Leishman–Donovan bodies may be identified (fig. 373). There is some portal zone fibrosis [1]. The picture is similar in the American, Mediterranean or Oriental types [1].

REFERENCE

1. DA SILVA J.R. & DE PAOLA D. (1961) Hepatic lesions in American kala-azar: a needle-biopsy study. *Ann. trop. Med. Parasitol.* **55,** 249.

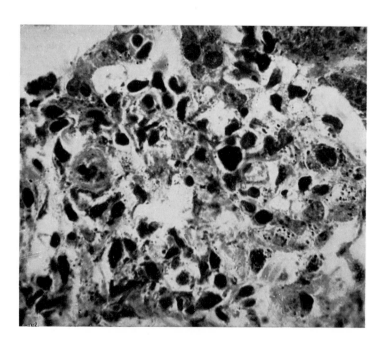

Fig. 373. Kala Azar. Leishman–Donovan bodies lying within histiocytic accumulations. Leishman, × 775.

HYDATID DISEASE

Hydatid disease is due to the larval or cyst stage of infection by the tapeworm, *Echinococcus granulosus*, which lives in dogs. Man, sheep and cattle are intermediate hosts and the dog is the common definitive host.

BIOLOGY (fig. 374)

Man is infected by contact with the excreta of dogs often during childhood. The dog is infected by eating the viscera of sheep, which contain hydatid cysts. Scolices, contained in the cysts, adhere to the small intestine of the dog and become adult taenia which attach to the intestinal wall. The terminal segment of the worm, the proglottis, contains about 500 ova when shed into the lumen of the bowel. The infected faeces of the dog contaminate grass and farmland, and the contained ova are ingested by sheep, pigs, camels or man. The ova adhere readily to the coats of dogs, so man is infected by handling dogs, as well as by eating contaminated vegetables.

The ova have chitinous envelopes which are resistant to physical agents, but are dissolved by gastric juice. The liberated ovum burrows through the intestinal mucosa and is carried by the portal vein to the liver, where it develops into an adult cyst. Most of the cysts are caught in the hepatic sinusoids and, in fact, 70% of eventual hydatid cysts are in the liver. A few ova pass through the liver and right side of the heart and are held up in the pulmonary capillary bed and so give rise to pulmonary hydatid cysts. A few ova reach the general systemic circulation, giving rise to cysts in such organs as spleen, brain and bone.

THE DEVELOPMENT OF THE HEPATIC CYST (fig. 375)

In the course of its slow development from the ovum, the adult cyst provokes a cellular response in which three zones can be distinguished—a peripheral zone of fibroblasts, an intermediate layer of endothelial cells, and an inner zone of round cells and eosinophils. The peripheral zone, derived

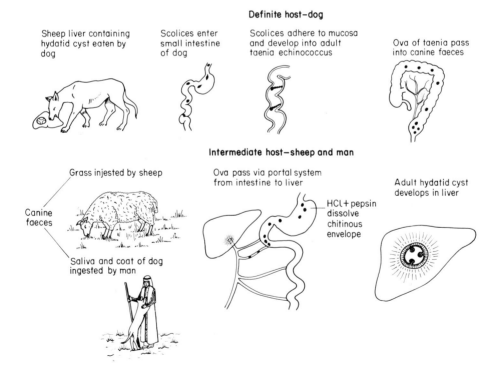

Definite host–dog

Sheep liver containing hydatid cyst eaten by dog

Scolices enter small intestine of dog

Scolices adhere to mucosa and develop into adult taenia echinococcus

Ova of taenia pass into canine faeces

Intermediate host–sheep and man

Grass injested by sheep

Canine faeces

Saliva and coat of dog ingested by man

Ova pass via portal system from intestine to liver

HCL + pepsin dissolve chitinous envelope

Adult hydatid cyst develops in liver

Fig. 374. The life cycle of the hydatid parasite (Douglas 1948).

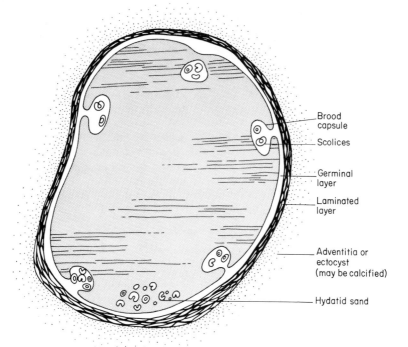

Fig. 375. The basic constitution of a hydatid cyst.

from the tissues of the host, becomes the *adventitia* or *ectocyst*, a thick layer which may eventually calcify. The intermediate and inner zones become hyalinized (the *laminated layer*). Meanwhile, vacuolation occurs and the cyst becomes lined with a single layer of nucleated epithelium (the *germinal layer*).

The nucleated germinal layer gives rise to nodes of multiplying cells, which become vacuolated and pedunculated and project into the lumen of the cyst as *brood capsules*. Scolices develop from a thickening of the lining of the brood capsule and eventually indent it. The attachment of the brood capsule to the germinal layer becomes progressively thinner until the capsule bursts, releasing the scolices into the fluid of the cysts. These fall to the bottom by gravity and are sometimes termed *hydatid sand*. When ingested by the dog, the cycle begins again.

Daughter cysts, and even grand-daughter cysts, develop by fragmentation of the germinal layer. The majority of cysts in adult patients are thus multilocular.

ENDEMIC REGIONS

This disease is common in sheep-raising countries, where dogs have access to infected offal. The endemic regions include South Australia, New Zealand, Africa and South America. It is becoming less common in Iceland, and almost all cases in the United States occur in immigrants. It is frequent in southern Europe, especially Cyprus and Greece, Spain and in the Middle and Far East. The disease is rare in Britain apart from some areas in Wales [5]. The disease in Alaska and Northern Canada may be more benign.

THE DISTRIBUTION OF CYSTS IN THE LIVER

Hydatid cysts usually involve the right lobe on its antero-inferior or postero-inferior surface. If the right lobe is involved anteriorly, the costal margin is pushed forward; if posteriorly, the diaphragm is pushed upwards. When the left lobe is involved, it is usually anterior and the swelling presents in the epigastrium.

CLINICAL FEATURES

These depend on the site of the cyst, the stage of development and whether it is alive or dead.

The rest of the liver hypertrophies and hepatomegaly is pronounced.

The *uncomplicated hydatid cyst* may be silent and found incidentally at autopsy. It should be suspected if a rounded, smooth swelling, continuous with the liver, is found in a patient who is not obviously ill. The only complaints may be a dull ache in the right upper quadrant and sometimes a feeling of abdominal distension. The tension of the cyst is always high and fluctuation is never marked.

COMPLICATIONS

Rupture

Intraperitoneal rupture is most frequent and leads to secondary dissemination throughout the peritoneal cavity.

Rupture into bile ducts may lead to cure or to cholestatic jaundice. The clinical picture is of recurrent cholangitis.

Colonic rupture leads to elimination *per rectum* and to secondary infection.

The cysts may adhere to the diaphragm, rupture into the lungs resulting in expectoration of daughter cysts. Alternatively, the lungs may be involved secondarily to erosion into hepatic veins.

Infection

Secondary invasion by pyogenic organisms nearly always follows rupture into the biliary passages. This leads to the death of the parasite. The picture is of a pyogenic abscess.

Occasionally the entire content of the cyst undergoes aseptic degeneration, leading to death of the parasite. This amorphous yellow debris is distinct from the pus produced by secondary infection.

Other organs

Associated cysts can occur in lung, kidney, spleen, brain or bone, but mass infestation is rare in man and usually the liver is the only organ involved. If a hydatid cyst is found in another site, such as lung or spleen, there is always concomitant infestation of the liver.

Hydatid allergy

Hydatid fluid contains a foreign protein which sensitizes the host. This may lead to severe anaphylactic shock, but more commonly it manifests itself as recurrent urticaria or 'hives'.

DIAGNOSIS

Serological tests

Hydatid fluid contains specific antigens, leakage of which sensitize the patient with the production of antibodies.

The Casoni skin test [4] has been abandoned because of non-specificity and difficulty in obtaining satisfactory test fluid.

The indirect haemagglutination test and complement fixation tests are positive in about 85% of patients.

Results may be negative for all tests if the cyst has never leaked, if it contains no scolices or if the parasite is dead.

Radiological changes

These include a raised, poorly moving right diaphragm, hepatomegaly and calcification. Calcium is laid down in the ectocyst as a distinct round or oval opacity (fig. 376) or merely as shreds in the liver area. Other rare causes of hepatic calcification include haemangioma, primary liver cancer, tuberculoma, intra-hepatic gall-stones, amoebic abscess and gumma. It is also necessary to consider calcification in such adjacent structures as suprarenal, kidney, gall bladder, peritoneum, diaphragm, costal cartilages and in an old subphrenic abscess.

Floating bodies are occasionally seen within hydatid cysts, indicating the presence of free-moving daughter cysts. Infected gas-containing cysts may show a fluid level.

Hepatic cysts may cause displacement of adjoining structures such as the stomach or hepatic flexure of the colon.

Characteristic radiological changes may be seen in the lungs, spleen, kidney or bone.

Splenic venography may show compression of the portal venous branches or a filling defect within the liver [7].

Selective coeliac angiography shows stretching and elongation of the hepatic arteries in the arterial phase and avascular areas in the hepatogram [9].

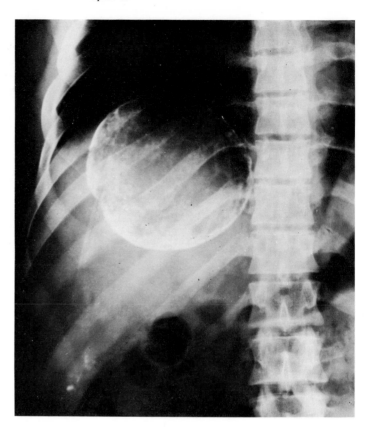

Fig. 376. X-ray of the abdomen shows a calcified hydatid cyst in the liver.

Hepatic scanning and ultrasound are invaluable methods of localizing the cyst and of following the course and effects of treatment (fig. 377).

Eosinophilia. This is not specific but may strengthen clinical suspicion sufficiently to perform a serological test.

Exploratory aspiration is a dangerous procedure, which may lead to widespread peritoneal dissemination or fatal anaphylaxis.

PROGNOSIS

The uncomplicated, hepatic hydatid cyst carries a reasonably good prognosis. The risk of complications is, however, always present. Intraperitoneal or intrapleural rupture is grave, but rupture into the biliary tree is not so serious because spontaneous cure may follow the biliary colic. Infection used to be fatal, but the outlook is now improved by chemotherapy. Calcification is unwelcome if surgery is attempted, because of the difficulty in collapsing the cyst cavity.

TREATMENT

Dogs are denied access to infected offal, and hands are washed after handling dogs. Dogs in affected areas must be regularly de-wormed.

The risks of rupture and secondary infection are so great that, unless small and multiple, hepatic hydatids should be treated surgically [1, 8] if the patient's general condition permits. The object is to remove the cyst completely, without soiling and infection of the peritoneum, and with complete obliteration of the resulting dead space. Complete removal of the cyst with its adventitia from the liver is virtually impossible. This is the ideal form of excision to avoid spilling the contents. In order to sterilize the contents, alcohol or 20% saline should be injected into the cyst before it is handled. Uninfected unilocular cysts may be removed and the adventitial pouch sutured without drainage. If infected, the parasite is removed and the edges of the adventitial pouch marsupialized for drainage. Eventual healing is by secondary intention. Radical removal of postero-superior cysts is

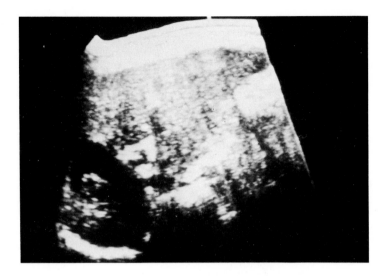

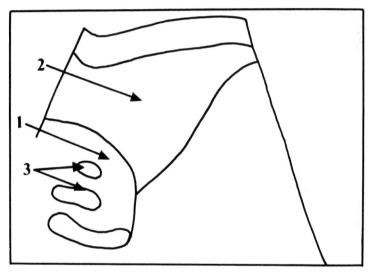

Fig. 377. Ultrasound shows a hydatid cyst (1) in the right lobe of the liver (2). Daughter cysts (3) can be seen inside the larger cyst.

usually impossible because of the proximity to hepatic veins and inferior vena cava. In some instances partial hepatectomy or hepatic lobectomy may be necessary.

Cholangitis is treated by biliary drainage and evacuation of any cysts. The technical problem is great.

Rupture into the peritoneal cavity

The cyst contents are removed from the peritoneal cavity as far as possible by sucking and swabbing.

The scolices, however, usually settle down in the peritoneal cavity and form daughter cysts so that recurrence is almost inevitable.

MEDICAL TREATMENT

Mebendazole is a benzimidazole derivative under trial for the treatment of *E. granulosus* infection. It diffuses through the cyst membrane and interferes with glucose metabolism and microtubular function in the parasite. 400–600 mg three times a day for 21–30 days leads to clinical improvement with fall in specific echinococcal IgE [3]. Ultrasound and CT scanning show reduction in cyst size [2]. However, sometimes, at later operation, the parasite has been shown not to have been killed by the drug. Penetration into large cysts is also not consistent. Side-effects include gastric irritation, pruritus, rash and transient abnormalities in liver function tests.

REFERENCES

1. BARROW J.L. (1978) Hydatid disease of the liver. *Am. J. Surg.* **135**, 597.
2. BEARD T.C., RICKARD M.D. & GOODMAN H.T. (1978) Medical treatment for hydatids. *Med. J. Aust.* **1**, 633.
3. BEKHTI A., SCHAAPS J-P., CAPRON M. *et al* (1977) Treatment of hepatic hydatid disease with mebendazole: preliminary results in four cases. *Br. med. J.* ii, 1047.
4. CASONI T. (1911) La diagnosi biologica dell'echinococcosi umana mediale l'intra dermoreazione. *Folia clin. chem. Micr. Salsomaggiore* **4**, No. 5.
5. COOK B.R. (1964) The epidemiology of *Echinococcus* infection in Great Britain. II. The incidence of *Echinococcus granulosus* and some other cestodes in farm dogs in mid-Wales. *Ann. trop. Med. Parasitol.* **58**, 147.
6. DOUGLAS D.M. (1948) Hydatid disease. *Edinb. med. J.* **55**, 78.
7. GILSANZ V., GALLEGO M. & CALLE YUSTE P. (1961) Portal circulation in hydatid cyst of the liver. *Arch. intern. Med.* **108**, 540.
8. LEWIS J.W.J., KOSS N. & KERSTEIN M.D. (1975) A review of echinococcal disease. *Ann. Surg.* **181**, 390.
9. McNULTY J.G. (1968) Angiographic manifestations of hydatid diseases of the liver; a report of two cases. *Am. J. Roentgenol.* **102**, 380.

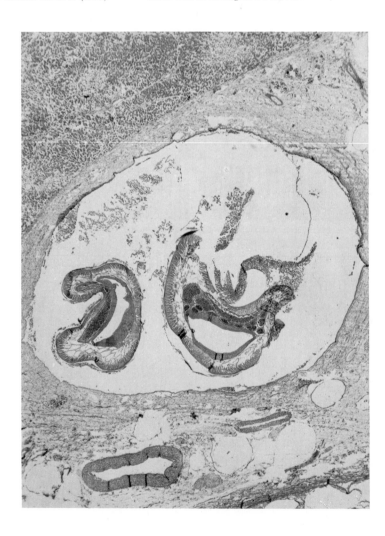

Fig. 378. Section shows a dead ascaris in an intra-hepatic blood vessel in a portal zone. There is surrounding fibrous tissue reaction. H & E, ×40.

ASCARIASIS

The roundworm *Ascaris lumbricoides* is a large worm 10–20 cm long and usually too big to enter the biliary passages. Occasionally, however, it lodges in the common bile duct and produces partial bile duct obstruction and secondary cholangitic abscesses [3]. This is particularly common in the Far East. Biliary obstruction with hepatic ascariasis has been reported in 788 cases in five years from Peking Children's Hospital [5]. The ascaris may be the nucleus for gall-stone formation [5]. The worm usually dies in the bile ducts and may even calcify there when it can be demonstrated in a plain X-ray of the abdomen. Intravenous or operative cholangiography may show the ascaris as a linear filling defect (fig. 378). Endoscopic retrograde cholangiography may be useful. Haemobilia may complicate biliary ascariasis with hepatic abscess formation [4].

Hepatic granulomas have been associated with ascaris infection [1, 2]. These are presumably related to ova and larvae. This suggests possible auto-infection. The ova segment in the liver. The ova may have reached the liver via the portal vein or possibly by retrograde flow in the bile ducts. Eggs, giant cells and a granulomatous reaction with dense surrounding eosinophil infiltration may be seen (fig. 379).

The *diagnosis* is rarely made before operation, the condition being confused with a gall-stone in the common duct.

The *treatment* is surgical, with removal of the worm.

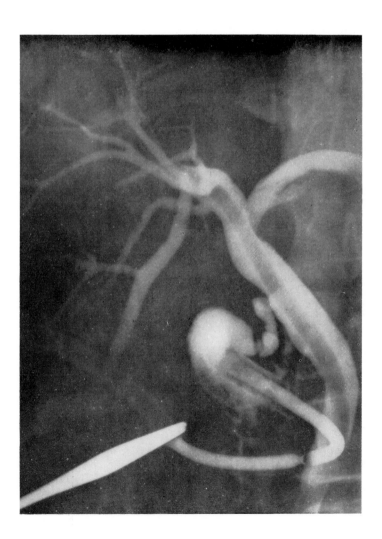

Fig. 379. Operative cholangiogram through the gall bladder showing an ascaris in the common bile duct.

REFERENCES

1. DRURY R.A.B. (1962) Larval granulomata in the liver. *Gut* **3**, 289.
2. KHALEQUE K.A. & ALAM K.S. (1963) Hepatic granuloma caused by *Ascaris* ova. *J. trop. Med. Hyg.* **66**, 249.
3. PFEFFERMANN R., FLOMAN Y. & ROZIN R.R. (1972) Ascariasis of the biliary system. *Arch. Surg.* **105**, 118.
4. ROSENBAUM J.M. & JOHNSTON C. (1966) Hemobilia with multiple liver abscesses and ascariasis. *Am. J. Dis. Child.* **112**, 82.
5. TEOH T.B. (1963) A study of gall-stones and included worms in recurrent pyogenic cholangitis. *J. Pathol. Bact.* **86**, 123.

TRICHINIASIS

This disease is caused by the eating of raw infected pork with subsequent dissemination of trichinella larvae throughout the body.

Hepatic dysfunction is shown by an abnormal bromsulphthalein retention. Hepatic histology may show invasion of hepatic sinusoids by trichinella larvae and also fatty change [1].

Diagnosis is difficult unless it occurs in an epidemic. The presence of eosinophilia is suggestive. Muscle pain and tenderness may warrant muscle biopsy.

Treatment is by emetine, and laparotomy is indicated if the biliary tract is obstructed. Treatment, on the whole, is unsatisfactory.

REFERENCE

1. GUATTERY J.M., MILNE J. & HOUSE R.K. (1956) Observations on hepatic and renal dysfunction in trichinosis. Anatomic changes in these organs occurring in cases of trichinosis. *Am. J. Med.* **21**, 567.

TOXOCARA CANIS (VISCERAL LARVA MIGRANS)

This parasite is spread by cats and dogs. The second stage can infect the liver of man, forming granulomas. Hepatomegaly, recurrent pneumonia, eosinophilia and hypergammaglobulinaemia are associated findings. The serum fluorescent antibody test is positive.

REFERENCE

1. ZINKHAM W.H. (1978) Visceral larva migrans. *Am. J. Dis. Child.* **132**, 627.

LIVER FLUKES

Cysts are consumed and larvae develop in the duodenum and eventually reach the bile ducts. Their route is uncertain. They might invade the biliary passages from the duodenum but would then have to proceed against the direction of biliary flow. The flukes probably invade the liver through its peritoneal coat and are carried via the parenchyma to the bile ducts. During the migratory phase they cause fever and eosinophilia. When they reach the biliary passages they may cause obstruction, the clinical picture simulating a stone in the common bile duct with complicating suppurative cholangitis.

The Chinese liver fluke (*Clonorchis sinensis*) is found mainly in eastern Asia. It is also seen in immigrant Chinese. It gains access to the body by the ingestion of cysts contained in improperly cooked or raw fish. In uncomplicated cases the changes are confined to the walls of the bile duct with abundant adenomatous formation; fibrosis increases with time [2]. Malignant change in the adenomatous tissue is a serious consequence and accounts for at least 15% of the incidence of primary carcinoma of the liver seen in Hong Kong [1]. Complications arise from obstruction to the main bile ducts with secondary infection, usually by *E. coli*, followed by intra-hepatic stone formation, cholangitis and multiple abscess formation. Percutaneous cholangiography has been used to show the flukes [4]. There is no direct relationship to cirrhosis [2].

The common sheep fluke (*Fasciola hepatica*) is found mostly in mid and western Europe and in the Caribbean. The animal infestation rate in Britain is high: 30–90% of all sheep and cattle excrete the ova. This increases in wet summers when the intermediate host, the snail *Lymnaea trunculata*, is also more numerous [5]. The encysted cercariae from these snails survive on herbage and patients are affected usually by eating contaminated watercress.

The clinical picture in the acute stage is of cholangitis with fever, right upper quadrant pain and hepatomegaly. Eosinophilia and a raised serum alkaline phosphatase are noted. The picture may simulate choledocholithiasis.

Liver biopsy shows infiltration of the portal zones with histiocytes, eosinophils and polymorphs. Hepatic granulomas and ova in the liver may occasionally be seen [3].

Diagnosis is suspected by finding the clinical picture of biliary tract disease with eosinophilia [3]. It is confirmed by finding ova in the faeces. These however, may not be detected until twelve weeks after the infection when parasites have attained sexual maturity. They disappear later. The serum fasciola complement fixation test is positive [3].

Treatment is by bithionol (2,2′–thiobis (4,6-dichloraphenol)) [3].

REFERENCES

1. Hou P.C. (1956) The relationship between primary carcinoma of the liver and infestation with *Clonorchis sinensis. J. Pathol. Bact.* **72,** 239.
2. Hou P.C. & Pang L.S.C. (1964) *Clonorchis sinensis* infestation in man in Hong Kong. *J. Pathol. Bact.* **87,** 245.
3. Jones A.E., Kay J.M., Milligan H.P. *et al* (1977) Massive infection with fasciola hepatica in man. *Am. J. Med.* **63,** 836.
4. Okuda K., Emura T., Morokuma K. *et al* (1973) Clonorchiasis studied by percutaneous cholangiography, and a therapeutic trial of toluene-2,4-diisothiocyanate. *Gastroenterology* **65,** 457.
5. Taylor A.W. (1961) Liver-fluke infection in man. *Lancet* ii, 1334.

JAUNDICE OF INFECTIONS

BACTERIAL PNEUMONIA

Nowadays jaundice is an unusual complication of pneumonia. It is, however, still frequent in African negroes where it may be related partly to haemolysis in those deficient in glucose 6-phosphate dehydrogenase [4]. The jaundice is also both hepato-cellular and cholestatic.

Liver biopsy by light microscopy shows non-specific changes; electron microscopy [3] shows bile canalicular dilatation with loss of microvilli, suggesting cholestasis. There is also evidence of toxic liver injury. Increased numbers of fat-storing lipocytes are seen during the acute stage.

SEPTICAEMIA

Jaundice is a rare complication. Infection can be by Gram-negative or Gram-positive organisms and is often post-operative. It may be cholestatic [5]. Haemolytic and hepato-cellular components are also present.

Itching is rare, there is no pain, and the liver is enlarged.

Serum bilirubin can be up to 15 mg/dl; serum alkaline phosphatase is also raised. Serum enzymes are normal. Liver biopsy shows only a non-specific hepatitis with occasional focal necrosis, fatty change and cholestasis, polymorphs and periportal cell infiltrates [1, 2]. Cultures of liver biopsy are usually sterile.

Urinary tract infections are a commoner cause of jaundice in children than in adults (Chapter 23). When they cause it in the older patient, septicaemia usually co-exists.

REFERENCES

1. Bernstein J. & Brown A.K. (1962) Sepsis and jaundice in early infancy. *Pediatrics* **29,** 873.
2. Miller D.J., Keeton G.R., Webber B.L. *et al* (1976) Jaundice in severe bacterial infection. *Gastroenterology* **71,** 94.
3. Theron J.J., Pepler W.J. & Mekel R.C.P.M. (1972) Ultrastructure of the liver in Bantu patients with pneumonia and jaundice. *J. Pathol.* **106,** 113.
4. Tugwell P. & Williams A.O. (1977) Jaundice associated with lobar pneumonia. *Q. J. Med.* **46,** 97.
5. Zimmerman H.J., Fang M., Utili R. *et al* (1979) Jaundice due to bacterial infection. *Gastroenterology* **77,** 362.

Chapter 28
Hepatic Tumours

The liver is affected by both simple and malignant growths (table 67). The simple ones are anatomical curiosities of no clinical importance. Malignant disease of the liver, however, is common, secondary deposits in the liver being much more common than primary cancers.

Table 67. Primary tumours of the liver.

Origin	Tumour
Liver cells	Benign adenoma
	Primary hepatocellular carcinoma
Bile ducts	Benign cholangioma
	Bile duct carcinoma
Connective tissue	Benign fibroma
	Sarcoma
Blood vessels	Haemangioma
	Malignant haemangio-endothelioma

PRIMARY HEPATO-CELLULAR CARCINOMA

The frequency of primary liver cancer depends on the geographic area for which statistics are taken (table 68). In temperate climates it is a rare condition, being found in under 1% of autopsies. In the East African Bantu, however, four out of every five autopsies show hepato-cellular cancer. The highest frequency is in the African and oriental races in whom there is nearly always an associated cirrhosis. It is the second commonest cancer encountered in South East Asia. The condition is, however, increasing in the West [12], and in California the frequency has multiplied three times in 20 years [69].

EXPERIMENTAL LIVER CANCER

A bewildering number of carcinogens can cause tumours in animals, but their relevance to man is

Table 68. World-wide incidence rates of primary liver cancer reported by cancer registries (Doll *et al* 1966).

Area	Rate per 100 000 males per year
Group 1	
Mozambique	98.2
China	17.0
South Africa	14.2
Hawaii	7.2
Nigeria	5.9
Singapore	5.5
Uganda	5.5
Group 2	
Japan	4.6
Denmark	3.4
Group 3	
England and Wales	3.0
USA	2.7
Chile	2.6
Sweden	2.6
Iceland	2.5
Jamaica	2.3
Puerto Rico	2.1
Colombia	2.0
Yugoslavia	1.9

uncertain. They include *p*-dimethyl-amino-azo-benzene (butter yellow), nitrosamines, aflatoxin and senecio alkaloids.

There are great species differences in the experimental production of neoplasms. Moreover, many so-called 'hepatomas' do not have the malignant characteristics of hepato-cellular carcinoma in man. The age, sex and endocrine status of the animal are important in determining the development of cancer. The activity of the carcinogen may be associated with the activity of the drug metabolizing enzymes.

The carcinogen is always bound to a macromolecule before a tumour is induced.

MYCOTOXINS

The most important mycotoxin is aflatoxin produced by a contaminating mould, *Aspergillus*

Table 69. Aflatoxin ingestion and hepatoma incidence
(Linsell *et al* 1977).

Country	Locale	Aflatoxin intake (ng/kg/day)	Hepatoma rate (per 10^5/year)
Kenya	High altitude	3.5	1.2
Thailand	Songkhla	5.0	2.0
Swaziland	Highveld	5.1	2.2
Kenya	Mid altitude	5.9	2.5
Swaziland	Midveld	8.9	3.8
Kenya	Low altitude	10.0	4.0
Swaziland	Lebombo	15.4	4.3
Thailand	Ratburi	45.0	6.0
Swaziland	Lowveld	43.1	9.2
Mozambique	Inhambane	222.4	13.0

flavus. It is highly carcinogenic to the rainbow trout, the mouse, the guinea-pig and monkey. There is variation in the susceptibility of different species. Aflatoxin and similar toxic moulds can readily contaminate food such as ground nuts or grain especially when stored in tropical conditions.

Estimated minimum aflatoxin intake from foods in various areas of Africa correlates with the frequency of primary liver cancer [53] (table 69). However, a five-year follow-up of patients suffering from aflatoxin poisoning failed to reveal cirrhosis or cancer in the survivors.

It is possible that aflatoxin acts as a co-carcinogen with hepatitis B. It is also possible that aflatoxin suppresses the cellular immune response and may increase the hepatitis B carriage rate, and hence the risk of development of primary liver cancer [55].

RELATION TO CIRRHOSIS

It is understandable how carcinoma arises in a cirrhotic liver. The nodular hyperplasia progresses to multiple carcinomas. Liver cell *dysplasia* marked by cellular enlargement, nuclear pleomorphism and multinucleate cells affecting groups of cells or whole nodules may be an intermediate step [5]. The cirrhosis is usually of large nodule type. In one series of 1073 primary carcinomas of the liver 658 (61.3%) also showed cirrhosis.

In about 30% of African patients with hepatitis B infection and primary liver cancer cirrhosis is not present [43].

There are pronounced geographical differences in the frequency of cancer in cirrhotic livers [22]. There is a particularly high association in South Africa and Indonesia, where cancer is reported in more than 30% of cirrhotic livers, whereas frequencies of 10–20% are reported from India, Britain and North America. Primary carcinoma is less common in alcoholics but may be increasing. Malignant cholangiocarcinoma is not usually preceded by cirrhosis.

RELATION TO HEPATITIS B

In 1970 a positive association was reported between primary liver cell cancer and a positive hepatitis B test [76]. World wide, the problem of hepatitis B carriage correlates with frequency of primary liver cancer. In Britain, for instance, the mortality for primary liver cancer is 1–2 per 100 000 and the carriage rate for hepatitis B surface antigen is 0.1 per 100 000, whereas in China the primary liver cancer mortality is approximately 17 per 100 000 and the hepatitis B antigen carrier rate 7.5–14 per 100 000 (table 70). In the nine geographical areas of Greece, the primary liver cancer mortality strongly correlates with the prevalence of hepatitis B antigenaemia [86].

Populations with a high incidence of HBsAg carriage and primary liver cancer migrating to low incidence areas continue to show evidence of hepatitis infection and a high liver cancer mortality. This has been shown particularly in Chinese-Americans [85].

HBsAg titres tend to be low in patients with primary liver cancer and an even higher association is found if anti-HBc is sought. This marker is shown in 95% of African and Asian patients with primary liver cancer [62]. Markers for hepatitis B can be shown by immunofluorescence in liver tissue adjoining the tumour and even in the tumour cells themselves [94].

Table 70. Association of HBV with hepatoma
(Lutwick 1979).

Country	Test(s)	Hepatoma associated with HBV (%)	Control associated with HBV (%)
Uganda	HBsAg	40	3
Taiwan	HBsAg	80	15
USA	HBsAg	21	0.4
Senegal	Anti-HBc	93	42
Hong Kong	Anti-HBc	70	36
USA	Anti-HBc	24	4
Uganda & Zambia	HBsAg, anti-HBs, anti-HBc	96	63
USA	HBsAg, anti-HBs, anti-HBc	74	20
Senegal	HBsAg, anti-HBs, anti-HBc	61	11*

*Control group age and sex matched with either cancer or no cancer.

HBsAg = hepatitis B surface antigen; anti-HBs = antibody to hepatitis B surface antigen; anti-HBc = antibody to hepatitis B core antigen.

Pre-cancerous changes, particularly dysplasia, have a strong association with HBsAg [5]. The viral genome may be integrated into cancer cells [1, 11, 37, 82]. Relation to hepatitis B is probably not only through cirrhosis as primary liver cancer may be found in non-cirrhotic carriers of hepatitis B [77].

American woodchuck (groundhog) hepatitis is an animal model for hepatitis B. The causative agent resembles the hepatitis B virion and the woodchucks develop hepato-cellular carcinoma [83].

RELATION TO ALCOHOL

An appreciable number of patients with hepato-cellular carcinoma give a history of alcoholism and cirrhosis. Hepatitis B and alcohol may act synergistically, producing the cirrhosis and primary liver cancer [70].

SEX HORMONE THERAPY

See page 313.

GENETIC FACTORS

Despite the frequency in Chinese and black people in Africa, there is no clear evidence of a genetic predisposition. In particular, HLA antigens fail to show predisposition either to hepato-cellular carcinoma or to hepatitis B infection [45].

MISCELLANEOUS FACTORS

Hepato-cellular carcinoma can complicate massive immuno-suppressive therapy in patients having renal transplants [6].

Clonorchiasis may be followed by hepato-cellular and cholangio-cellular carcinoma.

The relationship between schistosomiasis and liver cancer has not been established.

Primary liver cancer is a frequent cause of death in haemochromatosis.

Pathology

In the massive type, a single tumour occupies the right lobe, and in the nodular type many small tumours are seen. The tumour is usually white, sometimes necrotic, bile stained or haemorrhagic. Large hepatic or portal veins within the liver are often thrombosed and contain tumour.

Hepato-cellular carcinoma (figs. 380, 381)

The cells resemble normal liver, with compact finger-like processes or solid trabeculae. The tumour simulates normal liver with varying degrees of success. The cells sometimes secrete bile and contain glycogen. There is no intercellular stroma and the tumour cells line the blood spaces.

The tumour cell is usually smaller than the normal liver cell; it is polygonal, with granular cytoplasm. Occasionally, atypical giant cells are found.

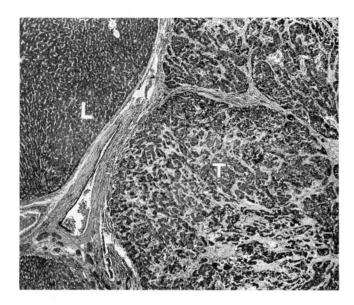

Fig. 380. Hepato-cellular carcinoma. The tumour cells (T) are arranged in trabeculae simulating normal liver which is seen on the left of the section (L). H & E, × 22.

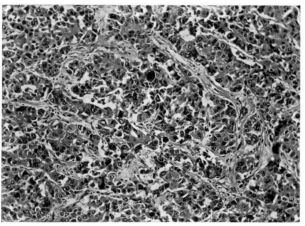

Fig. 381. Hepato-cellular carcinoma. The tumour cells are smaller than normal with granular cytoplasm and large hyperchromatic nuclei. Mitoses are conspicuous. A typical giant cell may be seen. Stroma is scanty and the tumour cells have blood spaces between them. H & E, × 90.

The cytoplasm is eosinophilic, becoming basophilic with increasing malignancy. The nuclei are hyperchromatic and vary in size. Predominantly eosinophilic tumours may sometimes be seen. The centres of the tumours are often necrotic. Periportal lymphatic involvement with malignant cells is an early feature. PAS positive, diastase resistant globular inclusions are found in about 15%, usually in those with high α-fetoprotein levels [18]. They may represent hepatocyte-produced glycoproteins. α_1 anti-trypsin and α-fetoprotein have also been shown.

In young people fibrosis arranged in lamellar fashion around tumour cells may be seen [20]. This type has a better prognosis and operability rate is greater than in ordinary hepato-cellular carcinoma.

It may be extremely difficult to differentiate simple from malignant hepatic tumours. All gradations exist from benign to malignant hepato-cellular tumours. Dysplasia is an intermediate appearance [5].

Electron microscopy. 'Cytoplasmic' hyaline is described in human hepato-cellular carcinoma cells [42]. The cytoplasmic inclusions are filamentous bodies and also autophagic vacuoles [24].

Bile duct carcinoma (fig. 382)

This is a glandular type of tumour arising from

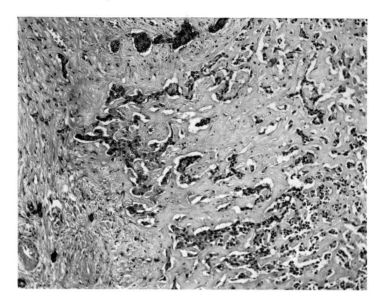

Fig. 382. Bile duct carcinoma. The tumour cells are arranged in tubular fashion simulating bile ducts. The cell type is columnar. Stroma is dense, fibrous avascular. H & E, ×90.

intra-hepatic bile ducts. The tumour cells arrange themselves in tubules, resembling bile ducts. Sometimes they have a papillary arrangement. There is no bile secretion. The stroma is different from that of malignant hepatoma; it consists of fibrous or connective tissues with little or no capillary formation. The cell type is columnar or cuboidal and periportal lymphatic permeation is also seen.

SPREAD

Intra-hepatic. Metastases in the liver may be multiple or in one lobe. Spread is by the blood vessels, for the tumour cells abut on vascular spaces, which they readily penetrate. Lymphatic permeation and direct infiltration also occur.

Extra-hepatic. Involvement of small or large hepatic or portal veins or the inferior vena cava may be seen. Tumour emboli result in pulmonary thrombosis. Systemic spread results in deposits anywhere, but especially in bone.

Regional lymph glands at the porta hepatis are frequently involved, and the mediastinal and cervical chains of glands can also be infiltrated.

Large pulmonary metastases are rare. The tumour may involve the peritoneum with resulting haemorrhagic ascites; this may be terminal.

The histology of metastases. The secondary tumour may faithfully reproduce the structure of the primary, even forming bile. Sometimes, however, the cell type diverges widely from the pri-

mary. Bile or glycogen in cells of a metastasis suggests an hepatic primary.

Clinical features

Age. All ages are affected. In races such as the Chinese and the Bantu the sufferers are often below 40 years old. In temperate climates the patients are usually over 40 years.

Sex. Males exceed females in a ratio of 4–6:1.

Associated cirrhosis must be established. Primary carcinoma of the liver should be suspected if a patient with cirrhosis deteriorates for no obvious reason or if a local lump can be palpated in the liver. It should be considered if there is no improvement when ascites or pre-coma is adequately treated.

Rapid decline in a patient with haemochromatosis or with chronic liver disease and a positive HBsAg also suggests a complicating carcinoma.

The patient complains of malaise and abdominal fullness. He loses weight. The temperature is rarely higher than 38°C.

Pain is frequent but rarely severe and is felt as a non-specific, continuous dull ache in the epigastrium, right upper quadrant or back. Severe pain is due to perihepatitis or involvement of the diaphragm.

Gastro-intestinal symptoms such as anorexia, flatulence and constipation are common.

Dyspnoea is a late symptom and may be due to the large size of the tumour compressing or

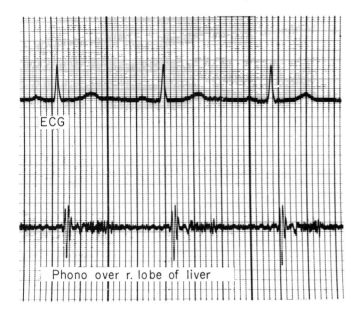

Fig. 383. Hepato-cellular carcinoma in the right lobe. Phonogram of the right lobe of the liver showing a systolic murmur (Clain *et al* 1966).

directly involving the diaphragm, or to pulmonary metastases.

Jaundice is by no means constant and never deep. The depth has little relation to the extent of hepatic involvement. Very rarely the tumour may invade main bile ducts [2, 11].

The liver is enlarged, not only downwards into the abdomen but also upwards into the thorax. A hard irregular lump may be felt in the right upper quadrant, continuous with the liver. If the left lobe is involved, the mass is epigastric. Sometimes multiple masses are palpable, but they are not usually tender. However, tenderness may be so severe that the patient cannot tolerate palpation.

A friction rub, due to perihepatitis, is occasionally heard over the tumour. An arterial murmur (fig. 383) [16] is due to increased arterial vascularity. In the absence of acute alcoholic hepatitis such a murmur is diagnostic of hepato-cellular carcinoma.

Ascites is found in about half the patients. The protein content is high. Malignant cells may be found but interpretation of these in peritoneal fluid is difficult. LDH and carcino-embryonic antigen may be increased. The fluid may be blood stained. Rupture causes haemoperitoneum. This may present insidiously or as an acute abdomen with severe pain. Prognosis is very poor [68].

Portal vein thrombosis adds to ascites. *Hepatic vein* block may occur.

Haemorrhage from oesophageal varices is frequent and usually terminal.

CLINICAL FEATURES OF METASTASES

Lymph glands may be felt, especially in the right supra-clavicular region. *Pulmonary metastases* may result in a pleural effusion. Massive pulmonary embolization may lead to dyspnoea. *Osseous metastases* may appear in ribs and vertebrae. *Brain secondaries* give the features of a brain tumour.

SYSTEMIC EFFECTS [60]

Florid endocrine changes are associated more often with the embryonic hepatoblastoma of childhood than with adult primary liver cell carcinoma.

Painful gynaecomastia [84] with increased secretion of oestrogen may be seen.

Hypercalcaemia [60], due to pseudo-hyperparathyroidism, has been reported on a number of occasions. The tumour may contain a parathormone-like material, and serum parathormone levels are raised.

Hypoglycaemia can be found in up to 30% of patients [58]. This may be due to demand for glucose by an enormous tumour mass and so is often associated with an undifferentiated rapidly progressing tumour. Rarely the hypoglycaemia is seen with a well-differentiated slowly progressive cancer. In this type glucose 6-phosphatase and phosphorylase are reduced or absent in the tumour while the glycogen content in tumour and adjacent tissue is increased. This suggests an acquired glycogen storage disease as the mechanism of the hypoglycaemia. In this group control is difficult even with an enormous carbohydrate intake. Methyl prednisolone and diazoxide are ineffective [49].

Insulin-like production by the tumour has been reported [75]. This is an unlikely explanation of the hypoglycaemia for plasma insulin or insulin-like activity are not increased when the blood glucose level is low.

Hyperlipidaemia is rare [74], but about a third have increased serum cholesterol levels when maintained on a low cholesterol diet [4]. In one patient, the hyperlipidaemia and the hypercholesterolaemia were caused by production of an abnormal lipoprotein with β mobility [74].

The hypercholesterolaemia has also been related to the absence of a negative-feedback system whereby cholesterol feeding inhibits hepatic cholesterol synthesis.

BIOCHEMICAL CHANGES

These may be only those of cirrhosis. The serum alkaline phosphatase is markedly elevated and serum transaminase levels increase.

Electrophoresis of serum proteins may show a γ and an α_2 component. A serum macroglobulin of myeloma type is a rare finding [88].

Polyclonal gammopathy, with marked plasmacytosis, can be related to primary hepato-cellular carcinoma [26].

Immunological tests

SERUM α_1 FETOPROTEIN [91]

α_1 fetoprotein (AFP) is a normal component of plasma protein in human foetuses older than six weeks, and reaches maximum concentration at between 12 and 16 weeks of foetal life. A few weeks after birth it disappears from the circulation but reappears in the blood of patients with primary liver cancer and can be shown in the tumour by indirect immunofluorescence [4, 28, 64]. AFP is also present in the serum of patients with embryonic tumours of ovary and testis and in embryonic hepatoblastoma. It may also be present

with carcinomas of the gastro-intestinal tract with hepatic secondaries.

AFP was originally detected by a simple, non-sensitive, immuno-diffusion method. Positivity by this technique was virtually equivalent to a diagnosis of primary liver cell cancer. Positivity in patients with primary liver cancer in different geographic areas differed: in Great Britain it was about 30%, in Greece 60%, in the United States 50%, in Hong Kong 59% and in South Africa 78%. The method was usually positive with the larger, more undifferentiated tumours.

A more sensitive immunoassay method led to detection in 90% of primary liver tumours but also in other conditions. AFP has even been detected in the serum of normal persons. It is found during late pregnancy. AFP is raised in acute viral hepatitis and in a wide variety of patients with chronic liver disease. The increases are usually modest and transient [23]. Values of 2000 ng/100 dl are diagnostic of primary liver cancer; below this level rising values have to be shown to be diagnostic.

Serum AFP falls if a patient has the primary liver cancer removed or has an orthotopic liver transplantation. Persisting low levels indicate residual tumour and increases indicate rapid tumour growth. Serial values are useful in assessing therapy (fig. 384).

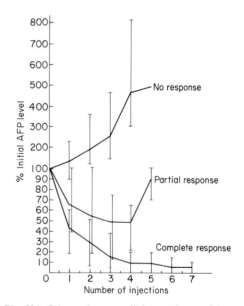

Fig. 384. Primary hepato-cellular carcinoma. Mean and range of AFP levels expressed as a percentage of the level at presentation in patients showing complete, partial and no response to adriamycin therapy (Johnson *et al* 1978).

Serum AFP is a valuable screening procedure for primary liver cancer in a patient with cirrhosis. It may also be used for population surveys. Between 1975 and 1978, 242911 inhabitants of Shanghai were screened and 39 cases of primary liver cancer were discovered (16/100 000). Earlier diagnosis resulted in more cases being suitable for resection and hence in longer survival.

OTHER TUMOUR MARKERS

Carcinoembryonic antigen is present in most forms of chronic liver disease. Values are particularly high with hepatic metastases [47]. Because of lack of specificity, it is of little value in diagnosis of primary liver cancer. Lack of specificity also applies to the serum α_1 *anti-trypsin* and α-*acid glycoprotein* which are sometimes associated with primary liver cancer.

Serum ferritin is increased and to a greater extent than the aspartate transaminase. This suggests the increase is due to production of ferritin by the tumour rather than to liver necrosis [14]. The ferritin:transaminase ratio may be used to monitor progress of primary liver cancer.

Serum vitamin B_{12} binding protein may be very high [41] and this probably arises from the tumour. The serum B_{12} level is increased as is the unsaturated vitamin B_{12} binding capacity.

HEPATITIS B MARKERS

Tests for HBsAg should always be performed. Titres may be low and radio-immunoassay is essential. Other markers such as anti-HBc may be positive and this increases the likely relationship to hepatitis B.

Haematological changes

The leucocyte count is usually raised to about 10000 per mm^3 with 80% polymorphonuclears. Eosinophilia is an occasional finding. The platelet count may be high.

The erythrocyte count is usually normal and anaemia is mild. Erythrocytosis is suggested if the haemoglobin level exceeds 16 g; it is seen in 11%. It is probably due to increased erythropoietin production by the tumour [63, 74]. Leucocytosis and thrombocytosis are absent, so excluding polycythaemia rubra vera.

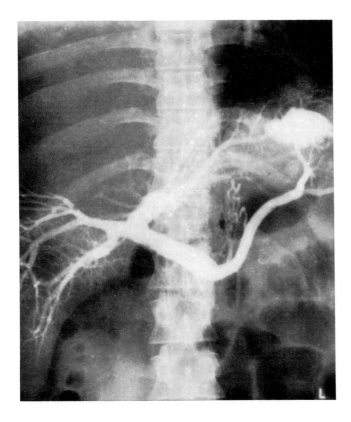

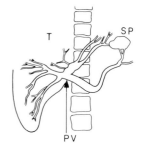

Fig. 385. Primary hepatic carcinoma. Splenic venogram showing a pool in the spleen (SP), depression and bifurcation to the left of the portal vein (PV) and a non-filled area in the superior aspect of the right lobe representing the tumour (T).

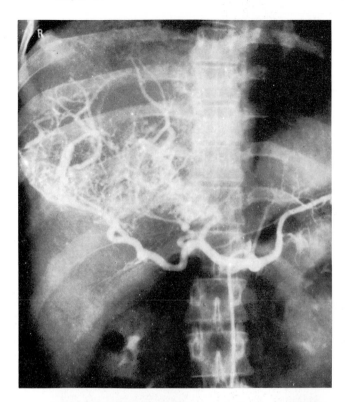

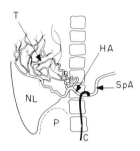

Fig. 386. Same case as
fig. 385. Selective coeliac
arteriogram showing
catheter in the coeliac axis
(C), the splenic artery (SpA)
and the hepatic artery (HA).
An abnormal arterial pattern
(T) is shown in the tumour.
The normal liver (NL) is not
outlined by contrast media.
P is pyelogram.

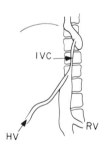

Fig. 387. Same case as
fig. 385. Inferior vena cava-
gram showing the renal vein
(RV), reflux in the right hepatic
vein (HV) and the inferior
vena cava (IVC) displaced to
the left and narrowed by the
tumour.

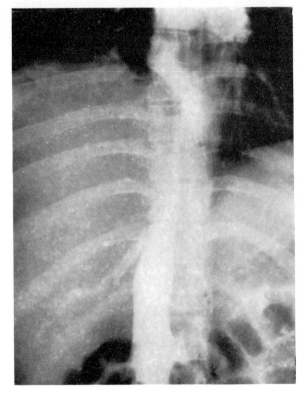

Blood coagulation may be disturbed. Fibrino-lytic activity tends to be decreased [51]. This may be due to liberation by the tumour of an inhibitory substance. Increase in plasma fibrinogen levels may be secondary to this effect.

Dysfibrinogenaemia may represent reversion to a foetal form of fibrinogen [33]. Ground-glass cells in hepato-cellular carcinoma may contain fibrinogen and be producing it [81].

Tumour localization

VASCULAR RADIOLOGY

Hepatic angiography

This is very valuable for localization, for diagnosis, to determine operability and to follow the effects of therapy. The tumour is supplied by the hepatic artery, and selective coeliac and superior mesenteric arteriography results in filling of the lesion (fig. 386). The appearances can be related to the gross anatomy of the tumour [67]. The arterial pattern is bizarre with pooling, stretching and displacement of vessels. The vessels may be sclerosed, have an irregular lumen and be fragmented. Arteriovenous shunts can be shown often with retrograde filling of the portal trunk [66]. There may be delayed emptying of the lesion. The portal vein may be distorted if there is tumour invasion (fig. 386).

Splenic venography

This shows displacement of the main portal veins by the tumour. It demonstrates whether the portal

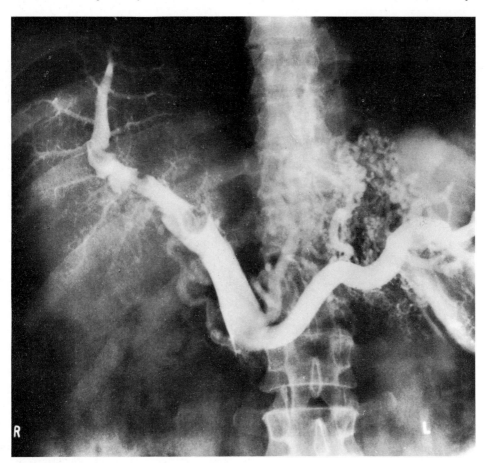

Fig. 388. Primary hepato-cellular carcinoma. Splenic venogram shows filling defects in the portal vein due to tumour invasion. Gastro-oesophageal collaterals are also seen.

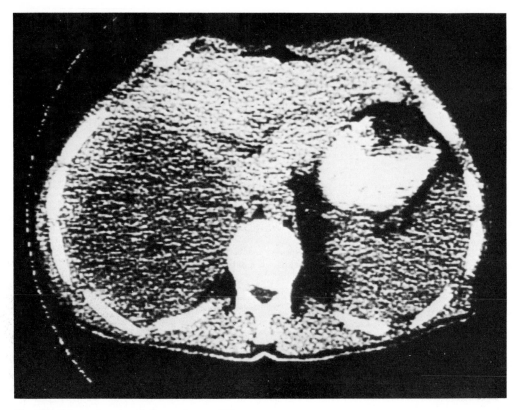

Fig. 389. Primary hepato-cellular carcinoma. CT scan shows filling defect in the right lobe of the liver.

vein is patent or obstructed by tumour. In the hepatogram phase the tumour shows as a non-filled zone (fig. 385).

Inferior vena cavagrams are useful in showing displacement or obstruction of the inferior vena cava. Retrograde filling of the hepatic veins may be noted (fig. 387).

Retrograde hepatic venography has been used to demonstrate filling defects and distortion of hepatic venous radicles by tumour.

HEPATIC SCANNING

Isotope scans show the tumours as filling defects (see fig. 44). Lesions larger than 2 cm in diameter are shown. Isotopes providing a positive uptake such as ^{67}gallium confirm that the lesion is a primary liver carcinoma [37] (see fig. 45). Abscesses of the liver or elsewhere, however, do take up gallium.

Computerized axial tomography may also show the tumour (fig. 389).

NEEDLE LIVER BIOPSY (page 471)

Diagnosis

Increased awareness of the condition has improved the accuracy of diagnosis. Although the likelihood is greater in such areas as Africa or South East Asia, primary liver cancer is being increasingly recognized world wide. In one series of 75 patients, 63% were diagnosed definitely ante-mortem and a further 20% clinically suspected [44]. Abdominal pain or weight-loss with hepato-megaly or ascites were the common presentations. Deterioration in a patient with known chronic liver disease arouses suspicion. A rising serum AFP is suspicious; a positive (> 2000 ng/100 dl) is diagnostic, but elevations are not constant. The demonstration of a space-filling lesion by scanning or radiology is helpful, and final confirmation comes from hepatic histology obtained by needle biopsy.

Occasionally a plain X-ray of the abdomen shows calcification (sunburst lesion) (fig. 390).

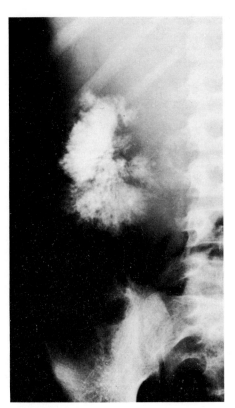

Fig. 390. Primary liver cancer. A plain X-ray of the abdomen shows calcification (sunburst lesion).

Prognosis

The outlook is hopeless and the course is shorter in those with cirrhosis or who are HBsAg positive [27]. The duration of chronic liver disease to the presentation of primary liver cancer is less if the disease is HBsAg-associated [50]. The final illness is usually about seven months, although occasionally, with a slow growing tumour, survival is two to three years. The massive type of carcinoma runs a shorter course than the nodular. Tumours with a thick fibrous capsule may be slower growing and more susceptible to resection [65].

TREATMENT

Prevention

If hepatitis B infection could be controlled by a vaccine (Chapter 15) the incidence of primary liver cancer would fall world wide but especially in areas with high prevalence of hepatitis B carriage.

Better agricultural methods and improved storage and transport of cereals will reduce contamination by mycotoxins.

Resection

The liver has a remarkable capacity for regeneration [79, 80]. After partial resection DNA synthesis increases and the remaining liver cells become larger (hypertrophy) and undergo increased mitosis (hyperplasia). Multiple factors control this process. Substances in portal blood are important. Some of these *hepatotrophic factors*, such as insulin and glucagon, are of pancreatic origin. Inhibitory growth factors must also exist, and the liver may produce its own growth control factor.

The resectability rate for all hepatic tumours is very low [29]. Resection is possible in less than 1%. Better results are obtained in the paediatric age group and where cirrhosis is absent, for the cirrhotic liver does not regenerate [52]. Surgery must, however, be considered in any patient with a malignant primary tumour confined to one lobe. The localization must be confirmed by scanning and hepatic arteriography, and at laparotomy there must be no evidence of extra-hepatic spread. The left lobe is resected with relative ease. The right lobe is more difficult. Up to 90% of the liver may be removed with eventual survival [57]. Operative mortality is about 20%. The best prognosis is in the single, fairly well differentiated tumour of childhood or in sex hormone-related liver cancer. Resection for metastatic cancer cannot be recommended [30].

Chemotherapy

Adriamycin (Doxorubicin). This drug induces remissions in about one-third of patients with primary liver cancer [39]. Grade A patients, that is those without jaundice, ascites or high transaminase values, have a survival after treatment of 43% compared with grade B patients of 18% (fig. 391). Hepatitis B antigen-negative patients may respond better than those who are positive. Therapy is monitored by α-fetoprotein levels (fig. 384).

The dose is 60 mg/m^2 body surface (diluted with 5% dextrose) given intravenously every three weeks. The maximum dose is 550 mg. The dose is reduced by half if the serum bilirubin level is raised, if the white cell count is less than 2000 or if the platelets are less than 100 000. An electrocardiogram is taken before each dose. Side-effects

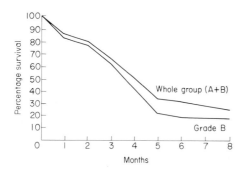

Fig. 391. Treatment of 44 patients with primary hepato-cellular carcinoma by adriamycin. Simple actuarial survival curves for all patients (grades A—good prognosis; and B—poor prognosis) and for grade B patients alone (Johnson *et al* 1978).

include mild nausea, vomiting, haematuria and alopecia (the hair regrows later). Marrow depression and cardiotoxicity are possibilities but are very rare.

Quadruple therapy [17]. Improvement in survival is small, symptomatic improvement rarely impressive and side-effects common. Drugs used include combinations of methotrexate, 5-fluorouracil, actinomycin D and cyclophosphamide.

NON-OPERATIVE HEPATIC ARTERIAL THERAPY

The tumour is largely supplied by the hepatic artery, and ligation has been used in treatment but with limited success.

Chemotherapeutic agents such as 5-fluorouracil have been delivered directly to the tumour through a catheter inserted either percutaneously via a femoral artery and coeliac axis or directly at operation. This allows a high concentration of agent to be delivered to the tumour. Results seem little better than when the drug is given systemically. The more vascular the tumour the better the result with hepatic arterial therapy [48].

Hepatic arterial branches supplying the tumour can be embolized using gelfoam via a catheter in the hepatic artery [92]. The portal vein must be patent. Embolization can be followed by chemotherapy. The procedure usually requires general anaesthesia and antibiotic cover is given. It is often painful. Abscess formation, fever and misplaced injections are other complications. The tumour rapidly acquires a fresh arterial circulation via alternative vessels.

Embolization has its best result in the treatment of hepatic *carcinoid tumours* [3]. There is a marked reduction in symptoms and the tumours shrink. Therapy can be repeated.

Radiotherapy

Radiotherapy up to a total of 3000 rads to the liver has resulted in a few instances of tumour regression with palliation of pain and hepatomegaly. Side-effects include radiation hepatitis and hepatic-venous obstruction (Budd–Chiari syndrome).

Hepatic transplant [78]

Hepatic transplantation has been used in these patients but with generally unsatisfactory results (Chapter 23). If the patient survives the surgery, the immuno-suppression necessary to prevent rejection favours recurrence and metastasis.

OTHER PRIMARY TUMOURS

Primary sarcoma of the liver

This is an extremely rare tumour and difficult to distinguish from a highly anaplastic liver cell carcinoma. Spread of a sarcoma arising in a nearby structure such as the thoracic cage or diaphragm must be excluded. About 100 cases have been reported. Primary leiomyosarcoma is very rare [61].

The histology is typical of sarcoma. Reticulin stains show the uniform distribution of fibres characteristic of sarcoma.

About a third of sufferers also have cirrhosis. The condition is most frequent in children. The prominent clinical features are pyrexia and an abdominal mass. Hypoglycaemia may develop. The course is rapidly downhill.

Malignant haemangio-endothelioma (haemangioblastoma)

This very rare and highly malignant tumour is difficult to distinguish from primary hepato-cellular cancer. The liver is enlarged and full of knobbly cavernous growths.

Histologically, blood-filled cavernous sinuses are lined with layers of highly malignant, anaplastic, endothelial cells which in parts may resemble the earliest stages of embryonic vascular development. Many well-differentiated tumours resemble peliosis hepatis. They may have a Kupffer cell origin; indeed needle biopsies from the lesion may show only Kupffer cell hyperplasia and be difficult to interpret [59].

The clinical course is rapidly downhill with cachexia and blood-stained ascites. A bruit may be heard over the liver. The tumour is sometimes radio-sensitive. Platelets may be consumed in the tumour and disseminated intravascular coagulation has been reported [87]. Occasionally the course is chronic with ascites and hepatomegaly over many years [15, 38]. The condition may present in infancy (Chapter 23).

Thorotrast consists of a colloidal solution of thorium dioxide with the isotope radiothorium which is mainly an α-ray emitter and has a half-life of 1.39×10 years. It was formerly used as a contrast medium in radiology. Primary hepatic tumours have developed years after intravascular administration [38]. Hepato-cellular or bile duct carcinoma has a latent period of about 20 years and haemangio-endothelioma about 15 years. Plain X-ray of the abdomen shows continued presence of the isotope in liver and spleen and this is confirmed by autoradiographs of liver tissue. Total body counting may be used to quantitate radioactivity in the patient's body. Microradiology has been used to demonstrate deposition of thorium in the liver at autopsy. Cirrhosis can develop even without liver tumours.

Other aetiological factors in angiosarcoma [54] include vinyl chloride (page 300), arsenic (page 303) and androgenic–anabolic steroids [25] (page 317) (see fig. 288).

Simple tumours of the liver

ADENOMA (page 314)

This is very rare. They present as right upper quadrant masses or as acute intraperitoneal haemorrhage. They have an association with sex hormone therapy (Chapter 17) and with pregnancy.

CHOLANGIOMA

This is a very rare, simple tumour of bile duct origin. It has the structure of a cystadenoma and it must be distinguished from a simple cyst or polycystic disease of the liver. A mixed type of tumour

is also recorded with both proliferating bile ducts and hepatic cells.

HAEMANGIOMA

This is the commonest simple tumour of liver, being found in about 5% of autopsies. It is usually single and small but occasionally may be multiple or very large. Two forms occur in the liver—the *cavernomous*, which is the commoner and is due to dilatation of existing blood channels; it is often found by chance at autopsy. The other is the *true haemangioma*, a tumour due to proliferation of the remains of vascular embryonic tissue.

The tumour is commonly subcapsular, on the convexity of the right lobe of the liver, and is occasionally pedunculated. On section it appears round or wedge-shaped, dark red in colour and has a honeycomb pattern, with a fibrous capsule which may be calcified. Histologically, the cavernoma shows a communicating network of spaces containing red blood corpuscles, whereas the true haemangioma is composed entirely of newly formed arterioles.

Clinically, a vascular hum may be heard over the tumour in the liver. Spontaneous rupture may be fatal. Occasionally the tumour may be very large, causing symptoms by pressure on adjacent viscera [34].

Thrombocytopenia may develop, presumably due to adhesion of platelets to the vascular lining of the tumour [19].

Needle liver biopsy is contraindicated if the diagnosis is suspected although it is usually uneventful.

Peritoneoscopy is diagnostic.

Radiology

A plain X-ray may show the calcified capsule. Coeliac angiography [32] shows space-filling lesions which displace large hepatic arterial branches to one side. The hepatic arteries are not enlarged, taper normally and divide to normal small vessels before filling the vascular spaces. The spaces tend to adopt a circular or 'C' shape due to the central fibrosis. Haemangiomas may show prolonged opacification even up to 18 seconds. They may be recognized incidentally during angiography for another condition.

Scanning shows a filling defect in the liver.

Treatment is not usually indicated, for the only risks are carcinomatous change and haemorrhage and these are very rare. Attempts at surgical removal are fraught with difficulties, and if the tumour is diagnosed at laparotomy, it is better left alone.

Corticosteroids may be helpful in the infant, particularly if complicated by congestive heart failure. Radiation therapy may be useful, about 1500 rads being given over two weeks.

Non-metastatic hypernephroma [89]

Hepatosplenomegaly with reduction in serum albumin, increased serum globulins and alkaline phosphatase can complicate hypernephroma without hepatic metastases. Liver biopsy shows non-specific cellular infiltration. The changes may regress if the renal tumour is resected. The mechanism of the hepatic changes is unknown.

HEPATIC METASTASES

The liver is the most frequent site of blood-borne metastases, irrespective of whether the primary is drained by systemic or portal veins. It is involved in about a third of all cancers, including half of those of stomach, breast, lung and those arising from the portal territory.

Pathogenesis [13, 93]

Invasion from tumours in adjacent organs, retrograde lymphatic permeation and extension along the lumen of blood vessels are all unusual.

Portal emboli come from malignant neoplasms arising in the organs of the portal vascular territory. Primary tumours in the uterus and ovaries, prostate or bladder, may involve contiguous tissue drained by the portal vein and hence give embolic metastases to the liver; these are extremely rare.

Microscopically, hepatic arterial embolization is difficult to identify, because the picture is confused by the succeeding intra-hepatic metastases. The high incidence of arterial emboli causing hepatic tumours is evidence that the liver provides favourable soil for malignant growth.

Pathology

There may be only one or two microscopic nodules or the whole liver may be enormous and full of metastases. Liver weights of 5000 g are not unusual and one liver is said to have weighed 21 500 g. The deposits are usually white and well demarcated. Occasionally the centre may be soft, necrotic and haemorrhagic. On the surface of the liver they show characteristic umbilication; this results from necrosis of the centre, which has outgrown its blood supply. Perihepatitis may be seen over peripheral lesions.

The tumour cells metastasize rapidly and widely through the liver, both by perivascular lymphatics and by direct invasion of the portal venous radicles.

Injection studies show that, in contrast to hepato-cellular carcinoma, metastases may have a decreased rather than increased blood supply from

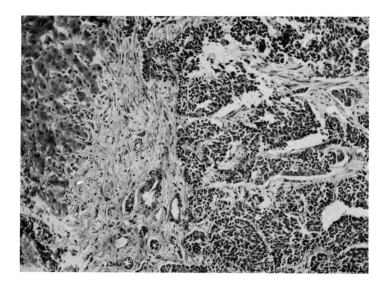

Fig. 392. Anaplastic secondary carcinoma of the liver. The tumour is composed of sheets of undifferentiated malignant cells. Normal liver cells are seen to the left. There was a small bronchial primary growth which was not revealed by chest X-ray. H & E, × 110.

the hepatic artery. This is particularly so in those of gastro-intestinal origin [36].

Histology

The secondary deposits in the liver may reproduce the histology of the primary lesions. However, this is not necessarily so, and in many instances the primary tumour may be well differentiated, while the secondary deposits in the liver may be extremely anaplastic and give no hint of their origin (fig. 392).

Clinical features

These may be due to the hepatic metastases, to the distant primary growth or more usually to a combination of both.

The patients complain of malaise, lassitude and loss of weight. Abdominal distension and a dragging sensation are due to the enlarged liver. Occasionally the pain is sharp and intermittent, simulating biliary colic. Fever and sweats may occur.

Depending upon the weight loss, the patient may be emaciated, with an enlarged abdomen. The liver may be normal sized or so large that it protrudes visibly in the right upper abdomen. The tumour deposits are hard and may be umbilicated. Friction may be heard over them. The deposits are not vascular, so an arterial bruit is not heard. Splenomegaly is frequent, even in those with a patent portal vein. Jaundice is mild and may be absent. Deep jaundice implies invasion of major bile ducts.

Oedema of the legs with dilated veins coursing upwards over the abdominal wall suggests that the inferior vena cava is obstructed as it runs on the posterior aspect of the liver.

Glands in the right supra-clavicular region may be involved.

A pleural effusion may indicate pulmonary metastases and similar localizing signs may provide clinical evidence of the primary growth.

Ascites reflects peritoneal involvement and occasionally a thrombosed portal vein. Bleeding may be secondary to portal hypertension.

Rarely obstructive jaundice may be seen with metastases from breast [71] or colon [90]. Haemobilia is another unusual complication [31].

Secondary malignant deposits are by far the commonest causes of a really large liver.

Hypoglycaemia is a rare complication. The primary is usually a sarcoma [95].

When malignant carcinoid of the small intestine or bronchus is associated with vaso-motor abnormalities and pulmonary stenosis, there are always many hepatic metastases.

The *urine* shows excess of urobilin; bile pigments are only present if the patient is deeply jaundiced.

Unless the bile ducts are completely obstructed, the *stools* are well coloured, and if the primary lesion is in the alimentary tract they may give a positive reaction for occult blood.

Laboratory investigations

BIOCHEMICAL TESTS

Even with an enormous liver, sufficient functioning tissue remains. The smaller intra-hepatic bile ducts may be compressed yet no jaundice develops. The area with uninvolved ducts may excrete the bilirubin from the occluded areas. A slight increase in the proportion of serum conjugated bilirubin may be the only abnormality. Serum total bilirubin values greater than 2 mg/100 ml suggest involvement of major bile ducts at the hilum.

Serum alkaline phosphatase, lactic dehydrogenase and *transaminase* levels are often increased.

Serum albumin concentration is normal or slightly decreased. The *serum globulin* level may be normal, slightly raised or even, occasionally, very high. Electrophoresis may show a raised α_2- or γ-globulin.

Serum carcino-embryonic antigen may be present [56].

The ascitic fluid shows increased protein, occasionally the presence of carcino-embryonic antigen and increases in lactic dehydrogenase three times over the serum value.

HAEMATOLOGY

A polymorph leucocytosis is fairly common: even values up to 40 000–50 000 per mm^3 are sometimes recorded. There may be a mild anaemia.

NEEDLE LIVER BIOPSY

The intercostal approach should be used unless a palpable nodule can be biopsied directly. Tumour tissue is characteristically white and friable. If a cylinder of tissue is not obtained it is worth examining any blood clot or debris for malignant cells. Histology will not always enable the site of the primary to be detected especially if the tumour is undifferentiated (fig. 392). Cytological examination of aspiration fluid and touch preparations of the biopsy may slightly increase the yield of cancer cells [7].

The chance of obtaining a positive result increases with the extent of tumour, size of liver, and the presence of a palpable nodule. Localization of the tumour by scanning, ultrasound or peritoneoscopy [40] increases the positivity, for it allows the needle to be directed into the tumour. General anaesthesia increases the chances of a positive biopsy [10]. If liver metastases are suspected, a preoperative needle biopsy is well worth while. A positive may prevent an unnecessary laparotomy.

PERITONEOSCOPY

The liver surface is seen, metastases identified and any suspicious nodule biopsied. This increases positivity over blind needle biopsy.

RADIOLOGY

A *plain film* of the abdomen demonstrates the large liver. The diaphragm may be elevated and its contour irregular. *Calcification* in hepatic tumours is rare but is noted with primary cancer or haemangiomas and in secondaries, for instance from the colon [46] or the breast [73].

Chest radiograph may show associated pulmonary metastases.

Barium swallow may show oesophageal varices and the *meal* displacement to the left and rigidity of the lesser curve of the stomach. *Barium enema* may reveal depression of the hepatic flexure and transverse colon. The barium meal, follow-through, enema and fibroptic endoscopy are helpful in demonstrating any primary tumour.

Scanning, selective coeliac arteriography and *splenic venography* are useful in localizing the malignant deposits. Unless serum biochemical tests are abnormal routine scans are of little value in the detection of metastases.

Special diagnostic problems

The patient with a known primary growth may be suspected of having liver secondaries but they cannot be confirmed clinically. Suggestive evidence includes slightly increased serum bilirubin, transaminase and alkaline phosphatase levels. If the serum alkaline phosphatase and transaminases are

normal there is a 90% chance of there being no hepatic metastases. Aspiration needle biopsy, scanning and peritoneoscopy are useful.

The other problem, of more academic interest, is obvious involvement of the liver when the primary is unknown [21]. Breasts, thyroid and lungs must be considered as possible primaries. Positive stool blood suggests gastro-intestinal cancer, and fibroendoscopy, sigmoidoscopy, barium meal and enema are useful. Removal of skin tumours and the presence of melanomas suggest malignant melanoma. Suspected carcinoma of the body of the pancreas merits ERCP and angiography. Needle liver biopsy is usually positive and may indicate the site of the primary. However, even this may show only the presence of a squamous, scirrhous, columnar or anaplastic growth, the site of the primary remaining unknown.

Prognosis

This depends on the site of the primary and the malignancy. In general, patients are dead within one year of diagnosis of hepatic metastases. Secondaries from tumours of colon and rectum have the best outlook. In these patients the survival rate is not influenced by the age of the patient, the location of the primary, or the type of palliative large bowel operation performed [8, 9].

Treatment

This remains very unsatisfactory. Those that have the best prognosis without therapy, for instance, secondaries from the rectum, do best with therapy. Most of the published results of therapy have no controls. Nevertheless, chemotherapy has to be considered, if only to offer the patient and his relatives some hope. Chosen treatment should be the one having the greatest prospect of slowing the progress and with the least undesirable side-effects.

5-fluorouracil (5-FU) has very few side-effects. The loading dose is 15 mg/kg intravenously every other day for 10 days to be followed by maintenance of 15 mg/kg intravenously once a week. The best results are in secondaries from the colon and rectum, but where objective methods such as scintiscanning are used for assessment, little value is shown.

Other chemotherapy includes quadruple, cyclophosphamide, methotrexate, vincristine and 5-FU, given in five-day courses with three weeks between. Side-effects are greater and results again uncontrolled. Breast secondaries seem to give the best results; those for colo-rectal metastases are less favourable.

Both the primary and secondary hepatic tumours are supplied by the hepatic artery, and cytotoxic drugs such as 5-FU given by this route can be delivered directly to the tumour. The catheter is inserted into the hepatic artery percutaneously and via the femoral artery. Treatment has been continued for up to 10 weeks. Acid peptic disease of the upper gastro-intestinal tract with massive haemorrhage is a complication. Some patients have shown symptomatic improvement with weight gain [35].

In the carcinoid syndrome, heroic surgery should be borne in mind. The tumours shell out rather easily. Embolization via the hepatic artery is also of value [3].

REFERENCES

1. ADEN D.K., FOGEL A., PLOTKIN S. *et al* (1980) Controlled synthesis of HBsAg in a differentiated human liver carcinoma-derived cell line. *Nature* **282**, 615.
2. AFROUDAKIS A., BHUTA S.M., RANGANATH K.A. *et al* (1978) Obstructive jaundice caused by hepatocellular carcinoma. Report of three cases. *Am. J. dig. Dis.* **23**, 609.
3. ALLISON D.J., MODLIN I.M. & JENKINS W.J. (1977) Treatment of carcinoid liver metastases by hepatic artery embolisation. *Lancet* ii, 1323.
4. ALPERT M.E., HUTT M.S.R. & DAVIDSON C.S. (1969) Primary hepatoma in Uganda. A prospective clinical and epidemiologic study of forty-six patients. *Am. J. Med.* **46**, 794.
5. ANTHONY P.P., VOGEL C.L. & BARKER L.F. (1973) Liver cell dysplasia: a premalignant condition. *J. clin. Pathol.* **26**, 217.
6. ARBUS G.S. & HUNG R.H. (1972) Hepatocarcinoma and myocardial fibrosis in an $8\frac{3}{4}$-year-old renal transplant recipient. *Canad. med. Assoc. J.* **107**, 431.
7. ATTERBURY C.E., ENRIQUEZ R.E., DESUTO-NAGY G.I. *et al* (1979) Comparison of the histologic and cytologic diagnosis of liver biopsies in hepatic cancer. *Gastroenterology* **76**, 1352.
8. BENGMARK S. & HAESTRÖM L. (1969) The natural history of primary and secondary malignant tumors of the liver. I. The prognosis for patients with hepatic metastases from colonic and rectal carcinoma by laparotomy. *Cancer* **23**, 198.
9. BENGMARK S. & HAFSTRÖM L. (1969) The natural history of primary and secondary malignant tumours of the liver. II. The prognosis for patients with hepatic metastases from gastric carcinoma verified by laparotomy and postmortem examination. *Digestion* **2**, 179.
10. BLEIBERG H., ROZENCWEIG M., MATHIEU M. *et al*

(1978) The use of peritoneoscopy in the detection of liver metastases. *Cancer* **41**, 863.
11. BRECHOT C., POURCEL C., ANNE LOUISE *et al* (1980) Pressure of integrated hepatitis B virus sequences in cellular DNA of human hepatocellular carcinoma. *Nature* **286**, 533.
12. BURNETT R.A., PATRICK R.S., SPILG W.G.S. *et al* (1978) Hepatocellular carcinoma and hepatic cirrhosis in the west of Scotland: a 25-year necropsy review. *J. clin. Pathol.* **31**, 108.
13. CAMERON G.R. (1954) The liver as a site and source of cancer. *Br. med. J.* i, 347.
14. CHAPMAN R.G., BATEY R. & SHERLOCK S. (1980) Serum ferritin in hepatocellular carcinoma. In press.
15. CHOWDHURY A.R., BLACK M., LORBER S.H. *et al* (1977) Hemangio-endotheliomatosis of the liver: a twelve year follow-up. *Gastroenterology* **72**, 157.
16. CLAIN D., WARTNABY K. & SHERLOCK S. (1966) Abdominal arterial murmurs in liver disease. *Lancet* ii, 516.
17. COCHRANE A.M.G., MURRAY-LYON I.M., BRINKLEY D.M. *et al* (1977) Quadruple chemotherapy versus radiotherapy in treatment of primary hepatocellular carcinoma. *Cancer* **40**, 609.
18. COHEN C. (1976) Intracytoplasmic hyaline globules in hepatocellular carcinomas. *Cancer* **37**, 1754.
19. COOPER W.H. & MARTIN J.F. (1962) Hemangioma of the liver with thrombocytopenia. *Am. J. Roentgenol.* **88**, 751.
20. CRAIG J.R., PETERS R.L., EDMONDSON H.A. *et al* (1979) Fibrolamellar carcinoma of the liver: a tumour of adolescents and young adults with distinctive clinicopathologic features. *Gastroenterology* **77**, A6.
21. DIDOLKAR M.S., FANOUS N., ELIAS E.G. *et al* (1977) Metastatic carcinomas from occult primary tumours. *Ann. Surg.* **186**, 625.
22. DOLL R., PAYNE P. & WATERHOUSE J. (1966) *Cancer Incidence in Five Continents*. International Union against Cancer and Springer-Verlag, Heidelberg.
23. ELETHERIOU N., HEATHCOTE J., THOMAS H.C. *et al* (1977) Serum alpha-fetoprotein levels in patients with acute and chronic liver disease. *J. clin. Pathol.* **30**, 704.
24. ENAT R., BUSCHMANN R.J. & CHOMET B. (1973) Ultrastructure of cytoplasmic hyaline inclusions in a case of human hepatocarcinoma. *Gastroenterology* **65**, 802.
25. FALK H., THOMAS L.B., POPPER H. *et al* (1979) Hepatic angiosarcoma associated with androgenic–anabolic steroids. *Lancet* ii, 1120.
26. FENOGLIO C., FERENCZY A., ISOBE T. *et al* (1973) Hepatoma associated with marked plasmacytosis and polyclonal hypergammaglobulinemia. *Am. J. Med.* **55**, 111.
27. FISHER R.L., SCHEUER P.J. & SHERLOCK S. (1976) Primary liver cell carcinoma in the presence or absence of hepatitis B antigen. *Cancer* **38**, 901.
28. FOLI A.K., SHERLOCK S. & ADINOLFI M. (1969) α_1-fetoprotein in patients with liver disease. *Lancet* ii, 1267.
29. FORTNER J.G., KIM D.K., MACLEAN B.J. *et al*

(1978) Major hepatic resection for neoplasia. *Ann. Surg.* **188**, 363.

30. FOSTER J.H. (1978) Survival after liver resection for secondary tumours. *Am. J. Surg.* **135**, 389.

31. GOLDNER F. (1977) Hemobilia secondary to liver disease. *Gastroenterology* **76**, 595.

32. GOOD L.I., ALAVI A., TROTMAN B.W. *et al* (1978) Hepatic hemangiomas: pitfalls in scintigraphic detection. *Gastroenterology* **74**, 752.

33. GRALNIK H.R., GIVELBER H. & ABRAMS E. (1978) Dysfibrinogenemia associated with hepatoma. *New. Engl. J. Med.* **299**, 221.

34. GREICO M.B. & MISCALL B.G. (1978) Giant hemangiomas of the liver. *Surg. Gynecol. Obstet.* **147**, 783.

35. GULESSERIAN H.P., LAWTON R.L. & CONDON R.E. (1972) Hepatic artery ligation and cytotoxic infusion in treatment of liver metastases. *Arch. Surg.* **105**, 280.

36. HEALEY J.E. Jr (1965) Vascular patterns in human metastatic liver tumors. *Surg. Gynecol. Obstet.* **120**, 1187.

37. HIRSCHMAN S.Z., VERNACE S.J. & SCHAFFNER F. (1971) D.N.A. polymerase in preparations containing Australian antigen. *Lancet* i, 1099.

38. JENNINGS R.C. & PRIESTLEY S.E. (1978) Haemangioendothelioma (Kupffer cell angiosarcoma), myelofibrosis, splenic atrophy and myeloma paraproteinaemia after parenteral thorotrast administration. *J. clin. Pathol.* **31**, 1125.

39. JOHNSON P.J., WILLIAMS R., THOMAS H. *et al* (1978) Induction of remission in hepatocellular carcinoma with doxorubicin. *Lancet* i, 1006.

40. JORI G.P. & PESCHLE C. (1972) Combined peritoneoscopy and liver biopsy in the diagnosis of hepatic neoplasm. *Gastroenterology* **63**, 1016.

41. KANE S.P., MURRAY-LYON I.M., PARADINAS F.J. *et al* (1978) Vitamin B_{12} binding protein as a tumour marker for hepatocellular carcinoma. *Gut* **19**, 1105.

42. KEELEY A.F., ISERI O.A. & GOTTLIEB L.S. (1972) Ultrastructure of hyaline cytoplasmic inclusions in a human hepatoma: relationship to Mallory's alcoholic hyalin. *Gastroenterology* **62**, 280.

43. KEW M.C. (1978) Hepatocellular cancer in southern Africa. In *Primary Liver Tumours.* Falk Symposium 25. MTP, Lancaster.

44. KEW M.C., DOS SANTOS H.A. & SHERLOCK S. (1971) Diagnosis of primary cancer of the liver. *Br. med. J.* iv, 408.

45. KEW M.C., GEAR A.J., BAUMGARTEN I. *et al* (1979) Histocompatibility antigens in patients with hepatocellular carcinoma and their relationship to chronic hepatitis B virus infection in these patients. *Gastroenterology* **77**, 537.

46. KHILNANI M.T. (1961) Calcified liver metastasis from carcinoma of the colon. *Am. J. dig. Dis.* **6**, 229.

47. KHOO S.K. & MACKAY I.R. (1973) Carcinoembryonic antigen in serum in diseases of the liver and pancreas. *J. clin. Pathol.* **26**, 470.

48. KIM D.K., WATSON R.C., PAHNKE L.D. *et al* (1977) Vascularity as a prognostic factor for hepatic tumours. *Ann. Surg.* **185**, 31.

49. KREISBERG R.A. & PENNINGTON L.F. (1970)

Tumor hypoglycemia: a heterogeneous disorder. *Metabolism* **19**, 445.

50. KUBO Y., OKUDA K., MUSHA H. *et al* (1978) Detection of hepatocellular carcinoma during a clinical follow-up of chronic liver disease. *Gastroenterology* **74**, 578.

51. KWAAN H.C., LO R. & MCFADZEAN A.J.S. (1959) Antifibrinolytic activity in primary carcinoma of the liver. *Clin. Sci.* **18**, 251.

52. LIN T-Y., LEE C-S., CHEN C-C. *et al* (1979) Regeneration of human liver after hepatic lobectomy studied by repeated liver scanning and repeated needle biopsy. *Ann. Surg.* **190**, 48.

53. LINSELL C.A. & PEERS F.G. (1977) Aflatoxin and liver cell cancer. *Trans. R. Soc. trop. Med. Hyg.* **71**, 471.

54. LOCKER G.Y., DOROSHAW J.H., ZWELLING L.A. *et al* (1979) The clinical features of hepatic angiosarcoma: a report of four cases and a review of the English literature. *Medicine (Baltimore)* **58**, 48.

55. LUTWICK L.I. (1979) Relation between aflatoxins and hepatitis-B virus and hepatocellular carcinoma. *Lancet* i, 755.

56. McCARTNEY W.H. & HOFFER P.B. (1976) Carcinoembryonic antigen assay in hepatic metastasis detection: an adjunct to liver scanning. *J. Am. med. Assoc.* **236**, 1023.

57. McDERMOTT W.V. Jr., GREENBERGER N.J., ISSELBACHER K.J. *et al* (1963) Major hepatic resection: diagnostic techniques and metabolic problems. *Surgery* **54**, 56.

58. McFADZEAN A.J.S. & YEUNG R.T.T. (1969) Further observations on hypoglycaemia in hepatocellular carcinoma. *Am. J. Med.* **47**, 220.

59. MacSWEEN R.N.M., VETTERS J.M., ROSS S.K. *et al* (1973) Haemangio-endothelial sarcoma of the liver. *J. Pathol.* **109**, 39.

60. MARGOLIS S. & HOMCY C. (1972) Systemic manifestations of hepatoma. *Medicine (Baltimore)* **51**, 381.

61. MASUR H., SUSSMAN E.B. & MOLANDER D.W. (1975) Primary hepatic leiomyosarcoma. *Gastroenterology* **69**, 994.

62. MAUPAS P., WERNER B., LAROUZE B. *et al* (1975) Antibody to hepatitis B core antigen in patients with primary hepatic carcinoma. *Lancet* ii, 9.

63. NAKAO K., KIMURA K., MIURA Y. *et al* (1966) Erythrocytosis associated with carcinoma of the liver (with erythropoietin assay of tumor extract). *Am. J. med. Sci.* **251**, 161.

64. NISHIOKA M., IBATA T., OKITA K. *et al* (1972) Localisation of α-fetoprotein in hepatoma tissues by immunofluorescence. *Cancer Res.* **32**, 162.

65. OKUDA K., MUSHA H., NAKAJIMA Y. *et al* (1977) Clinicopathologic features of encapsulated hepatocellular carcinoma. *Cancer* **40**, 1240.

66. OKUDA K., MUSHA H., YAMASAKI T. *et al* (1977) Angiographic demonstration of intrahepatic arterio-portal anastomosis in hepatocellular carcinoma. *Radiology* **122**, 53.

67. OKUDA K., OBATA H., JINNOUCHI S. *et al* (1977) Angiographic assessment of gross anatomy of hepatocellular carcinoma: comparison of celiac angiograms and liver pathology in 100 cases. *Radiology* **123**, 21.

68. Ong G.B. & Taw J.L. (1972) Spontaneous rupture of hepatocellular carcinoma. *Br. med. J.* iv, 146.

69. Peters R.L., Afroudakis A.P. & Tatter D. (1977) The changing incidence of association of hepatitis B with hepatocellular carcinoma in California. *Am. J. clin. Pathol.* **68**, 1.

70. Pettigrew N.M., Goudie R.B., Russell R.I. *et al* (1972) Evidence for a role of hepatitis virus B in chronic alcoholic liver disease. *Lancet* ii, 724.

71. Popp J.W. Jr, Schapiro R.H. & Warshaw A.L. (1979) Extrahepatic biliary destruction caused by metastatic breast cancer. *Ann. intern. Med.* **91**, 568.

72. Primack A., Vogel C.L. & Barker L.F. (1973) Immunological studies in Ugandan patients with hepatocellular carcinoma. *Br. med. J.* i, 16.

73. Saghatoeslami M., Khodarahmi K. & Epstein B.S. (1962) Calcified intra-hepatic metastases from carcinoma of the breast. *J. Am. med. Assoc.* **181**, 1139.

74. Santer M.A., Waldmann T.A. & Fallon H.J. (1967) Erythrocytosis and hyperlipemia as manifestations of hepatic carcinoma. *Arch. intern. Med.* **120**, 735.

75. Schonfeld A., Babbott D. & Gundersen K. (1961) Hypoglycemia and polycythemia associated with primary hepatoma. *New Engl. J. Med.* **265**, 231.

76. Sherlock S., Fox R.A., Niazi S.P. *et al* (1970) Chronic liver disease and primary liver-cell cancer with hepatitis-associated (Australia) antigen in serum. *Lancet* i, 1243.

77. Shikata T. (1976) Primary liver carcinoma and liver cirrhosis. In *Hepatocellular Carcinoma*, eds K. Okuda & R.L. Peters, pp. 53–71, Wiley, New York.

78. Starzl T.E., Koep L.J., Halgrimson C.G. *et al* (1979) Fifteen years of liver transplantation. *Gastroenterology* **77**, 375.

79. Starzl T.E. & Terblanche J. (1979) Hepatotrophic substances. In *Progress in Liver Disease*, vol. 6, p. 135, eds H. Popper & F. Schaffner. Grune and Stratton, New York.

80. Starzl T.E., Terblanche J., Porter K.A. *et al* (1979) Growth-stimulating factor in the regenerating canine liver. *Lancet* i, 127.

81. Strohmeyer F.W., Ishak K.G., Gerber M.A. *et al* (1980) Ground-glass cells in hepatocellular carcinoma may contain fibrinogen. *Am. J. Clin. Pathol.* **74**, 254.

82. Summers J., O'Connell A., Maupas P. *et al* (1978) Hepatitis-B virus DNA in primary hepatocellular carcinoma tissue. *J. med. Virol.* **2**, 207.

83. Summers J., Smolec J., Werner B.G. *et al* (1980) Properties and distribution of the Woodchuck hepatitis virus (WHV). In *Virus and Liver*, Falk Symposium 28. MTP, Lancaster.

84. Summerskill W.H.J. & Adson M.A. (1962) Gynecomastia as a sign of hepatoma. *Am. J. dig. Dis.* **7**, 250.

85. Szmuness W., Stevens C.E., Ikram H. *et al* (1978) Prevalence of hepatitis-B virus infection and hepatocellular carcinoma in Chinese-Americans. *J. infect. Dis.* **137**, 822.

86. Trichopoulos D., Tabor E., Gerety R.J. *et al* (1978) Hepatitis B and primary hepatocellular carcinoma in a European population. *Lancet* ii, 1217.

87. Truell J.E., Peck S.D. & Reiquam C.W. (1973) Hemangiosarcoma of the liver complicated by disseminated intravascular coagulation. *Gastroenterology* **65**, 936.

88. Viallet A., Benhamou J.-P., Berthelot P. *et al* (1962) Primary carcinoma of the liver and dysproteinemia. *Gastroenterology* **43**, 88.

89. Walsh P.N. & Kissane J.M. (1968) Nonmetastatic hypernephroma with reversible hepatic dysfunction. *Arch. intern. Med.* **122**, 214.

90. Warshaw A.L. & Welch J.P. (1978) Extrahepatic biliary destruction by metastatic colon cancer. *Ann. Surg.* **188**, 593.

91. Wepsic H.T. & Kirkpatrick A. (1979) Alphafetoprotein and its relevance to human disease. *Gastroenterology* **77**, 787.

92. Wheeler P.G., Melia W., Dubbins P. *et al* (1979) Non-operative arterial embolisation in primary liver tumours. *Br. med. J.* ii, 242.

93. Willis R.A. (1952) Secondary tumours of the liver. In *The Spread of Tumours in the Human Body*, p. 178. Butterworth, London.

94. Wu P-C. (1979) Patterns of hepatitis B surface antigen. *Arch. Pathol. lab. Med.* **103**, 165.

95. Younus S., Soterakis J., Sossi A.J. *et al* (1977) Hypoglycemia secondary to metastases to the liver. *Gastroenterology* **72**, 334.

Chapter 29
Gall-stones and Inflammatory
Gall Bladder Diseases

Composition of gall-stones

In the western world gall-stones are composed mainly of cholesterol (11–98%). Other constituents include calcium salts of bilirubin and trace amounts of fatty acids, phospholipids, bile acids and glycoproteins. Micro-analytical techniques allow analysis of as little as 35 mg gall-stone [76]. Crystallography confirms that the cholesterol is in monohydrate and anhydrous forms and is the major constituent, with calcium carbonate and phosphate, palmitate and amorphous material also identified [98]. Calcium salts and lipid are deposited alternately [8]. The nature of the nucleus of the stone is uncertain—pigment, glycoprotein and amorphous material have all been suggested.

The problem is to explain how, in normal persons, insoluble cholesterol is kept in solution in bile and what leads, in some people, to its precipitation to form gall-stones.

Composition of bile

Biliary cholesterol is in the free unesterified form. Concentration is unrelated to serum cholesterol level and depends only to a limited extent on the bile acid pool size and bile acid secretory rate.

Biliary phospholipids. These are insoluble in water and comprise lecithin (90%) with small quantities of lysolecithin (3%) and phosphatidyl ethanolamine (1%). Phospholipids are hydrolysed in the gut and there is no entero-hepatic circulation. Bile acids determine excretion and enhance synthesis.

Bile acids (fig. 393). The primary bile acids are the trihydroxy, cholic acid, and the dihydroxy, chenodeoxycholic acid. These are converted by bacterial action, usually in the colon, to the secondary bile acids, deoxycholic acid and lithocholic acid. Cholic, cheno- and deoxycholic acids are absorbed and undergo an entero-hepatic circula-

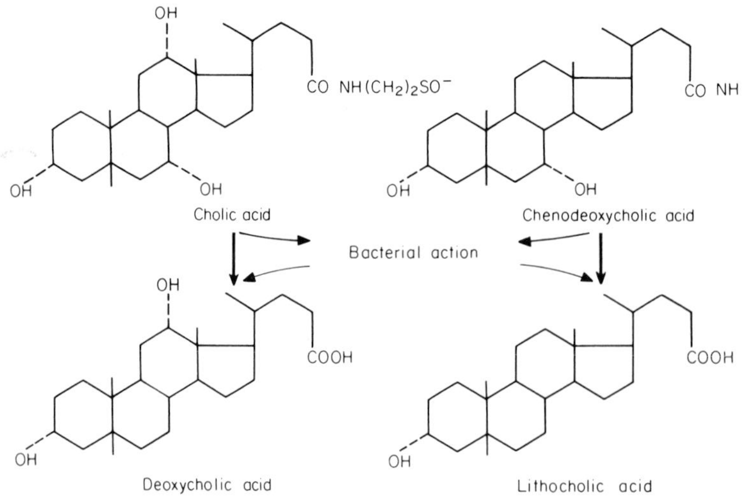

Fig. 393. The chemical structures of the primary (cholic and chenodeoxycholic) and secondary (deoxycholic and lithocholic) bile acids.

tion which takes place six to ten times daily [35]. Lithocholic acid is poorly absorbed and there is little to be found in the bile. The total bile acid pool is 3–5 g and the average daily production of cholic acid about 330 mg and chenodeoxycholic acid 162 mg.

The control of bile acid synthesis is complex; it is probably a negative feedback mechanism through the amount of bile salts and cholesterol reaching the liver from the gut. Bile acid synthesis is decreased by addition of bile salts and increased by interruption of the entero-hepatic circulation.

Factors in gall-stone formation (fig. 395)

ALTERED HEPATIC BILE COMPOSITION

Bile is 85–95% water. Cholesterol is insoluble in water and is maintained in solution by micelle formation (fig. 394). Above a certain level (the critical micellar concentration) bile acids coalesce to form micelles that have a hydrophilic external surface and a hydrophobic internal surface. Cholesterol is incorporated into the hydrophobic interior. Phospholipids are inserted into the walls of the micelles so that they are enlarged; these 'mixed micelles' are thus able to hold more cholesterol.

Using phase diagrams patients with cholesterol gall-stones can be shown to have excess cholesterol relative to bile salts and phospholipids, i.e. outside the micellar liquid zone (*lithogenic bile*) [2, 20]. Such super-saturated bile is necessary for cholesterol stone formation but not every patient with super-saturated bile forms gall-stones. Super-saturated bile can be found even in normal subjects during fasting [79].

Other factors must be involved. Cholesterol crystallization is probably a prerequisite [93]. Cholesterol crystals can be shown under the microscope in the bile of gall-stone formers. These cholesterol monohydrate crystals eventually grow and agglomerate, first into microscopic and then macroscopic stones. A nucleus is also required, and this may be anything from mucus to bacteria to bile pigments.

In the majority of patients, a diminished hepatic secretion rate of bile acids is the primary defect, and this is related to a reduced total body pool of bile acids [104]. The bile acids circulate more frequently within the entero-hepatic circulation, thereby suppressing synthesis. Alternatively, an over-sensitive feedback inhibition of bile salt synthesis is possible [73].

Patients with cholesterol gall-stones show a higher HMG-CoA reductase in liver biopsies, so increasing cholesterol synthesis [28]. At the same time, cholesterol 7α-hydroxylase is reduced, so reducing the synthesis of the primary bile acids.

Lithogenic bile also shows an increase of

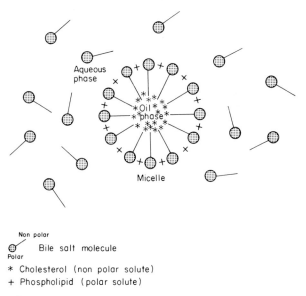

Fig. 394. The structure of micelles present in bile.

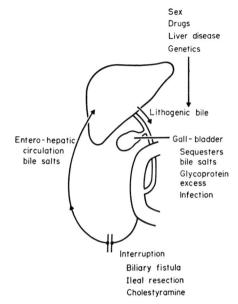

Fig. 395. Aetiological factors in the production of gall-stones.

viscosity favours stone formation. Desquamated epithelium and glycoprotein form the nucleus. A large, high-cholesterol layer exists close to the gall bladder wall and this could favour precipitation and allow the crystals to grow. A poorly contracting, diseased gall bladder would increase the likelihood of stone formation.

The bile remains lithogenic and the bile acid pool is unchanged after cholecystectomy [3]. Thus the position after cholecystectomy remains unaltered.

The gall bladder may have other parts to play in bile salt kinetics. It can sequester bile so that the entero-hepatic circulation of bile salts is interrupted and lithogenic bile is so produced. A diurnal variation in bile composition is known and during fasting the gall bladder undoubtedly accumulates bile.

With gall-stone disease the storage capacity of the gall bladder is impaired, contributing to the small bile salt pool. This reduction is unlikely to be the sole or even the major cause of gall-stones

dihydroxy over trihydroxy bile acids. Glycine conjugates, which solubilize cholesterol less efficiently than taurine ones, are in excess.

Hepatic bile having a constitution outside the micellar liquid zone has been shown in Indian and Caucasian patients with gall-stones in both the United States and the United Kingdom [94] and in gall bladder bile obtained at surgery from patients with stones.

BILIARY GLYCOPROTEIN

Glycoproteins comprise large-molecular-weight proteins (mucus, mucopolysaccharides and mucoproteins). Most gall-stones contain glycoproteins and most experimental models of lithogenesis are associated with excess glycoprotein in bile or biliary tract. Increased secretion precedes gall-stone formation. Their precise role in lithogenesis, however, remains uncertain. They could serve as a framework upon which the cholesterol crystals are laid down. In the gall bladder the increased viscosity could allow microspheroliths to be retained.

ROLE OF THE GALL BLADDER [62]

Although lithogenic bile comes from the liver, the stones are formed in the gall bladder. Increased

ROLE OF INFECTION

There is little to associate infection in the usual patient with uncomplicated gall-stones. The bile is often sterile and culture of the gall-stone yields no growth. Conceivably bacteria might deconjugate bile salts, making the bile more acid and less able to maintain cholesterol in solution. Infection in the gall bladder undoubtedly provides epithelial nuclei on which gall-stones may form.

AGE

There is a steady increase in gall-stone prevalence with advancing years. The presentation is usually in the 50s and 60s.

Gall-stones, not only of pigment but also cholesterol type, are reported in childhood [59].

SEX AND OESTROGENS

Gall-stones are twice as common in women as in men, and this is particularly so before the age of 50 [40].

The incidence is higher in multiparous than in nulliparous women. Incomplete emptying of the gall bladder in late pregnancy leaves a large residual volume and thus retention of cholesterol crystals, and this favours gall-stone formation [18]. Oestrogens also have a mildly cholestatic effect, with reduction of hepatic bile acid secretion and the production of more lithogenic bile.

The bile becomes more lithogenic when women are placed on birth control pills [11]. Women on long-term oral contraceptives have a two-fold increased incidence of gall bladder disease over controls [15]. Post-menopausal women taking oestrogen-containing drugs have a highly significant (2.5 times) increase in gall bladder disease [16].

OBESITY

This seems to be commoner among gall-stone sufferers than in the general population. Obesity is associated with increased cholesterol synthesis and excretion [91].

GEOGRAPHICAL PREVALENCE

American Indians have the highest known prevalence. This is related to super-saturation of the bile with cholesterol with consequent reduction of the circulating bile salt pool [105]. Gall-stones are also very frequent in the United States generally, in the United Kingdom, France, Germany, Sweden and indeed in the whole western world. Africans are largely free of cholelithiasis. The incidence, however, is rising as westernized diets and improved standards of living spread.

CIRRHOSIS OF THE LIVER

There is a strong association of cirrhosis, including primary biliary cirrhosis [77], with gall-stones, about 30% having gall-stones [17]. Although the bile acid excretion is reduced the stones are usually pigmented ones. The bile acid pool is reduced but phospholipid secretion and cholesterol excretion are also lowered so that the bile is not lithogenic. It has greater cholesterol binding powers than in controls [106].

OTHER FACTORS [10]

Ileal resection breaks the entero-hepatic circulation of bile salts, reduces the total bile salt pool and is followed by gall-stone formation.

Long-term cholestyramine therapy results in frequent bile salt loss, a reduced bile acid pool and gall-stone formation.

Cholesterol-lowering diets high in unsaturated fat and plant sterols but low in saturated fats and cholesterol result in increased gall-stone formation [96].

Clofibrate enhances biliary cholesterol excretion and makes the bile more lithogenic [81].

Cancer of the gall bladder (see Chapter 32).

Summary

The formation of gall-stones depends on the production of bile in which cholesterol cannot be maintained in micellar form (*lithogenic bile*). This might be related to increased secretion of cholesterol or perhaps to reduction in total bile acid pool. The gall bladder is important in providing nuclei for stone formation and acting as a reservoir allowing growth of the stone. Infection in the gall bladder provides nuclei for stones and alters the chemical composition of the bile, favouring precipitation. Changes in reservoir function of the gall bladder may be important in altering the total bile acid pool.

Pigment gall-stones [95]

This term is used for black or dark brown stones containing less than 25% cholesterol. They are 2–5 mm in diameter, irregular or smooth, amorphous, or crystalline on cross-section. They consist of calcium salts of bilirubin, phosphate, carbonate and other ions and have been divided to calcium carbonate-containing and non calcium carbonate-containing groups. They represent some 27% of gall-stones removed at cholecystectomy. About a half are radio-opaque. They cannot be dissolved by chenodeoxycholic acid.

In some patients the concentration of unconjugated bilirubin relative to bile salts in bile is increased. This may be due to accelerated hydrolysis of bilirubin conjugates excreted in bile. Pigment stones show an increased prevalence with haemolysis, especially hereditary spherocytosis, sickle cell disease, and mechanical destruction of erythrocytes on prosthetic heart valves [65].

They may be found in elderly patients in the United States, especially males, undergoing cholecystectomy. The aetiology is unknown but is not infective.

They show an increased prevalence with all forms of cirrhosis including biliary [17, 97]. This is probably related to haemolysis and a low biliary excretion of bile acids.

Pigment gall-stones are frequent in oriental countries where they tend to be associated with parasitic infestations of the biliary tract such as *Clonorchis sinensis* or *Ascaris lumbricoides*. Well-to-do urbanized Japanese have mainly cholesterol stones, whereas the labouring classes develop mainly pigment stones [75]. Stones are frequently intra-hepatic. In Japan, *E. coli* is frequently cultured from pigment stones and bacterial beta-glucuronidase may be important in stone formation [69].

Radiology of gall-stones (see Chapter 6)

Only about 10% of gall-stones are radio-opaque, compared with 90% of renal calculi. Visualization is due to the calcium content of the stone. Mixed stones may or may not have sufficient calcium to be rendered visible.

Gall-stones are usually multiple and faceted, although occasionally a single, rounded, ring stone fills the whole gall bladder (fig. 396).

They usually have a peripheral rim of calcium and a clear centre. Occasionally the structure is laminated due to alternate deposition of cholesterol and calcium bilirubin. Rarely gall-stones contain gas which shows as stellate, translucent areas (*Mercedes-Benz sign*) [50].

Cholecystography with tomography will demonstrate about half the 90% of gall-stones not shown in the straight film of the abdomen. Failure may be associated with a non-functioning gall bladder, less often with the contrast material concealing the stones or with hepato-cellular dysfunction.

The stones appear as negative shadows which move with changes of posture. In the erect position they may float on the contrast medium as a translucent layer (floating gall-stones) (fig. 397) [84].

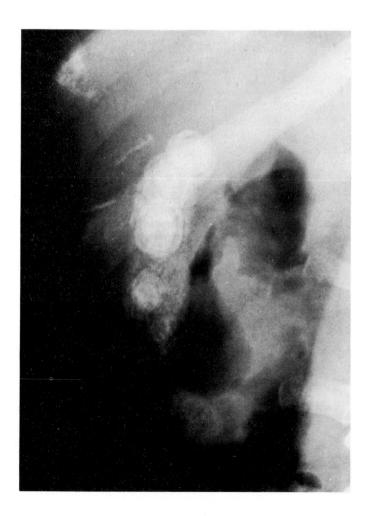

Fig. 396. Plain X-ray of the abdomen shows calcified gall-stones with alternate deposition of cholesterol and calcium salts. These stones would not be suitable for medical dissolution.

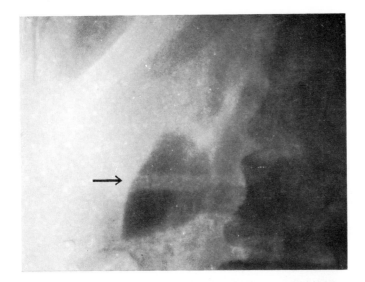

Fig. 397. Floating gall-stones. Cholecystogram. Patient erect. The radio-translucent gall-stones form a layer across the gall bladder which is indicated by an arrow.

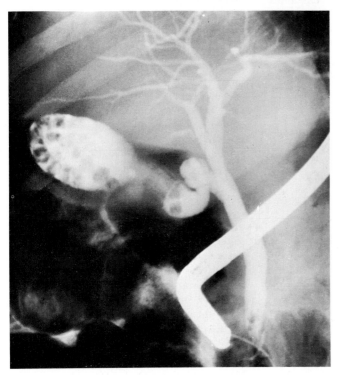

Fig. 398. Endoscopic retrograde cholangiography shows gall-stones in the gall bladder and at the lower end of the common bile duct.

ERCP is more satisfactory than intravenous cholangiography in the diagnosis of both gall bladder stones and bile duct stones (fig. 398) [80].

Ultrasound or CT scanning may show a thickened gall bladder wall and the presence of stones (see fig. 50) [68]. It is particularly valuable in the acute situation.

The natural history of gall-stones (fig. 399)

Disease of the gall bladder is rare unless it complicates gall-stones.

Stones in the gall bladder are symptomless (*silent gall-stones*) unless they migrate into the

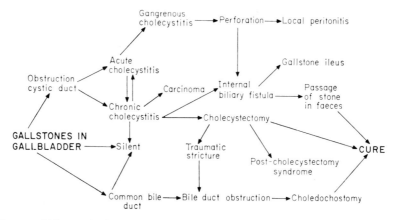

Fig. 399. The natural history of gall-stones.

neck of the gall bladder or into the common bile duct.

Migration of the stones to the neck of the gall bladder causes *obstruction of the cystic duct* resulting in chemical irritation of the gall bladder mucosa by the retained bile, and this is succeeded by bacterial invasion. According to the severity of the changes, *acute* or *chronic cholecystitis* results. Acute cholecystitis may gradually subside or progress to acute gangrene and perforation of the gall bladder or to empyema.

If it subsides spontaneously, chronic inflammatory changes persist with subsequent acute exacerbations.

Chronic cholecystitis can be silent. Usually, however, there are dyspeptic symptoms, and the patient may eventually come to cholecystectomy. This is usually curative, but may rarely lead to the *post-cholecystectomy syndrome* or the unfortunate sequel of *traumatic stricture of the bile duct.*

Internal biliary fistula follows the migration of a gall-stone from the acutely, or more usually chronically, inflamed gall bladder into an adjacent viscus. The stone may be passed in the faeces, or impact in the alimentary tract, causing *gall-stone ileus.*

Gall-stones traversing the common bile duct may pass uneventfully into the duodenum, or remain clinically silent in the duct, but usually result in partial *obstruction to the common bile duct* with intermittent obstructive jaundice. Infection behind the obstruction is common, with consequent *cholangitis,* and this may ascend to the liver, giving rise to abscesses.

'Silent' gall-stones

Gall-stones may be symptomless and diagnosed by chance from an X-ray or during an operation for some other condition. The future course of action is controversial. One school believes that the stones should be removed even if they are not causing symptoms. Follow-up studies, however, show that only a small proportion—about 15%—develop symptoms and require cholecystectomy [25] and gall-stones are a frequent incidental autopsy finding. Symptomatic gall-stones have a different prognosis. Within 11 years, about one-third will develop complications necessitating cholecystectomy [109].

Cholecystectomy should not be done unless symptoms can definitely be ascribed to gall bladder disease. If gall-stones are removed for vague indigestion, the patient's post-operative condition is likely to be worse than before. The risk of subsequent cancer of the gall bladder is small, for carcinoma is rare compared with the incidence of gall-stones and is usually preceded by symptoms of cholecystitis for many years.

MEDICAL DISSOLUTION OF GALL-STONES

CHENODEOXYCHOLIC ACID

The total bile salt pool is reduced in gall-stone patients. Attempts at expansion and at increasing bile salts in bile might therefore be of use in dissolving gall-stones. The bile salt usually given is chenodeoxycholic acid [30, 99, 100]. This lowers biliary cholesterol by reducing hepatic synthesis and biliary secretion of cholesterol [4]. Chenodeoxycholic acid becomes the predominant bile acid in bile.

Radiolucent stones (< 15 mm diameter) in a functioning gall bladder can be expected to dissolve in 60% of patients. The dose is 13–15 mg/kg body weight given as a single dose at bedtime [54, 71]. Obese subjects may need 18–20 mg/kg body weight [55].

Dyspepsia decreases rapidly on starting therapy. Small stones (< 5 mm diameter) show signs of dissolution at six months. Large stones (> 10 mm diameter) may take up to two years to disappear. Progress is assessed by an oral cholecystogram performed at six-month intervals. Pigment stones will not dissolve.

Unfortunately about 30% of patients, one year after gall-stone dissolution, will show a recurrence. Low dose, intermittent chenodeoxycholic acid therapy has been suggested for prophylaxis in these patients.

The most frequent side-effect is diarrhoea, which is dose-related. Chenodeoxycholic acid is converted by colonic bacterial action to lithocholic acid, which is potentially hepato-toxic. However, man eliminates this bile acid by efficient sulphation and conversion to ursodeoxycholic acid [88]. Hepato-toxicity has not been shown [61]. Transient rises in serum transaminases, however, are usual after starting therapy. As with other drugs, chenodeoxycholic acid should not be taken during pregnancy.

OTHER AGENTS

Ursodeoxycholic acid. This is derived from the Japanese white collared bear. It is the 7-beta epimer of chenodeoxycholic acid and reduces cholesterol saturation in bile by inhibiting hepatic HMG-CoAR. It dissolves cholesterol gall-stones [70, 103]. It has several advantages over chenodeoxycholic acid: smaller doses (10 mg/kg body weight) are required; dissolution is more rapid; diarrhoea and an increase in serum transaminases are absent. It is, however, much more expensive.

Rowachol. This mixture of essential oils lowers the cholesterol content of bile and can dissolve gall-stones, including those in the common bile duct [9, 34]. Its place in the long-term management of gall-stone disease has not yet been established.

The disadvantages of medical dissolution of gall-stones include restriction to non-calcified stones and the possible side-effects. These must be weighed against the established advantages of surgery. At the present time it should be reserved for those who will co-operate and have small, non-calcified, incapacitating gall-stones in a functioning gall bladder and in whom general health, age or associated conditions prevent cholecystectomy.

ACUTE CHOLECYSTITIS

AETIOLOGY

In 96% of patients the cystic duct is obstructed by a gall-stone (fig. 400). The imprisoned bile salts have a toxic action on the gall bladder wall. Lipids may penetrate the Rokitansky–Aschoff sinuses and exert an irritant reaction. The rise in pressure compresses blood vessels in the gall bladder wall; infarction and gangrene follow.

Pancreatic enzymes may also cause acute cholecystitis, presumably by regurgitation in the presence of obstruction of a common biliary and pancreatic channel. Such pancreatic regurgitation may account for some instances of acute

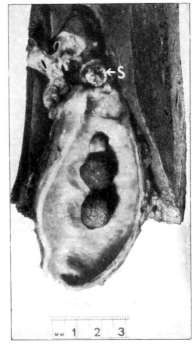

Fig. 400. Three gall-stones lie in a greatly thickened, chronically inflamed gall bladder. A further calculus (S) is lodged in the cystic duct. Scale is in cm.

cholecystitis developing in the absence of gall bladder stones.

Bacterial inflammation is an integral part of acute cholecystitis. Bacterial deconjugation of bile salts may produce toxic bile acids which can injure the mucosa.

PATHOLOGY

The gall bladder is greyish-red in colour with a lustreless surface. There are vascular adhesions to adjacent structures. The gall bladder is usually distended, but after previous inflammation the wall becomes thickened and contracted. It contains turbid fluid which may be frankly purulent (*empyema of the gall bladder*). A gall-stone may be lodged in the neck (fig. 400).

Histology shows haemorrhage and moderate oedema reaching a peak about the fourth day and diminishing by the seventh day. As the acute reaction subsides it is replaced by fibrosis.

Related lymph glands at the neck of the gall bladder and along the common bile duct are enlarged.

Bacteriology. Cultures of both gall bladder wall and bile usually show organisms of intestinal type, including anaerobes, in about three-quarters of cases. The liver is rarely culture-positive.

CLINICAL FEATURES

These vary from those of mild inflammation to fulminating gangrene of the gall bladder wall. The acute attack is often an exacerbation of underlying chronic cholecystitis.

The sufferers are often obese, female and over 40, but no type, age or sex is immune.

Pain often occurs late at night or in the early morning. It is most common in the right upper abdomen or epigastrium and is referred below the angle of the right scapula, the right shoulder, or rarely to the left side. It may simulate angina pectoris.

The pain usually rises to a plateau and can last 30–60 minutes without relief, unlike the short spasm of biliary colic [39]. Attacks may be precipitated by late-night, heavy meals or fatty foods, or even by such simple acts as abdominal palpation or yawning. The wretched, perspiring sufferer lies motionless in a curled-up posture, preferably with local heat applied to the abdomen.

Distension pain is due to the gall bladder contracting to overcome the blocked cystic duct. It is

transmitted by stimulation of splanchnic and phrenic nerve endings in the gall bladder wall [45]. This visceral pain is deep seated, central and unaccompanied by muscular rigidity and superficial or deep tenderness.

Peritoneal pain is due to irritation of the overlying parietal peritoneum which has a segmental innervation. This pain is superficial with skin tenderness, hyperaesthesia and muscular rigidity. The fundus of the gall bladder is in apposition to the diaphragmatic peritoneum, which is supplied by the phrenic and last six intercostal nerves. Stimulation of the anterior branches produces right upper quadrant pain and of the posterior cutaneous branch leads to the characteristic right infrascapular pain.

The spinal nerves extend a short distance into the mesentery and gastro-hepatic ligament around the major bile ducts, and stimulation of these nerves is interpreted as pain and referred to the back and right upper quadrant. This explains the pain of stones in the common bile duct and of cholangitis.

Digestive system. Flatulence and nausea are common, but vomiting is unusual, unless there is a stone in the common bile duct.

EXAMINATION

The patient appears ill, with shallow, jerky respirations. The temperature rises with bacterial invasion. Jaundice usually indicates associated stones in the common bile duct [107].

The abdomen moves poorly. Spread of infection to peritoneal surfaces leads to gastric and duodenal distension. Hyperaesthesia is maximal in the 8th and 9th right thoracic segments, and the right upper abdominal muscles are rigid. The gall bladder is usually impalpable; occasionally a tender mass of gall bladder and adherent omentum may be felt. Murphy's sign is positive. The liver edge is tender.

The *leucocyte count* is raised to about 10 000/mm³, with a moderate increase in polymorphs.

A plain film of the abdomen should be taken.

Intravenous or isotopic scanning is of considerable value (Chapter 5). A completely normal gall bladder rules out acute cholecystitis, whereas a well-opacified common bile duct without filling of the gall bladder is reasonable evidence of an obstructed cystic duct (see fig. 47).

Ultrasound or CT scanning may show a thickened gall bladder wall and the presence of stones (see fig. 50) [68]. Either technique may be of particular value in the acute situation.

DIFFERENTIAL DIAGNOSIS

Acute cholecystitis is liable to be confused with other conditions which may cause sudden pain and tenderness in the right hypochondrium. These include referred pain from muscular and spinal root lesions.

Below the diaphragm, acute retrocaecal appendicitis, intestinal obstruction, a perforated peptic ulcer or acute pancreatitis may be confusing.

Diaphragmatic pleurisy may be associated with tenderness in the gall bladder area and this is also characteristic of Bornholm disease. Myocardial infarction should always be considered.

PROGNOSIS

The acute fulminating disease is becoming less common because of earlier antibiotic therapy and more frequent cholecystectomies for recurrent gall bladder symptoms. Spontaneous recovery follows disimpaction of the stone in 85% of patients [36].

After the acute inflammation has subsided, the gall bladder remains shrunken, fibrotic, full of stones and non-functioning. Recurrent acute cholecystitis may follow, but there may be surprisingly long, clinically silent periods.

Rarely, acute cholecystitis proceeds rapidly to gangrene or empyema of the gall bladder, fistula formation, hepatic abscesses or even generalized peritonitis.

TREATMENT

General measures include bed rest, intravenous fluids, a light diet and relief of pain with pethidine (demerol) and buscopan. Antibiotics prevent such complications as peritonitis, cholangitis and septicaemia. If operation takes place within 24 hours of the onset, 30% of gall bladder cultures are positive. This rises to 80% after 72 hours [107]. In one series, 46.7 of 501 unselected cholecystectomy specimens showed positive bacterial cultures, usually *E. coli*, klebsiella, enterococci, clostridia or staphylococci. Where wound infection ensued, it was often with the same organism as cultured from the gall bladder [41]. Anaerobes include bacteroides and fusobacteria [38].

Choice of antibiotic [7]. In the presence of acute inflammation and biliary obstruction, antibiotics may not achieve satisfactory levels in the bile and diseased tissues. Concurrent hepatic disease affects biliary excretion and dangerous blood levels can develop.

The penicillins, cephalosporins and cefamycins achieve therapeutic biliary levels. Amino glycosides, such as gentamycin, do not reach useful biliary levels.

Erythromycin is excreted mainly in the bile, but has the wrong spectrum for most biliary infections.

Metronidazole is largely excreted in the urine, but satisfactory biliary levels are achieved. It is of value for the anaerobic infections.

The tetracyclines, ampicillin, cefotoxin, metronidazole and cotrimoxazole are satisfactory antibiotics for use in acute cholecystitis.

Surgery. With antibiotics the acute inflammation usually subsides within three days and elective cholecystectomy can be performed later. If the patient does not improve, or shows obvious deterioration, then surgery is indicated. Cholecystectomy is never a 'middle of the night' operation by an inexperienced surgeon. Facilities for operative cholangiography must be available. If performed during the first three days, cholecystectomy is the operation of choice and has a mortality of about 0.5% [51]. If operation is performed later or the patient's condition is poor or, at the time of operation, there are difficulties in anatomical definition, cholecystostomy is the procedure of choice. It has to be followed by definitive cholecystectomy later on.

About 10% of patients with acute cholecystitis will have associated common duct stones. These indicate exploration of the common duct unless inflammation around the porta hepatis renders dissection and identification of structures difficult.

Acute gangrenous cholecystitis

Acute calculous cholecystitis may proceed to complete necrosis of part of the gall bladder wall and perforation [85]. This is hastened by increased intravesical pressure due to a stone in the cystic duct with vascular obstruction and infarction of the gall bladder wall, or a gall-stone may erode the necrotic wall. Alternatively, dilated, infected, Rokitansky–Aschoff sinuses may provide a weak point for rupture.

Rupture is at the relatively avascular fundus. Adhesions form between adjacent organs with local abscess formation. Rupture into the free peritoneal cavity is unusual. Rupture into adjacent viscera leads to internal biliary fistulae.

This complication usually occurs in elderly men when symptoms may be inconspicuous and diagnosis difficult. Younger men on steroid or immuno-suppressive therapy are also affected. The illness commences as an ordinary cholecystitis but, instead of subsiding in 48 hours, the symptoms progressively increase. Localized right upper quadrant pain is constant, a tender gall bladder mass is palpable and the patient looks toxic and ill.

The temperature may be high, normal or subnormal. The leucocyte count is usually raised.

Prognosis. This is poor, with a mortality of 17% [85].

Treatment. Following massive antibiotic therapy and restoration of the fluid balance, the gangrenous gall bladder wall is removed or drained as an emergency and any abscess drained.

Acute emphysematous cholecystitis

The term is used to denote infection of the gall bladder with gas-producing organisms, *E. coli*, *Clostridium welchii* or aerobic and anaerobic streptococci. The clinical picture is that of a severe, acute cholecystitis. This may be related to obliterative vascular disease in the cystic artery and hence be important in male diabetics [72].

Radiology is diagnostic. In the plain film of the abdomen the gall bladder is seen as a sharply outlined pear-shaped gas shadow. Occasionally air may be seen infiltrating the wall and surrounding tissues. Gas is not apparent in the cystic duct which is blocked by a gall-stone. In the erect position, a fluid level is seen in the gall bladder; this is never seen with an internal biliary fistula.

Antibiotics are given in large doses. Cholecystostomy is the simplest procedure compatible with free drainage.

CHRONIC CALCULOUS CHOLECYSTITIS

This is the commonest type of clinical gall bladder disease. The association of chronic cholecystitis with stones is close—and indeed almost constant.

Aetiological factors, therefore, include all those responsible for the formation of gall-stones (page 477). The chronic inflammation may follow

acute cholecystitis, but more usually develops insidiously.

PATHOLOGY

The gall bladder is usually contracted with a thickened, sometimes calcified, wall but may be cystic. The contained bile is turbid with a sediment of debris, sometimes called biliary mud. The contained stones are seen lying loosely embedded in the wall or in meshes of an organizing fibrotic network. One stone is usually lodged in the neck (fig. 400). The mucosa is ulcerated and scarred. Histologically the mucosa is thickened and congested with lymphocytic infiltration and occasionally complete destruction of the mucosa.

CLINICAL FEATURES

Chronic cholecystitis is difficult to diagnose because of the ill-defined symptoms. A familial incidence of gall-stones, previous attacks of jaundice, multiparity and obesity form a suggestive background. Rarely, episodes of acute cholecystitis punctuate the course.

Abdominal distension or epigastric discomfort, especially after a fatty meal, may be temporarily relieved by belching. Nausea is common, but vomiting is unusual unless there are stones in the common bile duct. Apart from a constant dull ache in the right hypochondrium and epigastrium, pain may be experienced in the right scapular region substernally or at the right shoulder. Postprandial pain may be relieved by alkalis.

Local tenderness over the gall bladder and a positive Murphy sign are very suggestive of gall bladder disease.

INVESTIGATIONS

The temperature, leucocyte count, haemoglobin and erythrocyte sedimentation rate are within normal limits. A plain X-ray of the abdomen may show gall-stones. Cholecystography, cholangiography or ultrasonography may reveal gall-stones. The gall bladder is usually non-functioning. ERCP is helpful in demonstrating stones in the gall bladder and the size of the common bile duct and any stones in it.

DIFFERENTIAL DIAGNOSIS

Fat intolerance, flatulence and post-prandial discomfort are common symptoms. Even if associated with radiological evidence of gall-stones in a well-functioning gall bladder, the calculi are not necessarily responsible, for stones are frequently present in the symptom free.

Other disorders producing a similar clinical picture must be excluded before cholecystectomy is advised, otherwise symptoms persist post-operatively. These include peptic ulceration, hiatus hernia, chronic urinary tract infections and functional dyspepsias. A careful appraisal of the patient's psychological make-up is necessary.

The oral cholecystogram is only 90–95% accurate so that 5–10% of patients with normal cholecystograms have gall-stones. There is a possibility that symptomatic gall bladder disease may not only be over-diagnosed but may sometimes be unrecognized.

PROGNOSIS

This chronic disease is compatible with a good life expectancy. Acute exacerbations of cholecystitis are possible. Rarely, gall bladder cancer may develop in an organ which is the seat of chronic calculous cholecystitis.

TREATMENT

Medical measures may be tried if the diagnosis is uncertain and a period of observation is desirable. This is especially so when indefinite symptoms are associated with a well-functioning gall bladder. The general condition of the patient may contraindicate surgery. The place of medical means for dissolving radiolucent stones has already been discussed (page 482).

Obesity should be corrected. Fat intake will depend upon the functional state of the gall bladder: if it is non-functioning, a low-fat diet is advisable. Cooked fats are badly tolerated and should be avoided.

Cholecystectomy

This is indicated if calculous cholecystitis has been diagnosed and the patient's symptoms continue. It is the most commonly performed, elective, abdominal operation. The operation demands adequate assistance, exposure, illumination and the facilities for operative cholangiography.

The common bile duct should be explored if stones have been visualized either pre-operatively or by operative cholangiography. Other indica-

tions include a past history of jaundice, the aspiration of turbid bile, palpable stones, a dilated, thickened duct and the presence of multiple small stones in the gall bladder. A bile duct of small calibre should never be explored.

The T-tube is in position in the common bile duct for not longer than two days as a longer time increases morbidity [110]. Culture of the bile is done for post-operative deaths are often due to septicaemia [22].

Intravenous fluids are not usually necessary as fluids may be taken by mouth almost immediately and a light diet on the second day.

Slight and transient increases in serum bilirubin and alkaline phosphatase levels can be expected in the normal post-operative cholecystectomy course [89]. Greater increases indicate such complications as mild peritonitis or injury to the bile ducts. Pancreatitis is another post-operative complication [57].

NON-CALCULOUS CHOLECYSTITIS

Only 2–10% of acute cholecystitis develops without coincident gall-stones.

Acalculous cholecystitis may complicate bacteraemia from elsewhere. It was recorded in Vietnam with bacteraemia following extensive injury and after severe burning [66, 74].

Other causes of cholecystitis without gall-stones include clostridia (emphysematous cholecystitis with diabetes), polyarteritis, steroid treatment and trauma.

TYPHOID CHOLECYSTITIS

Circulating typhoid bacilli are filtered by the liver and excreted in the bile. The biliary tract, however, is infected in only about 0.2% of patients with typhoid fever.

Acute typhoid cholecystitis is becoming very rare. Signs of acute cholecystitis appear at the end of the second week or even during convalescence, and are sometimes followed by perforation of the gall bladder.

Chronic typhoid cholecystitis and the typhoid carrier state. The typhoid carrier passes organisms in the faeces derived from a focus of infection in the gall bladder or biliary tract. Chronic typhoid cholecystitis is symptomless and can be present without any history of an acute attack of typhoid fever. A gelatine capsule on a nylon string is a

satisfactory method of obtaining culture of duodenal specimens [43].

The carrier state is not cured by antibiotic
therapy. Cholecystectomy is successful if there is
not an associated infection of the biliary ducts.
Chronic typhoid cholecystitis is not an important
aetiological factor in the production of gall-stones.

Biliary carriers of other salmonellae have been
reported [32] and treated with ampicillin and
cholecystectomy.

ACTINOMYCOTIC CHOLECYSTITIS

Actinomycosis localized to the mucosa of the gall
bladder is excessively rare. It should be treated by
cholecystectomy.

Giardiasis can result in biliary dysfunction [49].

CHOLESTEROSIS OF THE GALL BLADDER
(STRAWBERRY GALL BLADDER)

Cholesterol esters and other lipids are deposited
in the submucosal and epithelial cells as small, yellow, lipid specks and, together with the intervening
red bile-stained mucosa, give the appearance of a
ripe strawberry (fig. 401). The deposits are at first
found only on the mucosal ridges but later they

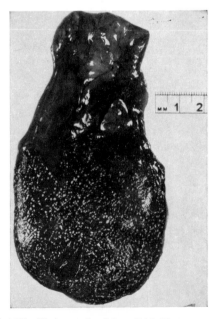

Fig. 401. Cholesterosis of the gall bladder
(strawberry gall bladder). Scale is in cm.

extend into the troughs. As more lipid is deposited,
it projects into the lumen as polyps which may
become pedunculated. The change is confined to
the gall bladder and never extends to the ducts.

The lipid is seen in reticulo-endothelial xanthoma cells of the mucosa, which is not inflamed. The cholesterosis is related to the biliary,
not blood cholesterol concentration.

There are no symptoms and the cholecystogram
shows a normally functioning organ. Occasionally
filling defects may be noted [23]. Cholesterol gall-
stones develop in about half the patients.

Post-cholecystectomy problems

Poor results after cholecystectomy can be expected
in about one-third of patients. These may be due
to wrong diagnosis. About 95% of those *with gall-
stones* are freed of symptoms or improved post-
operatively [13]. Results are thus good if stones are
present but if none is found this questions the
original diagnosis. The patients may have been
suffering from a psychosomatic or some other
disorder.

Symptoms may be related to technical difficulties at the time of surgery. These include *traumatic biliary stricture* (Chapter 30) and *residual
calculi*.

A *cystic duct remnant*, greater than 1 cm, is very
frequent after cholecystectomy [13]. It is an infrequent cause of symptoms in the absence of common duct stones [52]. These are the only patients
to benefit from removal of the cystic duct or gall
bladder remnant.

Amputation neuromas can be demonstrated in
some patients with post-cholecystectomy symptoms. However, removal offers no relief and this
seems unlikely to be the cause [13].

Fibrosis or stenosis of the sphincter of Oddi may
or may not be associated with jaundice or bile duct
stones. It is very rare and is treated by endoscopic
or surgical sphincterotomy.

Chronic pancreatitis, a common association of
choledocholithiasis, may persist post-operatively.

Post-cholecystectomy syndrome. Biliary dyskinesia may persist or even originate after cholecystectomy. These changes are responsible for the
term post-cholecystectomy syndrome. The existence of biliary dyskinesia is in some doubt partly
because it has been loosely used to cover persistent
symptoms probably unrelated to gall bladder
disease.

Cholangiography. Intravenous with tomography, endoscopic, or percutaneous, have proved of particular value in the investigation of symptoms after cholecystectomy. Residual calculi, stricture, ampullary stenosis, a cystic duct stump or normal appearance are significant findings.

Gall-stones in the common bile duct (choledocholithiasis)

The majority of stones in the common bile duct have migrated from the gall bladder and are associated with calculous cholecystitis. Secondary stones that are not of gall bladder origin usually form following partial biliary obstruction due to such changes as residual calculus, traumatic stricture or sclerosing cholangitis.

Stones are single or multiple, oval and conforming to the long axis of the duct. They tend to impact in the ampulla of Vater and may project into the duodenum.

EFFECTS OF COMMON BILE DUCT STONES

Silent stones. Rarely the common bile duct can be full of stones, but without symptoms.

Bile duct obstruction is usually partial, for the calculus exerts a ball-valve action at the lower end of the common bile duct.

Cholangitis. The stagnant bile is readily infected, probably from the intestines. The bile becomes opaque and dark brown (*biliary mud*). Rarely the infection is more acute and the bile is purulent. The common bile duct is thickened and dilated, with desquamated or ulcerated mucosa, especially in the ampulla of Vater. The cholangitis may spread to the intra-hepatic bile ducts and, in severe and prolonged infections, cholangitic abscesses are seen. The cut section of liver shows cavities containing bile-stained pus, communicating with the bile ducts. *E. coli* is the commonest infecting organism. Others include bacteroides, streptococci, lactobacilli and clostridia.

Acute or chronic pancreatitis may result from stones in the ampulla of Vater, with bile regurgitation along the pancreatic duct.

CLINICAL PICTURE

The clinical features are those of cholestatic jaundice with cholangitis.

The classical picture is of an elderly, obese woman with a previous history of flatulent indigestion, fat intolerance and mid-epigastric pain, presenting with the triad of jaundice, abdominal pain, chills and fever.

The cholestatic jaundice is usually mild, but is occasionally deep or absent. The bile duct obstruction is rarely complete and the amount of pigment fluctuates in the stools.

Pain occurs in about three-quarters of the patients. It is always severe, colicky, intermittent and needing analgesics for its relief. Sometimes it is a constant, sharp, severe, mounting pain. The site may be right upper quadrant or epigastric. It radiates to the back and to the right scapula. It is associated with vomiting. Palpation of the epigastrium is painful. *Fever* occurs in about a third of the patients, ranging from a continuous pyrexia to occasional spikes of 38–38.5°C.

Faeces usually contain stercobilinogen although in reduced amounts. *Urine* contains excessive amounts of urobilinogen and bilirubin when the patient is jaundiced. It is also infected when the patient is febrile.

The bile obtained by duodenal aspiration shows a mixed growth of intestinal organisms, predominantly *E. coli*. The bacterial overgrowth in the small intestine is confirmed by a positive bile salt 'breath' test which confirms that deconjugating bacteria are present [56].

The *serum* shows the findings of cholestatic jaundice. The serum conjugated bilirubin conjugation is raised to about 3–10 mg/100 ml.

If the stones obstruct the main pancreatic duct, the serum amylase concentration may rise sharply.

Haematological changes. The leucocyte count may be raised, with an increase in the polymorphs; the level depends on the acuteness and severity of the cholangitis. The erythrocyte sedimentation rate is raised.

Blood culture should be performed repeatedly during the febrile period and the antibiotic sensitivity of any organism determined. Although the usual organisms encountered are the intestinal ones such as *E. coli* and anaerobic streptococci, other unusual ones such as the aeromonas species must be sought [31].

X-rays of the abdomen may show calculi in the gall bladder, and more medially and posteriorly in the common bile duct. Endoscopic retrograde cholangiography may confirm the presence of stones (fig. 398).

Ultrasound may show dilated intra-hepatic ducts although more often these are undilated.

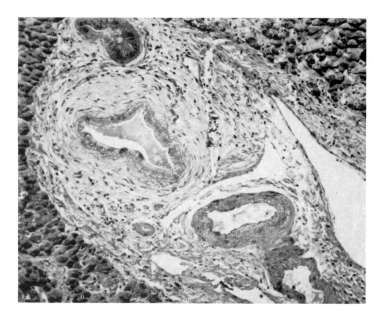

Fig. 402. Portal zone from operative liver biopsy of a patient with sclerosing cholangitis secondary to choledocholithiasis. The duct wall shows concentric fibrosis and the whole portal area is fibrosed. PAS, × 126 (Sherlock 1965).

NEEDLE LIVER BIOPSY

This is rarely necessary for diagnosis. In the anicteric, hepatic histology is normal or associated with slight lymphocytic and polymorph infiltration. In the icteric it shows cholestasis.

If there is cholangitis, an abscess containing Gram-negative organisms may be shown.

Prolonged intermittent biliary obstruction due to choledocholithiasis is a cause of biliary cirrhosis. The bile ducts show concentric scarring (fig. 402). This results in secondary sclerosing cholangitis.

DIAGNOSIS

This is not difficult if jaundice follows abdominal colic and febrile episodes. Too often, however, there is only vague indigestion, no fever, no gall bladder tenderness and an unhelpful white blood count. Alternatively, the patient may present with painless jaundice. The condition must then be differentiated from other forms of cholestasis, including neoplastic, and acute virus hepatitis (table 29). The bile in total biliary obstruction due to carcinoma is rarely infected [90].

PROGNOSIS

Mortality is 5–6%—much higher than the overall figure of 1.7% for operations performed for other non-malignant disease of the biliary tract [47].

Prognosis is good if all stones can be removed, but complications follow residual calculi. Rarely, stricture of the lower end of the common bile duct follows ulceration of the mucosa by impacted stones.

The biliary cirrhosis and cholangitis will regress if the obstruction is relieved.

MANAGEMENT OF COMMON DUCT STONES

Antibiotics are only temporarily effective in controlling the cholangitis if the bile duct remains obstructed. Other pre-operative measures include control of fluid and electrolyte balance, correction of anaemia and intramuscular vitamin K_1 if the patient is jaundiced.

In the severely ill, pre-operative biliary drainage for a few days either by the percutaneous transhepatic route (Chapter 32) or by endoscopic cannulation of the common bile duct with drainage of bile trans-nasally is useful [27, 33, 37]. Drainage is combined with intensive antibiotic therapy both systemic and directly into the bile ducts. The patient is thus brought to surgery or endoscopic sphincterotomy in a much better condition.

The common bile duct must be explored and all calculi removed. The chronically infected gall bladder should also be removed to prevent further migration of stones into the bile ducts. A transduodenal sphincterotomy may or may not be in-

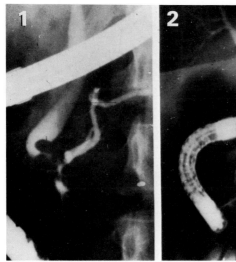
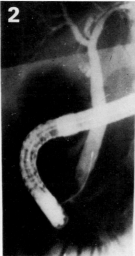
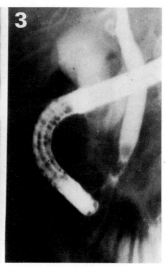

Fig. 403. Endoscopic sphincterotomy. Endoscopic retrograde cholangiography shows (1) a residual gall-stone at the lower end of the common bile duct, (2) the electrocautery is in position at the lower end of the common bile duct, (3) post-sphincterotomy the stone has passed and air bubbles are seen in the common bile duct.

cluded. The bile duct is drained with a T tube of adequate size (no. 16 French).

The operative recognition of stones in the bile duct is difficult. Percutaneous and endoscopic cholangiography are valuable pre-operative procedures. Stones can be missed by simple palpation, but probing with bougies is uncertain and carries the risk of causing a false passage to the duodenum. Stenosis of the sphincter of Oddi may result. If stones are present at the lower end of the common bile duct, the duodenum should be opened and the papilla examined from below.

Direct cholangiography should be performed routinely at the time of operation and again post-operatively before removal of the tube draining the common duct.

Residual bile duct calculi

Approximately 15% of patients operated upon for gall-stones will have stones in the bile duct [46]. More than 1% of those having a cholecystectomy will have a retained common bile duct stone during the immediate post-operative period. Such stones usually result from failure to perform operative cholangiography. Calculi in the hepatic ducts are especially liable to be overlooked.

Residual bile duct calculi may be suspected if the patient experiences pain when a T tube drain-

ing the bile duct is temporarily clamped. Cholangiography reveals filling defects (fig. 403). Sepsis and cholangitis occur post-operatively.

TREATMENT

Small stones, less than 0.5 cm in diameter, will probably pass into the duodenum spontaneously. If a T tube is *in situ*, the stones can be removed through it [24]. Under TV monitoring a controllable catheter is manipulated into the bile duct. A Dormia basket is advanced through it into the common bile duct and the stone extracted (fig. 404). Sometimes the stone can be pushed through the papilla to the duodenum.

Choledochoscopy with direct visualization may be useful [12].

Complications include perforation of the sinus tract and bile duct and fever [19].

Stones may also be dissolved by the instillation of agents into the biliary system via the T tube. Sodium cholate was first employed [108], but this caused diarrhoea; then heparin was used [21]. The most recent is mono-octanoin, a commercial emulsifying agent [102]. This is given for 3–25 days continuously using a battery-operated portable pump. It can also be perfused directly into the common bile duct by trans-nasal catheterization, usually after endoscopic sphincterotomy [19, 27].

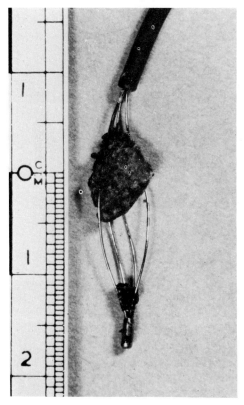

Fig. 404. Dormia basket containing a gall-stone which has been extracted from the common bile duct via a T tube.

Endoscopic sphincterotomy [24, 26, 87, 113]

Following fibroptic endoscopic cannulation of the common bile duct a sphincterotomy of the ampulla of Vater may be performed. This is done with a wire snare and a high frequency diaphragm current (fig. 405). It is performed under fluoroscopic control and with diazepam sedation. The technique is 90% successful in removing common duct stones. The valve-like function of the ampulla is, however, destroyed, allowing reflux of air and duodenal contents into the biliary system (fig. 403). The pressure in the common bile duct falls [42]. Small stones pass spontaneously; larger stones can be removed by a Dormia basket or a catheter loop [112].

Complications include haemorrhage, acute pancreatitis, cholangitis and duodenal perforation. The complication rate is about 10% and the mortality 2%. The procedure is cost effective and only two to three days of hospitalization are necessary.

Endoscopic sphincterotomy should be offered to patients presenting with common bile duct stones after cholecystectomy, particularly if elderly and frail. Emergency sphincterotomy must be considered in patients who have gall bladders *in situ* but have common bile duct stones complicated by severe cholangitis, septicaemia or biliary pancreatitis. Surgical operation may be safer in the average young fit patient with retained stones, but this is not yet established. A patient may prefer the simpler procedure. No significant adverse effects have yet been revealed in follow-up studies. However, the possibility of long-term complications dictates the need for caution in offering this procedure to young patients who are fit for re-operation [26].

Cholangitis

This is usually associated with partial biliary obstruction due to choledocholithiasis, biliary stricture, sclerosing cholangitis and, rarely, neoplastic biliary obstruction [14].

Malaise and fever are followed by shivering and sweating (*Charcot's intermittent biliary fever*). Malaise, fever, pain, vomiting and pruritus increase with the jaundice. In those previously anicteric the urine darkens and the stools may become pale. The syndrome is due to oedema of the bile duct mucous membrane, so that partial biliary obstruction becomes complete. There is septicaemia with a positive blood culture for *E. coli* and other intestinal organisms. As the oedema subsides so the partial biliary obstruction is relieved and the temperature falls. Associated renal failure may be related to endotoxins.

Multiple abscesses may develop in the liver (Chapter 27).

ACUTE OBSTRUCTIVE CHOLANGITIS

This is the most severe form of cholangitis. In addition to the classical symptoms of cholangitis the patient is lethargic, prostrated and shocked. Purulent material accumulates under increasing pressure in the biliary tract. A Gram-negative septicaemia is associated with endotoxic shock.

Treatment. Emergency decompression of the common bile duct is mandatory even in the apparently moribund [48]. This can be transhepatic, endoscopic or surgical.

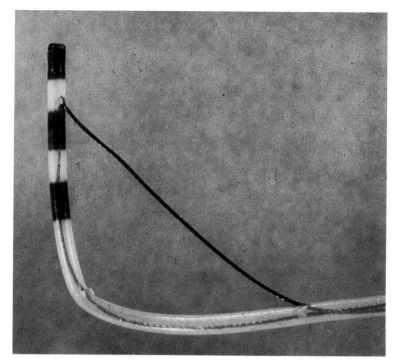

Fig. 405. Catheter and electrocautery used for endoscopic sphincterotomy.

Intra-hepatic gall-stones

Stones in the intra-hepatic ducts are particularly common in certain parts of the world such as the Far East and Brazil [75] where they are associated with parasitic infestation [67]. Gall-stones form in chronically obstructed bile ducts due to such conditions as traumatic biliary stricture, primary sclerosing cholangitis, or Caroli's disease (see fig. 66). They are usually of pigment type and are associated with stones in the common bile duct. Secondary hepatic infection results in multiple abscesses.

Intra-hepatic calculi are difficult to treat and recurrence is frequent. Lavage of the duct is often performed after T tube drainage of the common bile duct. In some instances choledocho-intestinal anastomosis or even hepatic lobectomy may be necessary [92].

Biliary fistulae

EXTERNAL

These follow procedures such as cholecystostomy, trans-hepatic biliary drainage or T tube choledo-chotomy. Very rarely they follow gall-stones, carcinoma of the gall bladder or trauma.

Bile has a higher sodium and bicarbonate content than plasma. Patients with external biliary fistulae run a risk of severe hyponatraemic acidosis and rise in blood urea levels [60].

INTERNAL

These may follow cholecysto-enterostomy. In 80% they are due to longstanding calculous cholecystitis. The inflamed gall bladder, containing stones, adheres and ruptures into a segment of the intestine, usually into the duodenum and less often the colon. The ejected gall-stones may be passed or cause intestinal obstruction (*gall-stone ileus*), usually in the terminal ileum.

Post-operative biliary strictures, especially after multiple efforts at repair, may be complicated by fistula formation, usually hepatico-duodenal or hepatico-gastric. The fistulae are short, narrow and liable to block.

Biliary fistulae may also follow rupture of a chronic duodenal ulcer into the gall bladder or common bile duct. Fistulae may also develop between the colon and biliary tract in ulcerative colitis or regional ileitis, especially if the patient is receiving corticosteroid therapy [29].

Rarely, in a patient with duct stones, a fistula can develop between the hepatic duct and portal vein with massive bilaemia, shock and death [5].

Clinical features. There is a long history of biliary disease. The fistula may be symptomless and, when the gall-stones have discharged into the intestine successfully, the fistula closes. Such instances are often diagnosed only at the time of a later cholecystectomy.

About one-third give a history of jaundice or are jaundiced on admission [86]. Pain may be absent or as severe as biliary colic. The features of cholangitis may be present. In cholecysto-colic fistula the common bile duct may be filled with calculi, putrefying matter and faeces, which cause the severe cholangitis. Bacteria deconjugate in the colon producing severe diarrhoea. Weight loss is profound.

Radiological features [83] include gas in the biliary tract (see fig. 59) and the presence of a gall-stone in an unusual position. A barium meal, in the case of a cholecystoduodenal, or a barium enema, in the case of a cholecysto-colic fistula may fill the biliary tree. Small bowel distension may be noted.

ERCP may be diagnostic [53].

TREATMENT

Fistulae due to gall bladder disease must be treated surgically. Adherent viscera are separated and closed and cholecystectomy and drainage of the common bile duct performed. The operative mortality is high being about 13% [86].

Gall-stone ileus

If a gall-stone over 2.5 cm in diameter enters the intestine it causes obstruction, usually of the ileum, less often of the duodeno-jejunal junction, duodenal bulb, pylorus or even colon. The impacted gall-stone may excite an inflammatory reaction in the intestinal wall, or cause intussusception.

Gall-stone ileus is very rare. The patient is usually an elderly, afebrile female possibly with a preceding history suggestive of chronic cholecystitis. The onset is insidious, with nausea, occasional vomiting, colicky abdominal pain and a somewhat distended but flaccid abdomen. Finally, a complete intestinal obstruction leads to rapid physical deterioration.

A plain film of the abdomen (fig. 406) may reveal loops of distended bowel with fluid levels and possibly the obstructing stone. Gas may be seen in the biliary tract and gall bladder [6], indicating a biliary fistula. Leucocytosis is not usual unless there is associated cholangitis with pyrexia.

The prognosis is poor. An accurate pre-operative diagnosis is unusual.

Treatment should be surgical after the patient's general condition has been restored by fluids and electrolytes. Exploration should be thorough, for more than one gall-stone may be present. Reported mortality is about 26.1%. Occasionally

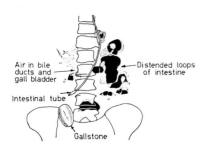

Air in bile ducts and gall bladder

Distended loops of intestine

Intestinal tube

Gallstone

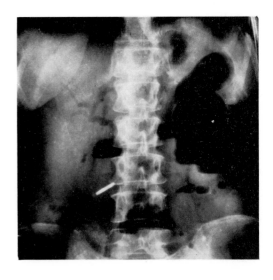

Fig. 406. Plain X-ray of the abdomen shows air in the biliary tree indicating a cholecyst-enteric fistula, a radio-opaque gall-stone just medial and to the right of the 5th lumbar vertebra and distended loops of small intestine indicating ileus.

the gall-stone passes spontaneously. Later elective cholecystectomy is essential.

Haemobilia [63]

Haemorrhage into the biliary tract may follow trauma, including surgical and needle liver biopsy, aneurysms of the hepatic artery or one of its branches, extra- or intra-hepatic tumours of the biliary tract, gall-stone disease, inflammation of the liver, especially helminthic or pyogenic, rarely varicose veins related to portal hypertension and sometimes in association with primary liver cancer.

Clinical features are pain related to the passage of clots, jaundice and haematemesis and melaena. Minor degrees may be shown only by positive occult blood tests in faeces. Fever or a palpable mass each occur in about 40% of patients.

Diagnosis is suspected whenever upper gastro-intestinal bleeding is associated with biliary colic, jaundice or a right upper quadrant mass or tenderness. Blood clot casts of the bile ducts found in gastric or duodenal aspirate, vomit or faeces are diagnostic. Angiography is useful for confirmation and anatomic definition of haemobilia. Excretory cholangiography of the bile ducts may also be helpful. ERCP or percutaneous cholangiography may show the clot in the ducts.

Treatment consists of exploring and draining the duct if the pain, bleeding and colic do not subside spontaneously.

Biliary peritonitis

AETIOLOGY

Post-cholecystectomy. Bile may leak from small bile channels between the gall bladder and liver or through an imperfectly ligated cystic duct. If the biliary pressure is raised, perhaps by a residual common duct stone, leakage is facilitated and the subsequent paraductal bile accumulation favours the development of stricture.

Rupture of the gall bladder. Empyema or gangrene of the gall bladder may lead to rupture and the formation of an abscess; this is localized by previous inflammatory adhesions.

Trauma. Crushing or gunshot wounds may involve the biliary tree. Needle biopsy of the liver or percutaneous cholangiography may rarely be complicated by puncture of the gall bladder or of a dilated intra-hepatic bile duct in a patient with

deep cholestasis. Oozing of bile rarely follows operative liver biopsy.

Spontaneous. Biliary peritonitis may develop in patients with prolonged, deep obstructive jaundice without demonstrable breach of the biliary tree. This is presumably due to bursting of minute bile ducts. It may also develop in infancy [64].

CLINICAL PICTURE

This depends on whether the bile is localized or free in the peritoneal cavity, sterile or infected. Free rupture of bile into the peritoneal cavity causes severe shock. Due to the irritant effect of bile salts, large quantities of plasma are poured into the ascitic fluid. The onset is with excruciating, generalized, abdominal pain. Examination shows a shocked, pale, motionless patient, with low blood pressure and persistent tachycardia. There is board-like rigidity of the diffusely tender abdomen. Paralytic ileus is a frequent complication. Biliary peritonitis should always be considered in any patient with unexplained intestinal obstruction. In a matter of hours secondary infection follows and the temperature rises while abdominal pain and tenderness persist. Anaerobic infection is common and increases the shock.

Laboratory findings are non-contributory. There may be haemoconcentration. Abdominal paracentesis reveals bile, usually infected. Serum bilirubin rises and this is followed by increase in alkaline phosphatase levels.

Prognosis is poor with a mortality of 60%.

TREATMENT

Fluid replacement is imperative. Paralytic ileus may demand intestinal intubation. Antibiotics are given to prevent secondary infection and the peritoneal cavity is drained.

The association of gall-stones with other diseases

PANCREATITIS

Three-quarters of females and one-third of males with chronic pancreatitis also have gall-stones.

Gall-stones and chronic cholecystitis may present as acute pancreatitis.

Small gall-stones in the ampulla allow bile to regurgitate into the pancreas and produce acute haemorrhagic pancreatitis [58]. Atrophy of the pancreas, with interstitial fibrosis, follows blockage of the main pancreatic duct by a gall-stone. Analysis of the faeces after an attack of acute pancreatitis associated with gall-stones shows small stones which have migrated and obstructed the pancreatic duct [1].

DIABETES MELLITUS

30.2% of all diabetics over 20 years old have gall-stones, compared with 11.6% of the general population of the same age. The older diabetic tends to be obese, an important factor in gall-stone formation. Chronic pancreatitis and gall-stones are associated and chronic pancreatitis can produce mild diabetes.

Patients with diabetes may have large, poorly contracting and poorly filling gall bladders. A 'diabetic neurogenic gall bladder' syndrome has been postulated [44].

REFERENCES

1. ACOSTA J.M. & LEDESMA C.L. (1974) Gallstone migration as a cause of acute pancreatitis. *New Engl. J. Med.* **290**, 484.
2. ADMIRAND W.H. & SMALL D.M. (1968) The physiochemical basis of cholesterol gallstone formation in man. *J. clin. Invest.* **47**, 1043.
3. ALMOND H.R., VLAHCEVIC Z.R., BELL C.C. Jr *et al* (1973) Effect of cholecystectomy on bile acid metabolism. *New Engl. J. Med.* **289**, 1213.
4. ANDERSON J.M. (1979) Chenodeoxycholic acid desaturated bile—but how? *Gastroenterology* **77**, 1146.
5. ANTEBI E., ADAR R., ZWEIG A. *et al* (1973) Bilemia: and unusual complication of bile duct stones. *Ann. Surg.* **177**, 274.
6. BALTHAZAR E.J. & SCHECHTER L.S. (1978) Air in gall bladder: a frequent finding in gall-stone ileus. *Am. J. Roentgenol.* **131**, 219.
7. BARRETT S.P. & WATT P.J. (1979) Antibiotics and the liver. *J. antimicrob. Chemother.* **5**, 337.
8. BEEN J.M., BILLS P.M. & LEWIS D. (1979) Microstructure of gall-stones. *Gastroenterology* **76**, 548.
9. BELL G.D. & DORAN J. (1979) Gall-stone dissolution in man using an essential oil preparation. *Br. med. J.* i, 24.
10. BENNION L.J. & GRUNDY S.M. (1978) Risk factors for the development of cholelithiasis in man. *New Engl. J. Med.* **299**, 1161.
11. BENNION L.J., GINSBERG R.L., GARNICK M.B. *et al* (1976) Effects of oral contraceptives on the gall bladder bile of normal women. *New Engl. J. Med.* **294**, 189.
12. BIRKETT D.H. & WILLIAMS L.F. (1980) Choledochoscopic removal of retained stones via a T-tube tract. *Am. J. Surg.* **139**, 531.
13. BODVALL B. (1973) The postcholecystectomy syndromes. *Clin. Gastroenterol.* **2**, 102.
14. BOEY J.H. & WAY L.W. (1980) Acute cholangitis. *Ann. Surg.* **191**, 264.
15. BOSTON COLLABORATIVE DRUG SURVEILLANCE PROGRAM (1973) Oral contraceptives and venous thromboembolic disease; surgically confirmed gall-bladder disease and breast tumours. *Lancet* i, 1399.
16. BOSTON COLLABORATIVE DRUG SURVEILLANCE PROGRAM (1974) Gallbladder disease, venous disorders, breast tumours: relation to estrogens. *New Engl. J. Med.* **290**, 15.
17. BOUCHIER I.A.D. (1969) Postmortem study of the frequency of gallstones in patients with cirrhosis of the liver. *Gut* **10**, 705.
18. BRAVERMAN D.Z., JOHNSON M.L. & KERN F. Jr (1980) Effects of pregnancy and contraceptive steroids on gall bladder function. *New Engl. J. Med.* **302**, 362.
19. BURHENNE H.J. (1980) Percutaneous extraction of retained biliary tract stones: 661 patients. *Am. J. Roentgenol.* **134**, 889.
20. CAREY M.C. & SMALL D.M. (1978) The physical chemistry of cholesterol solubility in bile: relationship to gallstone formation in dissolution in man. *J. clin. Invest.* **61**, 998.
21. CHARY S. (1977) Dissolution of retained bile duct stones using heparin. *Br. J. Surg.* **64**, 347.
22. CHETLIN S.H. & ELLIOTT D.W. (1971) Biliary bacteremia. *Arch. Surg.* **102**, 303.
23. CIMMINO C.V. (1960) Cholesterolosis. *Radiology* **74**, 432.
24. CLASSEN M. OSSENBERG F.W. (1977) Non-surgical removal of common bile duct stones. *Gut* **18**, 760.
25. COMFORT M.W., GRAY H.K. & WILSON J.M. (1948) The silent gall-stone: a ten to twenty year follow-up study of 112 cases. *Ann. Surg.* **128**, 931.
26. COTTON P.B. (1980) Non-operative removal of bile duct stones by duodenoscopic sphincterotomy. *Br. J. Surg.* **67**, 1.
27. COTTON P.B., BURNEY P.G.J. & MASON R.R. (1979) Transnasal bile duct catheterisation after endoscopic sphincterotomy: method for biliary drainage, perfusion and sequential cholangiography. *Gut* **20**, 285.
28. COYNE M.J., BONORRIS G.G., GOLDSTEIN L.I. *et al* (1976) Effect of chenodeoxycholic acid and phenobarbital on the rate-limiting enzymes of hepatic cholesterol and bile acid synthesis in patients with gall-stones. *J. lab. clin. Med.* **87**, 281.
29. CRAIG O. (1965) Hepato-colic fistula. *Br. J. Radiol.* **38**, 801.
30. DANZINGER R.G., HOFMANN A.F., THISTLE J.L. *et al* (1973) Effect of oral chenodeoxycholic acid on bile acid kinetics and biliary lipid composition in women with cholelithiasis. *J. clin. Invest.* **52**, 2809.
31. DE FRONZO R.A., MURRAY G.F. & MADDREY W.C. (1973) Aeromonas septicemia from hepatobiliary disease. *Dig. Dis.* **18**, 323.
32. DINBAR A., ALTMANN G. & TULCINSKY D.B. (1969) The treatment of chronic biliary salmonella carriers. *Am. J. Med.* **47**, 236.
33. DOOLEY J.S., DICK R., OLNEY J. *et al* (1979) Non-surgical treatment of biliary obstruction. *Lancet* ii, 1040.
34. DORAN M., KEIGHLEY R.B. & BELL G.D. (1979) Rowachol—a possible treatment for cholesterol gall-stones. *Gut* **20**, 312.

35. DOWLING R.H. (1972) The enterohepatic circulation. *Gastroenterology* **62**, 122.
36. DuPLESSIS D.J. & JERSKY J. (1973) The management of acute cholecystitis. *Surg. Clin. N. Am.* **53**, 1071.
37. FERRUCCI J.T. Jr, MUELLER P.R. & HARBIN W.P. (1980) Percutaneous transhepatic biliary drainage. *Radiology* **135**, 1.
38. FINEGOLD S.M. (1979) Anaerobes in biliary tract infection. *Arch. intern. Med.* **139**, 1338.
39. FRENCH E.B. & ROBB W.A.T. (1963) Biliary and renal colic. *Br. med. J.* ii, 135.
40. FRIEDMAN G.D., KANNEL W.B. & DAWBER T.R. (1966) The epidemiology of gallbladder disease: observations in the Framingham study. *J. chron. Dis.* **19**, 273.
41. FUKUNAGA F.H. (1973) Gallbladder bacteriology, histology and gallstones. *Arch. Surg.* **106**, 169.
42. FUNCH-JENSEN P., CSENDES A., KRUSE A. *et al* (1979) Common bile duct and Oddi sphincter pressure before and after endoscopic papillotomy in patients with common bile duct stones. *Ann. Surg.* **190**, 176.
43. GILMAN R.H., ISLAM S., RABBANI H. *et al* (1979) Identification of gall bladder typhoid carriers by a string device. *Lancet* i, 795.
44. GITELSON S., SCHWARTZ A., FRAENKEL M. *et al* (1963) Gall-bladder dysfunction in diabetes mellitus. The diabetic neurogenic gall bladder. *Diabetes* **12**, 308.
45. GLENN F. (1966) Pain in biliary tract disease. *Surg. Gynecol. Obstet.* **122**, 495.
46. GLENN F. (1974) Retained calculi within the biliary ductal system. *Ann. Surg.* **179**, 528.
47. GLENN F. & BEIL A.R. Jr (1964) Choledocholithiasis demonstrated at 586 operations. *Surg. Gynecol. Obstet.* **118**, 499.
48. GLENN F. & MOODY F.G. (1961) Acute obstructive suppurative cholangitis. *Surg. Gynecol. Obstet.* **113**, 265.
49. GOLDSTEIN F., THORNTON J.J. & SZYDLOWSKI T. (1978) Biliary tract dysfunction in giardiasis. *Am. J. dig. Dis.* **23**, 559.
50. HAY H.R.C. (1966) Gas in gall stones: a rare radiological sign in the acute abdomen. *Gut* **7**, 387.
51. HINCHEY E.J., ELIAS G.L. & HAMPSON L.G. (1965) Acute cholecystitis. *Surg. Gynecol. Obstet.* **120**, 475.
52. HOPKINS S.F., BIVINS B.A. & GRIFFEN W.O. Jr (1979) The problem of the cystic duct remnant. *Surg. Gynecol. Obstet.* **148**, 531.
53. HUNT D.R. & BLUMGART L.H. (1980) Iatrogenic choledochoduodenal fistula: an unsuspected cause of post-cholecystectomy symptoms. *Br. J. Surg.* **67**, 10.
54. ISER J.H., DOWLING R.H., MOK H.Y.I. *et al* (1975) Chenodeoxycholic acid treatment of gall-stones: a follow-up report and analysis of factors influencing response to therapy. *New Engl. J. Med.* **293**, 378.
55. ISER J.H., MATON P.N., MURPHY G.M. *et al* (1978) Resistance to chenodeoxycholic acid (CDCA) treatment in obese patients with gall-stones. *Br. med. J.* i, 1509.
56. JAMES O.F.W., AGNEW J.E. & BOUCHIER I.A.D.

(1973) Assessment of the ^{14}C-glycocholic acid breath test. *Br. med. J.* ii, 191.
57. KEIGHLEY M.R.B. & GRAHAM N.G. (1973) The aetiology and prevention of pancreatitis following biliary-tract operations. *Br. J. Surg.* **60**, 149.
58. KELLY T.R. (1976) Gallstone pancreatitis: pathophysiology. *Surgery* **80**, 488.
59. KIRTLEY J.A. Jr & HOLCOMB G.W. Jr (1966) Surgical management of diseases of the gallbladder and common duct in children and adolescents. *Am. J. Surg.* **111**, 39.
60. KNOCHEL J.P., COOPER E.B. & BARRY K.G. (1962) External biliary fistula: a study of electrolyte derangements and secondary cardiovascular and renal abnormalities. *Surgery* **51**, 746.
61. KOCH M.M., GIAMPIERI M.P., LORENZINI I. *et al* (1980) Effect of chenodeoxycholic acid on liver structure and function in man: a stereological and biochemical study. *Digestion* **20**, 8.
62. LAMORTE W.W., SCHOETZ D.J. Jr, BIRKETT D.H. *et al* (1979) The role of the gall bladder in the pathogenesis of cholesterol gall stones. *Gastroenterology* **77**, 580.
63. LARMI T.K.I. (1966) Hemobilia associated with cholecystitis, postcholecystectomy conditions and trauma: review of 12 cases. *Ann. Surg.* **163**, 373.
64. LEES W. & MITCHELL J.E. (1966) Bile peritonitis in infancy. *Arch. Dis. Childh.* **41**, 188.
65. LEVITT R.E. & OSTROW J.D. (1980) Hemolytic jaundice and gallstones. *Gastroenterology* **78**, 821.
66. LINDBERG E.T., GRINNANG L.B. & SMITH Z. (1970) Acalculous cholecystitis in Vietnam casualties. *Ann. Surg.* **171**, 152.
67. MAKI T., SATO T., YAMAGUCHI I. *et al* (1964) Treatment of intrahepatic gallstones. *Arch. Surg.* **88**, 260.
68. MARCHAL G.J.F., CASAER M., BAERT A.L. *et al* (1979) Gall bladder wall sonolucency in acute cholecystitis. *Radiology* **133**, 429.
69. MASUDA H. & NAKAYAMA F. (1979) Composition of bile pigment in gallstones and bile and their etiological significance. *J. lab. clin. Med.* **93**, 353.
70. MATON P.N., MURPHY G.M. & DOWLING R.H. (1977) Ursodeoxycholic acid treatment of gall-stones. *Lancet* ii, 1297.
71. MAUDGAL D.P., BIRD R. & NORTHFIELD T.C. (1979) Optimal timing of doses of chenic acid in patients with gall stones. *Br. med. J.* i, 922.
72. MAY R.E. & STRONG R. (1971) Acute emphysematous cholecystitis. *Br. J. Surg.* **58**, 453.
73. MOK H.Y.I., BELL G.D. & DOWLING R.H. (1974) Effect of different doses of chenodeoxycholic acid on bile-lipid composition and on frequency of side-effects in patients with gallstones. *Lancet* ii, 253.
74. MUNSTER A.M., GOODWIN M.N. & PRUITT B.A. (1971) Acalculous cholecystitis in burned patients. *Am. J. Surg.* **122**, 591.
75. NAGASE M., HIKASA Y., SOLOWAY R.D. *et al* (1980) Gallstones in western Japan: factors affecting the prevalence of intrahepatic gallstones. *Gastroenterology* **78**, 684.
76. NAKAYAMA F. (1968) Quantitative microanalysis of gallstones. *J. lab. clin. Med.* **72**, 602.
77. NICHOLAS P., RINAUDO P.A. & CONN H.O. (1972)

Increased incidence of cholelithiasis in Laennec's cirrhosis. A postmortem evaluation of pathogenesis. *Gastroenterology* **63**, 112.

78. NIELSEN M.L. & JUSTESEN T. (1977) Excretion of metronidazole in human bile. *Scand. J. Gastroenterol.* **12**, 1003.

79. NORTHFIELD T.C. & HOFMANN A.F. (1975) Biliary lipid output during three weeks and an overnight fast. I. Relationship to bile acid pool size and cholesterol saturation of bile in gallstone and control subjects. *Gut* **16**, 1.

80. OSNES M., GRØNSETH K., LARSEN S. *et al* (1978) Comparison of endoscopic retrograde and intravenous cholangiography in diagnosis of biliary calculi. *Lancet* ii, 230.

81. PERSEMLIDIS D., PANVELIWALLA D. & KIMBALL A. (1973) Effects of clofibrate and of oral contraceptives on biliary lipid composition and bile acid kinetics in man. *Gastroenterology* **64**, 782.

82. POMARE E.W. & HEATON K.W. (1973) Bile salt metabolism in patients with gallstones in functioning gallbladders. *Gut* **14**, 885.

83. ROMINGER C.J. & CANINO C.W. (1963) Internal biliary tract fistulae. *Am. J. Roentgenol.* **90**, 835.

84. ROMINGER C.J. & LOCKWOOD D.W. (1963) Floating gallbladder calculi. Their incidence in a review of one thousand cholecystograms. *Am. J. Surg.* **106**, 89.

85. ROSLYN J. & BUSUTTIL R.W. (1979) Perforation of the gall bladder: a frequently mismanaged condition. *Am. J. Surg.* **137**, 307.

86. SAFAIE-SHIRAZI S., ZIKE W.L. & PRINTEN K.J. (1973) Spontaneous enterobiliary fistulas. *Surg. Gynecol. Obstet.* **137**, 769.

87. SAFRANY L. (1977) Duodenoscopic sphincterotomy and gallstone removal. *Gastroenterology* **72**, 338.

88. SALEN G., TINT G.S., ELIAV B. *et al* (1974) Increased formation of ursodeoxycholic acid in patients with chenodeoxycholic acid. *J. clin. Invest.* **53**, 612.

89. SCHMIDT F.R. & MCCARTHY J.D. (1972) Variations in total serum bilirubin and alkaline phosphatase in the normal post-operative cholecystectomy course. *Am. J. Surg.* **124**, 794.

90. SCOTT A.J. & KHAN G.A. (1967) Origin of bacteria in bile duct bile. *Lancet* ii, 790.

91. SHAFFER E. & SMALL D.M. (1977) Biliary lipid secretion in cholesterol gallstone disease. *J. clin. Invest.* **59**, 828.

92. SIMI M., LORIGA P., BASOLI A. *et al* (1979) Intrahepatic lithiasis. Study of thirty-six cases and review of the literature. *Am. J. Surg.* **137**, 317.

93. SMALL D.M. (1980) Cholesterol nucleation and growth in gallstone formation. *New Engl. J. Med.* **302**, 1305.

94. SMALL D.M. & RAPO S. (1970) Source of abnormal bile in patients with cholesterol gallstones. *New Engl. J. Med.* **283**, 53.

95. SOLOWAY R.D., TROTMAN B.W. & OSTROW J.D. (1977) Pigment gallstones. *Gastroenterology* **72**, 167.

96. STURDEVANT R.A.L., PEARCE M.L. & DAYTON S. (1973) Increased prevalence of cholelithiasis in men ingesting a serum-cholesterol lowering diet. *New Engl. J. Med.* **288**, 24.

97. SUMMERFIELD J.A., ELIAS E. & HUNGERFORD G.D. *et al* (1976) The biliary system in primary biliary cirrhosis. *Gastroenterology* **70**, 240.

98. SUTOR D.J. & WOOLEY S.E. (1971) A statistical survey of the composition of gallstones in eight countries. *Gut* **12**, 55.

99. THISTLE J.L. & HOFMANN A.F. (1973) Efficacy and specificity of chenodeoxycholic acid therapy for dissolving gallstones. *New Engl. J. Med.* **289**, 655.

100. THISTLE J.L., HOFMANN A.F., OTT B.J. *et al* (1978) Chemotherapy for gall stone dissolution. I. Efficacy and safety. *J. Am. med. Assoc.* **239**, 1041.

101. THISTLE J.L. & SCHOENFIELD L.J. (1971) Induced alterations in composition of bile in patients having cholelithiasis. *Gastroenterology* **61**, 488.

102. THISTLE J.L., CARLSON G.L., HOFMANN A.F. *et al* (1980) Monooctanoin, a dissolution agent for retained cholesterol bile duct stones: physical properties and clinical application. *Gastroenterology* **78**, 1016.

103. TOKYO COOPERATIVE GALLSTONE STUDY GROUP (1980) Efficacy and indications of ursodeoxycholic acid treatment for dissolving gallstones: a multicenter double-blind trial. *Gastroenterology* **78**, 542.

104. VLAHCEVIC Z.R., BELL C.C. Jr, BUHAC I. *et al* (1970) Diminished bile acid pool size in patients with gallstones. *Gastroenterology* **59**, 165.

105. VLAHCEVIC Z.R., BELL C.C. Jr, GREGORY D.H. *et al* (1972). Relationship of bile acid pool size to the formation of lithogenic bile in female Indians of the southwest. *Gastroenterology* **62**, 73.

106. VLAHCEVIC Z.R., YOSHIDA T., JUTTIJUDATA P. *et al* (1973) Bile acid metabolism in cirrhosis. III. Biliary lipid secretion in patients with cirrhosis and its relevance to gallstone formation. *Gastroenterology* **64**, 298.

107. WATKIN D.F.L. & THOMAS G.C. (1971) Jaundice in acute cholecystitis. *Br. J. Surg.* **58**, 570.

108. WAY L.W., ADMIRAND W.H. & DUNPHY J.E. (1972) Management of choledocholithiasis. *Ann. Surg.* **176**, 347.

109. WENCKERT A. & ROBERTSON B. (1966) The natural course of gallstone disease. Eleven-year review of 781 nonoperated cases. *Gastroenterology* **50**, 376.

110. WILLIAMS C.B., HALPIN D.S. & KNOX A.J.S. (1972) Drainage following cholecystectomy. *Br. J. Surg.* **59**, 293.

111. WILSON I.D., DELANEY J.P., DUANE W.C. *et al* (1978) Choledocholithiasis. *Gastroenterology* **75**, 120.

112. WITZEL L., WOLBERGS E. & HALTER F. (1978) Removal of gallstones by a catheter loop after duodenoscopic sphincterotomy. *Lancet* ii, 296.

113. ZIMMON D.S., FALKENSTEIN D.B. & KESSLER R.E. (1975) Endoscopic papillotomy for choledocholithiasis. *New Engl. J. Med.* **293**, 1181.

Chapter 30
Benign Stricture of the Bile Ducts

Benign strictures of the common bile duct in 97% of cases follow biliary tract surgery, usually cholecystectomy. Various factors contribute. Oedema or haemorrhage surrounding the inflamed gall bladder, especially if contracted, makes the bile ducts difficult to distinguish from adjacent structures, and this may be heightened by aberrant anatomical relations. The bile ducts may thus be ligated, sectioned or perforated by suture material. Prolonged T tube drainage of the common bile duct, cholecystotomy, rough probing of the bile duct for calculi and attempts at operative cholangiography, especially with a normal sized duct, have resulted in stricture formation. A calculus in the common bile duct is an insufficient cause. Bile leakage after biliary operations may form periductal abscesses with constriction of the adjoining duct.

Excision of a choledochus cyst or a benign tumour of the bile ducts can be so difficult that stricture formation is inevitable.

A benign stricture can follow trauma, a perforated or penetrating duodenal ulcer, chronic sclerosing pancreatitis, benign bile duct tumours and primary sclerosing cholangitis (Chapter 14).

Anomalies of the right hepatic duct or cystic duct increase the risk of major bile duct injury.

PATHOLOGICAL CHANGES

The duct is usually partially injured, the occlusion develops slowly and a chronic obliterative cholangitis leads to a stricture about 2 cm long. The stricture is usually found in the common hepatic duct or right hepatic duct where the cystic duct has been adherent at the union of the cystic and common hepatic ducts (fig. 407) or less frequently in the supraduodenal portion of the duct.

The bile duct above the stricture is grossly dilated and thickened, and below, the duct is represented by a fibrous cord difficult to identify at operation. The bile duct dilatation extends into the liver and depends on the completeness of the obstruction.

The contained bile is viscid and usually infected, resembling biliary mud. Small calculi sometimes extend even into the intra-hepatic branches of the bile ducts (see fig. 66).

The liver shows cholestasis. Biliary cirrhosis develops with time. The spleen enlarges and shows chronic infection and portal hypertension.

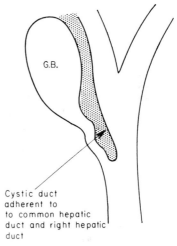

Fig. 407. Biliary stricture may be produced by dissection of adherent cystic duct from the common hepatic and right hepatic ducts.

CLINICAL FEATURES

The condition is commoner in females, because they have more biliary surgery. Seventy per cent are less than 50 years old.

If the main bile ducts have been completely divided, jaundice of cholestatic type appears three to seven days post-operatively. Alternatively, an external biliary fistula develops. Such a fistula, for even a few days, suggests that biliary stricture will follow. The fistula may drain intermittently, with episodes of jaundice when it is closed and subsidence of jaundice when it is draining. When the fistula finally closes, jaundice is continuous.

Post-operative biliary peritonitis with pain and fever is another early method of presentation.

More usually the bile duct injury is partial. Insidious jaundice develops early after operation. It may be three to four months before jaundice of variable intensity is apparent. This is the period of slow, constrictive cholangitis with stones forming above the stricture.

Intermittent attacks of cholangitis with or without jaundice accompany all grades of biliary stricture. The cholangitis is marked by pyrexia, sometimes very high, with a rigor, sweating and epigastric pain followed by pruritus, darkening of the urine, and pallor of the faeces (*Charcot's intermittent biliary fever*). Milder episodes are also seen which can be anicteric.

Sub-hepatic abscess after biliary surgery is another indication of developing stricture formation.

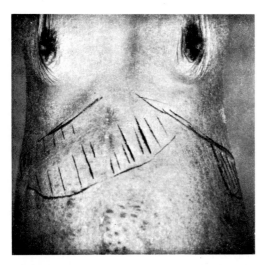

Fig. 408. Traumatic stricture of bile duct. Pigmented abdomen with scars of many surgical explorations. Hepatosplenomegaly.

Persistent dull pain may be experienced in the epigastrium.

With time, the patient becomes pigmented (fig. 408), with clubbing of the fingers. Skin xanthomas are a rare late development. The liver is firm, extending almost to the umbilicus. The old gall bladder incision is tender. The spleen becomes palpable.

Liver failure with deepening jaundice, ascites, oedema and encephalopathy is terminal. Gastro-intestinal bleeding due to portal hypertension is late. Peptic ulcers may bleed.

The patients become increasingly introspective as the months pass. They keep the most detailed notes of their symptoms and, perhaps understandably, become querulous and suspicious of their medical advisers.

INVESTIGATIONS

Serum biochemistry is that of intermittent, chronic cholestasis. The serum bilirubin level is moderately increased. The alkaline phosphatase (5'-nucleotidase) and bile acid levels may be raised even if the serum bilirubin value is normal; these are the best indicators of obstruction.

Radiology. A plain film may show air in the biliary tree (fig. 59), and sometimes the actual site

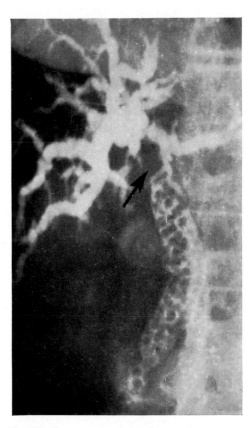

Fig. 409. Percutaneous cholangiogram shows dilated common bile duct, full of radio-translucent gall-stones. The stricture in the common hepatic duct is marked by an arrow. The intra-hepatic bile ducts are dilated and irregular.

of stricture. Intravenous cholangiography is usually unsuccessful. ERCP is very useful in diagnosis, but may fail following previous attempts at bile duct anastomosis with the duodenum or jejunum. Percutaneous cholangiography (figs. 409 and 66) should be attempted but may fail if the obstruction is partial, and the intra-hepatic ducts are sclerotic or contain stones. Such patients are usually anicteric between the attacks of cholangitis. Secondary sclerosing cholangitis is shown in longstanding cases (fig. 410).

Radiological demonstration of the anatomy of the biliary system is of inestimable value to the surgeon. If possible, barium meals should be avoided as the contrast material may regurgitate into the biliary tree and severe cholangitis can result.

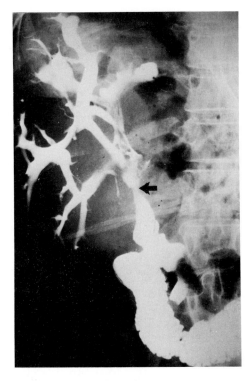

Fig. 410. Biliary stricture with patent choledocho-jejunostomy (arrow). Repeated attacks of cholangitis have led to secondary sclerosing cholangitis shown by irregular stenosis and dilatation of the intra-hepatic bile ducts.

Duodenal intubation reveals a heavy growth of *E. coli* and other enteric organisms. Similar organisms may be recovered from the blood and urine during a bout of cholangitis.

The heavy growth of organisms in the upper small intestine may lead to a 'blind loop' syndrome [9]. The breath test for bacteria in the small gut able to deconjugate bile salts is positive [7].

Haematological findings include a mild, normo-chromic, normocytic anaemia. A moderate leuco-cytosis accompanies the febrile episodes.

DIAGNOSIS

The distinction from residual or new bile duct calculi may be impossible; indeed, stricture, biliary sludge and stones may co-exist (fig. 409). Stones, usually pigment, form in the duct above the stricture related to bacteria which deconjugate bilirubin.

Distinction must be made from post-cholecystectomy functional symptoms. An elevated serum alkaline phosphatase level is a good index of continuing biliary obstruction.

Liver biopsy is also useful in confirming organic biliary obstruction. Histological changes range all the way from mild cholangitis to a fully developed biliary cirrhosis.

PROGNOSIS

This depends on whether a satisfactory surgical repair can be achieved. This is more likely the greater the length of duct available for anastomosis and, hence, strictures near the duodenum have a better prognosis than those near the hilum.

Surgeons who are especially experienced and skilled in the operation will achieve the best results. Operative and post-operative mortality is 13%, usually due to liver failure or haemorrhage [12]. Two-thirds are improved and, of these, one-third are cured [5]. The transected or ischaemic duct wall readily forms scar tissue and results in failure to achieve satisfactory operative results [4]. Re-stenosis is therefore frequent. If the patient remains symptom-free for four years post-operatively there is a 90% chance of complete cure. This happy result lessens with the number of operations, but *can* follow many attempts at repair.

The prognosis is worsened by prolonged obstruction, being best if suture is done soon after the injury. Secondary sclerosing cholangitis is usually irreversible (fig. 410). Secondary biliary cirrhosis should not be a contraindication to reconstructive procedures. Since hepato-cellular failure is late, liver function will improve and the portal venous pressure will fall if biliary obstruction can be relieved. If the patient is continuously jaundiced or suffering repeated attacks of cholangitis, cirrhosis is inevitable and death in liver failure follows in 5–12 years [11].

In general, re-operation *by an expert* should always be advised however apparently poor the operative risk and however many previous attempts at relief have been made.

TREATMENT

Prevention. The majority of strictures would be prevented if cholecystectomy were less popular, performed only by experienced surgeons, and if the ducts were not dissected in the presence of acute cholecystitis. No structure must be clamped or divided until the anatomy has been defined. If any doubt exists a cholecystotomy and biliary drainage are indicated. Important technical points include good exposure, adequate relaxation and a dry operative field. The cystic artery must be ligated *before* the cystic duct is tied. Traction on the gall bladder should be avoided. If diagnosed at the time of surgery the duct should be repaired by end-to-end anastomosis over a T tube [6]. If the length of duct is insufficient, a Roux-en-Y choledochojejunostomy may be performed.

The lateral aspect of the common or right hepatic duct is usually injured where the cystic duct has been dissected from it (fig. 407).

Medical. This is reserved for the patient with an inoperable stricture or with very mild symptoms. Antibiotics will largely be ineffective if there is cholangitis and biliary obstruction, and, with their continued usage, the causative organisms become resistant. Tetracycline, ampicillin, metronidazole and gentamycin should, therefore, be reserved for the acute attack of cholangitis or pre-operatively. Supplementary vitamins should include vitamins A, D and K, if necessary, intramuscularly and ascorbic acid orally. Anaemia should be corrected. If the patient has a biliary fistula, particular attention must be paid to the electrolyte balance.

Operative. Operations should be undertaken under antibiotic cover as soon as possible after the original bile duct injury, before obliterative cholangitis, adhesion formation and secondary changes in the liver have added to the risk and technical difficulties. The surgeon attempting the first repair carries a great responsibility because failure reduces the chance of subsequent cure. The best surgeon should therefore be the first to operate rather than each intervention being undertaken by one of greater skill and reputation than his predecessor.

The operation chosen will depend mainly on two factors—the site and length of the stricture and the amount of duct available for repair. Any operation must provide excision of the stricture with mucosal apposition between the duct lining and the intestinal mucosa. The anastomosis must be as large as possible and not under tension. An entero-anastomosis must be done if there is any risk of ascending infection from the bowel.

Even if sufficient duct is available proximally, excision of the stricture and end-to-end anastomosis of the duct is rarely performed. Deficiencies between the calibre of the duct above and below the stricture are too great for a satisfactory anastomosis to be achieved.

The best operation is choledocho-jejunostomy or, if the amount of duct available is too small, hepatico-jejunostomy (fig. 411). An entero-anastomosis is added to minimize reflux from the intestines causing cholangitis. Alternatively with

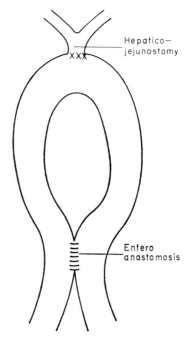

Fig. 411. Repair of high biliary stricture by hepatico-jejunostomy and entero-anastomosis.

high strictures of Roux-en-Y limb of jejunum may be brought up to the common hepatic duct. This operation can give satisfactory results over many years [1].

In cases of high stricture where hepatico-jejunostomy has been done a Y-shaped prosthesis is usually left in position, one limb in each hepatic duct and a vertical one in the jejunum. The duration of splinting is uncertain; some recommend at least six months and preferably 12; others put a limit of six weeks to three months [5]. The splint must be removed when the first sign of cholangitis appears. With low strictures T tube drainage is often done.

When no extra-hepatic ducts can be found for drainage, the left lobe of the liver may be amputated and a large intra-hepatic bile duct anastomosed to the side of a Roux-en-Y arm of jejunum [8] (*Longmire's operation*). The anastomosis usually closes fairly rapidly.

Strictures of the hepatic ducts can be repaired by Rodney Smith's procedure [10]. A latex tube with distal perforations is passed through the liver into a major bile duct at the hilum and hence into a loop of jejunum. The jejunum is drawn up to the hilum and its mucosa is sutured in intimate contact to the epithelium of the intra-hepatic bile ducts. This provides mucosa-to-mucosa approximation without compromising the blood supply.

Permanent silastic stents can be introduced through a stricture. This may be done by open operation, through the liver or via the endoscope from below (see page 514) [2, 3]. These stents tend to occlude from biliary sediment and stones. Chenodeoxycholic acid is unlikely to dissolve such pigment debris. However, it is now possible to change the stent without further surgery, either trans-hepatically or via the endoscope.

Peptic ulcer is a complication of hepaticojejunostomy.

Portal hypertension may be controlled by repairing the stricture, otherwise a porta-caval shunt must be performed later. This may be exceedingly difficult due to the adhesions from previous repairs and a splenorenal or mesentericocaval anastomosis may be the only ones possible.

The outcome following surgical correction of bile duct stricture depends on the degree of cholangitis, pericholedochitis and scarring and the quality of the duct to be anastomosed. It also depends on the number of previous corrective procedures and the time interval between the injury and the surgical repair. The higher the anatomic location of the stricture the less the chance of a successful result. The presence of hepato-cellular failure is ominous. Finally, the outcome depends on the experience and judgment of the surgeon in selecting and performing the most suitable corrective procedure.

REFERENCES

1. BISMUTH H., FRANCO D., CORLETTE M.B. *et al* (1978) Long term results of Roux-en-Y hepaticojejunostomy. *Surg. Gynecol. Obstet.* **146**, 161.
2. CAMERON J.L., SKINNER D.B. & ZUIDEMA G.D. (1976) Long term transhepatic intubation for hilar hepatic duct strictures. *Ann. Surg.* **183**, 488.
3. DOOLEY J.S., DICK R., OLNEY J. *et al* (1979) Nonsurgical treatment of biliary obstruction. *Lancet* ii, 1040.
4. GLENN F. (1978) Iatrogenic injuries to the biliary system. *Surg. Gynecol. Obstet.* **146**, 430.
5. HERTZER N.R., GRAY H.W., HOERR S.O. *et al* (1973) The use of T-tube splints in bile duct repairs. *Surg. Gynecol. Obstet.* **136**, 413.
6. HILLIS T.M., WESTBROOK K.C., CALDWELL F.T. *et al* (1977) Surgical injury of the common bile duct. *Am. J. Surg.* **134**, 712.
7. JAMES O.F.W., AGNEW J.E. & BOUCHIER I.A.D. (1973) Assessment of the ^{14}C-glycocholic acid breath test. *Br. med. J.* ii, 191.
8. LONGMIRE W.P. Jr & SANFORD M.C. (1949) Intrahepatic cholangiojejunostomy for biliary obstruction: further studies. *Ann. Surg.* **130**, 455.
9. SCOTT A.J. & KHAN G.A. (1967) Origin of bacteria in bileduct bile. *Lancet* ii, 790.
10. SMITH R. (1979) Obstructions of the bile duct. *Br. J. Surg.* **66**, 69.
11. TURNER M.D. & SHERLOCK S. (1962) The prognosis of biliary stricture. *Gut* **3**, 94.
12. WARREN K.W. & JEFFERSON M.F. (1973) Prevention and repair of strictures of the extra-hepatic bile ducts. *Surg. Clin. N. Am.* **53**, 1169.

Chapter 31
Diseases of the Ampulla of Vater
and Pancreas

CARCINOMA IN THE REGION OF THE AMPULLA OF VATER

The ampullary area is a common site for carcinomas which may arise from the mucosa of the lower end of the common bile duct, the main pancreatic duct, the pancreatic acini [10], the ampulla itself or rarely from the duodenal mucous membrane covering the biliary papilla.

Growths arising from any of these sites have the same overall effect (fig. 412) and will be considered as a group. They are often loosely termed 'cancer of the head of the pancreas'.

PATHOLOGY

The tumour rarely exceeds 3.5 cm in diameter. It may be difficult to recognize macroscopically. The site of origin is often obscure. Tumours arising from the ampulla itself tend to be polypoid and soft, whereas the acinar tumours are infiltrative, large and firm.

Histologically, the tumour is an adeno-carcinoma, whether arising from pancreatic duct, acini or bile duct. The ampullary tumours have a papillary arrangement and are often of low-grade malignancy; fibrosis is prominent.

Obstruction of common bile duct

This results from direct invasion causing a scirrhous reaction, from annular stenosis, and from tumour tissue filling the lumen. The duct may also be compressed by the tumour mass.

Functional obstruction due to involvement of nerves in the wall of the bile duct [4] may explain the occasional spontaneous relief of the jaundice. More likely is the fact that the surface of the growth becomes necrotic and sloughs, so that bile can again reach the duodenum.

The bile ducts dilate and the gall bladder enlarges. An ascending cholangitis in the obstructed ducts is exceedingly rare. The liver and other tissues show the changes of cholestatic jaundice.

Pancreatic changes

The main pancreatic duct may be obstructed as it enters the ampulla. The ducts and acini distal to the obstruction dilate and later rupture, causing focal areas of pancreatitis and fat necrosis. Later all the acinar tissue is replaced by fibrous tissue. Occasionally, particularly in the acinar type, fat necrosis and suppuration may occur in and around the pancreas.

Widespread venous thromboses (thrombophlebitis migrans) are reported in 27.6% of tumours of the head of the pancreas and 50% of the body and tail.

Glycosuria is related to interference with the escape of insulin from the pancreas.

Spread of the tumour

Direct extension in the wall of the bile duct and infiltration through the head of the pancreas is common with the acinar though not with the ampullary type. The second part of the duodenum may be invaded, with ulceration of the mucosa and secondary haemorrhage. The splenic and portal veins may be invaded and may thrombose with resultant splenomegaly. Peritoneal involvement is uncommon.

Involvement of regional nodes is found in approximately a third of operated cases. Perineural lymphatic spread was found in 84% of 83 cases of cancer of the pancreas [4]. Blood-borne metastases, with secondaries in liver and lungs, follow invasion of the splenic or portal veins.

CLINICAL FEATURES [2, 7]

Both sexes are affected, but males more frequently than females in a ratio of 2:1. The sufferer is usually between 50 and 69 years old.

The clinical picture is a composite one of cholestasis, pancreatic and biliary insufficiency, and the

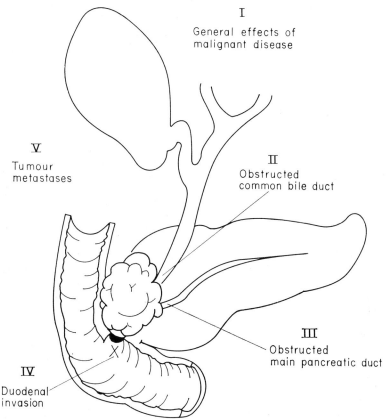

Fig. 412. The effects of carcinoma in the ampullary region. **I** General effects of malignant disease—weakness and weight loss. **II** Obstructed common bile duct. Dilated gall bladder and bile ducts—jaundice, hepatomegaly, pruritus. **III** Obstructed main pancreatic duct—fibrous atrophy of pancreas, steatorrhoea and occasional glycosuria. **IV** Duodenal invasion. Barium meal changes—occasional duodenal obstruction, positive stool occult blood, occasional melaena. **V** Tumour metastases. Nerves—back and epigastric pain; regional glands, liver, lungs, peritoneum.

general and local effects of a malignant tumour (fig. 412).

Jaundice is of gradual onset and progressively deepening but ampullary neoplasms can cause mild and intermittent jaundice. Cholangitis is unusual although occasionally fever does follow cholangitis above the obstruction.

Cancer of the head of the pancreas is not painless. Pain is experienced in the back, the epigastrium and right upper quadrant, usually as a continuous distress worse at night and sometimes ameliorated by crouching. It may be aggravated by eating.

Weakness and weight loss are progressive and have usually continued for at least three months before jaundice develops.

Although frank steatorrhoea is rare, the patient often complains of a change in the bowel habit, usually diarrhoea.

Vomiting and intestinal obstruction may follow invasion of the second part of the duodenum. More often ulceration of the duodenum can erode a vessel with haematemesis or, more commonly, occult bleeding. Ampullary lesions tend to present with jaundice, often intermittent. Tumours outside the ampullary area present early with vomiting of pyloric type but without jaundice [1].

Difficulty in making an accurate diagnosis may make the patient mentally depressed. It then becomes easy to believe, mistakenly, that the patient is psychoneurotic.

Examination. The patient is jaundiced and shows evidence of recent weight loss. Theoretically, the gall bladder should be enlarged and palpable (*Courvoisier's law*). In practice, the gall bladder is only felt in about half the patients, although at subsequent laparotomy a dilated gall bladder is found in three-quarters. The liver is enlarged with a sharp, smooth, firm edge. Hepatic metastases are rarely detected. The pancreatic tumour is impalpable.

The spleen is palpable if involvement of the splenic vein has caused thrombosis. Peritoneal invasion is followed by ascites.

General lymphatic metastases are more usual with cancer of the body rather than head of the pancreas. Occasionally, however, axillary, cervical and inguinal glands may be enlarged and Virchow's gland in the left supra-clavicular fossa may be palpable.

Occasionally, widespread venous thromboses simulate thrombophlebitis migrans.

Very rarely, small tender nodules of fat necrosis occur in the subcutaneous tissues, especially in the back of the neck. Release of pancreatic enzymes into the joints may simulate rheumatoid arthritis.

INVESTIGATIONS

Urine shows the features of cholestatic jaundice.

Glycosuria occurs in 15–20% and with it there is an impaired oral glucose tolerance test.

Faeces show steatorrhoea.

Tests for occult blood may be positive.

Blood biochemistry. The serum alkaline phosphatase level is greatly raised. The serum amylase and lipase concentrations are sometimes persistently elevated in carcinoma of the ampullary region. Hypoproteinaemia with, later, peripheral oedema may be found.

Duodenal intubation can be used to demonstrate the absence of bile and of pancreatic enzymes and the presence of blood.

Radiology

A barium meal [1] may show alterations in duodenal motility with deep indentations. To-and-fro churning of the contrast medium suggests partial obstruction. The duodenal mucosa may show constant irregularity due to infiltration by growth (fig. 413). A dilated common bile duct may produce a duodenal impression in the immediate post-bulbar region or in the bulb itself.

Stenosis of the duodenum may be total or partial and the proximal loop may be dilated (fig. 413).

The medial aspect of the second part of the duodenum may be deformed so that it looks like a reversed number three.

Enlargement and widening of the duodenal loop is uncommon. It suggests a large tumour which is more commonly acinar than ampullary. With large tumours, the stomach is displaced forwards and to the left, and the transverse colon downwards.

Coeliac angiography may reveal abnormal vessels in the pancreas.

Fibroptic duodenoscopy may be used to visualize the growth and allow a biopsy. *Retrograde endoscopic pancreatico-cholangiography* is also of value [11] and allows pancreatic duct cytology to be studied [6].

A chest radiograph may reveal metastases.

Aspiration liver biopsy is only necessary when the type of jaundice is in doubt.

Haematology. Anaemia is mild or absent. The leucocyte count may be normal or raised, with a relative increase in polymorphonuclear leucocytes. The erythrocyte sedimentation rate is usually raised.

DIFFERENTIAL DIAGNOSIS

The diagnosis must be considered in any patient over 40 years with progressive or even intermittent cholestasis. The suspicion would be strengthened by persistent or unexplained abdominal pain, weakness and weight loss, diarrhoea, glycosuria, positive faecal occult blood, hepatomegaly, a palpable spleen or thrombophlebitis migrans.

The distinction from jaundice due to other causes is presented in table 26.

PROGNOSIS

The prognosis of ampullary carcinoma is grave. The acinar type carries a worse prognosis than the ductal type, for the tumour is less operable and regional lymph glands are involved earlier. The ampullary type is smaller, it obstructs the common bile duct sooner and diagnosis is earlier. Carcinoma of the duodenum has the best prognosis.

If the early post-operative deaths are excluded, results of palliative or radical surgery show an average life expectancy for carcinoma of the head of the pancreas of 6.2 months, for carcinoma of the ampulla of Vater of 18.5 months, for carcinoma of the common bile duct of 12.7 months and for carcinoma of the duodenum 35 months. Earlier diagnosis is imperative. Duration of symptoms unfortunately gives little indication of the extent of disease.

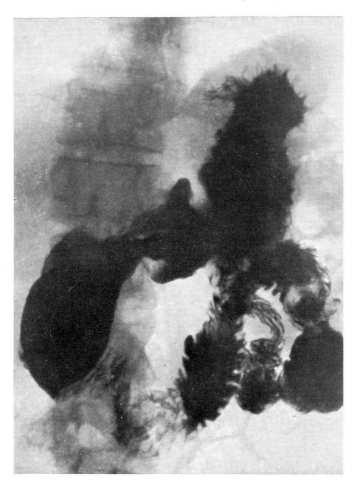

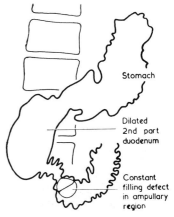

Fig. 413. Barium meal shows dilated duodenum and constant mucosal irregularity in the second part of the duodenum.

TREATMENT

The treatment of tumours of the ampullary region is surgical: either an attempted removal or palliative anastomosis between the gall bladder and gastro-intestinal tract. If the patient's general condition does not permit surgery, or if laparotomy reveals an inoperable growth, the treatment is that of chronic cholestasis (Chapter 14). Difficulties in removal arise because of the inaccessibility of the pancreas on the posterior wall of the abdomen in the vicinity of vital structures. The operability rate is therefore very low.

The usual procedure is *pancreatico-duodenectomy*, which is performed in one stage with removal of related regional lymph nodes, the entire duodenum and the distal third of stomach [16]. The continuity of the biliary passages is restored by anastomosis of the common bile duct with the jejunum. The continuity of the intestinal tract is restored by gastro-jejunostomy [8].

Frozen section examination of the resection margins is mandatory [5]. The survival is 20.3 months if all the tumour is removed, 12.9 months where resection margin shows tumour, and 6.2 months for a palliative bypass. If total pancreatectomy is possible the survival is 26 months [5]. A palliative operation if tumour is left behind is no better than a bypass.

The mortality of pancreatico-duodenectomy (Whipple's operation) for ampullary carcinoma is 8% [8]. Removal is most likely to be possible if the tumour is a small, papillary one situated at the ampulla.

Palliative procedures

Palliative surgery is indicated to relieve the intolerable pruritus and the jaundice. It also allows for the possibility that the obstruction is benign.

Choledocho-jejunostomy, with entero-anastomosis, is probably the most satisfactory procedure to prevent ascending cholangitis. Stenosis of the anastomosis by tumour is rare.

Trans-hepatic insertion of a prosthesis through the tumour into the duodenum (see fig. 416) or external biliary drainage must be considered as palliative procedures (see page 514) [3].

These palliative procedures do not prolong life.

Pruritus is relieved with cholestyramine or, if biliary obstruction is complete, by norethandrolone or methyl testerone.

Benign villous adenoma of the ampulla of Vater [14]

This leads to biliary colic and obstructive jaundice. It is usually confused with ampullary carcinoma and is diagnosed by frozen sections at surgery. It is treated by sub-mucosal excision.

CHRONIC PANCREATITIS

Pancreatitis, usually of alcoholic aetiology, can cause narrowing of the intrapancreatic portion of the common bile duct [12, 13, 15]. The resultant cholestasis may be transient during exacerbations of acute pancreatitis. It is presumably related to oedema and swelling of the pancreas. More persistent cholestasis complicates severe destructive pancreatitis when actual strictures of the lower common bile duct can be shown. Cysts of the head of the pancreas and abscesses can also cause biliary obstruction and persistent cholestasis.

Milder forms are shown by transient or prolonged rises of serum alkaline phosphatase without jaundice. Cholangitis is unusual.

Diagnosis is made by endoscopic retrograde cholangio-pancreatography (ERCP), which shows a smooth narrowing of the lower end of the common bile duct and a tortuous irregular, dilated, main pancreatic duct (see fig. 320). Calcification may be present in the pancreas.

Needle liver biopsy is used to distinguish acute alcoholic hepatitis. Portal zone fibrosis and inflammation in an alcoholic are also suggestive of chronic pancreatitis [9].

At surgery, if ERCP has not been performed, the distinction of chronic pancreatitis from pancreatic cancer can be exceedingly difficult. Multiple frozen sections offer the best chance of positive diagnosis.

TREATMENT

The patient must abstain completely from alcohol. Persistent cholestasis, with narrow strictures, is treated by surgery, usually choledocho-jejunostomy.

OBSTRUCTION OF THE COMMON BILE DUCT BY ENLARGED LYMPH GLANDS IN THE PORTAL FISSURE

Although the association is extremely rare, the enlarged glands are nearly always metastatic, frequently from a primary in the alimentary tract, lung or breast, or from a hepato-cellular carcinoma. Where malignant glands in the porta hepatis are associated with deep jaundice, the main bile ducts are usually being invaded rather than compressed. Alternatively, the secondary deposits in the hepatic parenchyma may invade the bile ducts, causing obstruction.

Portal fissure glands may be enlarged in non-malignant conditions, but the bile ducts usually escape compression. Jaundice in infections such as tuberculosis, sarcoidosis or infectious mononucleosis is not obstructive but due to direct hepatic involvement and to haemolysis.

Glandular enlargement in the reticuloses does, very rarely, cause obstruction to the common bile duct, but jaundice complicating these diseases is more often due to hepatic parenchymal involvement, to increased haemolysis or is of obscure cholestatic type.

OTHER CAUSES OF EXTRINSIC PRESSURE ON THE COMMON BILE DUCT

Duodenal peptic ulceration

This is an extremely rare cause of obstructive jaundice. Perforation so that the ulcer impinges against the bile duct or causes adhesive peritonitis may rarely cause biliary obstruction and this can also follow interstitial contraction as the ulcer heals.

Duodenal diverticulum

Diverticula of the duodenum are often found near the ampulla of Vater, but rarely cause obstruction to the bile ducts. When they do so, obstruction is partial and jaundice intermittent.

REFERENCES

1. BLUMGART L.H. & KENNEDY A. (1973) Carcinoma of the ampulla of Vater and duodenum. *Br. J. Surg.* **60**, 33.
2. COUTSOFTIDES T., MACDONALD J. & SHIBATA H.R.

(1977) Carcinoma of the pancreas and periampullary region: a 41 year experience. *Ann. Surg.* **186**, 730.

3. DOOLEY J.S., DICK R., OLNEY J. *et al* (1979) Nonsurgical treatment of biliary obstruction. *Lancet* ii, 1040.

4. DRAPIEWSKI J.F. (1944) Carcinoma of the pancreas: a study of neoplastic invasion of nerves and its possible clinical significance. *Am. J. clin. Pathol.* **14**, 549.

5. FORREST J.F. & LONGMIRE W.P. (1979) Carcinoma of the pancreas and periampullary region: a study of 279 patients. *Ann. Surg.* **189**, 129.

6. HALL T.J., BLACKSTONE M.O., COOPER M.J. *et al* (1978) Prospective evaluation of endoscopic retrograde cholangiopancreatography in the diagnosis of peri-ampullary cancers. *Ann. Surg.* **187**, 313.

7. HERMANN R.E. & COOPERMAN A.M. (1979) Current concepts in cancer. Carcinoma of the pancreas. *New Engl. J. Med.* **301**, 482.

8. MAKIPOUR H., COOPERMAN A., DANZI J.T. *et al* (1976) Carcinoma of the ampulla of Vater: review of 38 cases with emphasis on treatment and prognostic factors. *Ann. Surg.* **183**, 341.

9. MORGAN M.Y., SHERLOCK S. & SCHEUER P.J. (1978) Portal fibrosis in the livers of alcoholic patients. *Gut* **19**, 1015.

10. MORGAN R.G.H. & WORMSLEY K.G. (1977) Cancer of the pancreas. *Gut* **18**, 580.

11. REUBEN A. & COTTON P.B. (1979) Endoscopic retrograde cholangiopancreatography in carcinoma of the pancreas. *Surg. Gynecol. Obstet.* **148**, 179.

12. SARLES H. & SAHEL J. (1978) Progress report: cholestasis and lesions of the biliary tract in chronic pancreatitis. *Gut* **19**, 851.

13. SCOTT J., SUMMERFIELD J.A., ELIAS E. *et al* (1977) Chronic pancreatitis: a cause of cholestasis. *Gut* **18**, 196.

14. SOBOL S. COOPERMAN A.M. (1978) Villous adenoma of the ampulla of Vater: an unusual case of biliary colic and obstructive jaundice. *Gastroenterology* **75**, 107.

15. WARSHAW A.L., SCHAPIRO R.H., FERRUCCI J.T. *et al* (1976) Persistent obstructive jaundice, cholangitis, and biliary cirrhosis due to common bile duct stenosis in chronic pancreatitis. *Gastroenterology* **70**, 562.

16. WHIPPLE A.O. (1942) Present-day surgery of the pancreas (Bigelow Lecture). *New Engl. J. Med.* **226**, 515.

Chapter 32
Tumours of the Gall Bladder
and Bile Ducts

BENIGN TUMOURS OF THE GALL BLADDER

PAPILLOMA [18]

Multiple, small, papillomatous tumours, consisting of hypertrophied villi laden with cholesterol esters, may be found in as many as 80% of surgically removed gall bladders. They are often associated with cholesterosis.

Papillomas are seen in about 0.3% of cholecystograms. In a functioning gall bladder they appear as concave filling defects, pointing towards the centre on the lateral wall. They are about $\frac{1}{2}$–1 cm in diameter and may be multiple. Tangential views may show their point of attachment to the gall bladder wall. They are differentiated from gallstones by their fixed position.

ADENOMA

These very rare small, single tumours are usually fundal, where they form a semi-solid or cystic papillary mass. Adenoma is usually a symptom-free, incidental finding.

In cholecystograms, an adenoma is usually seen at the fundus as a small circular or semicircular translucent filling defect, the gall bladder being well filled.

CARCINOMA OF THE GALL BLADDER

This is an uncommon neoplasm. Gall-stones co-exist in over 90% and chronic cholecystitis is a frequent association. There is, however, no definite evidence of a causal relationship. Whatever causes gall-stones predisposes to cancer. The calcified (porcelain) gall bladder is particularly likely to become cancerous [25]. The common gall bladder papillomas are not pre-cancerous.

PATHOLOGY

Papillary adeno-carcinoma commences as a wart-like excresence. It grows slowly into, rather than through, the wall until a fungating mass fills the gall bladder. Mucoid change is associated with more rapid growth, early metastasis and gelatinous peritoneal carcinomatosis. *Squamous cell carcinoma and scirrhous* forms are recognized. *The anaplastic type* is particularly malignant.

The tumour usually arises in the fundus or neck, but rapid spread may make the original site difficult to locate. The rich lymphatic and venous drainage of the gall bladder allows rapid spread to related lymph nodes, causing cholestatic jaundice and widespread dissemination. The liver bed is invaded and there is local spread to the duodenum, stomach and colon resulting in fistulae or external compression.

Examination reveals a hard and sometimes tender mass in the gall bladder area. Intra-hepatic metastases are not usually palpable. The abdomen is distended and gelatinous peritoneal carcinomatosis may prevent individual organs being defined.

Serum, *urine* and *faeces* show the changes of cholestatic jaundice.

Liver biopsy shows the histological picture of biliary obstruction but does not indicate the cause, because intra-hepatic metastases are uncommon.

Plain film of the abdomen may show a gall bladder shadow or gall-stones.

ERCP may be helpful.

CT scanning and *ultrasound* [21] may be useful in defining the tumour.

Prognosis

This is hopeless because the majority are inoperable at the time of diagnosis. The only long-term survivors are those in whom the carcinoma was found incidentally at the time of cholecystectomy for gall-stones. In one series the mean survival was seven months from diagnosis [2]. The papillary type has the best prognosis as the growth is inwards rather than through the gall bladder wall and spread is later.

Treatment

Cholecystectomy has been recommended for all patients with gall-stones in an effort to prevent the development of carcinoma in the gall bladder. This seems drastic for a common condition, and could but lead to innumerable unnecessary cholecystectomies. The pre-operative diagnosis of carcinoma of the gall bladder should not preclude laparotomy although the results of surgical treatment are disappointing. In one series of 11 resected tumours only one patient survived five years [24].

Partial hepatectomy has been attempted but with unsatisfactory results.

BENIGN TUMOURS OF THE EXTRA-HEPATIC BILE DUCTS

These extremely rare tumours usually remain undetected until there is evidence of biliary obstruction and cholangitis [10]. They are rarely diagnosed pre-operatively.

Papilloma is a polypoid tumour which projects into the lumen of the common bile duct. It is a small, soft, vascular tumour, which may be sessile or pedunculated. The tumours may be single or multiple; they may be cystic [7]. Occasionally they undergo malignant change [19].

Adenoma can be found anywhere in the biliary tract. It is firm and well circumscribed and varies in size up to 15 cm in diameter.

Fibroma is small and firm and causes early bile duct obstruction.

Granular cell tumour is of mesenchymal origin. It largely affects black women, causing cholestasis [13].

The *treatment* is excision with end-to-end anastomosis of the bile ducts or more usually hepaticojejunostomy and entero-anastomosis.

CARCINOMA OF THE BILE DUCTS (CHOLANGIO-CARCINOMA)

Carcinoma may arise at any point in the biliary tree from small intra-hepatic bile ducts to the common bile duct. The histology of the tumour is the same whatever the site of origin. The clinical picture and treatment differ according to the site.

It is often difficult at surgery or autopsy to be sure of the exact origin.

ASSOCIATIONS

Bile duct cancers are associated with ulcerative colitis with or without sclerosing cholangitis usually involving extra-hepatic bile ducts [26] (Chapter 14).

All types of congenital cysts may be complicated by adeno-carcinoma. These include congenital hepatic fibrosis [8], cystic dilatation (Caroli's syndrome) [14], choledochal cysts [12], and polycystic liver [3]. Cholangio-carcinoma may be associated with biliary cirrhosis due to congenital biliary atresia [16].

The liver fluke infestations of the orient may be complicated by cholangio-carcinoma. In the Far East (China, Hong Kong, Korea, Japan), where *Clonorchis sinensis* is prevalent, cholangio-carcinoma accounts for 20% of primary liver tumours. These arise in the heavily parasitized bile ducts near the hilum.

In New York an association has been shown between hepato-biliary cancer and the typhoid carrier state [29]. Carcinogenic bile acids produced in infected bile have been postulated as the cause.

The role of gall-stones in pathogenesis is uncertain [20]. One woman taking oral contraceptives developed intra-hepatic cholangio-carcinoma [11].

Bile duct cancers are not closely associated with cirrhosis unless it is of the biliary type [20].

PATHOLOGY

The confluence of cystic duct with main hepatic duct or the right and left main hepatic ducts at the porta hepatis are common sites of origin and the tumour extends into the liver. It causes complete obstruction of the extra-hepatic bile ducts with intra-hepatic biliary dilatation and enlargement of the liver. The gall bladder is collapsed and flaccid. If the tumour is restricted to one hepatic duct, biliary obstruction is incomplete and jaundice absent. The lobe of the liver drained by this duct atrophies and the other hypertrophies.

In the common bile duct the tumour presents as a firm nodule or plaque which causes an annular stricture which may ulcerate. It spreads along the bile duct and through its wall.

Local and distant mestastases, even at autopsy, are found in only about half of the patients. They involve peritoneum, abdominal lymph nodes,

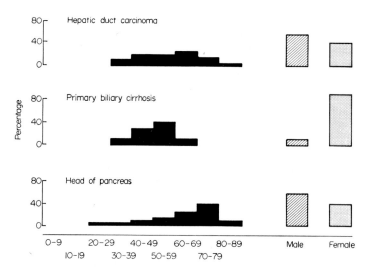

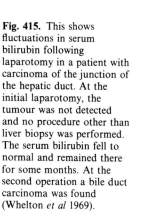

Fig. 414. Age distribution of hepatic duct carcinoma compared with primary biliary cirrhosis and carcinoma of the head of the pancreas (Whelton *et al* 1969).

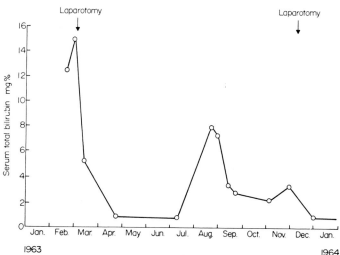

Fig. 415. This shows fluctuations in serum bilirubin following laparotomy in a patient with carcinoma of the junction of the hepatic duct. At the initial laparotomy, the tumour was not detected and no procedure other than liver biopsy was performed. The serum bilirubin fell to normal and remained there for some months. At the second operation a bile duct carcinoma was found (Whelton *et al* 1969).

diaphragm, liver or gall bladder [30]. Blood vessel invasion is rare and extra-abdominal spread is unusual.

Histologically the tumour is usually a mucus-secreting adeno-carcinoma with cuboidal or columnar epithelium and abundant fibrous stroma. Spread along neural sheaths may be noted.

CLINICAL FEATURES [30]

This tumour tends to occur in the older age group, patients being about 60 years old [30] (fig. 414). Slightly more males than females are affected.

Jaundice is the usual presenting feature, to be followed by pruritus—a point of distinction from primary biliary cirrhosis. Jaundice may be delayed if only one main duct is involved. The trend of the serum bilirubin level is always upward, but periods of clearing of jaundice are found in up to 50% [15] (fig. 415).

Pain, usually epigastric and mild, is present in about one-half of patients. Diarrhoea may be related to steatorrhoea. Weakness and weight loss, usually 14–28 pounds, are marked.

The condition may be associated with chronic ulcerative colitis [26], often following longstanding cholestasis due to sclerosing cholangitis.

Examination. Jaundice is deep. The patient is usually afebrile until terminally. Cholangitis is unusual until the bile ducts have been interfered with surgically [30].

The liver is very large and smooth, extending 5–12 cm below the costal margin. The spleen is not felt. Ascites is unusual.

INVESTIGATIONS

Serum biochemical findings are those of cholestatic jaundice. The serum bilirubin level is very high and fluctuations may reflect incomplete obstruction and primary involvement of one hepatic duct. Serum cholesterol is usually markedly increased.

The serum mitochondrial antibody test is negative and α-fetoprotein is not increased.

The *faeces* are pale and fatty and occult blood is often present. *Glycosuria* is absent.

Anaemia may be greater than that seen with ampullary carcinoma; the explanation is unknown—it is not due to blood loss. The leucocyte count is high–normal with increased polymorphs.

Hepatic biopsy shows the features of large bile duct obstruction. Tumour tissue is not obtained.

SCANNING

Isotope scans show a defect at the hilum of the liver resembling the palm of a hand with fingers extended (see fig. 46). This is mainly due to dilated intra-hepatic bile ducts and rarely to the tumour itself. *Ultrasound* is particularly helpful and shows dilated intra-hepatic bile ducts. It can sometimes identify the tumour mass.

CHOLANGIOGRAPHY

Endoscopic retrograde. The normal common bile duct and gall bladder are visualized and the obstruction at the hilum identified.

Percutaneous. This is usually successful. The obstruction is shown as a blunt or nipple-like termination (see fig. 64). Intra-hepatic bile ducts are always dilated. In some instances, intubation of both right and left duct systems may be necessary to outline the obstruction accurately.

Operative. This tends to be unreliable. Although the patency of the lower bile duct system is demonstrated, the intra-hepatic ducts may not be filled.

DIAGNOSIS (table 71, fig. 223)

Unless endoscopic or percutaneous cholangiography is performed in every patient with chole-

Table 71. Chronic cholestasis (Sherlock 1972).

Type	Diagnostic points	M test
Primary biliary	Females	
	Hepatic histology	+
Chronic chlorpromazine	Acute onset	
	Drug ingestion	
	Hepatic histology	±
Sclerosing cholangitis	Longstanding colitis	−
Carcinoma hepatic ducts	Deep jaundice	−
	Hepatic histology	
	Percutaneous and endoscopic cholangiography	

static jaundice the presumptive diagnosis is likely to be carcinoma of the ampullary region, which is the commoner condition. Even at operation after palpation of the hilum and after operative cholangiography through the common bile duct or gall bladder the diagnosis may still be in doubt. The significance of a large, green liver with a collapsed gall bladder may not be realized.

These patients may have had more than one laparotomy before the correct diagnosis is made. This may be due to failure to perform cholangiography whether retrograde, percutaneous or operative. Liver biopsy may not have been done or the results may have been misinterpreted by an inexperienced pathologist.

Primary biliary cirrhosis must be excluded (table 71). Careful interpretation of hepatic biopsies (needle and operative) together with the negative mitochondrial antibody usually makes the distinction possible.

Differentiation from chronic cholestatic drug jaundice depends on the history, the mode of onset and the hepatic histology.

Differentiation from primary sclerosing cholangitis can be extremely difficult particularly as the two conditions may co-exist (Chapter 16) [1]. Biopsy of the bile duct at operation may be necessary.

Hepato-cellular disease may be mimicked by the fluctuating jaundice [22].

PROGNOSIS

This is ultimately a fatal condition, but the tumour tends to be slow growing and metastasizes late so that survival is surprisingly long, particularly if the jaundice can be relieved. Mean survival in one series of 23 patients was 14.4 months [30]. It can be as long as five and a half years [1]. The tumour kills by its site, making it inoperable, rather than by its malignancy. Death is due to hepato-cellular failure and infection, usually suppurative cholangitis and septicaemia. Massive invasion of the liver by tumour or extra-hepatic metastases [15] rarely cause death. The prognosis is relatively good so that hepatic transplantation is not indicated.

TREATMENT

All patients should be operated on if the general condition permits. Operative cholangiography may be needed to define biliary anatomy and choledochoscopy to identify mutli-focal or radiologically inapparent neoplasms in the bile ducts [28].

Peripheral hepatic tumours should be removed by partial hepatectomy. However the liver must be non-cirrhotic and the tumour must be localized to one lobe. The number that is operable is exceedingly small.

Tumours of the lower bile duct may be resectable by a pancreatico-duodenectomy (Whipple's operation) with one year survival of about 60% [27].

Hilar tumours are rarely resectable—only six of 34 in one series [17]. A Roux loop of jejunum is anastomosed to the ducts in the hilum. Sometimes resection may be possible if the liver is split back to the vena cava [4]. Bilateral or single hepaticojejunostomies are then performed. However, many of these patients are old and frail and heroic surgery is rarely justified.

Usually palliation is all that can be offered, a prosthesis being introduced through the tumour into the bile ducts in the liver so allowing biliary drainage. This may be done from below at the time of surgery [6]. Alternatively a percutaneous transhepatic technique may be used, the endoprosthesis being introduced into the bile ducts over a guide wire (fig. 416) [5, 9, 23]. This palliative procedure can restore the patient to a good state of health for a remarkably long time [1, 30].

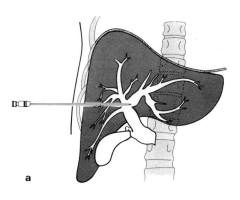

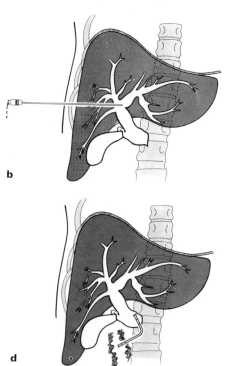

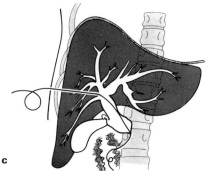

Fig. 416. Trans-hepatic insertion of biliary prosthesis (Dooley *et al* 1979). **a** The catheter over needle assembly is introduced under local anaesthesia into a selected major hepatic duct. **b** The needle is withdrawn and bile drains from the catheter confirming its position in a major bile duct. **c** A guide wire replaces the stillette and is passed further into the biliary system through the obstruction and into the duodenum. **d** Following dilatation of the stricture the endoprosthesis with lateral performation is advanced and, once in position, the guide wire and dilator are removed.

Radiotherapy (7000 rads) may be a useful adjunct to palliative procedures. Cytotoxic drugs are ineffective.

Symptomatic treatment is that of chronic cholestasis (Chapter 14).

REFERENCES

1. ALTEMEIER W.A., GALL E.A., CULBERTSON W.R. *et al* (1966) Sclerosing carcinoma of the intrahepatic (hilar) bile ducts. *Surgery* **60**, 191.
2. ARNAUD J-P., GRAF P., GRAMFORT J-L. *et al* (1979) Primary carcinoma of the gall bladder: review of 25 cases. *Am. J. Surg.* **138**, 403.
3. BLOUSTEIN P.A. (1977) Association of carcinoma with congenital cystic conditions of the liver and bile ducts. *Am. J. Gastroenterol.* **67**, 40.
4. BLUMGART L.H. (1978) Biliary tract obstruction: new approaches to old problems. *Am. J. Surg.* **135**, 19.
5. BURGHARTH F., JENSEN L.I. & OLESEN K. (1979) Endoprosthesis for internal drainage of the biliary tract: technique and results in 48 cases. *Gastroenterology* **77**, 133.
6. CAMERON J.L., GAYLER B.W. & ZUIDEMA G.D. (1978) The use of silastic transhepatic stents in benign and malignant biliary strictures. *Ann. Surg.* **188**, 552.
7. CATTELL R.B., BRAASCH J.W. & KAHN F. (1962) Polyploid epithelial tumours of the bile ducts. *New Engl. J. Med.* **266**, 57.
8. DAROCA P.J., TUTHILL R. & REED R.J. (1975) Cholangiocarcinoma arising in congenital hepatic fibrosis. *Arch. Pathol.* **99**, 592.
9. DOOLEY J.S., DICK R., OLNEY J. *et al* (1979) Nonsurgical treatment of biliary obstruction. *Lancet* ii, 1040.
10. DOWDY G.S. Jr, OLIOR W.G. Jr, SHELTON E.L. Jr *et al* (1962) Benign tumours of the extra-hepatic bile ducts. *Arch. Surg.* **85**, 503.
11. ELLIS E.F., GORDON P.R. & GOTTLIEB L.S. (1978) Oral contraceptives and cholangiocarcinoma. *Lancet* i, 207.
12. FLANIGAN D.P. (1977) Biliary carcinoma associated with biliary cysts. *Cancer* **40**, 880.
13. JAIN K.M., HASTINGS O.M., RICKERT R.R. *et al* (1979) Granular cell tumour of the common bile duct. *Am. J. Gastroenterol.* **71**, 401.
14. KAGAWA Y., KASHIHARA S., KURAMOTO S. *et al* (1978) Carcinoma arising in a congenitally dilated biliary tract: report of a case and review of the literature. *Gastroenterology* **74**, 1286.
15. KLATSKIN G. (1965) Adenocarcinoma of the hepatic duct at its bifurcation within the porta hepatis. An unusual tumour with distinctive clinical and pathological features. *Am. J. Med.* **38**, 24.
16. KULKARNI P.B. & BEATTY E.C. (1977) Cholangiocarcinoma associated with biliary cirrhosis due to congenital biliary atresia. *Am. J. Dis. Child.* **131**, 442.
17. LONGMIRE W.P. Jr, McARTHUR M.S., BASTOUNIS E.A. *et al* (1973) Carcinoma of the extra-hepatic biliary tract. *Ann. Surg.* **178**, 333.
18. LOITMAN B.S., CASSEL M.A. & HOLTZ S. (1962) Papillomas of the gall bladder. *Am. J. Roentgenol.* **88**, 783.
19. NEUMANN R.D., LIVOLSI V.A., ROSENTHAL N.S. *et al* (1976) Adenocarcinoma in biliary papillomatosis. *Gastroenterology* **70**, 779.
20. OKUDA K., KUBO Y., OKAZAKI N. *et al* (1977) Clinical aspects of intrahepatic bile duct carcinoma including hilar carcinoma: a study of 57 autopsy-proven cases. *Cancer* **39**, 232.
21. OLKEN S.M., BLEDSOE R. & NEWMARK H. (1978) The ultrasonic diagnosis of primary carcinoma of the gallbladder. *Radiology* **129**, 481.
22. PELLEYA-KOURI R., DUSOL M., ORTA D. *et al* (1976) Bile duct carcinoma mimicking chronic liver disease. *Arch. intern. Med.* **136**, 1051.
23. PEREIRAS R.V., RHEINGOLD O.J., HUTSON D. *et al* (1978) Relief of malignant jaundice by percutaneous insertion of a permanent prosthesis in the biliary tree. *Ann. intern. Med.* **89**, 589.
24. PIEHLER J.M. & CRICHLOW R.W. (1977) Primary carcinoma of the gallbladder. *Arch. Surg.* **112**, 26.
25. POLK H.C. (1966) Carcinoma and calcified gall bladder. *Gastroenterology* **50**, 582.
26. RITCHIE J.K., ALLAN R.N., MACARTNEY J. *et al* (1974) Biliary tract carcinoma associated with ulcerative colitis. *Q. J. Med.* **43**, 263.
27. STEPHENSON L.W., BLACKSTONE E.H. & ALDRETE J.S. (1977) Radical resection for periampullary carcinomas. *Arch. Surg.* **112**, 245.
28. TOMKINS R.K., JOHNSON J., STORM F.K. *et al* (1976) Operative endoscopy in the management of biliary tract neoplasms. *Am. J. Surg.* **132**, 174.
29. WELTON J.C., MARR J.S. & FRIEDMAN S.M. (1979) Association between hepatobiliary cancer and typhoid carrier state. *Lancet* i, 791.
30. WHELTON M.J., PETRELLI M., GEORGE P. *et al* (1969) Carcinoma at the junction of the main hepatic ducts. *Q. J. Med.* **28**, 211.

Chapter 33
Hepatic Transplantation

In 1955, Welch performed the first transplantation of the liver in dogs [28]. In 1963, Starzl and his group carried out the first successful hepatic transplant in man [21]. This Denver group has now reported 141 hepatic transplants, 42 of whom have survived one year; since 1976 the survival has been 50% [20]. The Kings–Cambridge Group are the other large group performing hepatic transplants and report that 18 of 94 patients have survived one year and that the rehabilitation of long-term survivors has been excellent [11]. The recipient of a new liver has about a 1 in 3 to 1 in 5 chance of surviving one year. These figures contrast strongly with those of renal transplant. The results, however, are improving.

Table 72. Organ transplant registry (cases reported to the Registry, July 1st 1977).

Update on liver transplantation in the world	
Transplant teams	43
Transplants	318
Recipients	302
Alive with functioning grafts	47
Longest survival with functioning graft	7.5 years
Longest current survival with functioning graft	7.5 years

At the present time hepatic transplantation should be done only in a few special centres where a highly motivated team of doctors (including hepatologists), nurses and technicians are available. The centre should be performing other organ transplants and facilities for organ removal and preservation and for immunological studies must be available.

Selection of recipients

General principles include the selection of patients aged less than 50 and with no evidence of infection outside the liver. The general state of the patient, such as psychiatric stability to carry through post-operative treatment and to attend regularly for fol-low-up, must be considered. An alcoholic with un-reliable behaviour or a mental defective would clearly be unsuitable.

Prognosis without transplant should be hope-less. The difficulty is that even patients with hepatic duct carcinoma have a mean survival of 14.6 months [30], which is more than for a recipient of an hepatic transplant. If the natural course of his illness would allow him to live longer than one year, the operation is not justified. The formula-tion of an exact prognosis in a patient with liver disease is made difficult by the remarkable powers of hepatic regeneration and because such compli-cations as haemorrhage from oesophageal varices cannot be predicted. The patient should not be moribund, but should be suffering from such severe liver disease that he is unlikely to be dis-charged from hospital. A team of hepatologists, preferably apart from the transplant team, should unanimously recommend the procedure.

NATURE OF THE LIVER DISEASE (table 73)

Primary hepato-cellular carcinoma. This might seem the ideal indication. The patients are often young and the tumour is usually unresectable. However, recurrence is 89%, perhaps due to the immuno-suppression needed to prevent rejection. The metastasis often 'homes' back to the graft [17]. Recurrence can be monitored by the serum α-feto-protein level [23]. However, despite the high rate

Table 73. Indications for liver transplantation 1963–1976 (ACS/NIH Organ Transplant Registry).

Biliary atresia	87
Cirrhosis	66
Malignant tumour	
primary	76
metastatic	7
Hepatitis	28
Hepatic necrosis	2
Wilson's disease	2
α_1 anti-trypsin deficiency	2
Budd–Chiari	2
Niemann–Pick	1
Sclerosing cholangitis	1

of ultimate tumour recurrence, long-term palliation can often be achieved [11].

Carcinoma of the large bile duct has proved an unsatisfactory indication as tumour recurrence is rapid in almost all cases.

Biliary atresia. Children are the best recipients of hepatic transplants [17]. Children with biliary atresia are crippled from birth. Society makes a great investment in their lives, from which no conceivable long-term benefit can be expected. They die at a very predictable time. It seems reasonable therefore to intervene with a clear conscience before the patients reach a moribund state. In the Denver series, biliary atresia has been the single most common reason for liver transplantation.

Chronic active hepatitis and cirrhosis. The operation must be performed before the patient is in a terminal condition with hypotension, bleeding, renal failure and systemic infection. If these are present, results are disastrous.

Hepatitis B-positive patients have been transplanted successfully. One patient survived 28 months post-transplant, succumbing to another infection. HBsAg was constantly present in the blood and at autopsy the transplanted liver showed chronic hepatitis [6]. If specific anti-HBs immunoglobulin is given during the anhepatic phase of the operation, patients may remain free of HBsAg after surgery [10].

A heterotopic transplantation with a child-donor liver has also been performed [8]. The patient has survived 28 months and the grafted liver is histologically almost normal although the patient's HBsAg remains positive.

Transplants have been successfully performed in the 'lupoid' type of chronic active hepatitis (with cirrhosis) and in cirrhosis of the alcoholic.

The most important future application of liver transplantation in adults probably lies in the group of cirrhotic patients [20].

In *primary biliary cirrhosis*, when deep jaundice has developed with bleeding varices and ascites, the life-expectancy is seldom more than one year. These patients are therefore suitable candidates for transplantation. In one series, four of 11 transplanted patients are alive and well after one to two years [11]. The mitochondrial antibody fluctuates post-operatively [16]. The relief of deep jaundice and pruritus is certainly worthwhile.

Inborn errors of metabolism. Two patients with Wilson's disease have survived over seven years post-transplant [20]. Serum caeruloplasmin rose. Seven patients in the end stages of homozygous

α_1 anti-trypsin deficiency have had liver transplants [7]. Four survived for one year. There was a change from the phenotype of the recipient to that of the donor. This supports the crucial role of the liver in this condition.

Other conditions transplanted have included congenital tyrosinosis, type IV glycogen storage disease and Niemann–Pick disease.

Hepato-renal syndrome. Three patients with end-stage renal failure associated with advanced chronic liver disease have been treated by hepatic homotransplantation. After two weeks, renal function was nearly normal [9]. Two have since died, 10 and 42 days post-operatively. The third survived 12 months after transplantation. This confirms that the renal failure of chronic liver disease is not related to structural abnormalities in the kidney but is secondary to the hepato-cellular failure.

Chronic portal–systemic encephalopathy. One patient with chronic portal–systemic encephalopathy had an hepatic transplant. There was marked neuropsychiatric improvement [13]. This implies that the organic cerebral changes of chronic portal–systemic encephalopathy are potentially reversible.

Budd–Chiari syndrome. Liver transplantation was successful in a woman with the Budd–Chiari syndrome of unknown aetiology [14]. The patient was alive 16 months later.

General preparation of the patient

A standard protocol must be filled in. The procedure is discussed fully with patients and relatives and consent given. Means of contacting the patient at any time, day or night, when a donor liver becomes available must be recorded [15].

The usual clinical, biochemical and serological investigation of any patient with liver disease is detailed and, in particular, such information as previous haemorrhages, pre-coma and ascites. The synthetic functions of the liver, such as serum albumin and prothrombin are helpful prognostically. HBsAg status is noted. Blood group and HLA antigens are recorded.

In patients with malignant disease, metastases must be sought as their presence would preclude transplantation.

Scanning is done to show size and site of any lesions. Arteriography shows the extent of any tumour infiltration and any vascular anomalies.

The portal vein must be shown to be patent by

splenic venography. In selected cases, the bile
ducts are shown by ERCP.

The donor

The problem is to find a suitable donor at the right
time. A state of irreversible coma (brain death)
must be diagnosed by a team independent of those
performing the transplant. Informed consent by a
legally responsible family member or members is
obtained. The donor should be less than 50 years
old, and not suffering from malignant or infectious
disease. The patient's condition should be similar
to that of kidney donor's with brain death, with
an intact circulation maintained on a ventilator [3,
20, 23].

The ABO blood group must be compatible. Detailed histocompatibility studies of the HLA type
are done, but results do not correlate with the clinical course [19, 31]. One long-term survivor had a
grade D mis-match, and one patient rejected at
two weeks with a grade A mis-match [19]. Two
long-term survivors had grade C matches [31].

In order to provide enough time for the transplant team to make adequate preparations, warn-
ing of a suitable donor must be given six hours
prior to switching off the ventilator.

The liver must not be too large for the recipient.
Children's livers have been transplanted into
adults.

The operative details are discussed elsewhere [3,
20]. The procedure is commenced while mechanical ventilation continues and the circulation
remains intact. The portal vein is perfused with
Hartmann's solution and the hepatic artery with
PPF solution to which heparin, hydrocortisone,
ampicillin, magnesium and potassium phosphate
have been added. Bile must be washed from the
large bile ducts and gall bladder to prevent subsequent sloughing of mucosa.

The liver is transported in a bowl containing ice-
cold saline. It can be preserved for up to 10 hours
by this simple method.

The recipient operation (fig. 417) [3, 20]

This is commenced shortly before the arrival of the
donor liver. The pre-operative systolic blood
pressure should be at least 100 mmHg as levels
below this are prognostically grave [3].

Portal vein and inferior vena cava are simultaneously occluded for between 50 and 90 minutes.
The portal veins of donor and recipient are anasto-

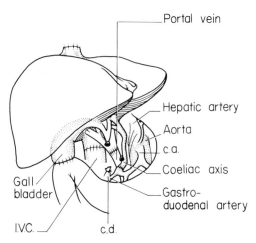

Fig. 417. The completed operation of hepatic
orthotransplantation in man. The anastomoses have
to be adapted to anatomical variations, particularly
in the hepatic artery. At the present time Roux-en-Y
loop anastomosis of the common bile duct to a loop
of jejunum is preferred to cholecystoduodenostomy
(Starzl *et al* 1968).

mosed. The inferior vena cava is reconstructed
above and below the liver. The homograft coeliac
axis or common hepatic artery is attached to the
donor common hepatic artery. Anatomical variations may necessitate a different arterial anastomoses. Femoral–femoral cardio-coronary bypass
may be useful in the anhepatic phase [5].

The method of maintaining continuity of the
biliary tract is crucial. Breakdown of biliary anastomoses leads to stricture, sludging, cholangitis
and abscesses, and is an important cause of later
death. Starzl [17] uses end-to-end common bile
duct anastomosis over an indwelling T tube. Calne
[3] uses a gall bladder conduit procedure, in which
the donor gall bladder is positioned between the
common bile ducts of donor and recipient, and
splinted by a T tube. Both procedures have
reduced post-transplant biliary complications.

Auxiliary 'heterotopic' hepatic homografts

Here the donor liver is transplanted but the
recipient's diseased liver is left *in situ* [8]. This
method of temporary hepatic assistance may be
useful in potentially reversible liver failure. It
avoids a technically exacting hepatectomy in a
gravely ill patient. Moreover, the retention of
autogenous liver tissue may be of value if the transplanted liver is rejected. The hepatic homograft
may undergo remarkable atrophy. This can be

related to maintenance of portal blood flow to the host liver, with none to the homograft. This again has been associated with deprivation of hepatic hepatotropic factors largely from the pancreas [18].

Immediate post-operative problems

These include all those discussed in Chapter 9 under acute hepato-cellular failure. In particular, hypoglycaemia, failure of blood clotting, and electrolyte abnormalities must be corrected. Albumin infusions may be useful over the first few post-operative days. Protein catabolism is high, but liver function usually satisfactory, so that normal or even high protein diets are given [12]. A combination of antibiotics is given for the first few weeks post-operatively.

Acute neurological complications—shown by decreased consciousness, fits, and occasionally akinetic mutism—are related to intra-operative cerebral air embolism [25].

IMMUNO-SUPPRESSION

For the first three days 500 mg hydrocortisone i.v. is given daily. This is followed by 200 mg prednisone daily, reducing to a maintenance dose of 60 mg daily. This is raised or lowered according to the presence or absence of rejection, in some patients it can be stopped. In the early stages the prednisone is combined with cyclophosphamide, 100 mg daily. After the first month, 150 mg azathioprine replaces the cyclophosphamide. Starzl also uses heterologous anti-lymphocyte globulin [17], but this is very costly.

The fungal metabolite cyclosporin A has proved very useful in organ transplantation [4]. No additional immuno-suppression is needed. Renal toxicity precludes its long-term use.

REJECTION

Immunologically, the liver is a privileged organ with regard to transplantation, having a higher resistance to immunological attack than other organs. The liver cell probably carries fewer surface antigens. Nevertheless, episodes of acute rejection are very common. These commence in the second week, and are marked by increases in serum bilirubin and transaminase values and, later, a dramatic rise in prothrombin time. Needle liver biopsy shows the rejection picture of graft-versus-host reaction, with massive infiltration of portal zones and sinusoids with lymphocytes and plasma cells, hepato-cellular necrosis and, particularly, damage to small bile ducts. Serum complement levels fall [26]. Acute rejection is treated by increasing the dose of prednisone. Azathioprine is not raised, as this drug requires adequate liver function for activity [29].

Chronic rejection is unusual. Histologically this is marked by intimal thickening of the hepatic arteries [22]. Immunofluorescent studies show deposition of complement in the arterial wall [2]. The process of rejection, if chronic, may proceed to hepatic fibrosis.

CHOLESTASIS

Cholestasis is multi-factorial. Rejection is associated with lesions of the small intra-hepatic bile ducts. Biliary complications include fistulas from anastomotic leaks or obstruction to the biliary tree by bile casts or calculi [24, 27, 31]. These can be demonstrated by percutaneous cholangiography, and can be repaired surgically [24].

Immuno-suppressant drugs, such as azathioprine, have hepato-toxic and cholestatic effects.

Infection plays a part. *E. coli* may be particularly important by deconjugating bilirubin and allowing pigment stones and sludge precipitation.

INFECTIONS

These generally result from biliary obstruction plus immuno-suppression. Enough therapy has to be given to prevent losing the new liver, but not so much that the patient dies of immunological invalidism. Septicaemias with Gram-negative organisms probably originate in the biliary obstructed liver or in large septic infarcts which follow uncontrolled rejection. Thrombosis of the right hepatic artery may be followed by sub-total hepatic gangrene and, again, the infarcted area may become infected. The infection is often with opportunist organisms, such as fungi.

The prognosis of cholestatic rejection with infection is very poor.

Repeated blood cultures are necessary. Hepatic scintiscanning is valuable in demonstrating abscesses within the liver. Percutaneous cholangiography using a fine needle is useful in diagnosing biliary complications. Needle biopsy of the liver is always useful.

The increased risk of new hepatic tumours,

particularly lymphomas, in transplant recipients is now well recognized and one probable case of reticulum cell sarcoma has been reported [31].

Summary

At the outset it was anticipated that acute rejection of the transplanted liver would be the major complication, but sepsis and biliary tract obstruction and fistulas have assumed equal importance. Research must continue, but at the present time the chances of long-term survival are not sufficiently high for the procedure to be generally recommended, except in a very few special cases and in well-organized centres.

REFERENCES

1. ACS/NIH ORGAN TRANSPLANT REGISTRY (1977) July Newsletter.
2. ANDRES G.A. *et al* (1972) Immunopathological studies of orthotopic human liver allografts. *Lancet* i, 275.
3. CALNE R.Y. (1978) Practical aspects of liver transplantation. *Ann. Chir. Gynaecol.* **67**, 39.
4. CALNE R.Y., ROLLES K., WHITE D.J.G. *et al* (1979) Cyclosporin A initially as the only immunosuppressant in 34 recipients of cadaveric organs: 32 kidneys, 2 pancreases and 2 livers. *Lancet* ii, 1033.
5. CALNE R.Y., SMITH D.P., McMASTER P. *et al* (1979) Use of partial cardiopulmonary bypass during the anhepatic phase of orthotopic liver grafting. *Lancet* ii, 612.
6. CORMAN J.L., PUTNAM C.W., IWATSUKI S. *et al* (1979) Liver allograft: its use in chronic active hepatitis with macronodular cirrhosis, hepatitis B surface antigen. *Arch. Surg.* **114**, 75.
7. HOOD J.M., KOEP L.J., PETERS R.L. *et al* (1980) Liver transplantation for advanced liver disease with alpha-1-antitrypsin deficiency. *New Engl. J. Med.* **302**, 272.
8. HOUSSIN D., FRANCO D., BERTHELOT P. *et al* (1980) Heterotopic liver transplantation in end-stage HBsAg-positive cirrhosis. *Lancet* i, 990.
9. IWATSUKI S., POPOVTZER M.M., CORMAN J.L. *et al* (1973) Recovery from 'hepatorenal syndrome' after orthotopic liver transplantation. *New Engl. J. Med.* **289**, 1155.
10. JOHNSON P.J., WANSBOROUGH-JONES M.H., PORTMANN B. *et al* (1977) Familial HBsAg hepatoma: treatment with orthotopic liver transplantation and specific immunoglobulin. *Br. med. J.* i, 216.
11. MACDOUGALL B.R.D., CALNE R.Y., McMASTER P. *et al* (1980) Survival and rehabilitation after orthotopic liver transplantation. *Lancet* i, 1326.
12. O'KEEFE S.J.D., WILLIAMS R. & CALNE R.Y. (1980) 'Catabolic' loss of body protein after human liver transplantation. *Br. med. J.* i, 1107.

13. PARKES J.D., MURRAY-LYON I.M. & WILLIAMS R. (1970) Neuro-psychiatric electroencephalographic changes after transplantation of the liver. *Q. J. Med.* **39**, 515.
14. PUTNAM C.W., PORTER K.A., WEIL R. *et al* (1976) Liver transplantation for Budd–Chiari syndrome. *J. Am. med. Assoc.* **236**, 1142.
15. SHERLOCK S. (1972) Selection and preparation of the patient for liver transplantation. In *Anaesthesia in Organ Transplantation*, p. 32. Karger, Basel.
16. SMITH M.G.M., WILLIAMS R., DONIACH D. *et al* (1971) Effect of orthotopic liver transplantation on serum-autoantibodies. *Lancet* ii, 1006.
17. STARZL T.E. (1978) Liver transplantation. *Johns Hopkins med. J.* **143**, 73.
18. STARZL T.E. & TERBLANCHE J. (1979) Hepatotropic substances in progress. In *Liver Disease*, vol. 6, p. 135, eds H. Popper & F. Schaffner. Grune & Stratton, New York.
19. STARZL T.E. *et al* (1969) Clinical and pathologic observations after orthotopic transplantation of the human liver. *Surg. Gynecol. Obstet.* **128**, 327.
20. STARZL T.E., KOEP L.P., HALGRIMSON C.G. *et al* (1979) Fifteen years of clinical liver transplantation. *Gastroenterology* **77**, 375.
21. STARZL T.E., MARCHIORO T.L., VON KAULLA K.N. *et al* (1963) Homotransplantation of the liver in humans. *Surg. Gynecol. Obstet.* **117**, 659.
22. STARZL T., PORTER K.A., SCHROTER G. *et al* (1973) Autopsy findings in a long-surviving liver recipient. *New. Engl. J. Med.* **289**, 82.
23. STARZL T.E., PORTER K.A., PUTNAM C.W. *et al* (1976) Orthotopic liver transplantation in ninety-three patients. *Surg. Gynecol. Obstet.* **142**, 487.
24. STARZL T.E., PUTNAM C.W., HANSBROUGH J.F. *et al* (1977) Biliary complications after liver transplantation: with special reference to the biliary cast syndrome and techniques of secondary duct repairs. *Surgery* **81**, 212.
25. STARZL T.E., SCHNECK S.A., MAZZONI G. *et al* (1978) Acute neurological complications after liver transplantation with particular reference to intraoperative cerebral air embolus. *Ann. Surg.* **187**, 236.
26. TORISU M. *et al* (1972) Serum complement after orthotopic transplantation of the human liver. *Clin. exp. Immunol.* **12**, 21.
27. WALDRAM R., KEMP A., WILLIAMS R. *et al* (1973) Bile secretion following liver transplantation in man. *Gut* **14**, 819.
28. WELCH C.S. (1955) A note on transplantation of the whole liver in dogs. *Transplant. Bull.* **2**, 54.
29. WHELAN G. & SHERLOCK S. (1972) Immuno-suppressive activity in patients with active chronic hepatitis and primary biliary cirrhosis treated with azathioprine. *Gut* **13**, 907.
30. WHELTON M.J., PETRELLI M., GEORGE P. *et al* (1969) Carcinoma at the junction of the main hepatic ducts. *Q. J. Med.* **38**, 211.
31. WILLIAMS R. *et al* (1973) Liver transplantation in man: the frequency of rejection; biliary tract complications and recurrence of malignancy based on an analysis of 26 cases. *Gastroenterology* **64**, 1026.

Index